Burnt Human Remains

Published and forthcoming titles in the Forensic Science in Focus series

Published

The Global Practice of Forensic Science
Douglas H. Ubelaker (Editor)

Forensic Chemistry: Fundamentals and Applications
Jay A. Siegel (Editor)

Forensic Microbiology
David O. Carter, Jeffrey K. Tomberlin, M. Eric Benbow, and Jessica L. Metcalf (Editors)

Forensic Anthropology: Theoretical Framework and Scientific Basis
Clifford Boyd and Donna Boyd (Editors)

The Future of Forensic Science
Daniel A. Martell (Editor)

Forensic Anthropology and the United States Judicial System
Laura C. Fulginiti, Kristen Hartnett McCann, and Alison Galloway (Editors)

Forensic Science and Humanitarian Action: Interacting with the Dead and the Living
Roberto C. Parra, Sara C. Zapico, and Douglas H. Ubelaker (Editors)

Disaster Victim Identification in the United States in the 21st Century: An Evolving Discipline
John A. Williams and Victor W. Weedn (Editors)

Anthropology of Violent Death: Theoretical Foundations for Forensic Humanitarian Action
Roberto C. Parra and Douglas H. Ubelaker (Editors)

Burnt Human Remains: Recovery, Analysis and Interpretation
Sarah Ellingham, Joe Adserias-Garriga, Sara C. Zapico and Douglas H. Ubelaker (Editors)

Forthcoming

Artificial Intelligence (AI) in Forensic Sciences
Katrin Franke and Zeno Geradts (Editors)

An Illustrated Guide to Forensic Skeletal Trauma Analysis
Donna C. Boyd

Burnt Human Remains

Recovery, Analysis, and Interpretation

EDITED BY

Sarah Ellingham
International Committee of the Red Cross, Geneva, Switzerland

Joe Adserias-Garriga
Mercyhurst University, Pennsylvania, USA

Sara C. Zapico
New Jersey Institute of Technology, New Jersey, USA
Smithsonian Institution, Washington, DC, USA

Douglas H. Ubelaker
Smithsonian Institution, Washington, DC, USA

AAFS AMERICAN ACADEMY OF FORENSIC SCIENCES

WILEY

This edition first published 2023

Registered Offices
John Wiley & Sons, Inc., 111 River Street, Hoboken, NJ 07030, USA
John Wiley & Sons Ltd, The Atrium, Southern Gate, Chichester, West Sussex, PO19 8SQ, UK

For details of our global editorial offices, customer services, and more information about Wiley products visit us at www.wiley.com.

Wiley also publishes its books in a variety of electronic formats and by print-on-demand. Some content that appears in standard print versions of this book may not be available in other formats.

A catalogue record for this book is available from the Library of Congress

Hardback ISBN:9781119682608; ePub ISBN: 9781119682745; ePDF ISBN: 9781119682646;
oBook ISBN: 9781119682691

Cover Image: Courtesy of Joe Adserias-Garriga
Cover Design: Wiley

Set in 10.5/13.5pt MeridienLTStd by Integra Software Services Pvt. Ltd, Pondicherry, India

C9781119682608_220523

Contents

About the Editors

Sarah Ellingham, PhD, is a Forensic Coordinator for the ICRC. Since joining the ICRC in 2016, she has worked in several contexts in Asia, Africa, and the Middle East in active and post-conflict settings. Sarah is a forensic anthropologist, certified by the Royal Anthropological Institute of Great Britain and Northern Ireland (Cert-FA-II), a Steering Committee Member of the British Association for Forensic Anthropology (BAFA), and an active member of the Interpol DVI Sub-Working Group for Anthropology and Pathology. Sarah obtained her PhD. on the biochemical analysis of burnt bone from Teesside University in 2015. She further holds an MSc in Forensic Anthropology, a BSc in Forensic Sciences, and is working towards an MSc in Psychology. Her research interests mainly focus on the analysis of burnt remains, disaster victim identification, and forensic humanitarian action. Sarah has authored several peer-reviewed scientific publications and was awarded the J.L. Angel Award for her research in 2016.

Joe Adserias-Garriga, PhD, DDS, D-ABFO, is a forensic anthropologist and odontologist from Spain. She received a Police Decoration for her contribution to casework from the Mossos d´Esquadra (Catalonian Police). Dr. Adserias-Garriga was involved in the identification of decedent border crossers as a forensic anthropologist at the Forensic Anthropology Center, Texas State University. She is a member of the ADA Standards Committee on Forensic Odontology and OSAC. Diplomate of the American Board of Forensic Odontology, member of the Board of Governors in the American Society of Forensic Odontology (ASFO), and ASFO President (2022). Member of the Board of Directors of the International Association of Coroners and Medical Examiners and a member of the INTERPOL DVI Odontology as well as Pathology-Anthropology Sub-Working Group. She is a Forensic Odontology consultant for the National Center of Missing and Exploited Children. Dr. Adserias-Garriga is an Assistant Professor of the Department of Applied Forensic Sciences at Mercyhurst University.

Sara C. Zapico, PhD, ABC-MB, is an assistant professor at the Department of Chemistry and Environmental Science at New Jersey Institute of Technology, Newark, New Jersey. She is also a research collaborator in the Department of Anthropology at the National Museum of Natural History, Smithsonian Institution in Washington, DC. Before NJIT, she was the graduate program director of the Professional Science Master's in Forensic Science (PSM-FS) and assistant teaching professor at Florida International University, in Miami, Florida. She also served as an associate at the International Committee of the Red Cross in Geneva, Switzerland. She has authored 30 peer-reviewed scientific publications and edited two books in the fields of biomedical sciences, forensic biochemistry, forensic anthropology, and humanitarian forensic action. Her research interests focus on the application of biochemical techniques to forensic anthropology issues such as age-at-death estimation and the determination of post-mortem interval, with implications on aging and biomedical sciences.

Douglas H. Ubelaker, PhD, D-ABFA, is a curator and senior scientist at the Smithsonian Institution's National Museum of Natural History in Washington, DC, and an adjunct professor at Michigan State University He has reported on over 980 forensic cases in his specialty of forensic anthropology and testified in numerous legal proceedings. Ubelaker has published extensively in the general field of human skeletal biology, with an emphasis on forensic applications and has served on the editorial boards of numerous leading scientific publications. He was the elected 2011–2012 President of the American Academy of Forensic Sciences and has received numerous honors from international organizations.

List of Contributors

Eric Bartelink, PhD, D-ABFA, is a Professor of Anthropology and co-Director of the Human Identification Laboratory at California State University, Chico. He is a Diplomate of the American Board of Forensic Anthropology, a certified instructor for California's Peace Officers Standards and Training, and current Vice-chair of the Organization of Scientific Area Committees' Anthropology Subcommittee under NIST. He is co-author of *Forensic Anthropology: Current Methods and Practice, Introduction to Physical Anthropology, Essentials of Physical Anthropology,* and co-editor of *New Perspectives in Forensic Human Skeletal Identification.*

John Berketa, PhD, is a senior forensic odontologist and scene team leader in Disaster Victim Identification in South Australia. Following the 2009 Victorian bushfire disaster he has conducted intensive research into maximizing post-mortem information of severely incinerated victims. He has attended many fire disaster scenes and has published various articles in national and international journals and book chapters. As well as a PhD., he has been recognized with various awards and is known as a global authority in the application of stabilization of incinerated dental remains. He is a postgraduate supervisor at the University of Adelaide, is on the scientific committee of International Organization of Forensic Odonto-Stomatology (IOFOS) and a peer reviewer of over a dozen forensic journals. He is a member of many forensic societies and regularly presents to both national and international organizations including Interpol, the Australian Society of Forensic Odontology, the American Academy of Forensic Science (AAFS) and the International Organization of Forensic Odonto-Stomatology (IOFOS).

Mary A. Bush, DDS, is an Associate Professor and Associate Dean for Students, Community, and Professional Initiatives at SUNY at Buffalo School of Dental Medicine. She is Past President of the American Society of Forensic Odontology and is a Fellow of the American Academy of Forensic Sciences. She is on the Editorial Board for the Journal of Forensic Science, has published numerous articles, has contributed to various textbooks, and lectures widely on the topic of forensic odontology, including an invited presentation at a congressional hearing on Capitol Hill. Dr. Bush has served on NIST's OSAC Odontology Subcommittee and the American Academy of Forensic Sciences Standards Board for Pattern Evidence.

Peter J. Bush, BS, is Director of the South Campus Instrument Center at the State University of New York School of Dental Medicine. He is a co-founder for the Laboratory for Forensic Odontology Research and a Fellow of the American

Academy of Forensic Sciences. He is a member of the Research Committee for the American Society of Forensic Odontology. Peter Bush has worked in many scientific fields, including Forensic Odontology. He has published over 80 articles and his work is referenced in numerous sources, including the NASA website.

Luis L. Cabo, PhD, received his Bachelor of Science degree in Biology, with a specialization in Zoology, from the University of Oviedo (Asturias, Spain). He also earned his master's degree in Biology, in addition to receiving his National Pedagogy and Teaching Certificate, from the University of Oviedo. His position as a researcher in both the Biology and Geology departments of The University of Oviedo provided Cabo with a vast amount of experience and knowledge in the fields of biology, paleoanthropology, archaeology, and geology. He has participated in over two dozen archaeological and paleontological field and laboratory projects. Cabo began his career at Mercyhurst, participating in the Summer Forensic Anthropology Short Courses. Since joining the Mercyhurst staff in 2003, Cabo, the Director of the Forensic and Bioarchaeology Laboratory, has assisted in the recovery and analysis of more than 200 forensic cases. He currently also serves as the primary graduate student research advisor.

Melina Calmon Silva, PhD, is a Brazilian forensic anthropologist. She is the vice-coordinator of the research group *Forensic Anthropology and Identification of Persons,* at the National Academy of Police, Federal Police of Brazil. She has worked as a Forensic Specialist for the International Committee of the Red Cross (ICRC) in Baghdad, Iraq, and as a Forensic Consultant for ICRC in Brazil. Dr. Calmon obtained her MA and PhD. in Anthropology from Tulane University in 2019, focusing on the role of forensic anthropology in the investigation of missing and unidentified persons cases. She is the Co-PI of the first taphonomy facility project in central Brazil. She holds the position of Executive Secretary at the Brazilian Association of Forensic Anthropology (ABRAF) 2020 / 2022 and is a member of the Anthropology Consensus Body at the American Academy of Forensic Sciences Standards Board. Dr. Calmon authored several peer-reviewed scientific publications and book chapters.

Rachael M. Carew, PhD, is a UK Certified Forensic Anthropologist (Cert-III) with the Royal Anthropological Institute and specializes in 3D printing skeletal models. Currently a lecturer in forensic science at Coventry University, Rachael gained her PhD. in Forensic Anthropology and Forensic Science from University College London (UCL) where she investigated the metrology and ethics of 3D printing for forensic anthropology evidence reconstruction. She also holds a BSc (Hons) in Forensic Science from University of the West of England (UWE), an MSc in Forensic Archaeology and Anthropology from Cranfield University, and is an Associate of the Chartered Society of Forensic Science and Secretary of the British Association for Forensic Anthropology (BAFA). With multiple publications in 3D reconstruction techniques, Rachael co-founded a 3D expert network group with the UK Forensic Capability Network to develop protocols for police casework. Rachael also consults internationally on 3D modelling and 3D printing research and applications in forensic science.

Eugénia Cunha, PhD, C-FASE, is a forensic anthropologist and the Director of the South Delegation of the National Institute of Legal Medicine and Forensic Sciences, Lisbon, Portugal. She has been a full professor at the University of Coimbra since 2003, where she created and co-coordinates the Laboratory of Forensic Anthropology. She is a co-founder and former President of FASE-Forensic Anthropology Society of Europe (2009–2016); Vice-President and founder member of ABRAF (Associação Brasileira de Antropologia Forense); Fellow of the American Academy of Forensic Sciences; Member of the Pathology and Anthropology Sub-group at the Interpol DVI Working Group; Roster member of JRR, Justice Rapid Response.

She has published extensively on forensic anthropology and skeletal biology. She has reported on about 500 forensic cases. To this date, 20 PhD. students have already completed their PhD. under her supervision. Her research interests include, among others, identification and age at death.

Cassandra M. DeGaglia, MA, is a PhD. student in the Department of Anthropology at Tulane University. She holds a BS in Biological Anthropology from the George Washington University and an MA in Anthropology from Mississippi State University. Additionally, she has been involved with research at the Smithsonian Institution's National Museum of Natural History in Washington, DC, since 2014. Her work spans a variety of topics in biological anthropology and includes projects relating to forensic anthropology, paleopathology, and paleodemography, and the ethical use of museum collections in anthropology.

Dennis C. Dirkmaat, PhD, D-ABFA, has been a board-certified forensic anthropologist since 1996. He was awarded the first (2020) Outstanding Mentor Award in the Anthropology Section of the AAFS. He is the 2021 winner of the AAFS' T. Dale Stewart Award for lifetime achievement in Forensic Anthropology. Dr. Dirkmaat is the Chair of the undergraduate program in Applied Forensic Sciences and the Master of Science in Anthropology graduate program at Mercyhurst University. Since 1986, Dr. Dirkmaat has conducted nearly 1000 forensic anthropology cases and has testified in court over 28 times as an expert witness. Chair of the Search and Recovery Committee of the Scientific Working Group-Disaster Victim Identification (SWG-DVI) group and co-chair of the Anthropology Committee of SWG-DVI (FBI, NIJ). Committee member of the Disaster Victim Identification Subcommittee OSAC. Dr. Dirkmaat has participated as a primary forensic anthropologist with the US Federal Government's Disaster Mortuary Operational Response Team (DMORT).

Peter Ellis, OAM, MB, FRCPA, is a forensic pathologist who has worked in Sydney and Queensland, Australia. He has extensive experience in all aspects of forensic pathology and is Adjunct Professor in Forensic Medicine and Pathology at Griffith University.

He has a special interest in identification science and has actively participated in numerous mass fatality incidents in Australia, New Zealand, and in SE Asia. He was the lead Australian pathologist for the Tsunami response in late 2004 and has also worked on forensic operations in Kosovo, East Timor, and Sri Lanka. He was the consulting forensic pathologist to the WW1 Fromelles mass grave project based in northern France. He has worked as the Chair of the Interpol DVI Pathology / anthropology sub-working group and has lectured extensively in Australia and SE Asia.

David Errickson, PhD, is a senior lecturer in forensic archaeology and anthropology at Cranfield University, United Kingdom. He is a certified forensic anthropologist (Cert-III) with the Royal Anthropological Institute of Great Britain and Northern Ireland (RAI), an Associate of the Chartered Institute for Archaeologists (ACIfA), and a lead archaeologist for Cranfield's Recovery and Identification of Conflict Casualties Team (CRICC) who partner with the Defense Prisoner of War / Missing in Action Accounting Agency (DPAA). David gained his PhD. from Teesside University, UK, where he investigated the application of 3D imaging to forensic anthropological context, including the display of information within the court. He further holds an MSc in Forensic Archaeology and Crime Scene Investigation, a BSc in Archaeology, and a Diploma in Professional Archaeology Studies. David has a substantial number of publications relating to 3D documentation in both anthropological and archaeological contexts.

Maria Teresa Ferreira, PhD, holds a PhD. in Anthropology, branch of Forensic Anthropology, and is Assistant Professor in the Department of Life Sciences at the University of Coimbra. At present, she is Coordinator of the Master of Forensic Anthropology and Vice-Coordinator for the branch of Forensic Anthropology of the PhD. in Anthropology; Vice-coordinator of the Center for Functional Ecology – Science for People and the Planet; Co-curator of the 21st Century Identified Skeletal Collection, Laboratory of Forensic Anthropology, Department of Life Sciences, University of Coimbra. She investigates mainly in the areas of Forensic Anthropology (namely, Forensic Taphonomy) and Bioarchaeology (in particular, slavery in the early days of Portuguese maritime expansion).

Hanna Friedlander, MA, is the Human Remains Analyst and Unidentified Remains Coordinator for the Michigan State Police (MSP), Missing Persons Coordination Unit. Her duties as the in-house forensic anthropologist include aiding federal, state, and local law enforcement in the search, detection, recovery, and identification of missing persons and unidentified remains within the State of Michigan. This includes cold case work, Native American (NAGPRA) repatriations, and the development and implementation of forensic anthropology trainings for law enforcement and other stakeholders. She is a responder for the Emergency Management Assistance Compact (EMAC) Program through the MSP Emergency Management Homeland Security Division and Forensic Anthropological Consultant for Kenyon International Emergency Services. She completed her MA in Biological Anthropology at the University of Alberta. Her interests include heat-related bone alteration, trauma analysis, 3D technology pertaining to trauma analysis, and skeletal marker assessment utilized for the identification of unidentified remains.

Alison Galloway, PhD, D-ABFA, is Professor Emerita, University of California, Santa Cruz and a board-certified forensic anthropologist. Her research focuses on time since death, effects of traumatic injury, and the consequences of thermal damage to human remains. She is co-editor of *The Evolving Female: A Life History Perspective, Broken Bones: Anthropological Analysis of Blunt Force Trauma,* and *Forensic Anthropology and the U.S. Judicial System*. She continues to practice forensic casework in central California.

David Gonçalves, PhD, is a biological anthropologist at the Portuguese Directorate-General for Cultural Heritage. At the Archaeosciences Laboratory, he currently undertakes research in human bioarchaeology and provides expertise on the management of archaeological activity involving human remains. He has dedicated most of his research career to the study of burnt human bones and teeth and is the co-developer of the first ever reference collection composed of experimentally burnt skeletons which is housed at the Laboratory of Forensic Anthropology of the University of Coimbra. By combining macroscopic with physical-chemical analyses, David has been attempting to find new and more reliable methods of retrieving relevant information from human bones and teeth subjected to heat.

Denice Higgins, PhD, is a researcher and forensic odontologist at the University of Adelaide. She received her doctorate in forensic biology on DNA identification from degraded human teeth. Dr. Higgins also holds a Bachelor of Dental Surgery and a Graduate Diploma in Forensic Odontology. She is the Director of the Forensic Odontology Unit in Adelaide, providing services to Australian Government and Policing Agencies. She worked on several large-scale DVI events and further coordinates and teaches a Graduate Diploma course in Forensic Odontology and supervises research students. She chairs the Medical Sciences Scientific Working Group for the National Institute of Forensic Science, Australia and New Zealand Policing Advisory Agency and is the President of both the Australian Society of Forensic Odontology and the South Australian Branch of the Australian and New Zealand Forensic Science Society. Dr. Higgins is a fellow of both the International

College of Dentists and the Pierre Fauchard Academy and is a member of the Australian Dental Association and the International Society for Forensic Genetics.

Kalyna Horocholyn, MA, was born and raised in Winnipeg, MB. From a young age, she has always been fascinated with stories, the connections between people, and the different ways that life histories are shared. Kalyna completed her Bachelor of Science in Bioarchaeology at the University of Winnipeg in 2010. She completed her Master of Arts in Anthropology at the University of Alberta in 2013, with her research focus on examining cremated remains for the purpose of microscopically identifying human remains from other larger mammalian remains. She attended McMaster University in Hamilton, ON, and obtained the title of PhD. Candidate before seeking new ways of connecting with people, as her interest in the dead had waned and she yearned to work with the living once more. Kalyna lives in Kitchener, ON, with her wife, Erin Horocholyn, and their three cats and one dog. Kalyna is now pursuing a professional career in social work with ambitions to become a counselor.

Ashley Kendell, PhD, is an Associate Professor of Anthropology and the Coordinator for the Certificate in Forensic Science at California State University, Chico. Having worked as a death investigator for five years, she offers extensive experience in medicolegal death investigation and her research spans the sub-disciplines of bioarcheology and forensic anthropology. She is also a certified POST instructor, teaching homicide investigation courses to regional and state law enforcement. Currently, she is a co-editor of a volume focused on wildfire response and victim recovery, which is nearing completion.

Haley Khosrowshahi, MA, is a museum professional living in Washington, DC. Her work at the Smithsonian National Museum of Natural History in the Anthropology Department under forensic anthropologist Dr. Douglas H. Ubelaker fostered a passion for research and further exploring the forensic contributions to human rights. After finishing a BA in Archaeology at the George Washington University, Haley moved to California to pursue an MA in Museum Studies at the University of San Francisco. Her studies focused on cultural heritage, museum law, and different ways museums could engage visitors. Her thesis titled: "Transparency through Display: Using Orphaned Collections to Reconnect with Museum Audiences," focused on how museum objects with unclear ownership could still be informative and tell a compelling narrative that museums should explore with new curatorial models.

Alexandra R. Klales, PhD, D-ABFA, is an Associate Professor of Forensic Anthropology at Washburn University and is the founder / director of the Washburn University Forensic Anthropology Recovery Unit (WU-FARU), which conducts forensic anthropological casework in Kansas and Missouri. She earned a BA in Anthropology from the University of Pittsburgh, MS in Forensic and Biological Anthropology from Mercyhurst University, and a PhD. in Anthropology from the University of Manitoba. Dr. Klales is a board-certified Diplomate (#123) of the American Board of Forensic Anthropology, a Member of the Anthropology Section of the American Academy of Forensic Sciences, and editor of the journal Forensic Anthropology. Her research focuses on improving biological profile methods, understanding skeletal sexual dimorphism, and developing protocols for the forensic archaeological recovery of human remains. She teaches courses in biological anthropology, forensic anthropology, human skeletal biology, and forensic archaeology at Washburn University and as continuing education forensic anthropology short courses.

Calil Makhoul, MSc, is PhD. student in Anthropology, branch of Forensic Anthropology, in the University of Coimbra. He is an invited lecturer in the Superior Institute for Social and Political Sciences at the University of Lisbon. Currently, he is a forensic autopsy technician and a member of the DVI Portuguese team in the National Institute of Legal Medicine and Forensic Sciences, Center Branch, in Coimbra. He is a level II certified forensic anthropologist of FASE-Forensic Anthropology Society of Europe. He investigates mainly in the areas of Forensic Anthropology (namely, commingled Human Burnt Remains) and Forensic Entomology (in particular, successional entomofauna).

Pamela Mayne Correia, MA, Pamela completed her MA at the University of Alberta. She is an academic at the University of Alberta, Anthropology Department. Her research interests are in the area of the analysis of cremated human skeletal material, trauma analysis, bone taphonomy and in human identification, problems related to cremation, taphonomy, and the identification of human remains using traditional histological methods. She is curator for the three museum collections managed by the Department of Anthropology. Pamela provides the core courses and instruction in forensic anthropology. She was the Chair of the Anthropology / Medical / Odontology Section of the Canadian Society of Forensic Sciences for ten years. She is a consulting forensic anthropologist for the Office of the Chief Medical Examiner and has contributed to numerous cases for the RCMP, Medical Examiner, and Archaeological Survey since 1989. As part of this work, Mayne Correia is involved in the Missing Children / Persons and Unidentified Human Remains Project in Alberta, as well as ongoing identification of human remains.

Alexandria McDaniel, MS, holds a BS in Anthropology with a minor in Criminal Justice and an MA in Bioarchaeology from the University of Indianapolis. She is a Medicolegal Investigator I at the Office of Chief Medical Examiner in New York City. She believes that investigating the death of an individual is important in providing crucial information that is essential for the criminal justice system and public health, but also providing a voice for those who cannot speak for themselves. She has her ABMDI Board Certification. She studied low thermal alterations of pig bone at sub-ignition point.

Raymond Miller, DDS, is the forensic dental consultant to the Office of the Erie County Medical Examiner in Buffalo, NY, and a Clinical Associate Professor at the University at Buffalo School of Dental Medicine. He is a member of the Disaster Mortuary Operational Response Team and deployed to the World Trade Center, Hurricane Katrina, and the crash of Flight 3407. Dr. Miller is a retired Lieutenant Colonel and served as the Base Dental Surgeon for the 107th Attack Wing of the New York Air National Guard. He has served as the Odontology Section Chair of the American Academy of Forensic Sciences and is the Vice-chair of the American Dental Association's Standards Committee on Dental Informatics for Forensic Odontology. He has served as a forensic dental representative to the Disaster Victim Identification Subcommittee for the federal Organization of Scientific Area Committees and the American Academy of Forensic Sciences Standards Board.

Colleen Milligan, PhD, D-ABFA, is Professor and Chair of the Department of Anthropology at California State University, Chico. She is also Co-Director of the Human Identification Laboratory at Chico State. Dr. Milligan is a Diplomate of the American Board of Forensic Anthropology and a certified instructor for California's Peace Officers Standards and Training. She has assisted California sheriff-coroner's offices, state agencies, and federal agencies in casework and field recoveries. She is also currently a co-editor of two upcoming volumes focused on wildfire response and mass fatality management, and a bioarchaeological study of an anatomical waste deposit in post-Civil War San Francisco.

Megan Moore, PhD, D-ABFA, is an Associate Professor of Anthropology at Eastern Michigan University in Ypsilanti, Michigan. She is Diplomate #140 of the American Board of Forensic Anthropology and she is the Forensic Anthropology Consultant for southeastern Michigan. She received the Ronald W. Collins Distinguished Faculty Teaching Award in 2019 and the Distinguished Honors Faculty Award in 2017. She completed her PhD. in Biological Anthropology at the University of Tennessee in Knoxville in 2008 and her MS in Biological Anthropology from the University of Oregon. Her research interests include skeletal biology, functional morphology, sexual polymorphism of the pelvis, and skeletal pathology and trauma analysis.

Allison Nesbitt, PhD, is an Assistant Teaching Professor in the Department of Pathology and Anatomical Sciences in the School of Medicine at the University of Missouri in Columbia, Missouri. She earned a master's degree in Anthropology with a concentration in Forensic and Biological Anthropology from Mercyhurst

University in Erie, Pennsylvania and a master's and PhD. in Anthropology from Stony Brook University in Stony Brook, New York. Her work focuses on the evolutionary and developmental variation of the human skull, anatomy education in the health professions, and improving diversity and inclusion in biological anthropology and anatomy.

Pier Paolo Petrone, MSc, is head of the Laboratory of Forensic Anthropology at the University Federico II of Naples, Italy. He carried out several archaeological excavations of pre-protohistoric and historical sites in Italy, North Africa, and Asia. His studies mainly focus on the effects and causes of death of the victims of the Vesuvius eruptions. Research on sites buried by the AD 79 and OBA Avellino Pumices events has provided useful information for the mitigation of the volcanic risk that affects three million people in metropolitan Naples. The results of these studies, published in prestigious journals (*Nature, PNAS, New England Journal of Medicine, PLoS ONE*), have been reported in the world press and are the subject of several scientific documentaries (Discovery Channel, BBC, History Channel, National Geographic, etc.). In 2019, his project: "Genetic Exploration of the Population of Herculaneum in AD 79" was funded by the National Geographic Society with a Research Grant.

Kassandra Pointer, BA, B.Ed, is a multidisciplinary educator and continuing-education specialist currently residing in Lethbridge, Alberta. Ms. Pointer completed her Bachelor of Arts in Biological Anthropology at the University of Alberta in 2015, having culminated her degree by partaking in a human osteological dig through the Slavia Foundation in Poland. During her Bachelor of Arts, Kassandra completed her undergraduate honor thesis on the histological analysis of cremated human bone, along with Pamela Mayne Correia. In 2019, she obtained her Bachelor of Education in Science Education from the University of Lethbridge, where her love of human anatomy melded with her adoration for teaching. She is now a substitute teacher in high school science and teaches adult courses at a continuing education center.

Elayne Pope, PhD, is a Forensic Anthropologist who researches how the human body burns, for application to fatal fire casework. She received her doctorate from the University of Arkansas in 2007 for: "The Effects of Fire on Human Remains." Dr. Pope has been a researcher and instructor for the San Luis Obispo Fire Investigation Strike Team (SLO FIST) Fatal Fire Death Investigation Course since 2008, where human cadavers are utilized to recreate fatal fire scenes (www.slofist.org). She worked as the Autopsy Supervisor and forensic anthropologist for six years at the Tidewater Office of the Chief Medical Examiner in Norfolk, Virginia. Dr. Pope is currently a forensic consultant and owner of Fatal Fire Forensics LLC.

(www.burnedbone.com) who specializes in legal / civil fatal fire case review and examinations, burn pattern analysis, skeletal trauma analysis, expert witness and testimony, training lectures and course instruction, and identification of fragmentary burnt bone (human vs. non-human / non-bone).

Julie Roberts, PhD, ChFA, is a Chartered Forensic Anthropologist (Cert FA-I) and archaeologist with over 20 years of practitioner experience in the excavation, analysis, and interpretation of burnt human remains. She received her PhD. from the University of Glasgow for her research into war crimes against children in Kosovo and Bosnia-Herzegovina in the 1990s. She is current Chair of the British Association for Forensic Anthropology, and the forensic anthropology coordinator for UK DVI, the national capability of the UK police service to respond to mass fatality incidents. She is company Scientific Advisor for Alecto Forensic Services, and a Visiting Research Fellow in the Faculty of Science at Liverpool John Moores University. Her research interests include analysis of factors which influence DNA success rates in mass fatality incidents, multidisciplinary approaches to improve identification rates in forensic and humanitarian contexts, and interpreting sequences of events in burnt and dismembered remains.

Christopher W. Schmidt, PhD, received his PhD. in Biological Anthropology from Purdue University in 1998. His research areas include the study of human teeth and the study of burnt human remains. His books include: *Long on the Tooth, Dental Wear in Evolutionary and Biocultural Contexts*, co-edited with Jim Watson, and two editions of *Analysis of Burned Human Remains*, co-edited with Steve Symes. His primary area of research is dental microwear texture analysis, although he has published on a wide range of topics including Neandertal diet, paleopathology, historic cemeteries, bone tools, and tissue rehydration. The journals in which he has published are, likewise, diverse and include *Paleoanthropology, American Journal of Physical Anthropology, North American Archaeologist, Physics Today, Surface Topography: Metrology and Properties*, and the *Journal of Forensic Sciences*.

Austin A. Shamlou, MSc, attended The George Washington University and graduated with a Bachelor of Science in Biological Anthropology. During her time in Washington, DC, she volunteered at the National Museum of Natural History, assisting Dr. Ubelaker on a few of his projects. In the summers of 2017 and 2018 she participated in three field schools in Austria, Romania, and Poland, emphasizing her passions for osteology and bioarchaeology. Shamlou then attended Boston University School of Medicine and received her MSc in Forensic Anthropology. Her thesis research focused on frontal sinus variations as seen on computed tomography scans. Her current research interests are around human osteology and variation, digital data and distribution, as well as diversity and inclusion within the field.

Christophe Snoeck, PhD, is a Research Professor at the Vrije Universiteit Brussel (VUB, Belgium), and the head of the Brussels Bioarchaeology Lab (BB-LAB – www.bb-lab.be). He combines his multidisciplinary expertise in bioarchaeology and isotope geochemistry to answer key archaeological questions, with a particular focus on populations that practiced cremation. Since January 2018, he has also been the Scientific Coordinator of the CRUMBEL project - Cremation, Urns and Mobility: population dynamics in BELgium (www.crumbel.org), funded by the Belgian Excellence of Science program (EoS). And since 2021, with the start of his ERC Starting Grant LUMIERE (www.erclumiere.be), he aims to develop new proxies for the study of charred and calcined bone to answer questions of mobility and landscape use at the European level.

Rebecca Stone-Gordon, MSc, holds a BA in History and Anthropology and an interdisciplinary MS in audio technology and visual media from American University, in Washington, DC. She is currently working on an MA in Public Anthropology (Biological Anthropology and Archaeology) at the same university. Her research areas include feminist theory, disability studies, the history of anatomy, archaeology, and horror film and literature. She specializes in representations of anthropology, archaeology, and mummies in Anglo-American feature films. She is also involved in interdisciplinary forensic projects at the Smithsonian Institution. She is the director of volunteer management for the Museum of Science Fiction.

Tim J.U. Thompson, PhD, is Dean of Health and Life Sciences and Professor of Applied Biological Anthropology at Teesside University. He has been practicing, researching, and teaching forensic anthropology for over 20 years, and has published over 70 peer-reviewed papers, chapters, and books. He is an expert in the effect of burning on the skeleton and previously published *The Archaeology of Cremation*. He was Editor-in-Chief of the journal *Science & Justice* and the *Journal of Forensic & Legal Medicine*, is a Fellow of five professional bodies, and holds a prestigious National Teaching Fellowship for excellence in teaching and the support for learning. In 2021 he was appointed President Elect of the Chartered Society of Forensic Sciences.

Yara Vieira Lemos, MSc, holds a BSc in Medicine and MSc in Health Sciences. She is a Certified Specialist in Legal Medicine. She is a Medical Examiner at the Civil Police of Minas Gerais, working mainly at the Laboratory of Forensic Anthropology and Applied Thanatology. She is also a roster member of JRR (Justice Rapid Response) and Assistant Professor at the Medical Sciences College of Minas Gerais. She was elected 2020–2022 President of the Brazilian Association of Forensic Anthropology (ABRAF) and is also an associated editor of the *Brazilian Journal of Forensic Anthropology and Legal Medicine*.

P. Willey, PhD, D-ABFA, is Professor Emeritus of Anthropology at Chico State University, California. He is a Diplomate of the American Board of Forensic Anthropology. In retirement, he remains actively involved in forensic anthropology, analyzing cases, participating in search and recoveries, and penning chapters. He authored *Prehistoric Warfare on the Great Plains: Skeletal Analysis of the Crow Creek Massacre Victims*, co-authored *They Died with Custer: Soldiers' Bones from the Battle of the Little Bighorn*, as well as *Mystery of the Bones: Syphilis, the Lewis and Clark Expedition, and the Arikara Indians*, and co-edited *Health of the Seventh Cavalry: A Medical History*. His final co-edited volume concerns a post-Civil War San Francisco anatomical waste deposit and it nears completion.

Amanda N. Williams, PhD, is an instructor with Truckee Meadows Community College Anthropology Department. She received her BA (2010) in Anthropology and Sociology from the University of Tennessee, Knoxville (2010), and her MA (2013) and PhD. (2020) in Biological Anthropology from the University of Montana. Dr. Williams primarily serves as an instructor, but also works in cultural resource management, where she actively engages in fieldwork, lab work, and serves as an osteological consultant for several firms and federal agencies within the northern Nevada and northern California area. Dr. Williams's research interests focus on forensic anthropology and the taphonomic processes affecting the human body after death. She is primarily interested in how these processes can be used to answer broader questions surrounding time since death estimates and used to reconstruct in situ conditions of death events. Her current research focuses on developing a broader scoring system for analyzing burnt human remains. Her primary research interests include forensic anthropology, taphonomy, and archaeology.

Lauren Zephro, PhD, is a forensic anthropologist based in central California. Lauren is currently the Forensic Services Director for the Santa Cruz County Sheriff's Office where she oversees crime scene investigation, the forensic laboratory, the property and evidence section, and the County's multidisciplinary sexual assault response team. Lauren earned her MA in Anthropology from the University of Tennessee, Knoxville, and her PhD. in Anthropology from the University of California, Santa Cruz. She is a certified latent print examiner and a Fellow of the American Academy of Sciences Anthropology Section. Her research interests and publications are primarily focused on skeletal trauma, secular change, method and theory in forensic anthropology, and burnt bone.

Preface

Thermally altered remains continue to pose a particular challenge to forensic practitioners tasked with their analysis and interpretation; consequently, it is a highly dynamic aspect of forensic science, with constant development and innovation, both in the field and in the lab.

The idea of this book originally arose from a workshop titled: "Some like it hot: A forensic analysis of burnt remains," which we presented at the American Academy of Forensic Sciences' 70th annual meeting in Seattle, 2018. Each of us having spent a significant portion of our careers working with and researching burnt remains from the angle of our respective disciplines (forensic anthropology, forensic odontology, molecular biology, and analytical chemistry), our aim was to gather forensic specialists at the forefront of their métiers in the study of burnt human remains, to provide a fresh look at the complexities involved in their recovery, analysis, and interpretation, as well as to present the most cutting edge research trends to tackle these forensic puzzles.

The overwhelming interest and feedback we received after the workshop highlighted the potential relevance of an updated textbook on the subject matter. This volume does not aim to replace, but rather build on and complement the existing excellent books covering the topic of burnt remains, such as Schmidt and Symes' 2008/2015 *The Analysis of Burned Human Remains*, Thompson's 2015 *The Archaeology of Cremation: Burned Human Remains in Funerary Studies*, Symes and Dirkmaat's 2012 *Recovery and Interpretation of Human Remains*, and Fairgrieve's 2007 *Forensic Cremation: Recovery and Analysis*.

Understanding the changes undergone by bodies when subjected to fire is of paramount importance for not only the determination of identity, but also the reconstruction of the events leading up to incineration and the determination of cause and manner of death. Therefore this book takes a novel and multidisciplinary approach to tackle the subject of burnt human remains. It is divided into four main sections. After a review of the History of the Study of Burnt Remains (Chapter 1), the first section focuses on the Search and Recovery of Burnt Human Remains from the Fire Scene (Chapters 2–4), delving into aspects such as scene analysis and interpretation for crime scene and death investigators, as well as search and recovery techniques to preserve forensic anthropologically and odontologically relevant material, context, and information. The second section looks at the Examination and Identification of Burnt Human Remains (Chapters 5–10). This includes detailing traditional and new approaches to classifying the degree of burn trauma, discussing the application of forensic medicine to determining the cause and manner of death in burnt remains, skeletal alterations though thermal exposure and the resulting challenges for biological profile estimation. It further tackles the role of forensic odontology in the identification process of burn victims, as well as a review of novel and established approaches to trauma analysis on burnt skeletal remains. Section three looks at Analytical Approaches to the Analysis of Burnt Bone (Chapters 11–17). It covers the biochemical and structural alterations of bone subjected to fire and analytical techniques to observe and quantify them and correlating changes to temperature and exposure time, followed by a chapter on molecular changes and DNA profiling techniques from burnt bone, pointing out challenges, methods, and case examples. Further in this section, the classical approach of calorimetry to determine the degree of heat exposure is re-examined, as is the use of histology in order to distinguish human from non-human burnt bone fragments with a discussion on limitations to the technique. It elaborates how isotopic and elemental analysis on burnt bone can be used to reconstruct a person's mobility *in vivo*, as well as in some instances shed light on the burning conditions. A further chapter discusses the application of different imaging techniques, both 2D and 3D, which can be used for the analysis of heat-induced bone. The section closes with a presentation on the first reference collection of burnt remains, highlighting the availability of this skeletal assemblage for researchers, aiming to inspire more research in the field. The book finally concludes with a section on Case Studies (Chapters 18–22); following a statistical review of 44 years of forensic anthropology casework brought to the Smithsonian Institution in the Washington, DC area, four further chapters discuss the experience of their respective authors during casework in Brazil, the USA, and Afghanistan, giving not only practical, but furthermore international insights into the type of scenarios that law enforcement, medical examiners, and forensic anthropologists may find themselves confronted with regarding burned human remains. The final chapter constitutes an archaeological "cold case" – the analysis of the victims of the AD 79 eruption of Mount Vesuvius.

This book is intended to bridge the gap between research and practice. It is designed to be a "one-stop-shop" on the topic of burnt remains, and we are hoping it will become a valuable new resource for practitioners, academics, students, and the interested layperson alike. It is our aim to promote a multi- and interdisciplinary approach when facing burnt remains in case work and to inspire an increase in research in this ever-evolving field.

We would like to thank all contributing authors for agreeing to be part of this project and sharing their valuable insights and experiences. Thanks also to our editors at Wiley for their support and patience in the process of turning this project from an idea to a reality. And finally, thanks to you, our reader, for considering this book for your library. We hope it fulfills your expectations.

Sarah Ellingham
Joe Adserias-Garriga
Sara C. Zapico
Douglas H. Ubelaker

Series Preface

The forensic sciences represent diverse, dynamic fields that seek to utilize the very best techniques available to address legal issues. Fueled by advances in technology, research and methodology, as well as new case applications, the forensic sciences continue to evolve. Forensic scientists strive to improve their analyses and interpretations of evidence and to remain cognizant of the latest advancements. This series results from a collaborative effort between the American Academy of Forensic Sciences (AAFS) and Wiley to publish a select number of books that relate closely to the activities and Objectives of the AAFS. The book series reflects the goals of the AAFS to encourage quality scholarship and publication in the forensic sciences. Proposals for publication in the series are reviewed by a committee established for that purpose by the AAFS and also reviewed by Wiley.

The AAFS was founded in 1948 and represents a multidisciplinary professional organization that provides leadership to advance science and its application to the legal system. The 11 sections of the AAFS consist of Criminalistics, Digital and Multimedia Sciences, Engineering Sciences, General, Pathology/Biology, Questioned Documents, Jurisprudence, Anthropology, Toxicology, Odontology, and Psychiatry and Behavioral Science. There are over 7000 members of the AAFS, originating from all 50 States of the United States and many countries beyond. This series reflects global AAFS membership interest in new research, scholarship, and publication in the forensic sciences.

Zeno Geradts
University of Amsterdam
The Netherlands

Douglas H. Ubelaker
Senior Scientist
Smithsonian Institution
Washington, DC, USA

CHAPTER 1
History of the Study of Burnt Remains

Douglas H. Ubelaker[1], PhD, D-ABFA and Austin A. Shamlou[2], MSc
[1]*Curator, Smithsonian Institution National Museum of Natural History, Washington DC, USA*
[2]*Boston University School of Medicine, Boston, MA, USA*
Douglas H. Ubelaker, US Government employee, Curator, Department of Anthropology, National Museum of Natural History Smithsonian Institution, Washington, D.C.

Currently, many diverse and complex approaches are available for the analysis of burnt human remains, as documented in chapters of this book. However, these methods have been developed slowly over the last few decades. When the first author entered the field of forensic anthropology in the late 1960s and early 1970s relatively few methods were available. At that time, fragmentary burnt human remains were frequently discarded or ignored, with the sentiment that little information could be gleaned through analysis. That attitude has slowly evolved through recognition that although burning and skeletal fragmentation present limitations to analysis, a great deal can be learned with proper training and thoughtful selection of methods. As in other areas of forensic science, the problems presented by casework stimulated innovative research. That research led to new methods of analysis augmenting the information that can be extracted. This chapter examines the historical development of the casework and experimentation that have fed that intellectual and methodological progress. While the entire literature on this subject is too exhaustive to be presented fully, key publications marking that progress are highlighted.

1.1 Early Developments Prior to 1980

In 1949, Wilton Krogman (1903–1987) initiated experimentation on burnt remains in relation to his study of archaeologically recovered materials (Krogman, 1949). In his examination of burnt human remains recovered from a mound in Ohio, Krogman noted that fragments of specific bones could be recognized, but he became curious about the fracture patterns he observed. His curiosity led him to devise experiments to explain the patterns. Using body parts with intact flesh,

---

Burnt Human Remains: Recovery, Analysis, and Interpretation, First Edition. Edited by Sarah Ellingham, Joe Adserias-Garriga, Sara C. Zapico and Douglas H. Ubelaker.

fresh bone with flesh removed, and dry bone he examined fracture patterns resulting from burning utilizing an acetylene torch and a hickory wood fire. He concluded: "it is possible to completely destroy a human body by the use of fire" (Krogman, 1949:89). Key factors were the source of heat and context, exposure of the remains to maximum heat, and agitation of the calcined remains to promote fragmentation. While his complete destruction comment may have discouraged analysis and was subsequently challenged, his work opened the academic door for further research on burnt remains.

Five years later, Baby (1954) published similar research, also stimulated by study of archaeological samples from Ohio. Although offering few methodological details, he reported a "recent test" (Baby, 1954:4) suggesting a difference between dry bones exposed to fire and those exposed with flesh still present. The dry bones presented superficial checking, fine longitudinal striae, deep longitudinal fractures, splintering, and lack of warping. In contrast, those burned with flesh still presented displayed deep checking, diagonal transverse fracturing, and warping. These observations were reinforced by Binford (1963). Wells (1960) followed up this research with observations from modern cremations, noting fragmentation, "tubular curling" (p. 33) and the difficulty of estimating age and sex. In 1963, Gejvall also observed modern cremations and conducted experiments of reburning ancient, cremated bone, noting the resulting attributes of color, fragment size, and issues of determining the minimum number of individuals present.

Research by Van Vark (1970, 1974, 1975) provided more detail on burning effects on human bone. Controlled experiments revealed no shrinkage of bone at temperatures below 700°C. Progressive shrinkage was found at temperatures between 700°C and 900°C, with no further shrinkage at higher temperatures. With mandible samples, he found maximum shrinkage of 16.42%. He also noted that macroscopically, bone became progressively more brittle when exposed to temperatures up to 700°C and assumed a white color at higher temperatures. Microscopic features were less clear between temperatures of 400°C and 700°C, with loss of recognizable structure above 800°C. In similar experiments, Dokládal (1971) reported little shrinkage with the cranium and variation between 5% and 12% with other bones.

Richards (1977) furthered these temperature related experiments and noted the general sequence of soft tissue destruction and bone exposure with temperatures of 680°C and above. This work highlighted that soft tissue protects bone exposure to fire. In such cases, bone exposure and burning effects appear gradually as soft tissue is reduced. For this reason, the skeletal effects of fire exposure can vary with different bones of the body and even within individual bones. Also in 1977, Herrmann elaborated on microscopic changes, noting that above temperatures of 700–800°C bones display loss of organic matter, shrinkage, and fusion of bone mineral crystals. Then in 1978, Dunlop noted that color changes can also be affected by contact with metal, suggesting a correlation of pink color with copper, green with iron, and yellow with zinc.

T.D. Stewart's (1979) classic text, *Essentials of Forensic Anthropology: Especially as Developed in the United States*, summarized much of the research reported above, emphasizing how bones burned in the flesh could be distinguished from those burned as dry bone. He also noted that careful observation of patterns on different bones could reveal the position of the body during burning. This section of the text offered a guide not only for the analysis of forensic cases involving fire but also archaeological discoveries (e.g. Ubelaker, 1997).

1.2 Post-1980 Advanced Experimentation and Casework

In 1981, Thurman and Willmore devised an experiment involving burning of four human humeri with flesh present and four that were fresh but with flesh removed. Those with flesh revealed warping, serrated margins of fracture sites, transverse fractures, and diagonal cracking. The defleshed bone displayed minimal warping and fractures with parallel-sided margins.

Experimentation with burnt remains advanced in 1984 with the Shipman *et al.* (1984) study of mandible and astragalus samples from 60 sheep and goats. The bones were exposed to temperatures ranging from 185°C to 940°C, documenting color change, microscopic alterations, and shrinkage, as well as data from X-ray diffraction. The study further documented color changes and growth in the crystal size of hydroxyapatite. They also noted the importance of the difference between bone temperature and that of the heating device/source.

Also in 1984, Bradtmiller and Buikstra (1984) experimentally examined the effects of burning on human bone microstructure. Using a small electric oven, they exposed bone samples with and without flesh to temperatures up to 600°C for 30 minutes. They found that even at 600°C histological features were still visible. With increasing temperatures, the histological structures osteons increased in size, with a slight impact on age estimation using these structures.

Heglar (1984) emphasized the importance of a team approach to the recovery, analysis, and interpretation of burnt remains and the value of anthropological involvement. These themes also have been stressed subsequently by Bass (1984), Owsley (1993), McKinley and Roberts (1993), Owsley *et al.* (1995), Ubelaker *et al.* (1995), Ubelaker (1999), and Blau and Briggs (2011). Of course, the forensic pathologist also plays an important role (Shkrum and Johnston, 1992; Nelson and Winston, 2006). The matter of recovery of burnt human remains is further discussed in the following chapters of this volume: Pope (Chapter 2), Klales *et al.* (Chapter 3), Berketa and Higgins (Chapter 4).

Chandler (1987) published experimental results of the effects of burning on teeth. This study involved examination of the effect of increasing heat exposure to measurements of roots of mandibular premolars. The following percentages of shrinkage with increasing temperatures were found: 0.88% at 440°C, 1.52% at 525°C, 2.36% at 675°C, 16.9% at 800°C, and 14.0% at 940°C. They also detected variable crown destruction and some root curling. In an electron microscopy study of 60 human premolars and third molars, Wilson and Massey (1987) were able to recognize enamel and dentin structure up to 1000°C, but these tissues changed into a "globular form" with exposure over 800°C, for three hours. Duffy *et al.* (1991) later demonstrated the value of human pulp tissue for sex diagnosis after heat exposure. They also called attention to the key difference between overall fire temperature and that within the tooth. This research was built on more recently when Sandholzer *et al.* (2013) analyzed volumetric tooth shrinkage using high-resolution micro-CT scans, and found shrinkage to range from 4.78% at 400°C to 32.53% at 1000°C.

Recognizing that bone shrinkage following burning varied not only with temperature but also the type of bone, Holland (1989) reported experiments on eight cadavers burned at temperatures up to 500°C. Average shrinkage of the cranial base was less than 2%, indicating that this area of skeletal anatomy was still useful for identification after burning at that temperature. Cavazzuti *et al.* (2019) later reported that despite shrinkage, careful selection of measurements can be useful in estimating sex. Most recently, a systematic study by Rodrigues *et al.* (2021), who experimentally burned human bones at temperatures ranging from 450°C to 1050°C with exposure times of between 75 to 257 minutes, found that the scoring of morphological features for sex determination was already affected at low burning temperatures, whereas metric methodologies were more severely affected at higher burn intensities, but fairly reliable at low to medium intensity burns.

By the end of the 1980s, experience with burnt bodies led Eckert *et al.* (1988) to suggest a protocol for case management. They detailed an approach for inventory, construction of a biological profile, and recognition of variation in thermal effects. Glassman and Crow (1996) later suggested a standardized model for describing burn injuries in human remains. Quinn *et al.* (2014) noted the importance and complexity of related terminology. A revised scoring methodology for describing burnt human remains was described by Williams (Chapter 5).

1.3 The 1990s: New Methods and Case Applications

The 1990s ushered in examination of the use of DNA for identification in burn victims. Sajantila *et al.* (1991) reported successful DNA typing after amplification in ten charred bodies. Tsuchimochi *et al.* (2002) presented a technique for successful extraction of DNA from dental pulp, allowing sex determination from incinerated teeth. The possibilities and challenges of conducting DNA analyses from burnt remains are further elaborated in Zapico (Chapter 12).

With the temporal increase in commercial cremations, legal issues, usually relating to commingling, called for analysis. Murray and Rose (1993) presented an early case study, calling attention to the value of such factors as total weight of cremains, inclusions, container materials, and retention of medical and dental evidence.

Analysis of commercial cremations called for more data on the expected weight of cremains. Warren and Maples (1997) answered this call in 1997 with data from 100 individuals who had been commercially cremated. The weights of adult cremains ranged from 876 g to 3784 g. They found that cremains' weight represented an average of 3.5% of body weight in adults, 2.5% in children, and only 1% in fetuses. McKinley (2000) later described the importance of understanding the cremation process and noted that some pathological conditions can be recognized after cremation. Subsequently, Warren *et al.* (1999) described finding evidence of arteriosclerosis in cremated remains. Brooks *et al.* (2006) reported on the use of elemental analysis to distinguish between cremains and other materials, as did Ellingham *et al.* (2018) who discussed the use of SEM-EDX elemental analysis in cases of contested cremains. General recommendations for the analysis of commercial cremations are provided by Fairgrieve (2008) and Schultz *et al.* (2008).

Further advances involved new techniques of analysis and new technology. Grévin *et al.* (1998) emphasized the value of reconstruction to interpret burn cases. Quatrehomme *et al.* (1998) used scanning electron microscopy of maxillary/mandibular fragments to reveal correlations of exposure temperatures with the patterns observed with this instrument.

Although the fragmentation of bone exposed to fire can limit analysis, research indicates that traumatic injury still can be recognized. Herrmann and Bennett (1999) noted that although difficult, traumatic fractures not related to heat can be distinguished from heat-related fractures. Chop marks can be identified after incineration (De Gruchy and Rogers, 2002) as well as other type of trauma (Pope and Smith, 2004).

Interpretation of burn victims calls for understanding of the combustion process. DeHaan and Nurbakhsh (2001) called attention to the important factor of body fat of the victim in promoting combustion. The body itself, especially body fat, provides fuel for the fire, accelerating combustion from temperatures of 700°C upwards (Ellingham *et al.*, 2016). Other key factors include a porous, rigid char that functions as a wick and a sustained external flame. Christensen (2002) added that bone composition also can be a factor, with osteoporotic bone being more susceptible to fragmentation and color change.

By 2004, Thompson was able to define four stages of heat-induced transformation in bone: dehydration, decomposition, inversion, and fusion, and presented revised temperature ranges for these stages. He also identified the key changes known to take place with heat exposure: color change, weight loss, fracture formation, changes in strength, recrystallization, porosity change, and size change. The following year Thompson (2005) reported experimentation on 60 sheep, documenting these changes more thoroughly and noting that bone can involve both shrinkage and expansion.

In 2006, Bush *et al.* (2006) reported that composite resins in teeth can be detected after incineration. These resins can prove valuable to assist in identification efforts, which is further elaborated on in Bush *et al.* (Chapter 9).

Schmidt and Symes (2008) published an edited volume that summarized methods of analysis of burnt remains at that time. The volume presented many useful chapters, including discussion of changes related to both temperature and duration (Beach *et al.*, 2008), the impact of environmental conditions (Walker *et al.*, 2008), the association of bone color with depositional history (Devlin and Herrmann, 2008), analysis using isotope ratios (Schurr *et al.*, 2008), recovery procedures (Schmidt, 2008), bone destruction patterns (Symes *et al.*, 2008), and basic principles of fire interpretation (DeHaan, 2008).

In 2009, Piga *et al.* (2009) turned to X-ray diffraction analysis of 57 human bone sections and 12 molar teeth. They found that an increase in heat led to growth of hydroxyapatite crystallites.

Finally, several recent syntheses focusing on burnt remains set the academic stage for the chapters of this book. Ubelaker (2009) provided such a review summarizing 81 published works. Also in 2009, Thompson summarized methodology in burnt human remains, calling attention to his own important research, as well as that of others.

In 2015, Thompson edited a volume with the focus on burnt remains in funerary studies. In Thompson's volume, Garrido-Varas and Intriago-Leiva (2015) related a case from Chile requiring thermal interpretation. Ubelaker (2015) showed how recent research in thermal effects can be used effectively in forensic case interpretation.

Most recently, Cerezo-Román *et al.* (2017) published an edited volume with an archaeological focus. Chapters provide detail on archaeological approaches and analysis (Williams *et al.*, 2017).

1.4 Summary and Conclusions

Throughout the history of the analysis of burnt human remains several themes emerge. The problems and questions presented by casework lead to innovative research designs and experimentation. Results of that experimentation and the information gleaned are fed back into analysis protocols and approaches to new casework. Research is advanced by ideas and hypothesis testing, but also by new technology. The simple observational approaches utilized by such early workers as Krogman, Baby, and Stewart are now supplemented by X-ray diffraction, scanning electron microscopy, isotope analysis, and DNA amplification, just to name a few. Key observations are macroscopic in nature, but also include histological, microscopic, and chemical dimensions. Modern interpretation calls for careful recovery, consideration of context, understanding of the burning process, and then selection of the most appropriate methods of analysis from the many available. Terminology is important, but also complex and somewhat variable among different fields and practitioners. The research process continues and evolves with new technology and good ideas. Just a few decades ago, analysists were reluctant to study burnt remains, feeling that little could be learned. Research demonstrates that even fragmented, calcined remains offer a great deal of information. Such remains offer inviting challenges to contemporary forensic scientists.

References

Baby, R.S. (1954) Hopewell cremation practices. *Ohio Historical Society Papers in Archaeology*, **1**, 1–7.

Bass, W.M. (1984) Is it possible to consume a body completely in a fire? In: *Human Identification: Case Studies in Forensic Anthropology* (eds. T.A. Rathbun and J.E. Buikstra). Charles C. Thomas, Springfield, IL, pp. 159–167.

Beach, J.J., Passalacqua, N.V., and Chapman, E.N. (2008) Heat-related changes in tooth color: Temperature versus duration of exposure. In: *The Analysis of Burned Human Remains* (eds. C.W. Schmidt and S.A. Symes). Elsevier, San Diego, CA, pp. 137–144.

Binford, L.R. (1963) An analysis of cremations from three Michigan sites. *Wisconsin Archaeologist*, **44**, 98–110.

Blau, S. and Briggs, C.A. (2011) The role of forensic anthropology in disaster victim identification. *Forensic Science International*, **205**, 29–35.

Bradtmiller, B. and Buikstra, J.E. (1984) Effects of burning on human bone microstructure: A preliminary study. *Journal of Forensic Sciences*, **29**, 535–540.

Brooks, T.R., Bodkin, T.E., Potts, G.E., and Smullen, S.A. (2006) Elemental analysis of human cremains using ICP-OES to classify legitimate and contaminated cremains. *Journal of Forensic Sciences*, **51**, 967–973.

Bush, M.A., Bush, P.J., and Miller, R.G. (2006) Detection and classification of composite resins in incinerated teeth for forensic purposes. *Journal of Forensic Sciences*, **51**, 636–642.

Cavazzuti, C., Bresadola, B., D'Innocenzo, C., Interlando, S., and Sperduti, A. (2019) Towards a new osteometric method for sexing ancient cremated human remains. Analysis of Late Bronze Age and Iron Age samples from Italy with gendered grave goods. *PLoS ONE*, **14**, e0209423.

Cerezo-Román, J.I., Wessman, A., and Williams, H. (eds.). (2017) *Cremation and the Archaeology of Death*. Oxford University Press, Oxford, UK.

Chandler, N.P. (1987) Cremated teeth. *Archaeology Today*, **8**, 41–45.

Christensen, A.M. (2002) Experiments in the combustibility of the human body. *Journal of Forensic Sciences*, **47**, 466–470.

De Gruchy, S. and Rogers, T.L. (2002) Identifying chop marks on cremated bone: A preliminary study. *Journal of Forensic Sciences*, **47**, 933–936.

DeHaan, J.D. (2008) Fire and bodies. In: *The Analysis of Burned Human Remains* (eds. C.W. Schmidt and S.A. Symes). Elsevier, San Diego, CA, pp. 1–14.

DeHaan, J.D. and Nurbakhsh, S. (2001) Sustained combustion of an animal carcass and its implications for the consumption of human bodies in fires. *Journal of Forensic Sciences*, **46**, 1076–1081.

Devlin, J.B. and Herrmann, N.P. (2008) Bone color as an interpretive tool of the depositional history of archaeological cremains. In: *The Analysis of Burned Human Remains* (eds. C.W. Schmidt and S.A. Symes). Elsevier, San Diego, CA, pp. 109–128.

Dokládal, M. (1971) A further contribution to the morphology of burned bones. *Proceedings of the Anthropological Congress Dedicated to Ales Hrdlicka*. Czechoslovak Academy of Sciences, Prague, p. 561.

Duffy, J.B., Waterfield, J.D., and Skinner, M.F. (1991) Isolation of tooth pulp cells for sex chromatin studies in experimental dehydrated and cremated remains. *Forensic Science International*, **49**, 127–141.

Dunlop, J.M. (1978) Traffic light discoloration in cremated bones. *Medicine, Science, and the Law*, **18**, 163–173.

Eckert, W.G., James, S., and Katchis, S. (1988) Investigation of cremations and severely burned bodies. *The American Journal of Forensic Medicine and Pathology*, **9**, 188–200.

Ellingham, S.T., Thompson, T.J., and Islam, M. (2016) The effect of soft tissue on temperature estimation from burnt bone using Fourier transform infrared spectroscopy. *Journal of Forensic Sciences*, **61**(1), 153–159.

Ellingham, S.T., Thompson, T.J., and Islam, M. (2018) Scanning Electron Microscopy–Energy-Dispersive X-Ray (SEM/EDX): A rapid diagnostic tool to aid the identification of burnt bone and contested cremains. *Journal of Forensic Sciences*, **63**(2), 504–510.

Fairgrieve, S.I. (2008) *Forensic Cremation: Recovery and Analysis*. CRC Press, Boca Raton, FL.

Garrido-Varas, C. and Intriago-Leiva, M. (2015) The interpretation and reconstruction of the post-mortem events in a case of scattered burned remains in Chile. In: *The Archaeology of Cremation; Burned Human Remains in Funerary Studies* (ed. T. Thompson). Oxbow Books, Oxford and Philadelphia, PA, pp. 227–242.

Gejvall, N. (1963) Cremations. In: *Science in Archaeology* (eds. D. Brothwell and E.H. Higgs). Praeger, New York, pp. 379–390.

Glassman, D.M. and Crow, R.M. (1996) Standardization model for describing the extent of burn injury to human remains. *Journal of Forensic Sciences*, **41**, 152–154.

Grévin, G., Bailet, P., Quatrehomme, G., and Ollier, A. (1998) Anatomical reconstruction of fragments of burned human bones: a necessary means for forensic identification. *Forensic Science International*, **96**, 129–134.

Heglar, R. (1984) Burned remains. In: *Human Identification: Case Studies in Forensic Anthropology* (eds. T.A. Rathbun and J.E. Buikstra). Charles C. Thomas, Springfield, IL, pp. 148–158.

Herrmann, B. (1977) On histological investigations of cremated human remains. *Journal of Human Evolution*, **6**, 101–103.

Herrmann, N.P. and Bennett, J.L. (1999) The differentiation of traumatic and heat related fractures in burned bone. *Journal of Forensic Sciences*, **44**, 461–469.

Holland, T.D. (1989) Use of the cranial base in the identification of fire victims. *Journal of Forensic Sciences*, **34**, 458–460.

Krogman, W.M. (1949) The human skeleton in legal medicine: Medical aspects. In: *Symposium on Medicolegal Problems. Ser. 2* (ed. S.D. Levinson). Lippincott, Philadelphia, PA, pp. 1–92.

McKinley, J. (2000) The analysis of cremated bone. In: *Human Osteology: In Archaeology and Forensic Science* (eds. M. Cox and S. Mays). Cambridge University Press, Cambridge, UK, pp. 403–421.

McKinley, J.I. and Roberts, C. (1993) Excavation and post-excavation treatment of cremated and inhumed human remains. *Institute of Field Archaeologists Technical Paper Number*, **13**, 1–11.

Murray, K.A. and Rose, J.C. (1993). The analysis of cremains: a case study involving the inappropriate disposal of mortuary remains. *Journal of Forensic Sciences*, **38**, 98–103.

Nelson, C.L. and Winston, D.C. (2006) Detection of medical examiner cases from review of cremation requests. *The American Journal of Forensic Medicine and Pathology*, **27**, 103–105.

Owsley, D.W. (1993). Identification of the fragmentary, burned remains of two U.S. journalists seven years after their disappearance in Guatemala. *Journal of Forensic Sciences*, **38**, 1372–1382.

Owsley, D.W., Ubelaker, D.H., Houck, M.M., Sandness, K.L., Grant, W.E., Craig, E.A., *et al.* (1995) The role of forensic anthropology in the recovery and analysis of branch Davidian compound victims: techniques of analysis. *Journal of Forensic Sciences*, **40**, 341–348.

Piga, G., Thompson, T.J.U., Malgosa, A., and Enzo, S. (2009) The potential of X-ray diffraction in the analysis of burned remains from forensic contexts. *Journal of Forensic Sciences*, **54**, 534–539.

Pope, E.J. and Smith, O.C. (2004). Identification of traumatic injury in burned cranial bone: an experimental approach. *Journal of Forensic Sciences*, **49**, 431–440.

Quatrehomme, G., Bolla, M., Muller, M., Rocca, J., Grévin, G., Bailet, P., *et al.* (1998) Experimental single controlled study of burned bones: Contribution of scanning electron microscopy. *Journal of Forensic Sciences*, **43**, 417–422.

Quinn, C.P., Goldstein, L., Cooney, G., and Kuijt, I. (2014) Perspectives – Complexities of terminologies and intellectual frameworks in cremation studies. In: *Transformation by Fire* (eds. I. Kuijt, C.P. Quinn, and G. Cooney). The University of Arizona Press, Tucson, AZ, pp. 25–34.

Richards, N.F. (1977) Fire investigation – Destruction of corpses. *Medicine, Science, and the Law*, **17**, 79–82.

Rodrigues, C.O., Ferreira, M.T., Matos, V., and Gonçalves, D. (2021) "Sex change" in skeletal remains: Assessing how heat-induced changes interfere with sex estimation. *Science & Justice*, **61**(1), 26–36.

Sajantila, A., Ström, M., Budowle, B., Karhunen, P.J., and Peltonen, L. (1991) The polymerase chain reaction and post-mortem forensic identity testing: Application of amplified D1S80 and HLA-DQα Loci to the identification of fire victims. *Forensic Science International*, **51**, 23–34.

Sandholzer, M.A., Walmsley, A.D., Lumley, P.J., and Landini, G. (2013) Radiologic evaluation of heat-induced shrinkage and shape preservation of human teeth using micro-CT. *Journal of Forensic Radiology and Imaging*, **1**(3), 107–111.

Schmidt, C.W. (2008) The recovery and study of burned human teeth. In: *The Analysis of Burned Human Remains* (eds. C.W. Schmidt and S.A. Symes). Elsevier, San Diego, CA, pp. 55–74.

Schmidt, C.W. and Symes, S.A. (eds.). (2008) *The Analysis of Burned Human Remains*. Academic Press, San Diego, CA.

Schultz, J.J., Warren, M.W., and Krigbaum, J.S. (2008) Analysis of human cremains: Gross and chemical methods. In: *The Analysis of Burned Human Remains* (eds. C.W. Schmidt and S.A. Symes). Elsevier, San Diego, CA, pp. 75–94.

Schurr, M.R., Hayes, R.G., and Cook, D.C. (2008) Thermally induced changes in stable carbon and nitrogen isotope ratios of charred bones. In: *The Analysis of Burned Human Remains* (eds. C.W. Schmidt and S.A. Symes). Elsevier, San Diego, CA, pp. 95–108.

Shipman, P., Foster, G., and Schoeninger, M. (1984) Burnt bones and teeth: An experimental study of color, morphology, crystal structure and shrinkage. *Journal of Archaeological Science*, **11**, 307–325.

Shkrum, M.J. and Johnston, K.A. (1992) Fire and suicide: A three-year study of self-immolation deaths. *Journal of Forensic Sciences*, **37**, 208–221.

Stewart, T.D. (1979) *Essentials of Forensic Anthropology: Especially as Developed in the United States*. Charles C. Thomas, Springfield, IL.

Symes, S.A., Rainwater, C.W., Chapman, E.N., Gipson, D.R., and Piper, A.L. (2008) Patterned thermal destruction of human remains in a forensic setting. In: *The Analysis of Burned Human Remains* (eds. C.W. Schmidt and S.A. Symes). Elsevier, San Diego, CA, pp. 15–54.

Thompson, T. (2009) Burned human remains. In: *Handbook of Forensic Anthropology and Archaeology* (eds. S. Blau and D.H. Ubelaker). Left Coast Press Inc., Walnut Creek, CA, pp. 295–303.

Thompson, T. (ed.). (2015) *The Archaeology of Cremation: Burned Remains in Funerary Studies*, Vol. **8**. Oxbow Books, Oxford, UK.

Thompson, T.J.U. (2004) Recent advances in the study of burned bone and their implications for forensic anthropology. *Forensic Science International*, **146S**, S203–S205.

Thompson, T.J.U. (2005) Heat-induced dimensional changes in bone and their consequences for forensic anthropology. *Journal of Forensic Sciences*, **50**, 1008–1015.

Thurman, M.D. and Willmore, L.J. (1981) A replicative cremation experiment. *North American Archaeologist*, **2**, 275–283.

Tsuchimochi, T., Iwasa, M., Maeno, Y., Koyama, H., Inoue, H., Isobe, I., *et al.* (2002) Chelating resin-based extraction of DNA from dental pulp and sex determination from incinerated teeth with y-chromosomal alphoid repeat and short tandem repeats. *The American Journal of Forensic Medicine and Pathology*, **23**, 268–271.

Ubelaker, D.H. (1997) The Savich farm site cremations, Burlington County, New Jersey. *Bulletin of the Archaeological Society of New Jersey*, **52**, 88–92.

Ubelaker, D.H. (1999) *Human Skeletal Remains; Excavation, Analysis, Interpretation*, 3rd edn. Taraxacum, Washington, DC.

Ubelaker, D.H. (2009) The forensic evaluation of burned skeletal remains: A synthesis. *Forensic Science International*, **183**, 1–5.

Ubelaker, D.H. (2015) Case applications of recent research on thermal effects on the skeleton. In: *The Archaeology of Cremation; Burned Human Remains in Funerary Studies* (ed. T. Thompson). Oxbow Books, Oxford, UK and Philadelphia, PA, pp. 213–226.

Ubelaker, D.H., Owsley, D., Houck, M., Craig, E., Grant, W., Woltanski, T., *et al.* (1995) The role of forensic anthropology in the recovery and analysis of Branch Davidian Compound victims: Recovery procedures and characteristics of the victims. *Journal of Forensic Sciences*, **40**(3), 335–340.

Van Vark, G.N. (1970) *Some Statistical Procedures for the Investigation of Prehistoric Human Skeletal Material*. V.R.B. Offsetdrukkerij, Groningen.

Van Vark, G.N. (1974) The investigation of human cremated skeletal material by multivariate statistical methods I. Methodology. *International Journal of Skeletal Research*, **1**, 63–95.

Van Vark, G.N. (1975) The investigation of human cremated skeletal material by multivariate statistical methods II. Measures. *International Journal of Skeletal Research*, **2**, 47–68.

Walker, P.L., Miller, K.W.P., and Richman, R. (2008) Time, temperature, and oxygen availability: An experimental study of the effects of environmental conditions on the color and organic content of cremated bone. In: *The Analysis of Burned Human Remains* (eds. C.W. Schmidt and S.A. Symes). Elsevier, San Diego, CA, pp. 129–136.

Warren, M.W., Falsetti, A.B., Hamilton, W.F., and Levine, L.J. (1999) Evidence of arteriosclerosis in cremated remains. *The Journal of Forensic Medicine and Pathology*, **20**, 277–280.

Warren, M.W. and Maples, W.R. (1997) The anthropometry of contemporary commercial cremation. *Journal of Forensic Sciences*, **42**, 417–423.

Wells, C. (1960) A study of cremation. *Antiquity*, **34**, 29–37.

Williams, H., Cerezo-Román, J.I., and Wessman, A. (2017) Introduction: Archaeologies of cremation. In: *Cremation and the Archaeology of Death* (eds. J.I. Cerezo-Román, A. Wessman, and H. Williams). Oxford University Press, Oxford, pp. 1–26.

Wilson, D.F. and Massey, W. (1987) Scanning electron microscopy of incinerated teeth. *The American Journal of Forensic Medicine and Pathology*, **8**, 32–38.

PART I

Search and Recovery of Burnt Human Remains from the Fire Scene

CHAPTER 2

Fire Environments and Characteristic Burn Patterns of Human Remains from Four Common Types of Fatal Fire Scenes

Elayne Pope, PhD

Fatal Fire Forensics LLC. Researcher, Lecturer, and Forensic Consultant, Researcher and Instructor, San Luis Obispo Fire Investigation Strike Team (SLO FIST) Fatal Fire Death Investigation Course, CA

2.1 Introduction

Heat-related damage that is observed on burnt bodies from fatal fire scenes results from combinations of heat, duration, and, in many cases, the type of environment in which the fire occurred. The sequence of heat-related damage resembles the stages of decomposition, since soft tissue breakdown also occurs along a continuum that is affected by temperature, duration, and environment (Ubelaker, 1997). These same variables influence the physical condition of the burned body from a fatal fire scene. Thermal damage occurs rapidly over minutes to produce the physical characteristics that investigators observe at the scene and / or during the post-mortem examination at the Medical Examiner / Coroner's Office. The fire environment plays an important role in the creation of burn characteristics to the body's layered soft tissues of skin, subcutaneous fat, layered muscles, internal organs, bones, and dentition. This chapter introduces the importance of correlating the findings of the scene with burn pattern characteristics that can result from four common types of fatal fire scenes: structures, vehicles, confined space, and open space. Examples of each type of scene are presented, showing the full spectrum of heat-related damage that occurs to the body's layered tissues from start to finish through progressive diagrams with stages of thermal damage that occurs over time to the victim's body within the fire environment. Examples are given for what is expected to survive of the body after a devastating fire; the final burned condition of remains; and where / how to search for possible fragmentary bones within fire debris for each scene type. In addition to the normal heat-related changes that occur during the fire, examples of common

Burnt Human Remains: Recovery, Analysis, and Interpretation, First Edition. Edited by Sarah Ellingham, Joe Adserias-Garriga, Sara C. Zapico and Douglas H. Ubelaker.

post-fire fragmentation are also presented to help anthropologists distinguish fractures between the two post-mortem events.

2.2 Experimental Research of Fire and Human Bodies

The results presented in this chapter originated from over 12 years of experimental field observations (starting in 2008) from burning non-embalmed human cadaver bodies (n = 150+) in a variety of fire environments (n = 69 structures, n = 36 vehicles, n = 24 confined space, and n = 23 for outdoor scenes) to explore differences and similarities of burn patterns. This research was conducted with the San Luis Obispo Fire Investigation Strike Team (SLO FIST) during the annual Fatal Fire Death Investigation Course in San Luis Obispo, California (www.slofist.org). Non-embalmed cadaver bodies are placed into mock crime scenes (burn cells with fully furnished rooms, vehicles, trailers, outdoor brush piles, burn barrels, etc.), ignited, and then documented with digital photography, and thermocouples for temperatures during the fire, followed by post-fire photography and documentation of the burned body's final condition.

2.3 How the Human Body Burns

Fire and heat progressively alter the appearance and condition of the body's layered tissues, along with other combustible materials / fuels (furnishings) in the vicinity (Icove and DeHaan, 2009; DeHaan & Icove, 2012). Exposure to heat (direct / radiant) causes the body's soft tissues, primarily the skin surfaces to shrink and distort within minutes. Tissues of the body burn sequentially as layers of skin, subcutaneous fat, skeletal muscles, internal organs, bone and dentition (Adelson, 1954; DeHaan *et al.*, 1999; DeHaan and Icove, 2012; DeHaan and Nurbakhsh, 2001; Dolinak *et al.*, 2005; Fairgrieve, 2008; Icove and DeHaan 2009; Pope, 2007; Pope *et al.*, 2022; Spitz, 2006). Heat causes the charred skin surfaces to shrink and split into tapered ovoid openings which exposes the underlying subcutaneous fat layers (Adelson, 1954; Dolinak *et al.*, 2005; Fairgrieve, 2008; Pope *et al.*, 2022; Spitz, 2006; Pope, 2007). The underlying layer of subcutaneous fat renders from heat exposure into a liquefied grease that becomes a contributing fuel source during the fire (DeHaan *et al.*, 1999; DeHaan and Nurbakhsh, 2001). Rendered subcutaneous fat collects and pools at the body / floor junction, where it becomes absorbed and wicked into charred clothing and fire debris at the floor surface (DeHaan *et al.*, 1999; DeHaan and Nurbakhsh, 2001; Icove and DeHaan, 2009; DeHaan and Icove, 2012). Pooling and spattered grease are responsible for the spread of a rendered subcutaneous fat-fueled fire that can sustain flames burning around the body that can last for hours (DeHaan *et al.*, 1999; DeHaan and Nurbakhsh, 2001; Icove and DeHaan, 2009; DeHaan and Icove, 2012). The presence of clothing on the victim's body is an important variable since it protects the underlying skin surfaces from open flames that burn above in the fabrics during the early stages of the fire. Later as the charred clothing materials burn away and expose the underlying skin surfaces, the charred fabrics at the body-floor junction are ideal wicking materials for absorbing and burning the body's rendered subcutaneous fat as a contributing fuel source for the duration of the fire.

Under the subcutaneous fat layer are dense and fibrous muscle layers, which are a poor fuel source, that surrounds and protects the inner skeletal structures. Heat exposure causes the muscle fibers to shrink and contract, which initiates limb flexion and body movement during the fire that is commonly known as the pugilistic posture. Sites of early bone exposure correspond to thinner areas of overlying skin and soft tissues that stretch over these flexed joints. During the fire, the upper extremity exhibits heat-related burn patterns with exposed bone surfaces that occurs earliest on the dorsal surfaces of the flexed phalanges, metacarpals, carpals, and distal radius and ulna of the flexed hand and wrist, followed by exposure of the proximal ulna and distal humerus of the flexed elbow joint, followed by posterior and lateral exposure of the humeral midshaft, and lastly the lateral surfaces of the proximal humerus at the flexed shoulder joint (Pope *et al.*, 2022; Pope, 2007). Sites of early bone surface exposure for the lower extremity can include the dorsal surfaces of the flexed phalanges, metatarsals, tarsals (without footwear), anterior surfaces of the tibia midshaft, followed by exposure of the proximal tibia, patella, and distal femur of the flexed knee, then the anterior / lateral surfaces of the femoral midshaft, and lastly exposure of the lateral surfaces of the proximal femur at the flexed hip (Pope *et al.*, 2022; Pope, 2007). Pugilistic postural changes are best observed in the extremities but also occur for the torso, which results in an arched spine of the neck and lower back (Adelson 1954; Dolinak *et al.*, 2005; Icove and DeHaan, 2009; Pope *et al.*, 2022; Pope, 2007; Pope *et al.*, 2004; Spitz, 2006; Ubelaker 1997; Ubelaker, 2009; Spitz 2006). Upper limb repositioning causes the flexed arms to move outwardly above the floor / ground surface and then extending over the chest. Positional changes for the lower limb results in the spreading apart of the upper legs at the hip with outwardly flexed knees with the lower legs and heels drawn together at the ankles near the midline, and with the arched foot and ankle pointing downward (Pope *et al.*, 2022; Pope 2007). Longer durations of heat exposure results in the greater degrees of repositioning and flexion of the extremities for the observed pugilistic posture. Longer durations of burning can result in reduced charred muscle mass which can result in greater flexion of the joints and with increased exposure of the burned bone surfaces (Figure 2.1). Heat-related color changes of burned bones (charred and calcined) results from surfaces that were exposed the earliest and the longest to heat (Bohnert *et al.*, 1998; Pope *et al.*, 2022; Pope 2007).

Bone exposure was first observed over flexed joints of the extremities that resulted from skin splits and from the shrinking / retracting musculature. Once exposed directly to heat, the bone surfaces undergo patterned heat-related color changes. Heat exposure produces a sequence of color changes that results from

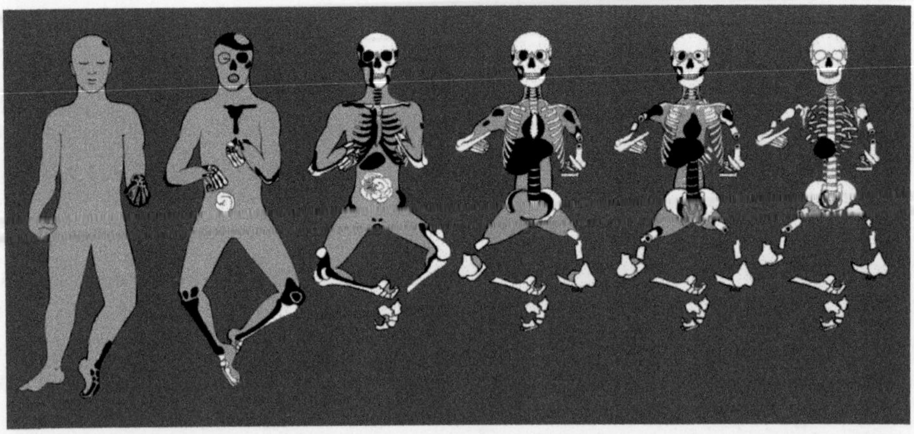

Figure 2.1 The sequence of the pugilistic posture, progression of burn damage, and sites of bone exposure to heat.

the gradual pyrolysis of the organic components from the bone's surface. The heat-related color changes are transient on the exposed bone surfaces during the fire which can result from skin splits over the flexed joints (fingers / wrist / elbow) or from the gradual retraction of charred musculature along surfaces of the bone. The continuum of heat-related color and texture changes begins with the exposure of the unburned light yellow bone that transitions into a thin fluid white / brown linear heat border that contours the charred muscles, next follows the development of a progressively darker band of greasy translucent tan / yellow / brown bone that borders the greasy black charred bone, and later can later transition into the brittle dried white / gray calcined bone from prolonged heat exposure. (Bradtmiller and Buikstra, 1984; Shipman *et al.*, 1984; Buikstra and Swegel, 1989; Goncalves *et al.*, 2015; Mayne, 1990; Mayne Correia, 1997; 2009; Pope *et al.*, 2004; Pope, 2007; Pope *et al.*, 2022; Thompson, 2004; Ubelaker, 1997). Exposed charred and especially calcined bone surfaces can develop heat-related fractures from shrinking of the cortical surfaces. Brittle charred and calcined bone becomes fragile and thermally weakened during the fire, which can break away under minimal pressure and may become separated from the main body and fall below into the fire debris substrate both during and after the fire (Pope *et al.*, 2022; Pope, 2007). Another common heat-related change is the fracture and separation / disarticulation of the flexed hand and wrist from the charred distal radius and ulna and may be referred to as 'fire amputation' of the extremities. Heat exposure causes the bulkier flexor muscles and tendons of the forearm to shorten which produces tension in the thermally weakened burned bone on the posterior surfaces of the distal radius and ulna that can fracture under strain. After the burned hand and wrist break away, they remain attached with the shrinking musculature and travel along the forearm. Separation of the burned hand and wrist can occur from heat-related fractures through the distal forearm bones or may occur along the natural joint surfaces above the wrist. Similar heat-related fractures can occur to the lower leg and ankle from the cumulative strain of the shortened lower leg (calf) muscles and Achilles tendon that stress and break the thermally weakened distal tibia and fibula, or may result in the separation of the foot and ankle along the natural joint surfaces. Later, when most of the long bones of the extremities have been exposed as charred and calcined structures, then they can become prone to fragmentation from the body during later the stages of partial to full cremation. This was observed in the distal ends of burned long bones that had fractured away from the body from the weight of the heavier charred musculature remaining around the flexed joints. These fractured segments of the extremities in charred and calcined bones occurred around sites of the distal radius and ulna, distal humerus, distal tibia and fibula, and distal femur. An understanding of how and where these burned skeletal fragments and dentition should be located and distributed can result in a more complete search and recovery of the burned human remains from the fatal fire scene.

2.4 Variables of Fire Environments

Fire environments are dynamic, with turbulent flames and fluctuations in temperatures (Icove *et al.*, 2009; DeHaan and Icove, 2012), unlike the artificial fire environments of crematoriums or muffle furnaces that have been traditionally used to model burnt human bone. Progressive changes in the fire's size begins first with ignition, followed by the stages of incipient growth, growth, fully developed / flashover, decay, followed by intentional / natural extinguishment (Icove and DeHaan, 2009; DeHaan and Icove, 2012). The duration of the fire correlates with the available fuel sources that burned around the body and the resulting extent of heat-related damage to the layered tissues of the body that burned within the surrounding fire environment (Bohnert *et al.*, 1998; Gonçalves *et al.*, 2015; DeHaan and Icove, 2012; Icove and DeHaan 2009; Pope *et al.*, 2004; Pope *et al.*, 2022).

Combustible fuels surrounding the body can also impact the degree of burn damage to the victim's body (Icove and DeHaan, 2009; DeHaan and Icove, 2012). These combustible fuels can include: natural materials such as wood, fibers, and fabrics; synthetic materials such as plastics, PVC, foam, and upholstery; and non-combustible materials such as metal, glass, ceramics, concrete / stone, drywall / gypsum board, and insulation (Icove and DeHaan, 2009; DeHaan and Icove, 2012). Any combination of these combustible materials and fuels may be encountered in common residential structural and some within vehicular fires. In addition to their spatial relationships with the body before, during, and after the fire, these burning materials can influence the body's degree of final pugilistic posturing and the heat-related burn patterns to soft tissues and bone. For example, a body that was originally lying on a couch surface can later fall to the floor as the the thermally weakened and charred wooden framework collapses under the weight of the victim's body – and if burning continues with heavy fire damage to the floor, the body may potentially fall through the living room floor and into the lower levels of a basement / crawl space. While burning on each item or surface, the body undergoes normal heat-related tissue changes of the layered soft tissues and bone along with positional changes in the body with flexion of the limbs. However, alterations can arise when the body makes contact with new objects / surfaces (such as fire debris on the floor) or later becomes partially protected / restricted by fire debris (ex: a structural beam or roof tiles falling on the body). Partial burial within fire debris also protects those surfaces from direct flame impingement. DeHaan (2008), outlined variables of fire exposure to human remains: (1) Size of the fire (a) Single item burning, (b) Multiple items burning, (c) Full-room involvement (flashover), (d) Sustained post-flashover burning. (2) Exposure of the body (a) On combustible floor for duration of fire, (b) On top of burning item(s), (c) On combustible floor that collapses during fire, (d) In suspension on a metal "framework" (e.g. car seat), (e) Exposed to fire on all sides. Most of these and other variables will be presented for the four common types of fatal fire scenes and the resulting burn patterns to the body.

2.5 Structure Fires

Residential structure fires begin as enclosed spaces that can involve variables of combustible and non-combustible furnishings; interior square footage of rooms; overall structure (manufactured home vs. a 2 story house), interior dimensions and layout (living room, hallways, bedrooms); the presence, number, and size of openings for ventilation (windows, doors); and the availability of various combustible construction materials (Icove and DeHaan, 2009; DeHaan and Icove, 2012). Common combustible furnishings in a residential structure fire can include beds, chairs, couches, recliners, or loveseats. These furnishings, in addition to other combustible fuels in the room (fabrics, wooden tables, cabinets, desks, dressers, etc.), can also contribute to the fire's growth and development around the body. Common household furnishings may be located under the body (couch / bed / recliner), next to the body (dresser / table / chairs), or have fallen on top of the body (bookshelf / cabinets) as fallen fire debris. Within a residential fire, the body can burn differently in various situations: burning directly on the floor, on furnishings (bed / recliner / couch), supported / suspended by floor joists under burned out floors, or falling through a thermally compromised floor into a lower level (basement or crawlspace) in and surrounded or partially buried in deeper fire debris layers. Partial or complete burial within layers of fire debris, (especially under burned gypsum board from collapsed walls and ceiling) not only protects those surfaces from direct flame impingement but also desiccates and dehydrates the charred muscle fibers on the burned surfaces, which can result in better preservation of the victim's body within the fatal fire scene, even when the fire damage to the structure is considered a total loss. Examples of each variable of the different fire environments are provided below, along with discussions of variables' influence on characteristic burn patterns to the layered soft tissues and heat-related burn patterns of exposed skeletal elements and dentition, the body's final burned condition, and when present, where the burned bone fragments may be distributed within the fire debris during the search and recovery for more heavily damaged burned bodies.

2.6 Burning Directly on the Floor

A body lying on a floor surface, from collapse or as their original position, burns distinctively. Any surface of the skin (face-up, face-down, or on the side) that are in direct contact with the floor remains protected from direct flame impingement, while the exposed surfaces of the layered soft tissues can burn from radiant / direct heat (Figure 2.2). Tight fitting clothing, belts, bras, and footwear that are in direct contact with the skin can delay burning of those protected areas until they become thermally compromised and burn away. During growth and development of the fire there is a continuum of heat-related changes that can occur to the layered soft tissues of skin, subcutaneous fat, layered muscles, organs, and exposed bone surfaces along with flexion of the extremities into the pugilistic posture are common heat-related transformations that can occur during burning. However, when the surrounding combustible fuels have been expended or extinguished, this arrests the heat-related changes to the body. When the victim is directly in contact with a solid floor surface of wood, tile, carpeted / tiled, or concrete slab, it protects and preserves that area of the body, which may include facial features, tattos, scars, or personal effects. Structure fires that burn for longer durations can result in deeper thermal damage to the layered soft tissues and bones of the victim's body. Burned shrunken and retracted muscles expose the once protected bone surfaces, directly to heat that undergoes thermal color changes until the fire is extinguished. Bodies with heavy fire damage and exposed burned bone surfaces may incur fragmentation during and / or after the fire which can result in smaller pieces distributed on the floor within the fire debris around and / or on the charred body (phalanges).

2.7 The Body on Furnishings: Couches and Chairs

Couches, recliners, and loveseats share a similar construction of a basic wooden framework with metal components of S-springs and / or metallic wires and hardware, foam cushioning, fabrics, and upholstery. Initially, the body remains elevated above the floor by the cushions and framework. As the fabrics and foam cushions burn away, portions of the underlying wooden

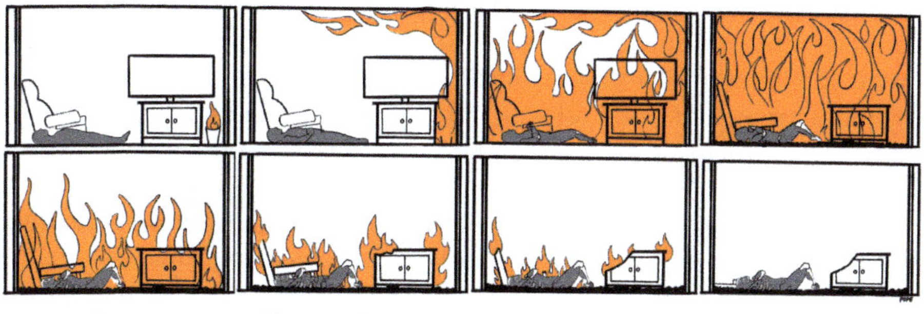

Figure 2.2 The sequence of heat-related changes of a body burning on the floor.

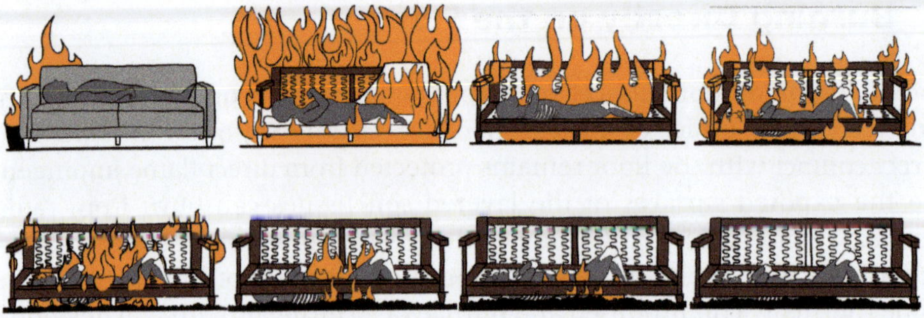

Figure 2.3 The sequence of heat-related changes of a body burning on a couch.

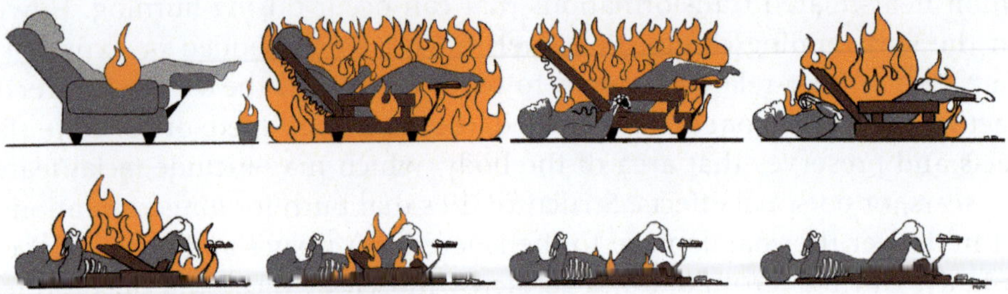

Figure 2.4 The sequence of heat-related changes of a body burning on a recliner.

framework becomes exposed directly to the fire. Surfaces of the body that are in direct contact with the fabrics / upholstery will initially remain protected from direct flame impingement, while the exposed surfaces will undergo heat-related changes to the layered soft tissues, bones, and the pugilistic positioning of the flexed extremities. As the flammable fabrics and cushion materials burn, the underlying wooden framework becomes exposed to flames and thermally weakened. The body sags and sinks into the burned wooden framework, from thermal fatigue of the metal S-springs sagging under the weight of the victim's body. (Figures 2.3 and 2.4). The weight of the body is then lowered to the floor surface into the fire debris layer which results in protection of those underlying surfaces from direct flame impingement. Victims that are seated in a thermally compromised recliner can collapse with the upper body extended through the charred seat back framework onto the floor. Bodies that were seated in basic wood or metal chairs (such as at a kitchen table) may slump over or sideways and may collapse onto the floor. For longer durations after flashover, the layered soft tissues of the body can continue burning from rendered subcutaneous fat as a fuel source that sustains smaller flames burning at the body-floor junction and can remain concentrated around the torso and upper thighs. After the fire, any burnt bone fragments that had fractured away from the body and fallen into the fire debris are likely to be found surrounding the body on the floor within the fire debris.

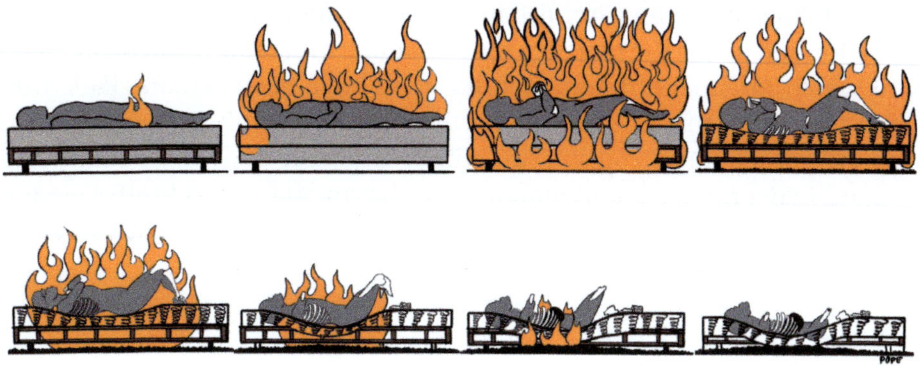

Figure 2.5 The sequence of heat-related changes of a body burning on a bed.

2.8 The Body on Furnishings: Bed

The structure of a bed (mattress and box springs) differs from the basic wood framework of couches and chairs. Mattresses that are constructed with uniform inner metal coil springs (not memory foam) keeps the body elevated and suspended above the floor during the fire. Surfaces of the body that are in direct contact with the bedding and mattress materials remain protected, while the exposed surfaces can become thermally damaged by flames and heat. As the flammable bedding fabrics and mattress materials burn away, the internal metal coil springs become exposed and supports the weight of the body for longer durations than the wooden frameworks of couches and recliners (Figure 2.5). The metal coil springs keep the body elevated within the fire environment and allows for more evenly distributed circulation of heat and flames that surround more surfaces of the body, which can result in more extensive burn damage to areas of layered soft tissues and exposed bone surfaces. The increased circulation of heat and flames around more / all surfaces of the body results in more evenly distributed burn patterns. Suspension of the body on top of the metal coil springs also results in rendered subcutaneous fat that drips below into the fire debris layer directly under the body that sustains a fuel source for open flames that burns both under the body and on the carbonized tissues of the decedent.

The annealed sagging metal coil springs (mattress / box springs) can cause the body's weight to shift position during the fire and this is also influenced by movements of the limbs and body from changes in the pugilistic posture. In some cases, the body may roll off bed and onto the floor during the fire. Exposed and burnt bones (charred and calcined ribs, phalanges, or cranial / long bones) may break away as the body moves and changes its position on the sagging burned mattress springs. Larger and more recognizable sections of the body often remain suspended during the fire, while the smaller burned bone fragments (charred and calcined portions of the fingers, hand, wrist, ribs, and / or cranial bones) can fall through the exposed metal springs and into the underlying fire debris. After the fire is extinguished, the search for burned human remains should include the identification of the larger recognizable portions of the body resting on top of the bedsprings followed by the careful hand an excavation and dry screening of the fire debris located under the mattress springs and the remaining burned bed framework to search for smaller fragments that may have detached and fallen during and after the fire event. In some cases, the carbonized soft tissues may become fused to the burned metal coil springs, which can make body removal more challenging and may produce additional post-fire fragmentation to the fragile burned bones during the manual separation and recovery process of the victim.

2.9 Loss of the Floor

Post-flashover conditions may result in the partial to total loss of walls, ceiling / roof materials, and, later may occur to thermally compromised areas of the floor. Burnt residential structures that have a lower-level crawl space or basement under the main house / manufactured home or that are multistory dwellings require extra considerations for the search and recovery process after a devastating fire. The potential for a thermally and structurally compromised floor around and under the body can introduce a new variable to the burning process, which can result in changes of the body's position, the extent of burn damage, and burn patterns to the body (Figure 2.6). Depending on the structure (single-story house, multistory house, apartments, or manufactured home, basement, crawl space the added variable of portions of the floor burning away is important to consider during the search and recovery process).

Wood floors (bare or carpeted) that burns from the surrounding fire environment later can become fueled by rendered subcutaneous fat that becomes absorbed and burns in the underlying charred wood surfaces. In more extreme cases, when areas of the floor have been breached by flames, these openings can allow for additional heat circulation and open flames around more surfaces of the body,

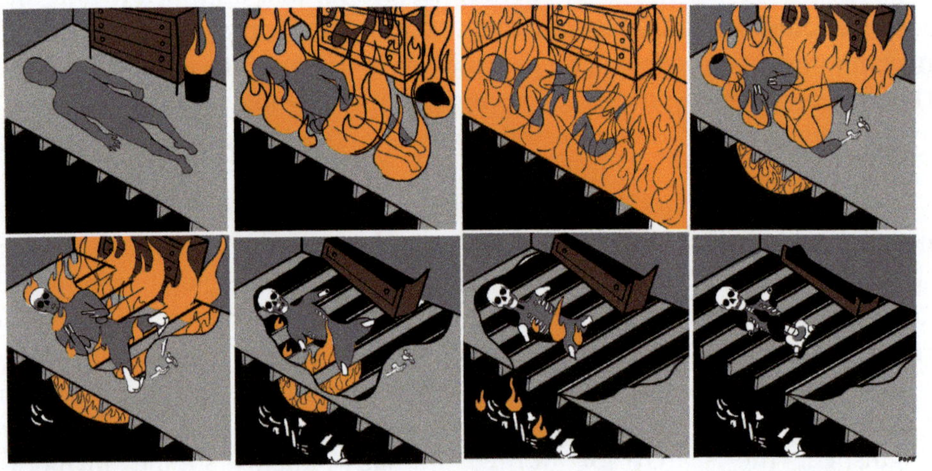

Figure 2.6 The sequence of heat-related changes of a body burning on floor joists.

especially if the victim is partially suspended and supported by the underlying floor joists and structural support beams. If portions of the burnt floor collapse, surfaces of the body may rest on the underlying floor joists / structural beams. The spacing of floor joists can support the victim's weight and at the same time allow for more evenly distributed heat circulation around the body as it remains suspended. Similar to the metal coil bed springs, the larger, more recognizable portions of the body often remain suspended on the structural floor joists while the smaller detached burned bone segments can fall into the fire debris of the lower level or onto the ground surface (manufactured home / crawl space).

2.10 Collapse into a Lower Level

If the floor has been thermally compromised, the charred floor joists may fail under the weight of the body and / or furnishings. Collapse of the floor and exposure into a lower level can introduce a new environment where the body may continue render and burn in the fire debris (Figure 2.7). If the body falls through the burnt floor joists, there's a potential for it getting caught in wiring, duct work, or other construction materials during the descent. Exposed and burnt bones can fracture from impact with any of these materials or from falling into the next layer itself can cause additional fragmentation of fragile burned bones and teeth. Larger fallen debris (charred joists, refrigerator, ductwork, roof tiles) can also crash down on top of fragile, burnt tissues of the body, which has the potential to increase burned bone fragmentation and distribution within the fire scene.

After descending into the next level, the new environment may also contain a burning / smoldering fire debris layer. This layer and any additional fallen fire

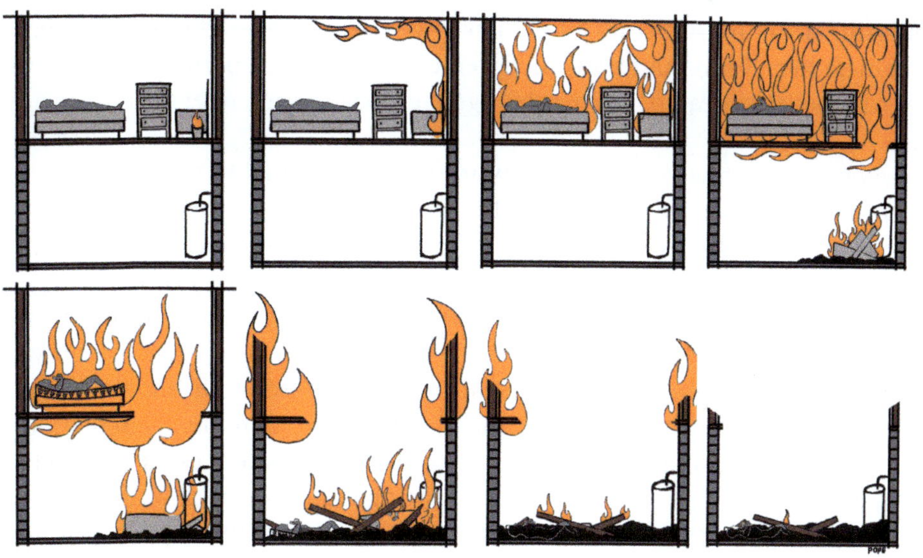

Figure 2.7 The sequence of heat-related changes of a body burning through the floor and having fallen into the basement.

debris (charred wood and drywall / gypsum board / construction materials) around and on top of the body can result in protection of these soft and skeletonized tissues of the body from direct flame impingement, thus results in preservation of the buried surfaces. In cases of partial burial within the fire debris, the exposed surfaces of the body above the debris line (face, arms, knees) can continue to burn, in contrast with the preserved and desiccated tissues that remain buried in smoldering fire debris and protected from open flames. Search and recovery may be more complex in these cases as layers of fire debris around and under the body should be searched and dry screened for identifying any fragmentary burned human remains (burned bones and teeth) along with any detached segments of the body (hands, feet, arms, legs, and cranial fragments). The distribution of skeletal fragments may be more complex, with smaller pieces scattered within the stratified layers of fire debris. In these cases, advanced archaeological techniques of careful hand excavation, and dry screening the fire debris around and under the body are necessary to ensure maximum recovery of the victim's remains.

2.11 Vehicle Fires

Compared to a structure fire, a vehicle fire occurs in a small, metal container. Vehicles have limited interior space and large amounts of synthetic combustible materials (plastics, fabrics, foam, and insulation) within the passenger compartment (Icove *et al.*, 2009; DeHaan and Icove, 2012). Vehicles can have elevated bucket seats for the front driver and passenger, and in some cases a broad metal bench for the backseat (some sedans / trucks), or bucket-style rear seating, which are more common in SUVs and minivans. Most of the vehicle's exterior and interior metal framework survives the fire, unlike most of the previously discussed wooden furnishings in structure fires that can experience thermal degradation and total loss. In a vehicle fire, these materials can produce unique burn patterns, depending on where the body is located: front passenger seat, back passenger seat, or inside the trunk.

The vehicle's smaller contained environment can quickly swell with flames if there is adequate ventilation during the fire's growth and development (from a cracked / opened window or door). Within minutes (or seconds, from an impact / collision or from use of ignitable liquids) the interior space can become a fully involved fire with turbulent flames surrounding the exposed surfaces of the victim's body (Icove *et al.*, 2009; DeHaan and Icove, 2012). The fire's size grows and extends through openings in the thermally compromised windshield, windows, or rear window, which provides additional ventilation and heat circulation that sustains the fire's growth and development. Initially, surfaces of the body that remain in direct or close contact with the seating materials, such as the backside of the torso and upper legs can remain better preserved than the exposed surfaces on the front of the body (seated position). As the seat covering materials (fabric, synthetic, leather) and cushioning burns away, these once protected areas become exposed to heat and flames. Areas of the body that remain in direct or close contact with flat surfaces of the doors, seats, floorboards, or other broad surfaces may be shielded from the turbulent flames and may have less burn damage when compared to the fully exposed front surfaces of the body.

As the fire's size diminishes, the smaller flames that are present within the passenger compartment space continue to burn in the front passenger compartment under the burnt dash from melted plastics and under the body from rendered subcutaneous fat accumulating in the floorboard that provides direct and radiant heat sources to the body. For some sedans / trucks, once the backseat cushioning materials have been thermally compromised, it exposes the internal metal framework dividing the rear passenger compartment and trunk with flames that can surround the upper body. A vehicle fire is a contained scene where any separated bone fragments fall into accumulated fire debris on the floorboard or base of the trunk.

2.12 Driver and Passenger Space

The body that is seated in the front driver or passenger bucket-style seats remains elevated above the floorboard surface during the fire. Common fuels in the passenger compartment of the vehicle can include carpet, upholstery (fabric, synthetic, leather), foam, plastics, rubber, and insulation materials. Within seconds or minutes, flames can engulf the interior that can produce direct and radiant heat damage on the front surfaces of the head, chest, abdomen, arms, and legs, while the backsides of the upper legs and torso remain temporarily protected by direct contact with the seat cushions. The arms can freely flex and move around the chest, while the bulkier upper legs spread apart from the flexed knees from the original seated position.

After the upholstery and foam cushions have been consumed, the remaining underlying wire framework of the bucket-style seat elevates and supports the body's weight throughout the duration of the fire. The back and base of the bucket-style seat consists of a metal frame work with wire springs that provides openings for circulation of heat around more surfaces of the body (Figure 2.8). This configuration is similar to the metal coil spring framework of a mattress and boxsprings, where the body remains elevated above the floor surface during the fire and receives more evenly distributed burn patterns on the exposed surfaces, particularly involving the upper body. Elevation by the metal framework of the bucket-style seat frame allows for the body's rendered subcutaneous fat to drip below into the fire debris layer directly under the body, both fueling the fire in the floorboard and burning as smaller flames on the body's carbonized tissues. This process can last for hours if the fire was not extinguished at an earlier point. The larger recognizable portion of the body often remains elevated in the seated position while smaller burned bone fragments may be present in fire debris in the floorboard in front of, under, and behind the seated victim.

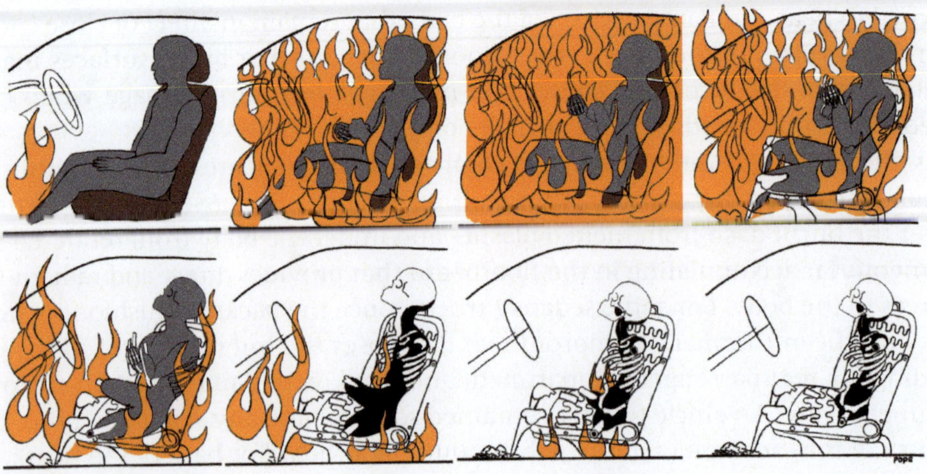

Figure 2.8 The sequence of heat-related changes of a body burning in the front passenger compartment.

2.13 Rear Passenger Space with Bench Seats

The rear passenger space receives the same amount of heat exposure in a vehicle fire when fully involved. Rear passenger seating construction can include an enlongated bench seat or elevated bucket-style seats. The bucket-style rear seats are similar in construction as the front passenger seats that keep the body elevated within the passenger compartment during the fire. For some vehicles, the rear seat may consist of a broad flat metal bench (under the cushions), which may be found in some sedans and trucks. Behind the cushioning, the upper back portion of the rear passenger seat is constructed of a metal framework of springs or perforated metal backing, which allows for direct flame impingement later during the fire that extends to the body from the trunk area once it is compromised by the flames. Burn patterns and soft tissue preservation for rear-seat victims may differ slightly from burn patterns and extent of thermal damage observed in the front passenger seats, sometimes with slightly better preservation of the lower body from remaining in direct contact with the metal bench seat. In this situation, the body does not remain elevated above the metal framework and there are no areas directly below the body for collecting rendered fat to burn as open flames except in the floorboard.

2.14 Trunk Environment

The trunk environment with a body inside is a smaller contained space when compared to the passenger compartment, with its enclosed and confined space (Figure 2.9). The trunk space is primarily a metal box that retains heat and flames

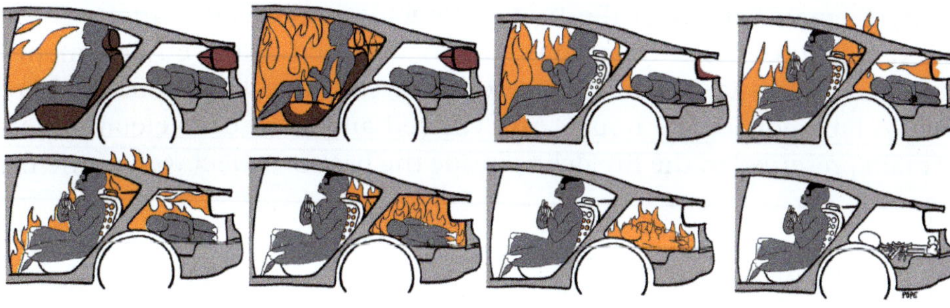

Figure 2.9 The sequence of heat-related changes of a body burning in the back seat and trunk.

after proper ventilation is available through the compromised upper back seat framework and melted taillight openings. In some cases, The body within may be partially flexed to fit the tight space. Before the flames penetrate through the trunk space, the interior remains protected from the main passenger compartment fire (unless it was the origin of the fire). Once the rear seat materials have become thermally compromised, heat and flames travel into the trunk space and surround the exposed surfaces of the body. Controlled ventilation through the openings of the tail lights results in concentrated flames passing over the body and into the interior back seat passenger compartment space. In cases of prolonged burning (hours), the overall mass of the body becomes reduced as charred and carbonized soft tissues and burned bones and fragmention. The presence or absence of a spare tire inside the trunk factors into whether the body remains in direct contact with the trunk base or partially elevated on the metal rim. The rubber tire is a fuel source that burns under and around the body. After the materials have been consumed, it can result in more evenly distributed heat circulation and exposure to flames around exposed surfaces of the victim's body. In contrast, a body that is lying in direct contact with the flat trunk base remains protected longer from lack of flame impingement while the exposed layered tissues continue to burn (longer preservation vs. quicker consumption). A body that remains partially elevated on the metal tire rim allows the rendered subcutaneous fat to drip and burn under the body in the fire debris within the wheel well.

Typically, a trunk fire burns later than the passenger compartment because the space needs proper ventilation and flames. After the upper backseat cushioning materials burn have through coupled with the presence of openings from the melted taillights, then cross ventilation occurs and combustible fuels in the trunk can ignite and become engulfed in flames around the body (similar to the conditions inside a commercial crematorium with an ideal forced gas / air mixture). Exposed surfaces of the body inside this confined space becomes a target object as the flames that travel through the smaller openings in the metal framework of the trunk, over the exposed surfaces of the body, and into the car's interior through the burned metal framework of the back seat, which can turn the trunk into a miniature crematorium with the proper combinations of heat, fuels, and controlled ventilation. These conditions in this confined space environment can render a body to partial or completely skeletonized charred and calcined bones if allowed to burn for several hours. Any charred and calcined skeletal fragments will remain preserved in the fire debris inside the base or wheel well of the trunk.

2.15 Confined Space Fires

Bodies that are burned inside tight spaces such as burn barrels, wood stoves / fireplaces, or trunks are subjected to a unique fire environment. Burning a body within these confined spaces requires adequate time, fuels, and often human activity to maintain the fire. Combustible fuels may already be present inside the space (trunk or burn barrel) or would need to be imported into the confined space (wood, ignitable liquids) in addition to the body inside. Burn barrels and wood stoves are smaller spaces; when a human body fills them, it doesn't burn very well initially (Figure 2.10). Inside a burn barrel or wood stove, the body occupies most of the space, with large surfaces of skin remaining in direct contact with the floor / base and walls. Also, burn barrels and wood stoves need a steady supply of fuel to begin rendering the body's fat – a slow process that requires the frequent addition of wood or fuels to maintain the fire. Inside, small flames burn in vacancies that are not occupied by the body's mass. Moderate attendance may be necessary at the site, to fuel and refuel each time the flames diminsh in size. As the fire debris layer grows deeper, it becomes a wicking material for the body's rendered subcutaneous fat to burn as small flames around the base.

Fuels may still be added repeatedly for hours afterward. However, the deliberate activities by the perpetrator of intentionally stoking and crushing the fragile burned bones and charred tissues can expedite the burning process since the smaller segments burn more efficiently and more space becomes available for the addition of more fuels around the body during the burning process. Gradually, the body's mass reduces in size, at which point the fire can be left to smolder for hours or days. The burn barrel / wood stove is a small, contained scene that retains the burnt skeletal fragments and teeth inside unless if there were

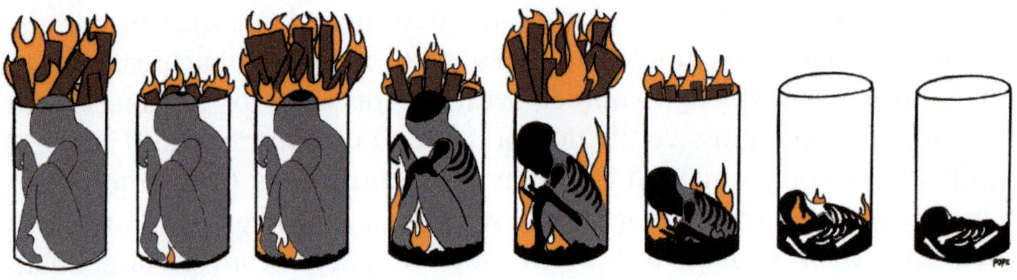

Figure 2.10 The sequence of heat-related changes of a body burning within a confined space environment.

openings in the side / bottom, or if the remains were transported to a different location.

2.16 Outdoor Space Fires

Fires that occur in outdoor environments, where the airflow is unlimited, can burn differently from the previously described enclosed environments of structures, vehicles, and confined spaces. The fire's size and duration depends on the types / amounts of fuels used, human involvement (in some cases), landscape environment (open / secluded), and weather conditions (dry, wind, rain). Naturally occurring wildfires or fires caused by lightening are also examples of outdoor fatal fire scenes.

Outdoor fatal fire scenes can also result when a perpetrator intentionally burns the victim's body to destroy evidence of a crime and / or personal identity. Individual outdoor incendiary fatal fire scenes can vary according to the size and types of combustible materials that were used as fuels for the debris pile – household furnishings, branches / logs, rubber tires, wood pallets, or the use of ignitable liquids alone. The landscape and surrounding environment are other variables that can influence the amount of burn damage – for example whether the fire occurs in a wide, open space (visible on the landscape) or in a secluded wooded / protected area with a fire that may go undetected, both of which can be affected by changes in winds and weather conditions. Previous or current wet conditions (precipitation) may hamper the fire's development and duration, whereas dry conditions and vegetation are more ideal combustible materials for burning.

2.17 Ignitable Liquids on Bodies

Bodies that are burned after being doused with ignitable liquids undergo a rapid set of heat-related changes before the liquid accelerants evaporate and burn away from the skin surfaces several minutes later. Ignitable liquids that are poured onto the body (and clothing) can produce a flammable vapor fire after ignition that can surround the body and, in some cases, can also burn surrounding vegetation, clothing, and / or proximate objects (tree / structure) depending on the size of the fire. The wicking properties of clothing retains ignitable liquids longer than naked skin alone. Ignitable liquids coats the skin and flows downward off the curved surfaces and pools at the body / ground junction around the victim's body. Clothing absorbed and retained the ignitable liquids that burned in the fabrics above the skin surface and temporarily provided protection from direct flame impingement. Superficial heat-related changes to the skin occur rapidly after ignition and can include scorched / singed skin, discoloration, blisters, skin splits, possible exposed and rendered subcutaneous fat, and early flexion of the extremities, beginning with the flexed finger joints. Minutes later, the flames diminish to several inches above the ground, burning primarily in charred clothing remnants around areas of the torso, thighs, shoulders, and neck at the body-ground junction. These smaller flames can self-extinguish or continue to burn if rendered subcutaneous fat is exposed and absorbed into charred clothing, dry vegetation, and fire debris which are wicking materials that sustain the burning process (DeHaan *et al.*, 1999; DeHaan and Nurbakhsh, 2001). After several minutes, the ignitable liquids on bare skin had expended (except in clothing / permeable materials protected under the body) and no longer contributed to the fire's development. Often with incendiary outdoor fires, ignitable liquids can be used to start the fire but have little effect on the body after several minutes of burning unless clothing or other wicking absorptive materials are present under and around the body to sustain the open flames.

2.18 Burning Outdoor Debris Piles

The arrangement of larger combustible fuels and the body's location within these materials is another important variable in an outdoor setting. The body can be buried lying on the ground underneath the debris pile (Figure 2.11) or positioned higher for more of a funeral pyre or bonfire configuration, where the body rests on top of or within the debris pile (Figure 2.12). Suspension on or within the debris pile (wood pallets, logs) during the fire allows for more evenly distributed heat exposure and thermal damage to the body's surfaces from heat circulation, which can be similar to the scenarios described earlier with the body partially elevated on the burned mattress springs and wireframe bucket-style seats in a vehicle.

If the body remains suspended within the burn pile during the fire, the rendered subcutaneous fat can wick into the charred wooden fire debris and burn under the body as well as on carbonized tissues. After the combustible fuels that were once supporting the body have burned away, the layered soft tissues of the body may continue to burn on the ground in the fire debris layer with smaller flames for hours from burning rendered subcutaneous fat. Additionally, any

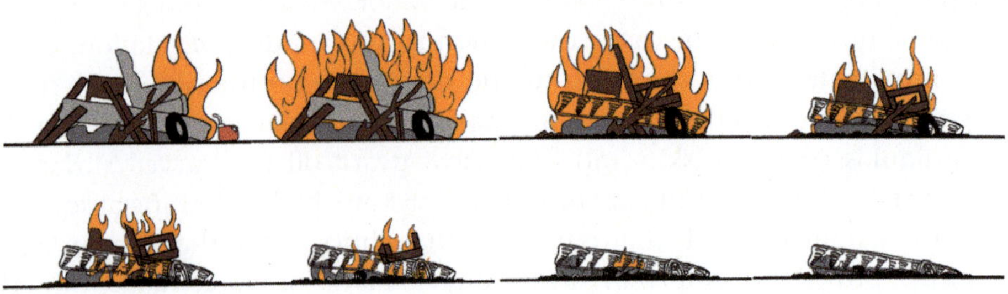

Figure 2.11 The sequence of heat-related changes of a body burning in an outdoor space buried under the fire debris.

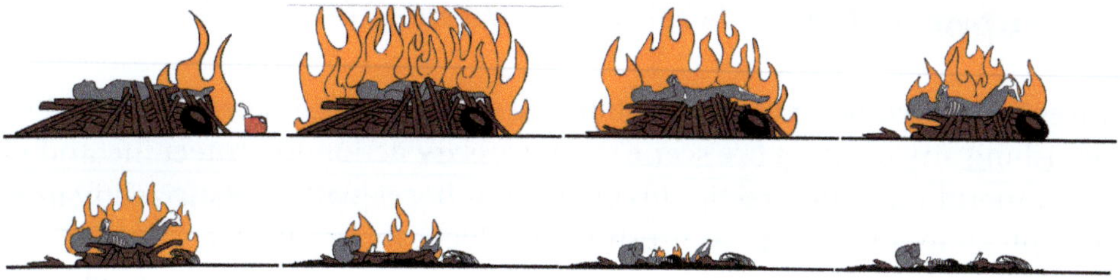

Figure 2.12 The sequence of heat-related changes of a body burning in an outdoor space on top of the fire debris pile.

human activity of tending to the fire by adding fuels and maintaining the fire can factor into the duration and extent of thermal damage to the burned body. Stoking the fire debris can cause additional fragmentation of burnt bones, leaving them present with in the fire debris around, on top of, and under the body. In contrast, a body that is buried under a large debris pile remains in direct contact with the ground which results in protected surfaces during the fire. In some cases, the extremities of the body may be restricted from movement into the pugilistic posture. For example if a mattress or large pieces of furnishings are on top of the body, these can pin or restrict the natural heat-related movements of the extremities, especially for flexion of the arms during the fire. On the other hand, a body that is located higher within the debris pile may lack such confining restrictions from attaining the pugilistic posture in the absence of heavy objects on top of the limbs. The main difference between the two locations within the burning debris pile is that a buried body may be restricted from fully developing the pugilistic posture and which may result in better protection and preservation of the victim's burned body when compared to the fire conditions involving the partially suspended body in the pyre or bonfire, that incurred earlier heat exposure to more surfaces of the body before falling into the protective layers of fire debris.

2.19 Post-Fire Fragmentation of Burnt Bones

This section introduces variables and pitfalls that can relate to activities of the search and recovery of burned human remains from residential structure fires, vehicle fires, outdoor spaces, and sometimes confined space fatal fire scenes. The activities associated with firefighting can potentially alter the body's original burnt condition. Several conditions can cause additional fragmentation of exposed and burnt bones that include normal exposure to heat as protective muscles burn away; movement and flexion of the limbs; crushing from any collapsed debris; damage from suppression; search and recovery methods; incomplete recovery, handling; and transport from the fatal fire scene to the Medical Examiner / Coroner's Office for forensic examination of the burned body.

2.20 Suppression

Fractures to burned bone can occur both during and in some cases after the fire. Extinguishing any burning fire scene is a necessary action to protect life and property. Common firefighting tactics involve using hoses with pressurized water as a method of extinguishment. A fire-hose nozzle can produce a straight stream (directly focused column of highly pressurized water), fogging (shower effect) or a graduated combination (Figure 2.13). There are notable differences between the two methods when considering physical evidence preservation of burnt human remains; however, it is not always known during firefighting efforts whether victims are inside the residence / vehicle. The straight stream method focuses a column of highly pressurized water that can cause extensive damage to the body if directly hit with force, which can cause fracturing, fragmentation, and dispersal of fragile burnt bone fragments on and around the body within the fire scene. Soft tissues and organs may also be affected when directly struck with the pressurized water stream and can result in damaged or projected internal organs outside of the abdominal cavity, and can result in disfigured charred muscles and soft tissues.

During suppression, portions of the fragile burnt bones can break away, not because of the temperature differential of cold water on a hot body, but instead from the direct force and impact of the pressurized water stream striking the surfaces of the victim's body. This suppression related damage is most commonly observed for the head, where the top of the cranial vault appears to be partially missing with the brain exposed and those smaller fragments be found distributed around the body within the fatal fire scene. The skull does not shatter or "explode" from internal heating or expansion of the brain by the fire, but instead the cranial bone fragments from being forcefully and directly struck with a pressurized water column. Also if furnishings under or surrounding the body are directly struck with the forceful water column from the straight stream method of extinguishment, this can cause shifting, collapse, and / or the deposit of additional fire debris (walls / ceiling) onto the victim's body. In contrast, the method of fogging or showering using the same pressurized water and results in better preservation

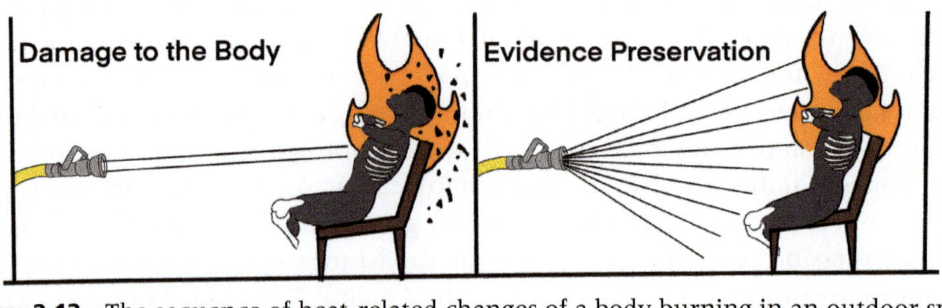

Figure 2.13 The sequence of heat-related changes of a body burning in an outdoor space buried under the fire debris. Suppression damage to the body from pressurized water from a fire hose: Straight stream directly impacts the tissues and burned bones, while fogging preserves evidence of burned human remains.

of the victim's burned remains as it essentially "rains" around the body, causing less post-fire damage to the burned soft and skeletonized tissues of the body.

2.21 Recovery and Transport from Fatal Fire Scenes

After the fire has been extinguished, the activities that are associated with overhaul and search through the fire scene has the potential to create additional crushing damage caused by heavy boots and dragging hoses. If the body is located this way, the post-fire damage to the burned body should be photographically documented and noted. Once a body is discovered, the process of scene documentation begins, using forensic methods of crime scene photography, archaeological gridding / mapping, careful hand excavation of fire debris, and dry screening of fire debris within the vicinity of the victim's body to ensure complete recovery. Certain types of fire debris can look similar to burnt human bones. For example the warped and curved pieces of drywall / gypsum board can look similar to the curved cranial bone fragments. Pieces of melted plastics can have a smooth outer surface that is similar to smooth cortical bone, with inner air bubbles that appear similar to trabecular bone. Door insulation from vehicles curls and may be confused with fragmentary calcined ribs.

Recovery entails removal of the body from its original in-situ context within the fire scene, which can produce additional damage to fragile burnt bones if handled improperly. In some cases, the largest and most recognizable portion of the body (charred armless, legless torso) is often removed, while leaving behind smaller burned bone fragments that can be subjected to crushing from investigators walking through the fire scene, or later discovered by family members returning later to salvage any personal belongings from their burned property. The level of experience and training of the body removal personnel can factor in the completeness of the recovery process. It is important to consider whether they have been trained in the forensic recovery techniques of fatal fire victims or if it was conducted by untrained personnel from a contracted body removal transport services. Another type of improper handling is when the fragile burnt bodies are moved by grabbing the wrists and ankles to drag or carry the victim outside of the fire scene, since there is a possibility of producing additional post-fire fractures to these burned and sometimes the unburned long bones of the distal extremities. If this does occur it is relatively easy to distinguish the post-fire break from improper handling versus perimortem traumatic injury, by examining the cross section at the fractured margins that are crisp, rich and brightly colored throughout. The post-fire cross sections of a fractured charred long bone can appear as a superficially blackened layer of the cortical surface, while underlying inner structures remain as fresh unburned yellow bone. Cross sections of calcined long bones can have a superficial gray/white layer of cortical bone with the underlying inner structures that remain charred black. Cross sections from the prolonged calcination of long bones transitions into a more uniform white/gray color throughout and can include heat-related fractures (surface and complete fractures) with possible shrinkage and warping. These layered heat-related color changes can also apply to post-fire fractures of cranial bone, the mandible, ribs, and other exposed burned bone surfaces. Another common mistake is when the body bag may be placed directly next to the fire victim before searching, removing, and sifting for burned bone fragments in the surrounding fire debris. Crushing can occur from boots of investigators or body transport service personnel while moving the body into the body bag, or additional fragmentation can result from pulverizing smaller burned bones under the weight of the victim's body during movement and placement into the body bag. If possible, any additional smaller burned bone fragments should be collected and transported within a rigid cardboard box or in other protective materials (loosely formed aluminum foil, evidence bags) and submitted along with the victim's body to the ME / Coroner's office for forensic examination. A majority of the time these smaller burned bone pieces are collected and then tossed directly into the body bag with the bulky victim's body inside and and then transported which can result in additional pulverization of those smaller bones.

Once the decedent is documented and sealed inside the body bag, carrying it through the scene can be problematic if the body bag sags or hits objects on its way out. Movement of a rigid and fragile burnt body within a flexible body bag may produce additional crushing damage to the exposed burnt bones. However, the use of a rigid backboard under the body supports and more evenly distributes the body's weight which can minimize the problem of excessive fragmentation of burned bones within the body bag. Also the use of the more durable disaster pouch body bags, which are constructed of a more rigid and heavier material, can produce unnecessary pressure points against the fragile burned structures of the cranial and facial bones, rib surfaces, forearms and wrist, and the flexed knees and lower legs during handling and transport. An alternative to this problem would be the use of a rigid and protective cremation box from a funeral home to safely transport the victim's fragile burned body. Strapping the victim's burned body onto the body removal gurney may cause localized crushing of the flexed arms, ribs, and flexed legs as the straps are tightly cinched down across the body to secure the remains for transport to the Medical Examiner / Coroner's Office. Before the forensic pathologist (or anthropologist) examines the victim's burned body, other types of handling and manipulations can occur during the process of receiving / transfer of victim's fragile burned body onto a morgue gurney followed by movement and rotation of the body for multiple radiographs, then the postmortem examination (rotating face up and face down), followed by the destructive autopsy procedures, all of which can occur before the forensic anthropologist conducts their examination of the burned bones. Understanding how and when these different heat-related and post-fire fractures occur can improve the analysis of burnt human remains regarding differentiating significant burn patterns from post-fire alterations that may be encountered in forensic anthropology casework involving burned human remains.

2.22 Conclusions

While the heat-related damage to bodies in fires can share similarities of the overall burn patterns, these are also influenced by variables (i.e. fuel loads, duration, interior dimensions, ventilation, furnishings, etc.) in the environment in which the body burned. The body's position during the fire – as lying face up or face down, remaining elevated during the fire or remaining in direct contact with surfaces of the the floor / ground / furnishings influences the areas of surface exposure and protection / preservation, overall burn patterns, and in some cases, the distribution of burned bone fragments located around the body within the fire debris at the fatal fire scene. Fragmentary remains of burnt bones and teeth can be recovered depending on the final condition of the body and scene within the surrounding fire debris. Recovery of these smaller burned skeletal fragments and in some cases, dentition along with the main body provides a more comprehensive picture of how the body burned. Finally, an awareness of the many post-mortem transformations that layered tissues of the body undergoes both during the fire (heat-related changes) and after (search, recovery, transport) can improve the forensic analysis of burnt human remains by the forensic anthropologist, especially for differentiating heat-related and post-fire fractures from any perimortem traumatic injury.

References

Adelson, L. (1954) Role of the pathologist in arson investigation. *Journal of Criminal Law, Criminology and Police Science*, **45**, 760 768.

Bohnert, M., Rost, T., and Pollak, S. (1998) The degree of destruction of human bodies in relation to the duration of the fire. *Forensic Science International*, **95**, 11–21.

Bradtmiller, B. and Buikstra, J.E. (1984) Effect of burning on human bone microstructure: A preliminary study. *Journal of Forensic Sciences*, **29**(2), 535–540.

Buikstra, J. and Swegel, M. (1989) Bone modification due to burning: Experimental evidence. In: *Bone Modification* (eds. R. Bonnichsen and H. Sorg). Center for the Study of the First Americans, University of Maine, Orono, ME, pp. 247–258.

DeHaan, J. (2008) Fire and bodies. In: *The Analysis of Burned Human Remains*, 1st edn. (eds. C. Schmidt and S. Symes). Elsevier Academic Press, San Diego, CA, pp. 1–13.

DeHaan, J., Campbell, S., and Nurbakhsh, S. (1999) Combustion of animal fat and its implications for the consumption of human bodies in fires. *Science and Justice*, **39**(1), 27–38.

DeHaan, J. and Icove, D. (2012) Fire related deaths and injuries. In: *Kirk's Fire Investigation*, 7th edn. Pearson, Boston, MA, pp. 611–654.

DeHaan, J. and Nurbakhsh, S. (2001) Sustained combustion of an animal carcass and its implications for the consumption of human bodies. *Journal of Forensic Sciences*, **46**(5), 1076–1081.

Dolinak, D., Matsches, E., and Lew, E. (2005) *Forensic Pathology Principles and Practice*. Elsevier Academic Press, Burlington, MA, pp. 239–246.

Fairgrieve, S. (2008) *Forensic Cremation: Recovery and Analysis*. CRC Press, Boca Raton, FL.

Gonçalves, D., Cunha, E., and Thompson, T. (2015) Estimating the pre-burning condition of human remains in forensic contexts. *International Journal of Legal Medicine*, **129**(5), 1137–1143.

Icove, D., and DeHaan, J.D. (2009) Fire deaths and injuries. In: Forensic Fire Scene Reconstruction, 2nd edn. Pearson Education Inc., Upper Saddle River, NJ, pp. 305–351.

Mayne Correia, P. (1997) Fire modification of bone: A review of the literature. In: *Forensic Taphonomy: The Postmortem Fate of Human Remains* (eds. W. Haglund and M. Sorg). CRC Press, Boca Raton, FL, pp. 275–293.

Mayne, P. (1990) *The Identification of Precremation Trauma in Cremated Bone*. Master Thesis, University of Alberta, Alberta, Canada.

Pope, E. (2007) *The Effects of Fire on Human Remains: Characteristics of Taphonomy and Trauma*. University of Arkansas, Fayetteville, AR.

Pope, E., Juarez, C., and Galloway, A. (2022). Refined classification system for thermally damaged human remains by body segment. *Forensic Anthropology*, **5**(1), 57–72.

Pope, E. and Smith, O. (2004) Identification of traumatic injury in burned cranial bone: An experimental approach. *Journal of Forensic Sciences*, **49**(3), 431–440.

Pope, E., Smith, O., and Huff, T. (2004) Exploding skulls and other myths about how the human body burns. *Fire and Arson Investigator*, **55**(4), 23–28.

Shipman, P., Foster, G., and Schoeninger, M. (1984) Burnt bones and teeth: An experimental study of color, morphology, crystal structure and shrinkage. *Journal of Archaeological Science*, **11**, 307–325.

Spitz, W. (2006) Fire and scalding injuries. In: *Spitz and Fisher's Medicolegal Investigation of Death Guidelines for the Application of Pathology to Crime Investigation*, 4th edn. CC Thomas Press, Springfield, IL, pp. 747–782

Thompson, T. (2004) Recent advances in the study of burned bone and their implications for forensic anthropology. *Forensic Science International*, **146**, S203–S205.

Ubelaker, D. (1997) Taphonomic applications in forensic anthropology. In: *Forensic Taphonomy: The Postmortem Fate of Human Remains* (eds. W. Haglund and M. Sorg). CRC Press, Boca Raton, FL, pp. 77–90.

Ubelaker, D. (2009) The forensic evaluation of burnt skeletal remains. *Forensic Science International*, **183**(1–3), 1–5.

CHAPTER 3

Recovery and Interpretation of Human Remains from Fatal Fire Scenes

Alexandra R. Klales[1], PhD, D-ABFA; Allison Nesbitt[2], PhD; Dennis C. Dirkmaat[3], PhD, D-ABFA and Luis L. Cabo[4], PhD

[1] *Associate Professor of Forensic Anthropology, Washburn University, KS*

[2] *Assistant Teaching Professor, Department of Pathology and Anatomical Sciences, School of Medicine, University of Missouri, MO*

[3] *Chair of the Department of Applied Forensic Sciences, Mercyhurst University, PA*

[4] *Director of the Forensic and Bioarchaeology Laboratory, Mercyhurst University, PA*

3.1 Introduction

Fatal fire scenes involve the death of one or more individuals in residences, non-residential buildings, vehicles, or as a result of outside fires. These scenes are complex due to thermal modification of the scene itself and the challenges of the subsequent scene investigation. The length of time the structure burned, risk of future fires, size and location of the burnt structure, topography of the site, weather, fire suppression techniques, size and number of debris and artifacts, and the number of deceased individuals are several factors that can impact the recovery and interpretation of a fatal fire scene. In addition, the investigation to determine the fire's cause by fire investigators and law enforcement and the identification and recovery of the deceased individuals by forensic anthropologists must be coordinated.

Historically, recovery protocols for fatal fire victims have been non-existent, poorly implemented, or vary greatly by jurisdiction, so much so that the United States National Institute of Justice (NIJ) funded a 2008 grant (Symes *et al.*, 2012a) to specifically develop uniform recovery protocols. In the years since this grant, the need for the integration of forensic anthropologists and forensic archaeological principles into these recoveries has been recognized within the fire investigation community, courses, and in fire investigation textbooks (e.g. National Fire Protection Association Standard 921, see text in the next section). This has resulted in better integration of a team-based approach and application of forensic

Burnt Human Remains: Recovery, Analysis, and Interpretation, First Edition. Edited by Sarah Ellingham, Joe Adserias-Garriga, Sara C. Zapico and Douglas H. Ubelaker.

archaeology to fatal fires or the direct involvement of a forensic anthropologist (or forensic anthropology team) in the recovery at these complex scenes.

A forensic anthropology team, or forensic anthropologist, integrated within a fire recovery team, can implement forensic archaeological recovery (FAR) protocols that are applicable to a variety of fatal fire scenes (Dirkmaat *et al.*, 2012). For instance, in a residential fire involving a two-story home with two adult individuals, a child, and a pet, the forensic anthropologist can easily locate the remains using FAR search techniques, differentiate the human from non-human remains, and recover the entirety of the remains while carefully documenting context and association. Forensic anthropologists possess a unique skillset that is needed in these complex scenes. They are specifically trained in fragmentary human osteology, comparative anatomy / osteology (human vs. non-human), and the recognition of taphonomically altered remains (e.g. thermal alterations and trauma timing). The forensic anthropologist, with a small team and using efficient methods, can systematically recover and document the human remains and associated evidence from the house in one or two days using efficient archaeologically based protocols (Dirkmaat *et al.*, 2012). In real time, identification of the human remains from the rest of the burnt debris and documentation of its location and associated evidence preserves the context of the scene and prevents misidentification of commingled individuals. In subsequent laboratory analyses, the forensic anthropologist can establish the biological profile (age, sex, ancestry, stature, individualizing traits) for each individual to aid in identification, sample bone for DNA analyses, assess the burn pattern of the remains, and interpret any taphonomic and traumatic modifications to the decedents. These methods and protocols can be applied to the systematic and documented recovery of human remains from outdoor, vehicle, and structure fire scenes by a forensic anthropologist or forensic anthropology team.

In this chapter, we summarize fatal fires, discuss the issues associated with their recovery when human remains are involved, and critique historic and widely applied recovery approaches. Next, we put forth recommendations and detailed step-by-step guidelines for the application of FAR principles to fatal fire recoveries. The protocols presented here are a combination of recommendations resulting from specific case experience (Dirkmaat and Adovasio, 1997; Bartelink *et al.*, 2020; de Boer, 2020), but are primarily based on published guidelines stemming from a three-year NIJ-funded research project on the use of forensic anthropology in fatal fire recoveries (Dirkmaat *et al.*, 2012; Symes *et al.*, 2012a). While improvements have occurred within the fire investigation community, such as the recognition for the need to integrate forensic anthropology since the grant results were published in 2012, more work needs to be done. Specifically, publishing about the use of recovery and identification protocols at fatal fire scene cases and on collaboration and communication between forensic anthropologists and fire investigators, law enforcement, and coroners / medical examiners (C / ME) is needed.

3.2 Summary of Fires in the USA

Fire scenes may be accidental, natural, or the result of mass disasters. In some instances they are set by perpetrators as a weapon in an attempt to prevent victim identification, or to destroy the scene and physical evidence related to the commission of a crime. In the USA, fires result in thousands of civilian deaths / injuries and billions of dollars of property damage per year. From 2010 to 2019, fire frequencies in the USA declined 3.2%; however, fire-related deaths rose 24.1% from 2010, with 3704 reported deaths in 2019 (U.S. Fire Administration, 2021). The National Fire Protection Association (NFPA) classifies three major categories of fires: structure (residential and nonresidential) fires, vehicle fires, and outside and other fires (Ahrens and Evarts, 2020). The most reported fires to which national fire departments respond are outside and other fires (45%), followed by residential and nonresidential structure fires (37%), and lastly vehicle fires (17%). While most reported fires in 2019 occurred outside / other fires, the majority (77%) of civilian deaths (n = 2870) in 2019 were in one- and two-family homes and apartment building residential structure fires, followed by vehicle fires (17%), with 644 total civilian deaths (Ahrens and Evarts, 2020). These statistics highlight the high number of fires, deaths associated with fire, and the potential demand for medicolegal recoveries of human remains from fatal fire scenes.

3.3 Statement of the Problem

Fatal fires are one of the most difficult scenes to recover, aside from mass disasters, especially if human remains are situated within the burnt debris. The complexity of the fatal fire scene is due to both the drastic modification to the contextual environment and the significant thermal modification that occurs to the body itself (see Dirkmaat *et al.*, 2012 for a more detailed discussion of body modifications). Recovery challenges include the large quantity of altered debris present, modifications to the scene by fire suppression efforts, disruption caused by first responder life-saving efforts, collapsed debris and safety concerns associated with structural integrity, and by homogenization (e.g. color) of the debris field and body (Dirkmaat *et al.*, 2012) (Figure 3.1). The human remains themselves are often highly fractured, friable, fragmented or missing, misshapen, and similarly colored to surrounding non-biological structures (Shipman *et al.*, 1984; Mayne Correia, 1997; Dirkmaat *et al.*, 2008, 2012; Symes *et al.*, 2008). Due to these challenges, human remains are often disturbed, missed, altered, misidentified, or even destroyed during the recovery and processing of scenes when using non-FAR protocols (Dirkmaat *et al.*, 2012; Symes *et al.*, 2012b). The recovery efficiency and completeness in turn impacts subsequent mortuary and laboratory analyses, including positive identification, analysis of perimortem trauma, and determination of cause and manner of death.

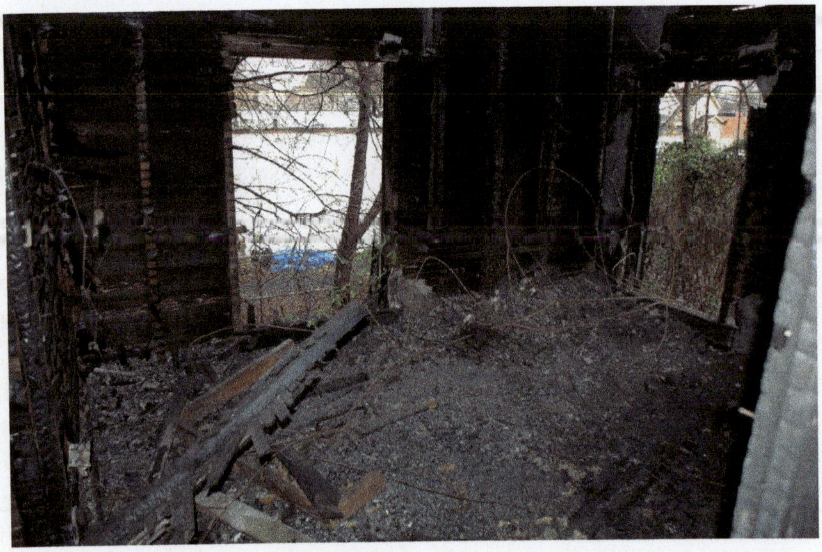

Figure 3.1 Residential structure fire with human remains showing homogenous coloration and large quantities of debris that complicate locating and recovering human remains in fatal fires when not using FAR.

Fatal fire scene recoveries and investigations vary considerably by region and can involve: first responders (emergency medical technicians, fire fighters, etc.), C / ME, medicolegal death investigators, law enforcement, fire / arson investigators, and forensic scientists such as crime scene investigators, forensic odontologists, forensic chemists, and / or forensic anthropologists. Proper and thorough investigation necessitates collaboration between these various specialties. First responders arrive at the scene with the intent to save lives above all else and their recovery efforts can modify the scene. If human remains are known or suspected to be contained within the fire, the C / ME has legal jurisdiction over the recovery of the body. A standard medicolegal death investigation involves photographic and written documentation, followed by a rapid recovery of the body into a body bag for transport to the mortuary facility. The information collected *should* minimally include the location, position, and orientation of the body in relation to the associated scene. In addition, the body should be treated and collected in a manner that prevents further destruction during transport. The C / ME is also later responsible for identifying the remains and certifying the cause (COD) and manner of death (MOD) following an investigation, which can include an inquest and autopsy. Fire investigators assist the death and criminal (if a homicide) investigations through determination of the fire cause and origin and through the collection and documentation of physical evidence at the scene. Law enforcement is responsible for investigating the circumstances surrounding any suspicious deaths or those deemed a potential homicide. The role of other forensic scientists varies from case to case, but can include a forensic chemist analyzing fire accelerants, forensic odontologists determining a positive identification from the dentition, and forensic pathologists completing an autopsy to certify COD / MOD. In some circumstances, albeit far too infrequently, forensic anthropologists assist with the analysis of the remains in the laboratory to facilitate identification and information related to the COD / MOD. Even less frequently, forensic anthropologists complete a FAR of the scene or are asked to aid in recovery efforts. However, we argue that, in association with law enforcement and investigators, forensic anthropologists are crucial to properly recover, identify, and assess trauma to human remains at fatal fire scenes due to their specialized training and unique skillset.

Fatal fire scene documentation is often incomplete without the use of a forensic anthropologist (or team), training / experience applying FAR techniques, and / or implementation of standardized recovery protocols. An analysis of fatal fire scene investigations completed in Ontario, Canada from 2000 to 2006 by an experienced fire marshal, as part of the aforementioned NIJ-funded research grant, revealed many missing qualitative and quantitative data fields / variables that should be collected to adequately document the fatal fire scene (Olson, 2009; Symes *et al.*, 2012a). Anecdotally, the authors of this chapter have also noticed a similar trend during active forensic casework conducted throughout the USA. For example, the amount of remains recovered from a fatal fire case scene excavation, notes or photographs of the recovery of the remains, or the pathology report were missing from the analyzed records of the Office of the Fire Marshal for the Province of Ontario during the period under examination. The notes, photographs, and pathology report should contain important information about body positioning and location, the contextual location of evidentiary information, identification of skeletal remains that help reconstruct the events of the fire. In addition, the rapid removal of the remains, common at most fatal fire scenes, and the resulting lack of documentation, often prevents subsequent reconstruction of this information, complicates the investigation, and creates additional post mortem modification to the already heavily modified body. Without proper documentation and removal, it is difficult or often impossible to answer important investigative questions such as:

- Why are certain elements missing or more altered?
- Where was the body originally placed and what relation does it have to evidence?
- What position was the body in and is the body position related to the COD / MOD?

Body position and location provide crucial information to the fire investigator on the death timeline and can provide MOD information (c.f. Fojas *et al.*, 2015). Improper collection and removal of the remains results in fragmentation and missing elements that in turn impede the forensic pathologist autopsy findings and the subsequent work of the forensic specialists involved (e.g. identification efforts). An experienced forensic anthropologist using FAR techniques can prevent loss of evidentiary material or human tissue (Harrison, 2019), reduce commingling and expedite scene processing (de Boer *et al.*, 2020), and preserve scene context and association (Dirkmaat, 2002; Ubelaker, 2009).

3.4 Current Fatal Fire Victim Recovery Protocols

"As a forensic science discipline, fire investigation is hampered by the amount of widespread, persistent, and problematic literature affecting the beliefs and the behavior of its practitioners."

(Lentini, 2006)

In the fire investigation world, emphasis in fatal fire recoveries has been on determining the cause and origin of the fire rather than on the recovery of the decedent and evidence. The Law Enforcement Assistance Administration published *Arson and Arson Investigation Survey and Assessment* in 1977 (Boudreau *et al.*, 1977) and the United States National Bureau of Standards (NBS) (now known as the National Institute of Standards and Technology, NIST) published the *Fire Investigator Handbook* in 1980 (Brannigan *et al.*, 1980). These publications were some of the very first attempts to standardize fatal fire recoveries; however, as Lentini (2006) note, they are based not on research but rather on experiential and anecdotal information, much of which has been debunked recently (see Lentini, 2006 for a more detailed discussion). Noticeably absent from the early versions of the NBS handbook are procedures for locating and recovering decedents in a systematic and scientific manner. Also lacking from these early editions is an adequate description of thermal modifications to the body and how to recognize and appropriately recover human remains that have been modified. Standard fire recovery protocols that are efficient and have been field tested with measurable and repeatable results continue to be desired (Harrison, 2019).

In 1985, the NFPA Standards Council appointed a technical committee to address these issues and in turn published the NFPA 921: *Guide for Fire and Explosion Investigations*. Section 25.5 *Investigating Fire Scenes with Fatalities* of NFPA 921 details the procedures that should be implemented when a fatality occurs. Sub-section 25.5.3 *Team Investigation* recommends contacting a forensic anthropologist in cases where the body is very badly burned or if foul play is suspected. The following protocols are recommended (NFPA, 2014):

- Utilizing a team-based approach
- Scene documentation (photographic, video, and sketching)
- Search of the entire scene (not just near the body) using a grid system
- Notation of stratigraphy
- Screening of removed debris
- Body removal

The guide uses vague generalities and does not provide detailed specifics on how the recovery operation should commence in a step-by-step fashion. *Kirk's Fire Investigation,* originally published in 1969, is on the 8th edition and closely aligns with the NFPA standards (Icove and Haynes, 2018). Unfortunately, in practice, these guidelines are ignored or not fully implemented and the frequency with which they are implemented is currently unknown. Also, many of these protocols have not been systematically tested in field and / or lab environments. Fast recovery has instead been the "priority because it reduces the psychological burden on survivors" (Cordner *et al.*, 2016). Mayne Correia and Beattie (2001), Dirkmaat *et al.* (2008), and Dirkmaat *et al.* (2012) provide a critical review of these fatal-fire recovery techniques, stressing the need for improvement due to the aforementioned issues with this approach.

Current fire investigator protocols (within the last five years) continue to focus on improving understanding of fire characteristics, the scene, evidence recovery, documentation protocols, all the while highlighting the importance of a collaborative approach (NFPA 921; Icove and Haynes, 2018; Lentini, 2019). These newer texts include short sections about post mortem changes to human remains, body position, search and grid recovery of human remains, debris stratigraphy (i.e. the order, position, and relation of layers), and scene and victim documentation (NFPA 921; Icove and Haynes, 2018; Lentini, 2019). While a vast improvement, these descriptions are often very brief and do not include detailed protocols of scene recovery, pictures, or descriptions of post mortem changes to human remains, or how to analyze perimortem bone trauma on burnt bone. Within the anthropological community, there has been more research into the impact of fire on human remains, understanding patterns of destruction, and documenting thermal alteration to human remains; however, much of this research has yet to be fully integrated into fire investigation recovery protocols. Given the expertise of forensic anthropologists, it is surprising that they still do not often have a larger role in the recovery and interpretation of fatal fire scenes as part of the recovery team. Perceived limiting factors and misconceptions that may be preventing forensic anthropologists from being integrated in the recovery efforts include time (takes too long), logistics, combined rescue and recovery efforts, availability in specific regions, and the associated costs (i.e. too expensive) (Symes *et al.*, 2008).

3.5 NIJ Protocols

Forensic archaeological recovery protocols and data collection can be implemented regardless of the region, jurisdiction, or command structure. Forensic anthropologists have already documented the importance and benefits of a forensic archaeological approach to fatal fire scenes (Dirkmaat and Adovasio, 1997; Dirkmaat, 2002; Dirkmaat *et al.*, 2012), in order to document the context, position, and association of the victims and evidence. These techniques include mapping (total station, global positioning system / GPS, scaled hand-drawn, three-dimensional scanning, and global navigation satellite systems / GNSS), written and photographic documentation of the physical evidence and human recovery process, and the excavation of the scene with systematic collection and recording of evidence (Dirkmaat and Adovasio, 1997; Mayne Correia and Beattie, 2001; Dirkmaat, 2002; Dirkmaat *et al.*, 2012). Early work by Dirkmaat (Dirkmaat and Adovasio, 1997; Dirkmaat, 2002) identifies the key components of a FAR and their specific benefits to fatal fire scenes.

To produce systematic, repeatable, efficient recovery procedures using field and lab tested methods and analyses, a NIJ grant-funded research project of burnt human remains was performed (#2008-DN-BX-K131) (Symes *et al.*, 2012a). The research project combined field and laboratory analyses to: 1) develop protocols and guidelines to recover burnt human remains from fire scenes; 2) describe typical patterns and characteristics of fire alteration to human remains and bone; and 3) describe and validate protocols for the analysis of sharp force trauma on burnt bone to differentiate sharp force trauma from thermal damage to bone. New protocols, search techniques, and data collection forms were developed to record data accurately, efficiently, and consistently at fatal scenes. These newer protocols were refined over the course of the grant, experimentally tested using six mock fatal fire scenes, and then implemented at actual fatal fire scenes (e.g. structure, vehicle, plane / train crash fires). A modular home or partially burnt home scene was typically processed in one working day, while a larger two-story residential structure was recovered in approximately two working days with a team of approximately ten people. The project was conducted in the USA (Pennsylvania) and Canada (Ontario) and illustrates that standardized scene protocols and standard operating procedures can be efficiently implemented regardless of the location, time, or weather. However, consistent implementation of these protocols and further documented effectiveness of them in practice is still missing from the current literature.

As with any forensic recovery, the goal is to elucidate behavior, determine the sequence of events, and establish context / association. The recovery process itself is a form of *controlled destruction* that must be completed in a systematic manner to adequately interpret and reconstruct the scene. The aforementioned intricacies of fatal fire scenes require a specific set of protocols, training, and experience to adequately recover the scene in a manner that preserves contextual information. The recovery efforts are best served using FAR protocols and using a forensic anthropological recovery team or integrated forensic anthropologist. The Bridgeville Fatal Fire Recovery Protocols, as they are now known, described in detail in the following paragraphs, were developed as part of the NIJ-funded grant and are the application of FAR techniques to the recovery of fatal fire scenes. The four phases of the FAR are modifications of those originally described by Dirkmaat and Adovasio (1997): 1) systematic and comprehensive search techniques; 2) determination of medicolegal significance; 3) documentation of context and forensic archaeological recovery; and 4) laboratory analysis and report preparation.

Prior to arrival at the scene, pre-planning efforts should include: securing the appropriate equipment, supplies, and personnel; gathering information on the structure, scene, or possible decedents; and gathering relevant data (aerial images, weather data, floor plans, blueprints, aircraft manifests, etc.). Once at the scene, a planning meeting including all relevant agencies (e.g. C / ME, forensic anthropologists, arson / fire investigator, etc.) should commence. If necessary, an incident command center should be established and jurisdictional matters should be resolved prior to beginning the recovery. Jurisdictional requirements vary by region, but typically the C / ME or law enforcement will contact the forensic anthropologist for assistance with processing the scene and recovering the human remains. The forensic anthropologist typically becomes involved in a fatal fire recovery either if human remains are suspected to be within the fire scene or when human remains have already been located (or potentially located).

Prior to starting the recovery, the scene should be secured and the fire should be fully extinguished. Appropriate personnel (e.g. fire fighters or investigators) must deem the scene and / or structure safe and sufficiently cooled before the recovery efforts can commence. Written, photographic, and geospatial documentation should begin upon arrival at the scene and should continue throughout the recovery (see Dirkmaat *et al.*, 2012). With fatal structure fires, it is especially important to note the stratigraphic profile of the debris pile and its corresponding relationship to the original structure.

In instances when remains have not yet been located, Phase I of the FAR commences: systematic and comprehensive search techniques. This involves a large-scale search beginning with non-intrusive methods. In instances of large structure fires involving many blocks or large-scale outside fires (e.g. forest fires), aerial reconnaissance using either aircraft or drones is helpful to assess the full scale and extent of the scene. Cadaver dogs can also be of utility provided they are specifically trained to locate burnt, decomposed, or skeletal remains and are trained to passively alert at a hit (e.g. sitting or calling rather than digging). In most instances, a large-scale pedestrian reconnaissance will be the most effective search approach. Searchers should be briefly trained and shown examples, where relevant, of the materials they are being asked to identify / locate. This should minimally include a description of what to expect regarding the human remains (e.g. high fragmentation, homogenous coloration, etc.) and the materials relevant to the fire / arson investigators' inquiry (e.g. black box in aircrafts, specific wires, electrical devices, etc.). The search pattern should be determined beforehand. In most cases a linear, grid, or quadrant / zone approach will work best, while spiral and wheel search methods should be avoided as they could potentially damage evidence. Corridors or quadrants should be determined and denoted prior to the search commencing. Searchers should align roughly shoulder to shoulder to ensure at least a 30% overlap in their field of vision. A line leader should be designated to monitor the forward progress of the group and ensure the search remains structured. The search should commence at the furthest perimeter of the immediate scene (e.g. one end of the structure) and rapidly progress in a straight line along the pre-determined corridors or zones. Searchers should flag anything deemed potentially significant; searches should not evaluate significance as this could potentially stall the progression of the search team. It may be necessary for searchers to remove larger overlying collapsed debris (e.g. portions of the roof or large appliances) to an area behind the search line. The entirety of the scene should be searched. A secondary team, consisting minimally of the forensic anthropologist and arson / fire investigator, then follows behind the larger search team, conducting the pedestrian reconnaissance to determine medicolegal significance (Phase II of the FAR) of any flagged materials.

Once the remains have been located and determined to be human, Phase III begins documentation of context and the FAR. A more thorough and detailed hands-and-knees search commences in the vicinity of the remains, if safe, starting approximately 2–3 meters out from the primary concentration and moving inward. Searches should consist primarily of 3–5 individuals familiar with forensic archaeological principles or who have prior experience with excavating human remains. The searches should be in tight formation and progress in either a straight line or in a concentric circle search pattern (moving in a collapsing circle inwards towards remains). Searching should still be fairly rapid until remains or evidence are encountered and the immediate perimeter of the remains is determined. The primary purpose of this more detailed and focused search is to identify materials located in the immediate crime scene, including biological tissues, personal effects, and associated evidence. Debris surrounding the body or associated evidence should be excavated by hand in a top-down fashion or using a trowel to cut perpendicularly through the sediment pile to the base. All materials should be collected in dust pans, put into buckets labeled with the appropriate corridor or quadrant label, and moved to outside the immediate scene for sorting.

The removed material is then rapidly hand sorted on tarps by a second team (2–3 individuals); thereby acting as an "early alert" system (Dirkmaat *et al.*, 2012). Any significant evidence or biological material found during this sorting should be noted, appropriately collected, and most importantly the hands-and-knee searchers should be immediately notified. Once notified, the hands-and-knees team should slow the pace of excavation and recovery. At this point, careful, fine excavation should commence in the immediate vicinity of the remains / evidence using archaeological principles. All debris surrounding the body and evidence should be excavated top-down using trowels, dust pans, brushes, and wooden tools as needed (Figure 3.2). Any significant stratigraphic layers in the debris pile should be noted to help interpret association and context of the remains in relation to the structure and evidence. Material excavated during this process should be screened through a ¼ inch mesh screen to ensure smaller biological material and evidentiary items are not missed. Again, provenience information (e.g. grid # / letter or zone) must be maintained for all material being removed from the scene for sorting and / or screening.

If the remains consist of a primary concentration and are mostly identifiable, they should be fully exposed from the top working downward and left *in situ* (Figure 3.3). Any loose or fragmentary materials can be stabilized with hardening spray or

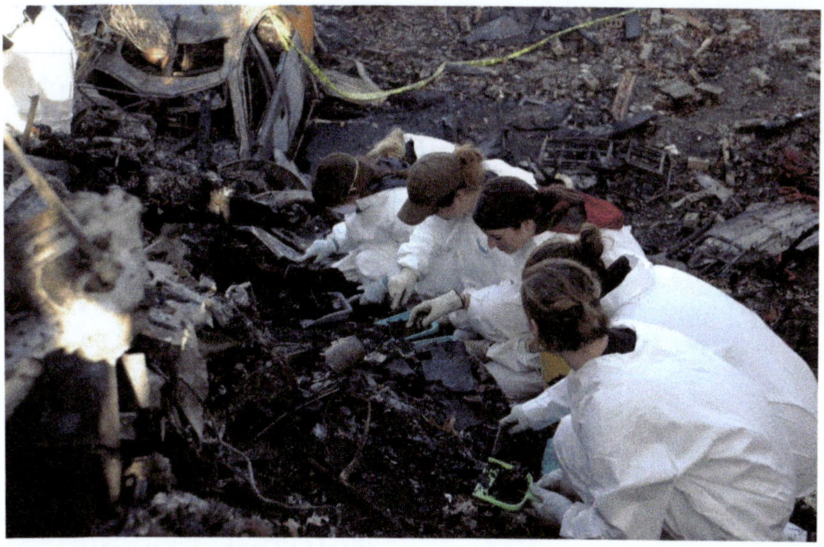

Figure 3.2 FAR excavation by hand in a top-down fashion through the debris pile to the base by moving in a collapsing concentric circle around the human remains.

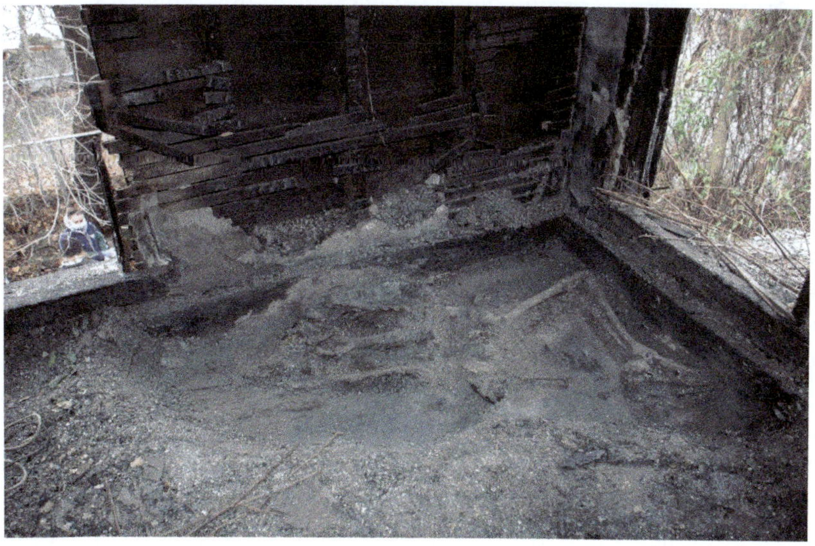

Figure 3.3 Remains excavated and fully exposed *in situ* at a residential structure fire after excavation using FAR protocols. Note: see "before" image of scene in Figure 3.1 above.

wrapped in heavy duty foil / plastic wrap or both. For example, exposed bone commonly found in the head, hand, feet, elbow, and knee regions should be stabilized to prevent further fragmentation during excavation, to ensure continuity of remains, and to prevent commingling (Figure 3.4). Once fully exposed the body should be documented (photo and written) and then mapped to document body position,

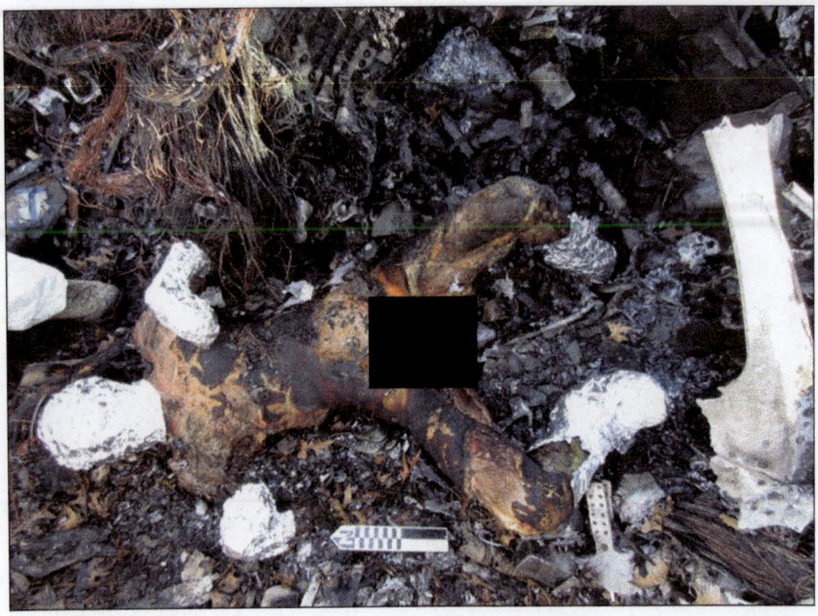

Figure 3.4 Fragmented and fragile areas stabilized prior to removal using heavy duty aluminum foil. Note: this is an example of the common "pugilistic posture" attained by fire victims whereby there is flexion of the elbows, knees, hips, and neck.

relationship of body to the scene, and evidence distribution. Mapping can be accomplished in a number of ways: three-dimensional scanning, scaled plan-view mapping and total station data collection, or GNSS geospatial collection to be paired with photographs (Figure 3.5). After the cessation of documentation, the remains and associated evidence are ready to be collected. The body should be stabilized and fully excavated (e.g. free of debris or entrapment) to ensure that it can be lifted as a cohesive unit directly into the recovery container. The goal is to lift and remove the body or body part straight up out of the debris pile, such that no portion of it is trapped under debris. If still entrapped, removal should never require pulling or tugging as it might result in leaving a body portion, or any human biological tissue behind. In this excavation manner, evidence and body parts not directly attached to the main portion of the body will be recovered and documented *in situ* and by the hypotheses of association, reconstruction of these disassociated parts to the main portion of the body occurs in the field. This will ensure that all biological tissues are noted *in situ*, and assigned the proper provenience designation, rather than having to be re-associated in the morgue using other means. Ideally, the body should be lifted directly onto a body board or hard surface (e.g. malleable plywood) and placed into a body bag. If necessary, the body should be loosely secured to the hard surface to prevent further fragmentation during transport. Associated fragments or debris containing biological tissues should be placed within the same body bag or appropriately labeled to ensure proper re-association in the morgue. This will save time and money by negating the need for re-association via DNA, which in some contexts may not even be possible due to the condition of the remains.

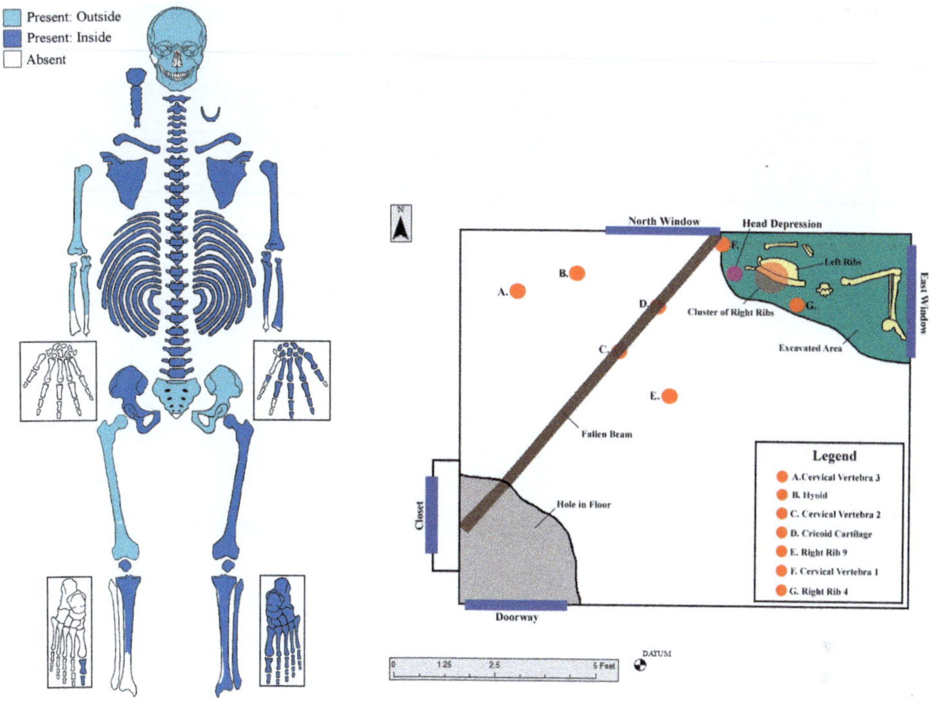

Figure 3.5 Left: skeletal homunculus of elements recovered at the scene by recovery location. Right: digitized scaled map created from geospatial data collected at the scene. Note: same residential structure fire from Figures 3.1 and 3.3 above.

If the remains are nearly cremated or highly fragmented and the body structure and position are not identifiable, all debris matrices should be collected for later sorting in more ideal laboratory conditions (Figure 3.6). Containers must be labeled with grid, coordinate, or zone information and geospatial data should be collected. More fine-toothed sorting and screening can be accomplished in the laboratory by hand or using geological sieves with finer mesh (Figure 3.7).

In total, the recovery of a single-story structure takes 1–2 days (approximately 8–10 hours) to process fully with a moderately sized team (~10 persons). Processing a multi-story house will increase the recovery time by an additional day or two, again depending on the size of the recovery team and personnel available. Vehicle fires can be processed in a single day with a smaller team (~4 persons) or at maximum two days if the debris field is larger from explosive materials and accelerants (see Special Circumstances section). Given that fire scenes are more complex than a regular crime scene, additional recovery time is expected and using the protocols already described does not add a significant number of days / labor hours.

The final phase (Phase IV) of the forensic archaeological recovery includes the laboratory analysis of the remains and report preparation. The forensic anthropologist's role in this phase will vary by jurisdiction, but in ideal scenarios the forensic anthropologist will be present for the post mortem autopsy examination. However,

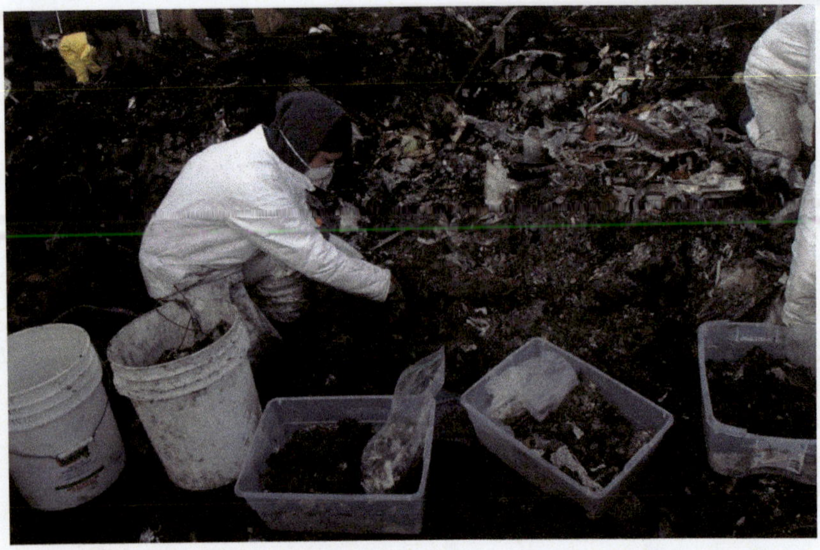

Figure 3.6 Cremated remains that are highly fragmented being excavated and collected in containers labeled with provenience information for later sorting in more ideal conditions.

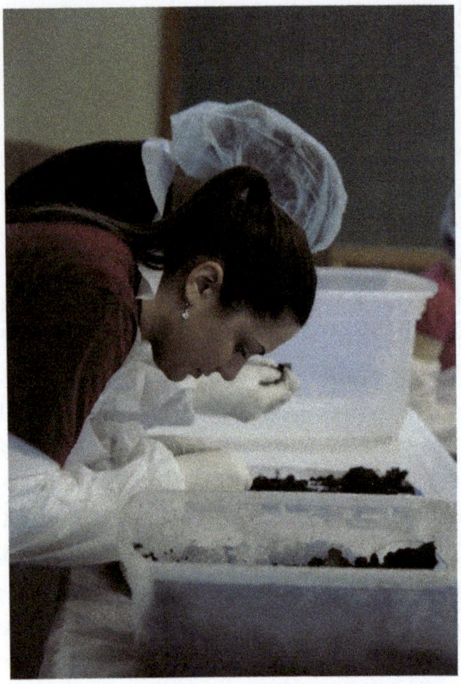

Figure 3.7 Forensic anthropologists hand sorting cremated human remains from the debris in the medical examiner's office. Note: same fire case in Figure 3.6 above.

in many instances the forensic anthropologist will receive the remains after the autopsy or documentation by the pathologist has been completed. In these scenarios, the forensic anthropologist may wish to request the scene and examination photos to see the condition of the remains after transport but prior to the examination; this is especially important if the forensic anthropologist was not involved in the recovery of the remains. At minimum, the forensic anthropology report involving thermal alteration should include an inventory, description, and interpretation of the burn pattern, and differentiation of perimortem trauma from postmortem head-induced alterations. See Dirkmaat *et al.* (2012: 126–129) for a more detailed discussion of fatal fire victim laboratory analyses and report preparation.

3.6 Special Circumstances

Special circumstances involving fires and motor vehicles, aircraft, or trains / subways involve slight modifications to the protocols described in the previous section. Vehicle fires are hybrid scenes with components of traditional indoor scenes (e.g. preserved structure and fixed reference points) and outdoor scenes (e.g. quantity of material, stratigraphy, taphonomic agents) (Klales *et al.*, 2016). There are also certain complexities unique to vehicle fires which warrant specific recovery protocols that differ from indoor scenes, outdoor scenes, or for the fatal structure fires already described. First, vehicle fires almost always have accelerants present, such as gasoline, that impacts how the vehicle burns. Second, components of the vehicle, such as the magnesium steering column, may create an exploding effect that mirrors the dispersal of materials more commonly encountered with bomb blasts or mass disaster scenes. Lastly, vehicle fires are more contained and are somewhat easier to process than structure fires due to their smaller size. Often, it is easier to identify the location of the human remains very quickly in vehicle fires.

Modifications to the protocols already described include preparing the vehicle prior to recovery efforts, adjusting the mapping system to accommodate the predefined compartments in a vehicle, and examining shielding effect (Klales *et al.*, 2016). The vehicle must be prepared beforehand to facilitate easier access to the remains. This entails removing the roof, trunk lid, and / or vehicle doors to facilitate access to the internal compartments of the vehicle. Next, a mapping system should be established that is most appropriate for the vehicle and body locations. Grid units by vehicle compartment (driver side front, passenger side rear, etc.) can be employed using the structural divisions of the vehicle itself. Alternatively, a baseline can be run along the length of the vehicle. In instances with multiple bodies (e.g. one in the trunk and front seats), it may be desirable to establish a secondary baseline perpendicular to the first. Excavation and recovery of the remains proceeds in the same fashion as already described: forensic archaeological principles used to expose the remains *in situ*, stabilization of loose elements, mapping / documentation, screening of recovered debris, recovery on back board into body bag for stabilization, and documentation / excavation of the area beneath the remains (Figure 3.8). With vehicle fires, it is common to have shielding effect whereby the remains protect the area underneath from thermal alteration (Figure 3.9).

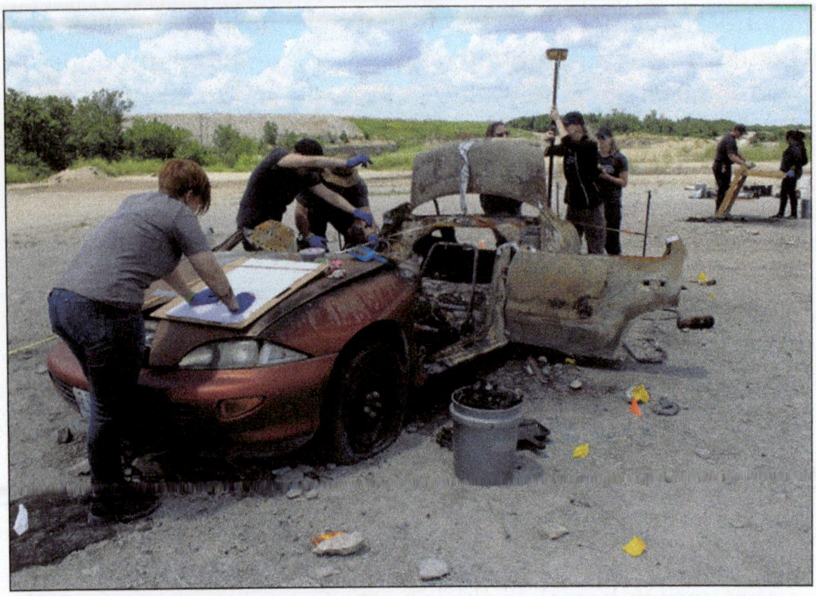

Figure 3.8 Scaled, hand-drawn, plan-view mapping of a vehicle fire scene using a baseline system, while geospatial data is being collected with a GNSS system, and excavated debris is being screened through ¼ inch mesh.

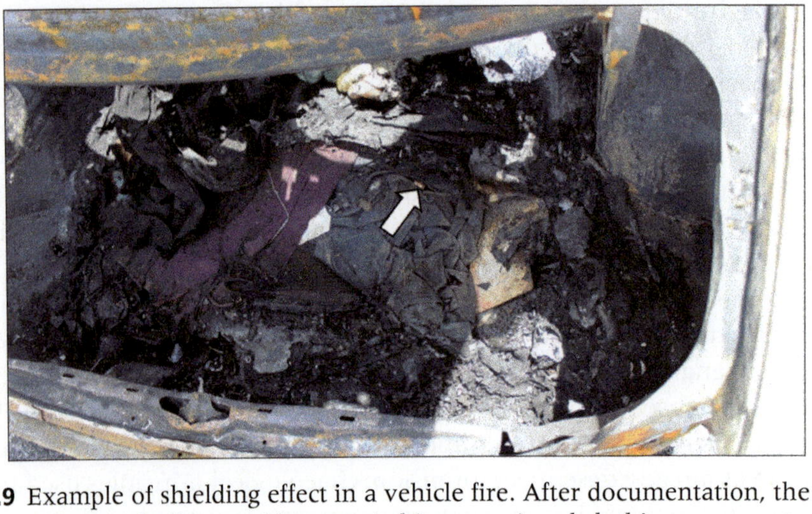

Figure 3.9 Example of shielding effect in a vehicle fire. After documentation, the body was recovered and a bullet cartridge case (white arrow) and clothing were protected from the fire because it was underneath the body.

The protocols and goals of a FAR when employed in larger situations involving multiple fire victims, such as train compartment fires and mass fatality incidents (MFI), are comparable to those used for structure and vehicle fires. Generally, these types of scenes are more complex and will take slightly longer to process, involve more inter-agency teamwork, and require more personnel / equipment. However, the four phases of the FAR and the steps described at the beginning of this section are still employed and recovery times are not significantly longer (e.g. an aircraft crash MFI recovery involving 50 decedents required only 29.5 total hours, see Case 2 in Box 3.1). Failure to use FAR protocols in these large-scale and multi-victim scenes impedes the ultimate goals of the recovery including determining the sequence of events, establishing an identity for each decedent or body element, and determining the cause and manner of death (see Box 3.1).

Box 3.1 A comparison of two scenes from the Department of Applied Forensic Sciences (DAFS) casework at Mercyhurst University, directed by Dr. Dennis Dirkmaat, D-ABFA, highlights the benefits of using the FAR protocols outlines above.

Case 1. Medicolegal investigators associated with a regional coroner's office recovered the remains of five decedents from a fatality scene involving a large-scale multiple vehicle crash. The main articulated biological tissue concentration, which consisted of primarily the torso and proximal appendages, of each of the five victims was removed from the scene. Careful notation of provenience for each of the five individuals was lacking and no information was gathered on the location of the individual or which seat the individual was potentially associated with. Very little effort was made to recover disassociated parts that were predictably in close proximity to the main concentration of each body. This included the burned and fragmented hands / feet, skull fragments, and portions of the lower appendages. As a result of the incomplete and hasty recovery, Dr. Dirkmaat and the DAFS forensic anthropology recovery team were requested the following day to ensure as close to 100% of the biological tissues as was possible were recovered. After a thorough search, the team discovered many skeletal elements in the cabin area where the victims had been previously recovered. However, these remains could not be associated with a particular individual because of the lack of provenience data collected for the primary concentration of each person. Even though all of the victims, that is their torsos and proximal appendages, were positively identified through dental and radiographic means, the extra elements and human bone fragments had to be submitted to DNA analysis for final association to a particular individual, adding considerable cost and time to the identification process. Use of the FAR protocols described already at the onset of the recovery would have mitigated this need and saved valuable time, resources, and money.

Case 2. In the recovery of the mass fatality (50 victims) Colgan Air Flight 3407 crash, in 2009 outside of Buffalo, NY, a comprehensive forensic archaeological excavation of the scene was directed by Dr. Dirkmaat and conducted by the DAFS forensic anthropology recovery team. The aircraft impacted a single residential structure, which resulted in a ruptured gas line that significantly burned both the structure and the aircraft. The focus of the FAR was the total excavation of the scene (decedents, personal effects, plane components, and house elements). All recovered biological tissues, ranging from nearly intact individuals to small isolated remains and skeletal elements, were properly documented (photo and written) and geospatial provenience data was collected via total station coordinate mapping. The forensic archaeological scene recovery protocols employed, now known as the Clarence Center Protocols, resulted in the notation of provenience of each primary body concentration and each set of unassociated biological tissue. Nearly complete individuals were excavated using the top-down approach, loose elements were stabilized, and the body was totally freed from entrapment prior to recovery. Use of these protocols ensured the remains were fully recovered and that loose elements associated with that individual were recovered in the field and did not require re-associating later. The recovery documentation and geospatial data, in combination with the DNA analysis of each biological tissue sample (i.e. body portions rather than partially complete individuals), allowed for association of all parts of each individual, regardless of level of fragmentation. Furthermore, the proveniencing of the biological tissues permitted a reconstruction of where each passenger was seated on the aircraft, using the plane manifest, at the time of impact. This precise provenience information of recovered elements proved to be extremely valuable when all identification attempts proved fruitless for one passenger out of the 50 known decedents. The comparison of: 1) the total station map with where each individual was located in the debris pile, and 2) the location of the gas line fire in the front center of the house which burned for 16 hours, were compared with the plane manifest of where each person was ticketed to be sitting on the flight (Figure 3.10). This reconstruction and analysis resulted in a defendable hypothesis that the unidentified individual was located in middle of the gas line fire area and was in turn totally cremated after the crash. The elements recovered in this area were thermally altered to such a high degree that after multiple attempts, no intact dental remains or usable DNA samples survived. Without the provenience information for the human remains located in this portion of the debris and the geospatial data and documentation (photo and written), it would not have been possible to reconstruct why a specific individual could not be identified via skeletal or dental remains.

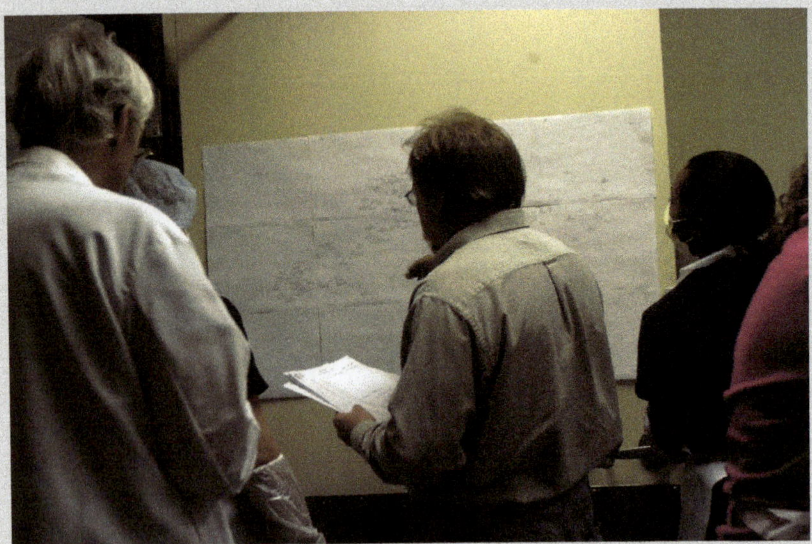

Figure 3.10 Comparison of the geospatial data collected during the FAR to the airline flight manifest to aid in identification of each decedent.

3.7 Conclusions

The scale of a fire scene is significantly larger than other types of recoveries and requires multi-agency collaboration, longer recovery periods, and more resources. However, as we have seen in the past, and has been extensively documented in Symes *et al.* (2012b), most fatal fire recoveries are completed in less time and the remains are often moved more quickly. The recovery of any scene is inherently destructive as the goal of the recovery is *controlled destruction* in a manner that is efficient, timely, and that allows you to reconstruct past events in detail (i.e. elucidate behavior and chain of events). In the years since the 2008 NIJ funded Recovery and Interpretation of Burned Human Remains grant (Symes et al. 2012a) grant, the role and expertise of the forensic anthropologist has been recognized (e.g. NFPA 921), but has failed to be widely applied in these types of cases. Forensic anthropologists possess skillsets essential to the fatal fire recovery, including the recognition and identification of human skeletal material that has been taphonomically altered or modified and the efficient and effective recovery of human remains. Forensic anthropologists' knowledge of taphonomy, human and comparative osteology, as well as scene evaluation, documentation, and recovery are important contributions to fire scene investigations (Mayne Correia and Beattie, 2001; Randolph-Quinney, 2014). Integrating a forensic anthropologist and utilizing forensic archaeology results in a near 100% recovery of recoverable remains and evidence, limiting damage, fragmentation, and disassociation of remains, and the scene is documented in a way that context and association can be interpreted. With any recovery, a team-based approach is best and flexibility is a must for the variety of scene types encountered. Minimally, the protocols already described and developed as part of an NIJ-funded grant should be employed in all fire scenes involving fatalities and fire-altered human remains. In an ideal scenario, a forensic anthropologist or forensic anthropology team would be involved at the onset of the recovery and could implement these FAR protocols during the recovery efforts.

Disclosure: Opinions or points of view expressed in this research represent a consensus of the authors and do not necessarily represent the official position or policies of the US Department of Justice or the National Institute of Justice. Any products and manufacturers discussed are presented for informational purposes only and do not constitute product approval or endorsement by the US Department of Justice or the National Institute of Justice.

References

Ahrens, M. and Evarts, B. (2021) NFPA's fire loss in the United States during 2019. National Fire Protection Association (NFPA). https://www.nfpa.org//-/media/Files/News-and-Research/Fire-statistics-and-reports/US-Fire-Problem/osFireLoss.pdf (accessed August 2, 2021).

Bartelink, E.J., Kendell, A.E., Galimany, J.L., Gardner, K., Hayes, L., Hegel, C.A., *et al.* (2020) Search and recovery protocols for fatal fire victims of the 2018 California Camp Fire. Proceedings American Academy of Forensic Sciences. Anaheim, CA.

Boudreau, J.F., Kwan, Q.Y., Faragher, W.E., and Fenault, G.C. (1977) *Arson and Arson Investigation: Survey and Assessment*. National Institute of Law Enforcement Assistance Administration, United States Department of Justice and Criminal Justice, Washington, DC.

Brannigan, F.L., Bright, R.G., and Jason, N.H. (1980) *Fire Investigation Handbook*, Vol. **134**. US Department of Commerce, National Bureau of Standards, Washington, DC.

Cordner, S., Coninx, R., Kim, H.-J., van Alphen, D., and Tindball-Binz, M. (eds.) (2016) *Management of Dead Bodies after Disasters: A Field Manual for First Responders*, 2nd edn. (Revised). Pan American Health Organization (PAHO), Washington, D.C.

de Boer, H.H., Roberts, J., Delabarde, T., Mundorff, A.Z., and Blau, S. (2020) Disaster victim identification operations with fragmented, burnt, or commingled remains: Experience-based recommendations. *Forensic Sciences Research*, **5**(3), 191–201. https://doi.org/10.1080/20961790.2020.1751385

Dirkmaat, D. (2002) Recovery and interpretation of the fatal fire victim: The role of forensic anthropology. In: *Advances in Forensic Taphonomy: Method, Theory, and Archaeological Perspectives* (eds. W.D. Haglund and M.H. Sorg). CRC Press, Boca Raton, FL, pp. 451–472. https://doi.org/10.1201/9781420058352-28

Dirkmaat, D.C. and Adovasio, J.M. (1997) The role of archaeology in the recovery and interpretation of human remains from an outdoor forensic setting. In: *Forensic Taphonomy: The Postmortem Fate of Human Remains* (eds. M.H. Sorg and W.D. Haglund). CRC Press, Boca Raton, FL, pp. 39–64.

Dirkmaat, D.C., Cabo, L.L., Ousley, S.D., and Symes, S.A. (2008) New perspectives in forensic anthropology. *American Journal of Physical Anthropology*, **137**(S47), 33–52. https://doi.org/10.1002/ajpa.20948

Dirkmaat, D.C., Olson, G.O., Klales, A.R., and Getz, S. (2012) The role of forensic anthropology in the recovery and interpretation of the fatal-fire victim. In: *A Companion to Forensic Anthropology* (ed. D.C. Dirkmaat). John Wiley & Sons, Ltd, Chichester, UK, pp. 113–135. https://doi.org/10.1002/9781118255377.ch6

Fojas, C.L., Cabo, L.L., Passalacqua, N.V., Rainwater, C.W., Puentes, K.S., and Symes, S.A. (2015) The utility of spatial analysis in the recognition of normal and abnormal patterns in burned human remains. In: *Skeletal Trauma Analysis* (eds. N.V. Passalacqua and C.W. Rainwater). John Wiley & Sons, Ltd, Chichester, UK, pp. 204–221. https://doi.org/10.1002/9781118384213.ch16

Harrison, K. (2019) The application of archaeological techniques to forensic fire scenes. In: *Forensic Archaeology* (eds. K.S. Moran and C.L. Gold). Springer International Publishing, Cham, Switzerland, pp. 153–162. https://doi.org/10.1007/978-3-030-03291-3_10

Icove, D. and Haynes, G. (2018) *Kirk's Fire Investigation*, 8th edn. Pearson, New York, NY.

Klales, A.R., Dirkmaat, D.C., and Cabo, L.L. (2016) New forensic archaeological recovery protocols for fatal vehicle fires. Proceedings American Academy of Forensic Sciences. Las Vegas, NV.

Lentini, J.J. (2006) *Scientific Protocols for Fire Investigation*, 0 edn. CRC Press, Boca Raton, FL. https://doi.org/10.1201/9781420003819

Lentini, J.J. (2019) Fire investigation: Historical perspective and recent developments. *Forensic Science Review*, **31**(1), 37–44.

Mayne Correia, P. (1997) Fire modification of bone: A review of the literature. In: *Forensic Taphonomy: The Postmortem Fate of Human Remains* (eds. W.D. Haglund and M.H. Sorg). CRC Press, Boca Raton, FL, pp. 275–293.

Mayne Correia, P. and Beattie, O. (2001) A critical look at methods for recovering, evaluating, and interpreting cremated human remains. In: *Advances in Forensic Taphonomy: Method, Theory, and Archaeological Perspectives* (eds. W.D. Haglund and M.H. Sorg), pp. 435–450. https://doi.org/10.1201/9781420058352-27

National Fire Protection Association. (2014) *NFPA 921: Guide for Fire and Explosion Investigations*. National Fire Protection Agency, Quincy, MA.

Olson, G.O. (2009) Recovery of human remains in a fatal fire setting using archaeological methods. DRDC CSS CR 2009-03. Defence Research and Development Canada Centre for Security Science, Ottawa. https://publications.gc.ca/site/eng/403087/publication.html (acccessed August 4, 2021).

Randolph-Quinney, P. (2014) Burnt human remains Part II: Identification and laboratory analysis. In: *Advances in Forensic Human Identification* (eds. X. Mallett, T. Blythe, and R. Berry). CRC Press, Boca Raton, FL, pp. 145–164. https://doi.org/10.1201/b165

Shipman, P., Foster, G., and Schoeninger, M. (1984) Burnt bones and teeth: An experimental study of color, morphology, crystal structure and shrinkage. *Journal of Archaeological Science*, **11**(4), 307–325. https://doi.org/10.1016/0305-4403(84)90013-X

Symes, S.A., Rainwater, C.W., Chapman, E.N., Gipson, D.R., and Piper, A.L. (2008) Patterned thermal destruction of human remains in a forensic setting. In: *The Analysis of Burned Human Remains* (eds. C.W. Schmidt and S.A. Symes). Academic Press, San Diego, pp. 15–vi. https://doi.org/10.1016/B978-012372510-3.50004-6

Symes, S.A., Dirkmaat, D.C., Ousley, S., Chapman, E., and Cabo, L. (2012a) Recovery and interpretation of burned human remains. Document (online) Grant #2008-DN-BX-K131. National Institute of Justice (NIJ), Washington, DC. https://www.ojp.gov/ncjrs/virtual-library/abstracts/recovery-and-interpretation-burned-human-remains

Symes, S.A., L'Abbé, E.N., Chapman, E.N., Wolff, I., and Dirkmaat, D.C. (2012b) Interpreting traumatic injury to bone in medicolegal investigations. In: *A Companion to Forensic Anthropology* (ed. D.C. Dirkmaat). John Wiley & Sons, Ltd, Chichester, UK, pp. 340–389. https://doi.org/10.1002/9781118255377.ch17

Ubelaker, D.H. (2009) The forensic evaluation of burned skeletal remains: A synthesis. *Forensic Science International*, **183**(1–3), 1–5. https://doi.org/10.1016/j.forsciint.2008.09.019

U.S. Fire Administration. (2021) U.S. Fire Statistics. U.S. Fire Administration (USFA) Federal Emergency Management Agency (FEMA). June 29, 2021. https://www.usfa.fema.gov/data/statistics/index.html

CHAPTER 4

Considerations to Maximize Recovery of Post-mortem Dental Information to Facilitate Identification of Severely Incinerated Human Remains

John Berketa, PhD and Denice Higgins, PhD
University of Adelaide, Australia

4.1 Introduction

Fire scenes in which victims have been severely burnt can vary from automobile accidents, aircraft or train crashes, commercial or domestic building fires, industrial fires, and, more frequently, wild fires. The number of deaths related to the scene incident may also vary from a single victim to hundreds of deceased. Forensic personnel involved at the scene not only obtain information to assist the evaluation of how and what happened, but also retrieve the remains of the victims so that they may be formally identified. Effective and reliable evidence collection from the scene requires following set standard operating procedures (SOP) with advanced preparation, training, and equipment (Kvaal, 2006; Berketa *et al.*, 2012; Lake *et al.*, 2012). Although each scene is different, with the necessity to adapt to each situation, there are certain set overall principles that should be followed. Each odontologist attending the scene should also have a good knowledge of the other personnel's roles and, importantly, work cohesively together to obtain the best result possible (McEntire, 2002).

4.2 Identification

If victims are burnt, visual identification is generally not possible as soft tissues vary from charred to totally incinerated. Hence, identification utilizing one or more of the three primary scientific methods of identification is required. Unfortunately, ridge pattern analysis is also usually not possible for victims of incineration due to tissue loss. With ongoing improvements of DNA sampling techniques and analysis,

Burnt Human Remains: Recovery, Analysis, and Interpretation, First Edition. Edited by Sarah Ellingham, Joe Adserias-Garriga, Sara C. Zapico and Douglas H. Ubelaker.

it is rare that identification with DNA is not possible. Deep tissues such as the bladder may be sufficiently insulated to remain a viable sampling option (Owen *et al.*, 2013). However, in the instance of intense or prolonged burning, readily useable DNA may not be available (Hartman *et al.*, 2011). As teeth are the most robust tissue in the body and some dental restorative materials are fire resistant, identification by dental means is frequently the most successful method in severe incineration (Woisetschläger *et al.*, 2011; Berketa, 2014). However, in these circumstances the dental structures are often rendered extremely fragile and are easily damaged and destroyed by inappropriate or non-ideal movement of the remains. Other methods of identification, including the retrieval of medical devices or implants (such as pacemakers and prosthetic implants), may assist identification (Ubelaker and Jacobs, 1995; Berketa *et al.*, 2015b). If no other method of identification is possible then circumstantial evidence is relied upon as a last resort.

If the burnt remains are fragmented and/or commingled, forensic experts such as odontologists who have trained with police scene officers under a SOP should be utilized at the scene (Bassed and Leditschke, 2011; Hill *et al.*, 2011). These experts are trained to identify dental remains and can document, photograph, stabilize, and collect remains for transportation to the mortuary. There may be a delay in recruiting the correct personnel to the scene and there is frequently media, political, and community pressure to recover the deceased as quickly as possible, but rushing the process of retrieval can often be self-defeating as evidence may be permanently lost or damaged. This loss of post-mortem information will lead to more uncertainty and further delays at the examination stage at the mortuary, hence delaying reconciliation and identification.

4.3 Documentation

When a forensic odontologist is notified that they are required to attend a scene of a fire, it is important that they note the details, including the time of the request, name, and contact number of who called, the address with details of the incident, and the name of who to report to at the scene. This information becomes a reference to remember facts in the ensuing chaos as these events are not part of a normal day's agenda. A proforma of a checklist to note this information, equipment required, together with safety reminders, creates order and minimizes the likelihood that important equipment and safety gear is forgotten. This documentation is also vital for the post incident debrief and answering any queries which might be asked at a review by coroners or other legal investigators. Safety concerns would include reviewing one's own current state to perform this important task of visiting the scene. (Was it a tiring day, has the odontologist been drinking alcohol, how far away is the scene, is the practitioner able to drive themselves, or is assistance required?) It would be prudent (if a second odontologist is available), to call them and ask that they attend as well, preferably with their own personal scene kit. Phone calls and outcomes should be documented.

4.4 Preparation

As well as scene clothing and personal protective equipment, comfortable clothing for travel to and from the site should be considered. As clothing may become soiled at the scene, a change of clothes and shoes for the return trip is advisable. A high visibility vest or jacket should be included, especially if the scene is likely to be in an area where machinery is operating or vehicle traffic is likely. The scene following a fire will usually be chaotic and possibly remote, so that as well as a prepared scene bag, items to take include: mobile phone with appropriate charger, nutrition bars, insect repellent, sunscreen, drinking water, and cleanser for hands and face.

4.5 Prepacked Scene Equipment

A prepacked transportable rucksack (Figure 4.1) or tool box containing all equipment and materials the odontologist requires to satisfactorily complete their tasks should always be at hand as it is difficult to predict if and when a deployment might occur. A light rucksack is preferable (as it should be easy to carry and allow freedom of your hands) as the scene may have to be approached from some distance on foot over rough terrain. Table 4.1 shows equipment that may be included.

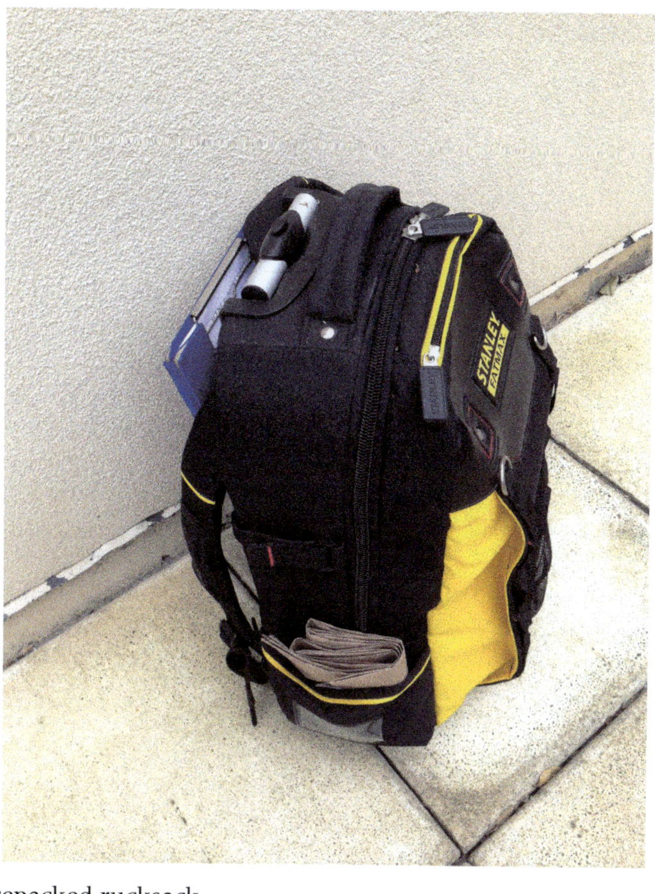

Figure 4.1 A prepacked rucksack.

Table 4.1 Prepacked contents of rucksack.

Equipment	Purpose
Paper documents, such as a running sheet, tooth and body charts, together with a stiff writing surface	Document all information whilst still recent
Writing pens and thick marker pen	Documentation and body bag marking
Magnifying or reading glasses	Detailed close-up work
Ski goggles that will fit over the top of reading glasses	Flying embers and dust necessitate eye protection
Hard hat	Protection from damaged structures and falling objects
Personal protective suit	Protects inner clothing and minimizes contamination
Robust gloves	Protection from sharp and hot objects when removing debris over remains
Thin examination gloves	Limit contamination
Face masks	Personal protection from aerosols and to limit DNA contamination
Robust foam kneeling board or knee pads	Protection of knees from sharp objects, hot objects, and liquid contamination
Head torch	Improve vision whilst keeping hands free
Flood light	As well as improving vision, a non-LED light will hasten the setting of stabilizing agents
Marker flags and string	Marking significant points of interest and gridding
ABFO No. 2 scale ruler	Assist with scene photography
Dental mirror, probe, and tweezers	Searching and collection of evidence
Small soft paint brush and trowel	Removing ash and soil
Clear gloss acrylic paint spray can or superglue	Stabilization of remains in non-suspicious events
Clag® glue or wheat paste mixture, gelatin granule pot	Stabilization of remains in possible suspicious events
Disposable small spray bottle	Spraying of stabilizing agent
Disposable mixing sticks	Mixing of stabilizing agent
Large paper bags	Enclosure of the head and collection of bones
Plastic specimen containers	Small object collection
Bubble wrap and cotton gauze	Protection of fragile remains
Masking tape and scissors	Sealing of paper bags and bubble wrap

4.6 Scene Arrival

Upon scene arrival, contact with the scene coordinator is essential. Again, note the time of arrival and the name of the coordinating officer on the running sheet/ deployment log. A discussion of the event should include: the nature of the event; the number of suspected deceased and their location. Most importantly, safety issues including identification of a safe passage through the scene to the deceased should be undertaken with the scene coordinator before any further action is undertaken.

4.7 Safety Issues

As well as safety aspects directly at the scene, the mental state of all attendees needs to be considered. A call out may occur without warning and often in the middle of the night. Hence a potential hazard is fatigue, including driving without adequate sleep both before and after attendance. If the scene is some distance from the office or home, provision of transportation by a third party, likely police, needs to be considered. Although unlikely, consideration should be made of the likelihood of an attendee having some emotional relationship (such as a relative or close friend) with possible victims, if known. If so, they may not be suitable for the task and the psychological well-being of the person needs to be considered. Also, symptoms of stress can occur at any time and a debrief of all participants following the incident is prudent; any concerns need to be discussed, with appropriate psychological assessment.

The physical safety of all persons at the scene is paramount. It is likely that the structures around the scene area will have been compromised by the fire event. Consideration should be given to the possibility of structures falling, unstable or sloped terrain, residual heat, sharp objects (such as broken glass, metal, and bone), passing traffic, dangerous wildlife, fine dust and ember particles, explosive devices, live electrical wires, asbestos, extreme heat, and chemical fumes. The gases from a fire event can include acrolein, acrylonitrile, benzene, formaldehyde, sulphur dioxide, hydrogen cyanide, polycyclic aromatic hydrocarbons, most certainly carbon dioxide, and most dangerously carbon monoxide. In a confined space, it is essential that the level of carbon monoxide is measured by portable alarmed monitors and deemed at a safe level to enter. As it is an odourless gas, it is undetectable without monitors and as it bonds to haemoglobin to exclude oxygen it can quickly affect people unless they are wearing appropriate breathing apparatus.

These hazards mandate discussion and understanding of all personnel who enter the scene and the use of appropriate personal protective gear including: sturdy, thick-soled work boots; long pants and long-sleeved shirts made of a thick non-synthetic material; face masks; safety glasses; high visibility vests; and

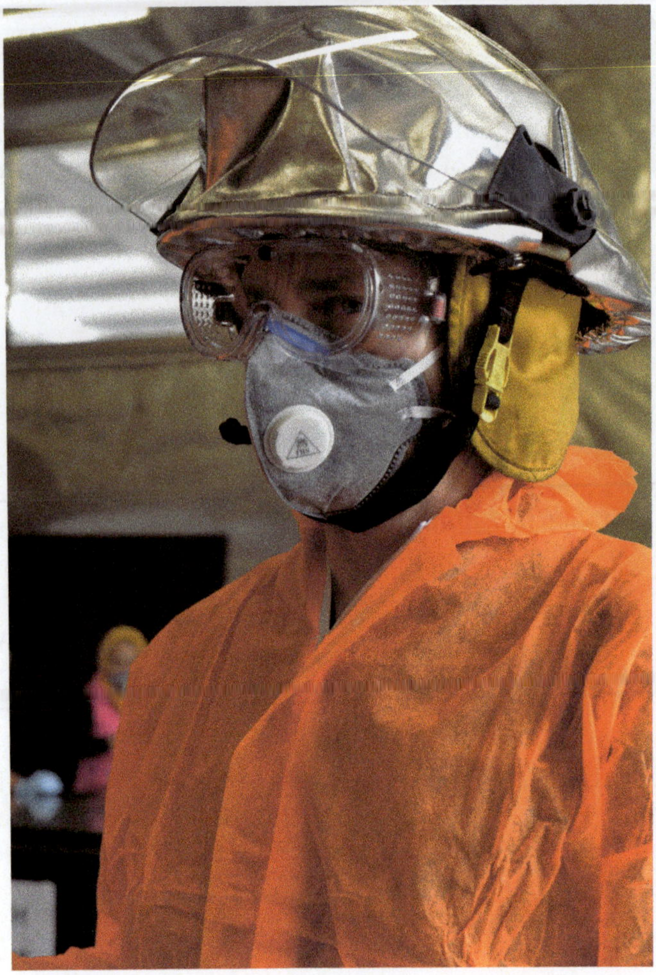

Figure 4.2 Safety apparatus to enter a building if no carbon monoxide or carbon dioxide is detected.

hard hats if required, as depicted in Figure 4.2. The wearing of a disposable personal protective suit will not only lend protection from ash but also limit contamination if trace testing is to be performed. The use of a head lamp, not only at night, but also in confined areas, allows good vision and frees up the use of both hands to identify and avoid hazards. Quite often at the scene there is debris around the victim, including sharp metal, hot surfaces, and broken glass. Hence, the wearing of heavy-duty gloves initially is recommended, together with the use of a kneeling mat. Examination gloves can be used to handle fine fragile evidence once the debris is removed. The retrieval of the body, once the remains have been stabilized, may require heavy lifting in a confined area, such as an upturned car. Thus, several personnel may be required to undertake the task safely. Prior training by specific recovery teams would minimize risk of personal injury and of damage to the remains. In motor vehicle incidents, it may be necessary for fire officers to remove some of the doors and struts first to allow access for successful retrieval.

4.8 Overall Scene Evaluation

The whole scene should be evaluated carefully. In a large event, the use of a drone, if available, would allow a safe overview without disrupting any evidence. A drawn map allows a quick summary and further clarifies the situation. The scene coordinator will organize a systematic wide search so that no body or important artifact is missed. A small peg with a flag helps in identifying these areas. Severely fragmented burnt remains scattered over a wide area may require systematic gridding with string so that every remain is collected. High impact incidents, such as vehicle accidents and building collapse, may produce scattered debris which could make discovery of human remains difficult. Distinctive features such as the bone suture pattern of the cranium can assist detection amongst the debris (as shown in Figure 4.3). The presence of the cranium would suggest that this area is likely to reveal additional victim remains.

On finding human remains it is important that correct processing occurs. This includes photographing the remains first and flagging the area if not processed immediately. A portrait, close-up photograph of the burnt head as shown in Figure 4.4 is particularly important as this can provide information regarding the number and position of teeth that may subsequently be lost during movement.

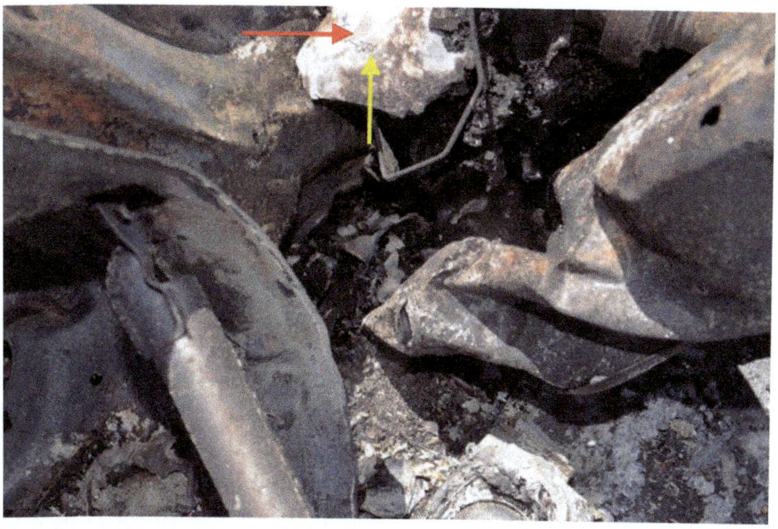

Figure 4.3 Distinct cranial suture pattern indicated by the red arrow.

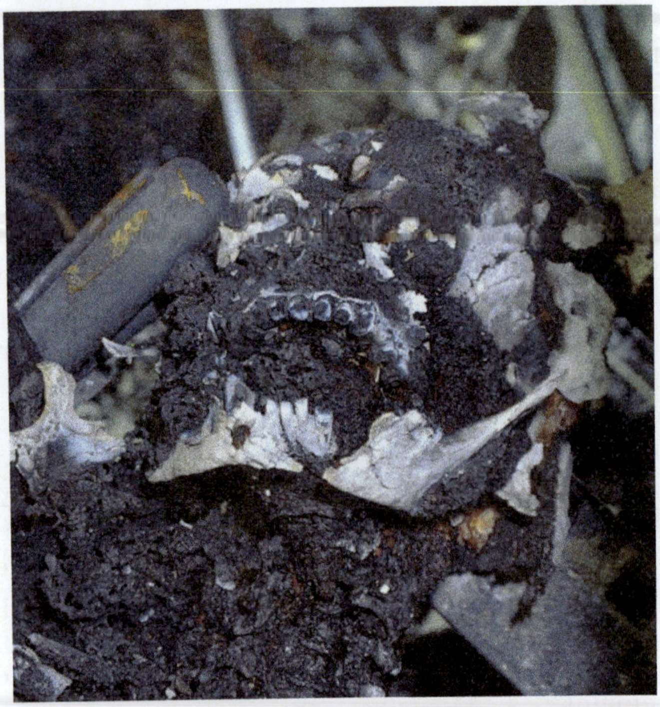

Figure 4.4 A close-up portrait photograph of the burnt head showing the position of the teeth before removal from the scene.

Teeth may be detached from the jaws; before stabilization or retrieval all remains should be photographed and the position documented as shown in Figure 4.5. Commingling can occur when multiple deceased are in close proximity and should be considered. The relationship of remains or loose prosthesis (such as dental implants) to each other should be photographed, drawn, and documented before removal. Ideally each body or part thereof, should be tagged and documented with a separate unique number. However, depending on the situation and the available resources, this may not be practical. This is a decision that will be made by the scene commander.

4.9 Considerations Regarding DNA Evidence

With the improvement of DNA sampling techniques and analysis, it is rare that identification by DNA analysis is not possible. Difficulties with analysis occurs if heat has led to degeneration of samples and if contamination occurs. Contamination by scene attendees might present a problem, so when working with remains, personal protective gear should be worn, as well as a face mask, since salivary micro droplets may contaminate the evidence. DNA sampling is best conducted not at the scene but in the controlled environment within the mortuary. Although

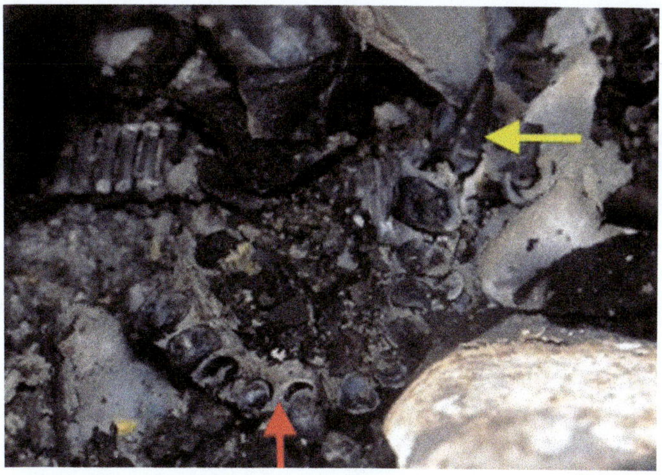

Figure 4.5 Burnt maxilla with displaced tooth (yellow arrow) and loose teeth (red arrow).

a DNA profile may be attainable, an ante-mortem sample may not be readily available, hence all evidence should be collected and all methods of identification including dental comparison must be considered.

4.10 Considerations Regarding Dental Evidence

Identification by dental evidence has been the main method of identification in a number of large-scale fires, such as the 2009 Victorian bushfires in Australia and the 2017 London Grenfell Tower fire in the UK. The matching of teeth, restorations, dental implants, and tooth morphology can all be utilized in identification (Berketa *et al.*, 2012). However, direct exposure to flame and extreme heat may render the teeth extremely fragile and susceptible to crumbling from minor forces, which can occur during collection and transportation to the mortuary.

To minimize damage, stabilization methods applied directly to the oral structures need to be employed. Mincer *et al.* reported that, whatever material was used, in all cases treated remains were better preserved than untreated remains (Mincer *et al.*, 1990). A consideration at this time is whether testing for volatiles is required. Even in a vehicle collision, non-accidental death circumstances may need to be considered. If the incident is deemed not suspicious, then clear gloss enamel spray paint makes an excellent material to stabilize the structures. It can set reasonably quickly, sets clear, is easy to apply, and is readily obtainable. If there is any doubt about the possibility of whether accelerants have been used and the immediate environmental temperature is high (≥32°C), then Clag® paste (wheat paste) can be diluted and applied as a spray. This mixture is, easily made, non-toxic, inexpensive, non-compromising to dental/radiographic examination, and free of volatiles (Berketa *et al.*, 2015a). It should be applied as a fine mist spray onto all the teeth until saturated. Unfortunately, the mixture does take some time to set fully, especially in cold conditions and in a moist environment. The utilization of a non-LED floodlight (generated by the police or fire brigade's portable generators) placed near the sprayed surfaces speeds up the setting process, but expect the mixture to take at least an hour to set. Also, in practice, it has been found that the mixture is often lumpy and does not spray to a fine even covering (Berketa and Higgins, 2021).

In a pilot study, Topoleski and Christensen suggested the use of gelatine solution as a stabilizing agent for burnt remains (Topoleski and Christensen, 2019). A study examining the use of agar and gelatine solutions as an alternative to Clag® paste (Berketa and Higgins, 2021) showed that although agar was impractical a gelatine solution takes only approximately ten minutes to set and emulates the effectiveness of Clag® paste. The setting time will be affected by temperature and humidity, so the environmental conditions need to be considered, with lower

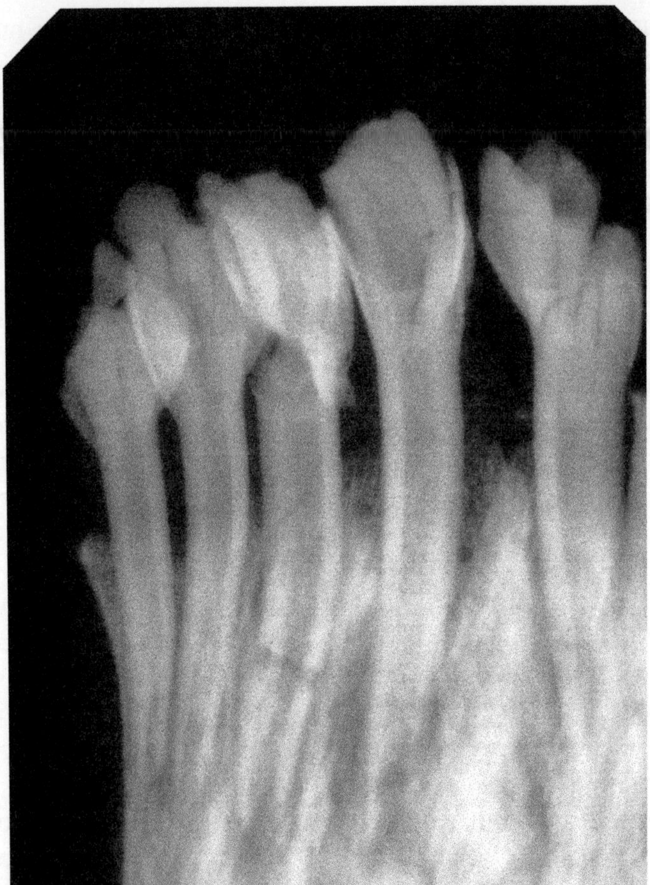

Figure 4.6 Radiograph of sheep teeth covered with gelatine.

temperatures speeding up the process. Usually with charred remains, it is difficult to distinguish restorations, with radiography being the best diagnostic method. The gelatine solution, similarly to acrylic spray, cyanoacrylate, and wheat paste, did not impede the visual imaging of radiographs, as can be seen in Figure 4.6.

Table 4.2 indicates suggestions of stabilizing materials in different situations.

Once a decision is made as to which stabilization material to use, place a foam knee mat next to the head for protection of the knees from sharps, glass, and hot embers, then document and photograph the oral structures before attempting to spray or move the head (Figure 4.7). When the sprayed stabilizing material is fully set, the head should be wrapped with cushioning material such as bubble wrap™ (Sealed Air Corporation, Charlotte, USA), then a paper bag or aluminum foil wrap can be placed over the entire wrapping to confine the contents, before moving the head.

4.11 Moving the Victim

Planning to remove the victim from the scene involves personnel that have specific training in the safe removal of the victims without danger to themselves. Obstacles in the way should be considered and this could include the removal of struts and doors of burnt motor vehicles. Care should be taken in buildings with fragile walls or material above the deceased, and hard hats must be worn. Once an exit path is discussed and established, a stiff board placed beneath the body prior to moving will support the remains, minimizing the shifting of structures towards a low point. If this is not feasible, many personnel are required to limit back injury to the lifters and minimize damage to the fragile remains, with one person specifically holding the head. Once the remains are in the body bag, make sure that the police have placed a numbered tag on the body. The board that was used previously can be switched to the outside of the bag to help lift the bag flat whilst carrying to the transport vehicle.

Table 4.2 Stabilizing materials.

	Short burning time	**No testing for accelerants required**	**High temperature, low humidity**	**All other situations**
Cyanoacrylate on upper teeth	★			
Clear gloss acrylic spray paint		★		
Wheat paste solution (Clag®)			★	
Gelatine solution				★

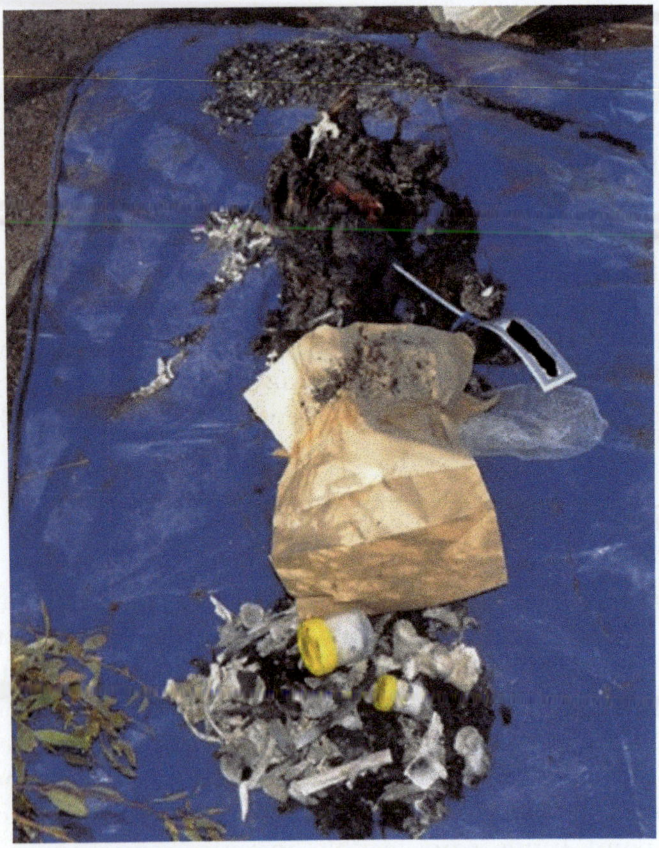

Figure 4.7 Head wrapped in bubblewrap and sealed within a paper bag.

Once the body is removed, a visit to the original scene site where the body was, is advisable. Further evidence, including loose teeth, implants, medical implants, watches, facial piercings, and other jewellery may be found. Documenting and photographing the collected objects is essential before placing them within the body bag. Even though medical implants such as hip and knee implants may appear totally charred, the identifying symbols can be recovered carefully in the mortuary (Berketa *et al.*, 2015b). Sieving the soil around the site might be beneficial, especially if the incident is historic and there have been significant weather events.

The outside of the body bag should be clearly marked at the head end with a permanent marker and labelled as "FRAGILE," "HEAD," "INCINERATED." Stabilization does not completely stop transportation damage and a personal reminder to the transporters of the fragility of the remains is beneficial. A phone call to the mortuary technician to give prior notice of the fragile condition of the remains can be undertaken as an added extra precaution. Bodies are usually robust, but not incinerated remains, and by advertising a particular interest in protecting these remains they may receive the special care needed. Discussion with the mortuary manager might also include the order in which examination of the remains takes place. The forensic pathologist or medical examiner might inadvertently damage the dental structures and an initial dental examination or joint examination with the medical examiner might be prudent.

Forensic scene officers, including odontologists and anthropologists, should undergo a scene debrief, discuss concerns, documenting important events and personnel involved at the scene whilst fresh in their memory, before leaving. Consider resting, if necessary, before travelling back home and note time of departure. Events can be documented in an official report in the following days, reflecting on the running sheet and the full debrief of all scene officers concerned. The scene equipment and materials should be restocked at a prompt convenient time, utilizing a checklist to be thorough.

4.12 Conclusions

To maximize post-mortem dental information following a fire event, attendance of trained and prepared forensic odontologists at the scene is advisable. Before entering the scene, an evaluation, including safety issues, is required. Discovered dental evidence should be documented and photographed, followed by appropriate stabilization, then cautious removal and careful transportation to the mortuary.

References

Bassed, R. and Leditschke, J. (2011) Forensic medical lessons learned from the Victorian Bushfire Disaster: Recommendations from the Phase 5 debrief. *Forensic Science International*, **205**(1–3), 73–76.

Berketa, J.W. (2014) Maximizing postmortem oral-facial data to assist identification following severe incineration. *Forensic Science, Medicine, and Pathology*, **10**(2), 208–216.

Berketa, J. and Higgins, D. (2021) The use of gelling agents to preserve burnt teeth within the dental alveoli for dental human identification – A study utilising sheep mandibles. *Forensic Science, Medicine and Pathology*, 1–6. https://doi.org/10.1007/s12024-020-00344-y.

Berketa, J.W., James, H., and Lake, A.W. (2012) Forensic odontology involvement in disaster victim identification. *Forensic Science, Medicine, and Pathology*, **8**(2), 148–156.

Berketa, J., James, H., Langlois, N., Richards, L., and Pigou, P. (2015a) Use of a non-volatile agent to stabilize severely incinerated dental remains. *Forensic Science, Medicine, and Pathology*, **11**(2), 228–234.

Berketa, J.W., Simpson, E., Graves, S., O'Donohue, G., and Liu, Y.-L. (2015b) The utilization of incinerated hip and knee prostheses for identification. *Forensic Science, Medicine, and Pathology*, **11**(3), 432–437.

Hartman, D., Drummer, O., Eckhoff, C., Scheffer, J.W., and Stringer, P. (2011) The contribution of DNA to the disaster victim identification (DVI) effort. *Forensic Science International*, **205**(1–3), 52–58.

Hill, A.J., Hewson, I., and Lain, R. (2011) The role of the forensic odontologist in disaster victim identification: Lessons for management. *Forensic Science International,* **205**(1–3), 44–47.

Kvaal, S.I. (2006) Collection of post mortem data: DVI protocols and quality assurance. *Forensic Science International,* **159**, S12–S14.

Lake, A., James, H., and Berketa, J. (2012) Disaster victim identification: Quality management from an odontology perspective. *Forensic Science, Medicine, and Pathology,* **8**(2), 157–163.

McEntire, D.A. (2002) Coordinating multi-organisational responses to disaster: Lessons from the March 28, 2000, Fort Worth tornado. *Disaster Prevention and Management: An International Journal,* **11**(5), 369–379.

Mincer, H.H., Berryman, H.E., Murray, G.A., and Dickens, R.L. (1990) Methods for physical stabilization of ashed teeth in incinerated remains. *Journal of Forensic Science,* **35**(4), 971–974.

Owen, R., Bedford, P., Leditschke, J., Schlenker, A., and Hartman, D. (2013) Post mortem sampling of the bladder for the identification of victims of fire related deaths. *Forensic Science International,* **233**(1–3), 14–20.

Topoleski, J.J. and Christensen, A.M. (2019 July) Use of a gelatin-based consolidant to preserve thermally-altered skeletal remains. *Journal of Forensic Science,* **64**(4), 1135–1138.

Ubelaker, D.H. and Jacobs, C.H. (1995) Identification of orthopedic device manufacturer. *Journal of Forensic Science,* **40**(2), 168–170.

Woisetschläger, M., Lussi, A., Persson, A., and Jackowski, C. (2011) Fire victim identification by post-mortem dental CT: Radiologic evaluation of restorative materials after exposure to high temperatures. *European Journal of Radiology,* **80**(2), 432–440.

PART 2

Examination and Identification of Burnt Human Remains

CHAPTER 5

Methods for Analyzing Burnt Human Remains

Amanda N. Williams, PhD
Department of Anthropology, Truckee Meadows Community College, Reno, Nevada, USA

Fatal fires involve the loss of life of one or more individuals. Most fire fatalities are either accidental in nature, or the result of suicide or homicide-related events (Parks *et al.*, 1989; Bonhert and Rothschild, 2003; Fanton *et al.*, 2006; Tumer *et al.*, 2012; Viklund *et al.*, 2013). Therefore, fire becomes a key component to the way individuals may have died. When fire is used in homicides, the body is set on fire with the intention to either destroy evidence or to damage the body to the extent that identification of the victim is unlikely (Fanton *et al.*, 2006; DeHaan, 2008; Symes *et al.*, 2008; Tumer *et al.*, 2012). Fires can alter human remains in various ways; however, complete destruction of a human body by burning is impossible and skeletal remains can almost always be recovered (Correia, 1997; DeHaan, 2012). Thus, some evidence of human remains will always exist. Fatal fires produce a range of physical alterations to the body, from blistering of soft tissue to the calcination of bones (DeHaan, 1999, 2012; Pope and Smith, 2004; Thompson and Chudek, 2007; Symes *et al.*, 2008). These physical alterations leave patterns that can be studied and analyzed to interpret perimortem events.

A variety of forensic professionals interact with and analyze these remains postmortem, which can lead to variation in how remains are described. While the medical literature tends to classify injuries by smoke inhalation (Prahlow, 2010) and categorical extent of thermal injuries to skin, that is, first, second, or third degree burns (Parks *et al.*, 1989; Mullins *et al.*, 2009; Giretzlehner *et al.*, 2013; Moore *et al.*, 2019), forensic anthropologists tend to focus on the condition of the skeleton. The variation in the way the forensic sciences record, describe, and analyze the same set of human remains poses challenges among forensic professionals. This chapter highlights the methods that have been developed for analyzing burnt human remains, while demonstrating the need for a more

Burnt Human Remains: Recovery, Analysis, and Interpretation, First Edition. Edited by Sarah Ellingham, Joe Adserias-Garriga, Sara C. Zapico and Douglas H. Ubelaker.

quantitative approach that can be defended in court. Additionally, this chapter also presents a new standardized method that would encompass all physical alterations of burnt remains and be more applicable to the broader forensic community. The new model is based on experimental observations from a variety of fire environments and represents a subset of fatal fire cases. A new classification system will provide forensic investigators with a novel tool for analyzing fatal fire cases and aid in building a legal case.

5.1 Anthropological Methods for Classifying Burnt Remains

Thermal alterations have been used in developing classification systems for burnt human remains. Three primary classification methods, Raymond Baby's (1954) model, Eckert and colleagues' (1988) classification system for cremated remains, and the Crow-Glassman Scale (CGS) (Glassman and Crow, 1996), have been used by anthropologists. The classification models were primarily created from descriptions of physical alterations, such as soft tissue loss, bone exposure, and fragmentation, observed on the human body. The design and development of the classification models contributes to their usage or applicability to the broader anthropological and forensic community. The earlier two methods, for example Baby (1954) and Eckert *et al.* (1988), developed classification systems based on cremated remains. Thus, the classification systems progress quickly through the burn process, capturing only the advanced stages of heat-related damage, and therefore are not widely used today. The third model does include additional thermal alterations; however, it still only captures a subset of the possible conditions that can be found, thus limiting its applicability and use today.

Baby (1954) devised a three-stage scale based on remains recovered from Hopewell burials; emphasis was placed on coloration, fragmentation, and fracturing. No other heat-related alterations were included in this system. The three stages include: complete incineration, incomplete incineration, and non-incinerated remains (Baby, 1954). Baby (1954) differentiated between levels by placing emphasis on differences in coloration and degree of fragmentation of remains. Burnt remains that exhibited a grey-blue coloration, warping, and fracturing were classified as complete. Remains that exhibited charring and a blackened coloration were classified as incomplete (Baby, 1954). A final and third stage in the system was created for non-incinerated remains, which described remains unaffected by the heat-related process (Baby, 1954). The three-stage model encompasses a range of variation, from no alterations to fragmentation and warping, limiting the applicability of this model to broader fire cases. Given the context of how this model was constructed, the stages are representative of advanced heat-related damage, for example bone exposure, fracturing, warping, and fragmentation. Thus, this model cannot be applied to remains where soft tissue, subcutaneous fat exposure, and muscle exposure may be present.

Eckert *et al.* (1988) derived a classification model from forensic case studies of remains with advanced stages of heat-related damage. The forensic cases used in developing this model exhibited a high percentage of fragmentation and calcination, with little to no soft tissue present (Eckert *et al.* 1988). Eckert *et al.* (1988) observed charring, fragmentation, soft tissue loss, and internal organ exposure. A four-stage model was developed for describing the severely burnt remains. The four stages include: complete, incomplete, partial, and charred (Eckert *et al.* 1988). The first two stages, for example complete and incomplete, are based on the degree of fragmentation present. The remains are considered complete if no bone fragments are present and considered incomplete if bone fragments can be found (Eckert *et al.* 1988). The latter two stages, for example partial and charred, assess physical alterations that occur in the earlier stages of the burn process. The partial stage assesses presence of soft tissue, while the charred stage refers to presence of internal organ exposure Eckert *et al.*, (1988). Most of the cases used in constructing this system exhibited incomplete fragmentation and charring. Thus, there were limited cases containing internal organ exposure or presence of soft tissue, creating limitations to its utility (Eckert *et al.* 1988).

A third model, the CGS, was developed to analyze burnt remains from the Branch Davidian Conflict in Waco, Texas (Glassman and Crow, 1996). This scale was developed to standardize the language used by forensic professionals charged with recovering and identifying burnt remains from the Branch Davidian conflict in Waco. This system was created post hoc, based on a specific set of conditions, and represents only a subset of the possible range of fire-related conditions. The CGS consists of the following five stages:

CGS Level #1: Blistering on body, some burning to head, body is still identifiable.
CGS Level #2: Body begins to exhibit various charring over total body surface area (TBSA), hands and feet begin to be severely damaged.
CGS Level #3: Severe damage to arms or legs, soft tissue loss, in some instances limbs are missing.
CGS Level #4: Severe charring to body, severe damage to skull, small portions of the arms and legs may be present.
CGS Level #5: No soft tissue remains, remains are almost in a cremated state, very fragmented, and identification is very difficult.

In its current form, the CGS is overly general, as it progresses quickly from blistering to fragmentation in only five stages, with no descriptions of times or temperatures that could have contributed to this process. The scale can also be subjective as it does not quantify surface area or percentage of body affected. The CGS describes additional soft tissue variables, for example blistering, charring, and soft tissue loss, making this model more applicable to the forensic community than previous models. The scale was created from a specific scenario in Waco, where the majority of remains were found in a highly fragmented state with limited soft tissue present, contributing to the development of the highly advanced stages found in the CGS. Thus, the scale fails to adequately capture the earlier stages of the burn process.

The lack of description of these earlier stages creates challenges for the applications of the CGS to a wide range of fire conditions, thereby limiting its use within the forensic community today. The classification models created capture a subset of the range of physical alterations that can be present on a set of remains. However, previous models failed to adequately encompass soft tissue alterations, creating limitations to applying these methods to forensic cases where soft tissue may be present.

5.2 Medicolegal Classification Methods

There are also inconsistencies among forensic professionals in how to describe and quantify the amount of heat-related damage. As such, descriptions of burnt bodies from pathologists and medical examiners are often inconsistent with those provided by forensic anthropologists in the bodily elements described, in the assessment of total body surface area (TBSA) affected, and in employing a variety of criteria to classify the burn injuries (Dunne and McMeekin, 1977; Martin-de las Heras *et al.*, 1999; Ahmed *et al.*, 2009; Fracasso *et al.*, 2009; Moore *et al.*, 2019). For example, TBSA is not analyzed in similar manner between disciplines. Pathologists follow the "rule of nines" when recording TBSA on human remains. The "Rule of Nines/Wallace Rule of Nines" is derived from the medical field and often used to classify burn injuries. Even though this method was created as a way for medical professionals to assess a patient's injuries, it is borrowed by pathologists and applied to fatal fire cases. The method was derived to provide medical professionals with a means to calculate the percentage of surface area burned on an individual, so they could in turn prescribe the proper treatment. Based on the "Rule of Nines," TBSA is calculated from nine predefined regions of the body. Each of the nine regions are given percentages based on proportion of surface area to body size (Martin-de las Heras *et al.*, 1999; Fracasso *et al.*, 2009; Giretzlehner *et al.*, 2013; Moore *et al.*, 2019). Within this model, percentages are assigned based on soft tissue injuries to the body. The model assesses burnt injuries to the head, trunk, and upper and lower extremities. Within each region, the percentages are broken down even further to account for differences between anterior and posterior, and within the chest and abdomen areas of the trunk. The "Rule of Nines" was created to help medical professionals make a quick assessment; however, there are some limitations. This model can be inaccurate by producing up to a 20% inter-observer error, as a large portion of the assessment is based on subjectivity and one's experience in handling these types of cases (Arora *et al.*, 2010; Giretzlehner *et al.*, 2013; Byard, 2018; Moore *et al.*, 2019). Giretzlehner and colleagues (2013) found that in contexts where burn injuries comprised less than 20% of the surface area, there was an increase in observer error, with a trend towards overestimating TBSA. Additionally, the model does not account for soft tissue changes in the hands or feet when deriving TBSA. The lack of inclusion of these elements has also been noted to have contributed to some of the inaccuracies in assessing TBSA.

Another method, often called the "Rule of Palms," is also sometimes referenced when calculating TBSA. This method was implemented as a means to better guide an observer to estimate TBSA (Arora *et al.*, 2010; Giretzlehner *et al.*, 2013; Byard, 2018; *Moore et al.*, 2019). This method often provides the observer with a benchmark for what one should consider a minimum of one percent surface area coverage. If the burnt area covers about the same surface area of one's palm, then it is marked at one percent. Overall, there have been recent advancements within the medical community to reduce this error by creating computer-based models that provide a better visual representation of each region. However, it should be noted these models are best applied to soft tissue changes, and are not applicable once bone is exposed, even to the hands/feet.

The forensic sciences lack a consistent, objective, and detailed scale to describe burn injuries or patterns in a variety of settings and conditions. Forensic anthropologists also analyze TBSA, but not according to the same guidelines. Instead, they calculate TBSA much more broadly and include the hands and feet in their analysis. Therefore, there is a need to develop an anthropological-based method that encompasses all thermal alterations and can be more broadly applied to a range of fire environments.

5.3 Need for New Model within the Forensic Sciences

Previous classification models were derived from specific contexts, like cremations, or the 1993 events at Waco, which made it more challenging to apply them to broader fatal fire cases. Given that these models were derived from specific environments, they do not include all aspects of the thermal alteration process, and therefore are not used today (Baby, 1954; Eckert *et al.*, 1988; Glassman and Crow, 1996). These models attempt to capture the burning process within five or less stages and provide little to no means of quantifying the amount of damage present on a human body. The lack of a more detailed model limits the applicability of previous models to modern-day fatal fire cases. Within anthropology, there is a need for a new classification model that assesses thermal alterations per bodily region and attempts to not only describe the amount of damage present but also seeks to quantify it. Previous models were primarily descriptive, with little or no attempt at quantifying the amount of thermal damage on a human body. The challenge at hand is to create a means to bridge the work between the forensic sciences and disciplines, all of whom may handle and examine the same cases.

Therefore, the following discussion introduces a new classification model with a more quantifiable approach that can be used to model the amount of heat-related damage and can be used to infer about *in situ* conditions. The new classification method aims to be more applicable to remains encountered in fatal fires and can be broadly used across disciplines to describe remains. This new method can aid investigators by providing additional information on the fire environment contributing to the bodily alterations observed and timing of injuries.

5.4 A New Classification System

Unlike previous models, a new classification system was developed based on experimental observations of burning human cadavers. Prior models (Baby, 1954 and Eckert *et al.*, 1988) were based on cremations or severely burnt cases, illustrating why there is a lack of soft tissue alterations represented in many of the descriptions. By using experimental observations, the entire thermal alteration process can be captured and incorporated into a new classification system. This model is based on experimental data of burnt human cadavers that comes from a range of fire environments, including structure, vehicle, confined space, and outdoor fires. Experimental observations were conducted as a part of the San Luis Obispo Fire Investigation Strike Team training (SLOFIST) course. Each year SLOFIST conducts a fatal fire death investigation course for forensic professionals in examining fatal fire deaths and scenes. The course involves the burning of donated human remains in vehicle, structure, outdoor, and confined space fire contexts. Vehicle fires comprised any individual placed in either the trunk or compartment seats. Structure fires consisted of any individual placed in a recreational vehicle (RV), shed, on a mattress, couch, or on the floor. Outdoor fires comprised scenarios where individuals were buried in a trench or placed in a tent. The confined space fires are characterized as any individual who was placed in a dumpster or environment with limited ventilation. The range of fire environments provided through the training course made it possible to collect a wide range of data on a variety of fire environments that may be more representative of burnt forensic cases. Data was collected during a four-year period and comprised 87 individuals. The burning process was recorded and documented, along with a visual assessment of the burned remains.

The progression of thermal damage to the human body was noted and formed the basis for the development of this new classification system. The classification system begins with a "fresh" stage or unburnt stage and progresses through the thermal alteration process. The lower scores on this new classification system represent the earliest stages of the burning process or those that are observed to occur first on a human body, like blistering, skin splitting, and subcutaneous fat exposure.

The later scores in the classification system reflect the latter stages of the burn process, including bone exposure, calcination, and fragmentation.

From these many observations, it was noted that the body does not burn equally among all regions, therefore this classification system is broken down by bodily region to account for this variability. Other experimental observations have noted that the hands and feet tend to be one of the first elements to burn and expose bone, followed by the frontal region of the skull (Pope and Smith, 2004; Thompson and Chudek 2007; DeHaan, 2008, 2012; Symes *et al.*, 2008). Unlike previous models, this classification system assesses thermal alterations from the skull/neck, trunk, long bones, and hands/feet. This new model covers the entire range of thermal alterations, from skin blistering to fragmentation in each bodily region. Each region is evaluated based on the progression of these alterations on the human body. Given the variation that is likely to exist in each region, it is unlikely that a body would be equally burned in all bodily regions, thus making it impossible to utilize previous models. The new classification system adds on to these descriptions and provides a means to quantify the amount of thermal damage on a set of remains.

The new model draws from taphonomic studies that utilize a similar quantitative method for describing the condition of remains during the decomposition process. Many of these studies draw upon physical changes in the condition of the body and use it to score the progression of changes that are present (Bass, 1984; Galloway *et al.*, 1989; Komar, 1998; Megyesi *et al.*, 2005). Accumulated models take the condition of the remains and provide a score per body region. Scores are added together to formulate an accumulated total body score. A similar approach was applied in the development of this new model, as it is more encompassing of the changes that can occur on a body regardless of fire environment. This new model accounts for all thermal alterations, and thus, rather than providing a percentage of surface area affected, provides an accumulated score summing all the regions. A summation of physical alterations more adequately captures the burning process and thus the variability that can occur.

The new classification system takes into consideration the limitations and challenges of previous models and demonstrates a more holistic approach to analyzing burnt human remains. The following method illustrates this new accumulated scoring model.

Categories/Scoring for Head and Neck = __________

1 = no charring, fresh body
2 = blistering and partial skin splitting is present
3 = skin splitting is widespread across head and neck, with less than 50% subcutaneous fat exposure
4 = subcutaneous fat exposure is widespread and muscles are exposed
5 = partial bone exposure and charring to cranial elements

6 = bone exposure, heat related fracturing, and partial calcination to cranial region
7 = widespread calcination and fragmentation

Categories/Scoring for Trunk = ________

1 = no charring, fresh body
2 = blistering and partial skin splitting is present
3 = skin splitting is widespread across the trunk, with partial charring of tissues, and less than 50% subcutaneous fat exposure
4 = widespread subcutaneous fat exposure and partial muscle exposure
5 = widespread muscle exposure and intestinal exposure
6 = partial bone exposure, with charring of bone
7 = widespread bone exposure, partial calcination, and heat-related fracturing
8 = widespread calcination and fragmentation

Categories/Scoring for Long Bones = ________

1 = no charring, fresh body
2 = blistering and some skin splitting is present (e.g. distal or proximal ends)
3 = skin splitting is widespread across all long bones, with partial charring of tissues, and less than 50% subcutaneous fat exposure
4 = widespread subcutaneous fat exposure, with partial charring of tissues
5 = widespread charring of tissues on all long bones, with muscle exposure
6 = pugilistic posture
7 = partial bone exposure and charring of bone
8 = widespread bone exposure, partial calcination, and heat-related fracturing
9 = widespread calcination and fragmentation

Categories/Scoring for Hands and Feet = ______

1 = no charring, fresh body
2 = blistering and partial skin splitting is present
3 = widespread skin splitting on both hands and feet, with less than 50% subcutaneous fat exposure
4 = widespread subcutaneous fat exposure, with partial charring of tissues
5 = widespread charring of tissues, with muscle exposure
6 = pugilistic posture
7 = partial bone exposure and charring of bone
8 = widespread bone exposure, partial calcination, and heat-related fracturing
9 = widespread calcination and fragmentation

= ______/33 pts (Possible)

5.5 Best Practices in Applying this New Model

This classification system can be best applied to remains that exhibit a variety of conditions, including soft tissue and skeletal alterations. When applying this new model, remains should be assessed independently per body region. Thus, this model is broken down into four main regions: the head and neck, trunk, long bones, and hands and feet. Scores are based on the stage or condition of the remains in that specific bodily region. When evaluating remains for skin splitting, subcutaneous fat exposure, and charring, to name a few, one must evaluate the alteration based on the percentage of surface area affected. One should examine each bodily region, noting what alterations are present and how much of the surface area is affected. For example, if the torso region exhibits widespread charring, muscle exposure, and intestinal exposure, then one would score the individual at a stage five. Given intestinal exposure was the highest thermal alteration observed, and no bone exposure was found, it would not be scored any higher on this new model. Each scoring stage encompasses terms such as partial and widespread to describe the amount of surface area covered. Partial represents alterations that cover less than 50% of the surface area, whereas widespread represents alterations that cover more than 50% of the surface area. If a region exhibits variability in physical alterations, one should always use the highest score that can be applied. For example, if the lower limbs exhibits charring and bone exposure, but the upper limbs do not, then the highest score that could be awarded would be a seven, due to bone exposure being present on the lower limbs.

Once scores are recorded for each region, they are added together to form a total body score (TBS). The following case studies illustrate how to best apply this new classification system.

5.6 Case Study #1

Case study #1 comprises an individual that was recovered from a vehicle fire. The new model described above was used in creating a total body score to describe the condition or state of the remains. This individual exhibited calcination on the mandible, the frontal portion of skull, the left zygomatic, and the left maxilla (see Figures 5.1 and 5.1b). Calcination was found on some regions of the skull, but not all, and did not comprise over 50% of the surface area. Given there were regions on the skull that did not have any calcination or bone exposure present, this individual was scored at a stage six on this new model.

When evaluating the trunk region, this individual had widespread muscle exposure from the sternum down through the ribs that covered more than 50% of the surface area. This individual also had widespread subcutaneous fat exposure and intestinal exposure (see Figures 5.1 and 5.1a), thus was scored at a stage five.

Given, there was no bone exposure present in this region, the trunk was not scored higher on this new model.

When evaluating the long bones, the arms exhibit widespread muscle exposure, with some bone exposure on the lower right arm (see Figure 5.1); whereas the legs exhibited muscle exposure and widespread charring (see Figures 5.1 and 5.1c). Given there was bone exposure on the right arm, this individual was scored at a stage seven. There was not enough widespread bone exposure or calcination on the limbs to be scored any higher.

When evaluating the hands and feet, the hands exhibited muscle exposure, charring, with the right hand exhibiting some bone exposure (see Figure 5.1). The feet exhibited widespread charring, with little to no bone exposure (see Figure 5.1c).

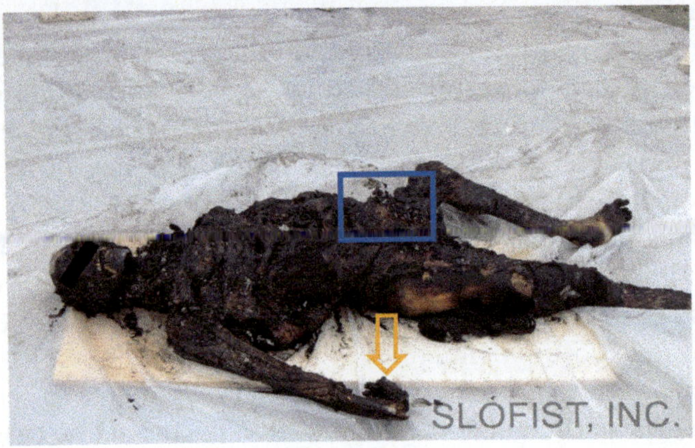

Figure 5.1 Individual #1 with intestinal exposure (highlighted in blue box above), and bone exposure on right hand (yellow arrow above).

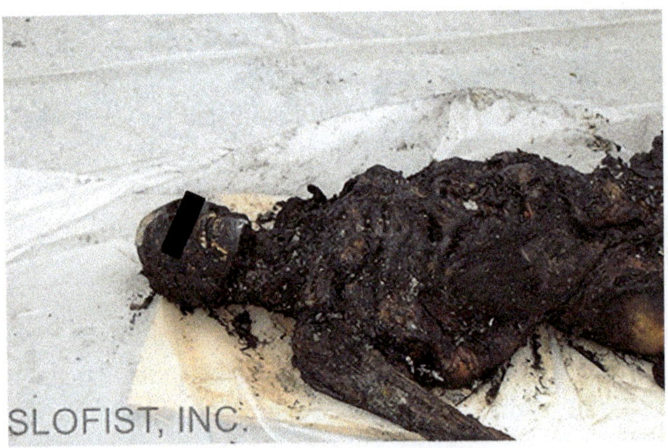

Figure 5.1a Individual #1 with widespread muscle exposure and intestinal exposure.

Given the right hand exhibits partial bone exposure and charring, this individual was scored at a stage seven. Scores from all regions were added together (6 + 5 + 7 + 7), and this individual was given a total body score of 25.

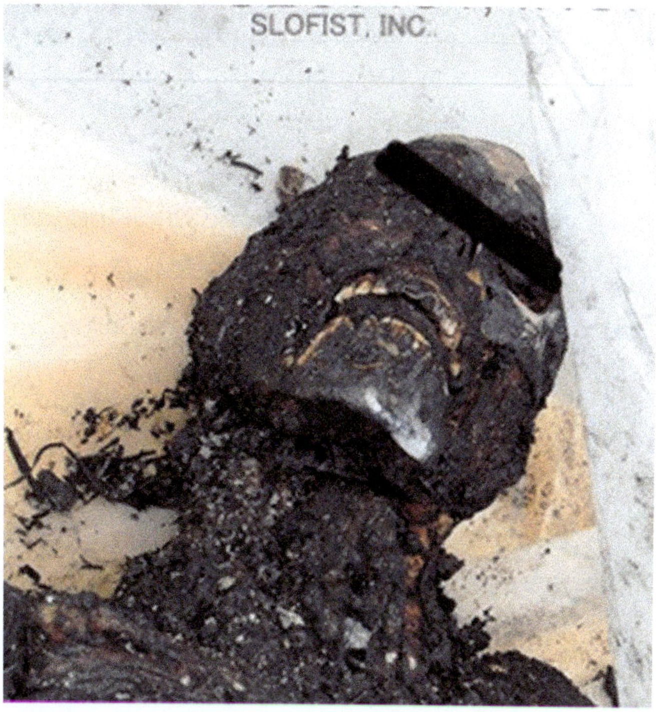

Figure 5.1b Individual #1 with calcination to frontal, mandible, and left zygomatic.

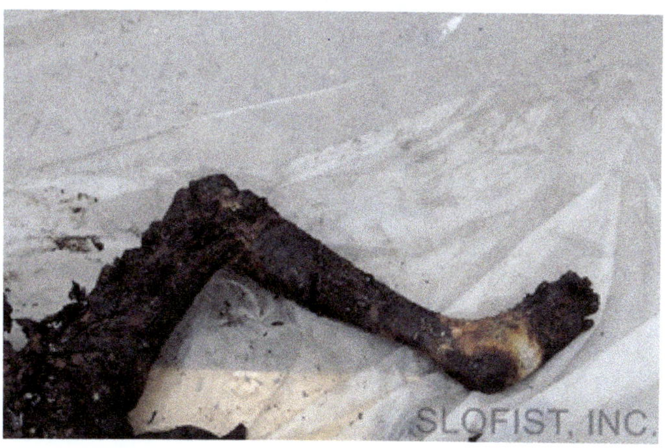

Figure 5.1c Individual #1 with charring and muscle exposure on left lower limb and foot.

5.7 Case Study #2

Case study #2 comprises an individual recovered from a structure fire. This individual exhibited calcination on the frontal, both parietal bones, and the temporal region of the skull (see Figures 5.2a). No calcination was observed on the mandible, maxilla, or the zygomatics. Given there is partial calcination and bone exposure, this individual was scored at a stage six in the head and neck region. There was not enough calcination and fragmentation to score this region any higher.

When evaluating the trunk, this individual exhibited an unburnt region that comprised more than 50% of the surface area on the left side of the torso (see Figures 5.2 and 5.2b), with partial charring of tissues on the right side. Given there is a portion of the torso that exhibits charring, this individual was scored at a stage three. There was not enough subcutaneous fat exposure, muscle exposure, or intestinal exposure to score this region any higher.

When evaluating the limbs, the legs exhibited widespread muscle exposure that comprised more than 50% of the surface area (see Figures 5.2 and 5.2c). The arms also comprised widespread muscle exposure, with some bone exposure and calcination to the right arm only (see Figures 5.2b and 5.2d). Given the presence of some bone exposure and calcination, this individual was scored at a stage eight.

When evaluating the hands and feet, the feet exhibit widespread muscle exposure and charring; whereas the hands exhibit bone exposure, calcination, and the pugilistic posture (see Figures 5.2c and 5.2d). Given the right hand exhibits

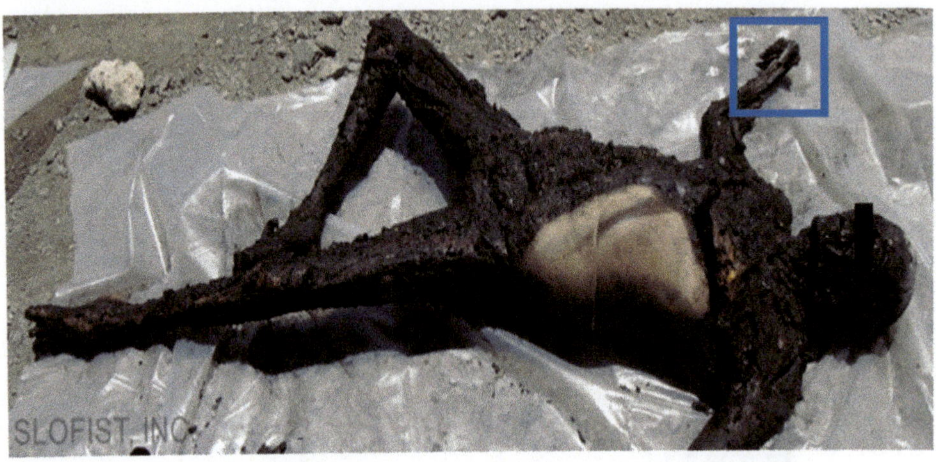

Figure 5.2 Individual #2 with calcination on skull and right hand (highlighted in blue box above).

calcination and fragmentation, this individual is scored at a stage eight. Scores from all regions were added together (6 + 3 + 8 + 8), and this individual was given a total body score (TBS) of 27.

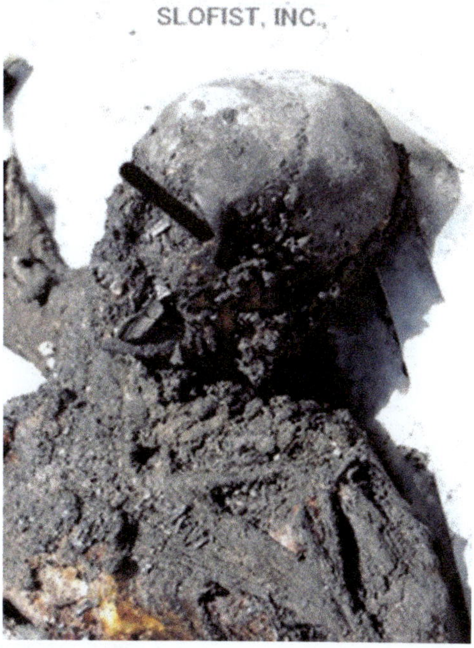

Figure 5.2a Individual #2 with calcination to frontal, both parietals,and a portion of the temporal bone; little to no calcination on mandible, zygomatics or maxilla.

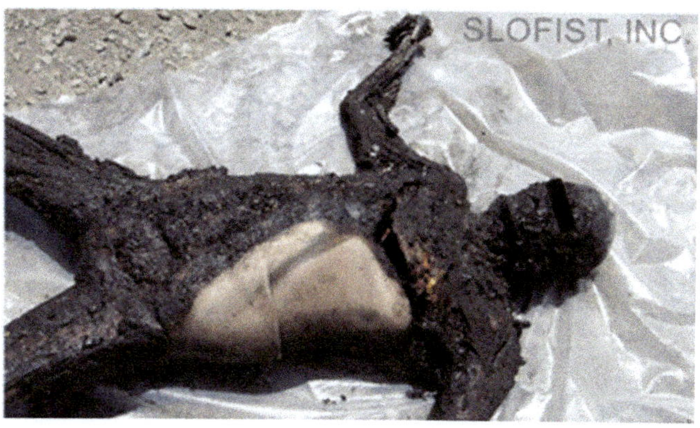

Figure 5.2b Individual #2 with partial charring on torso.

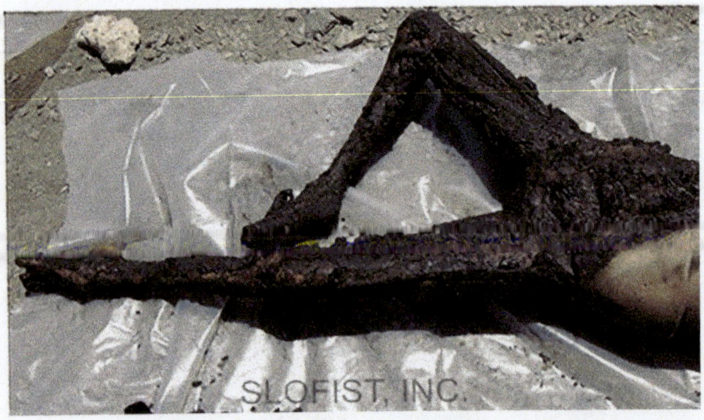

Figure 5.2c Individual #2 with muscle exposure and charring on lower limbs and feet.

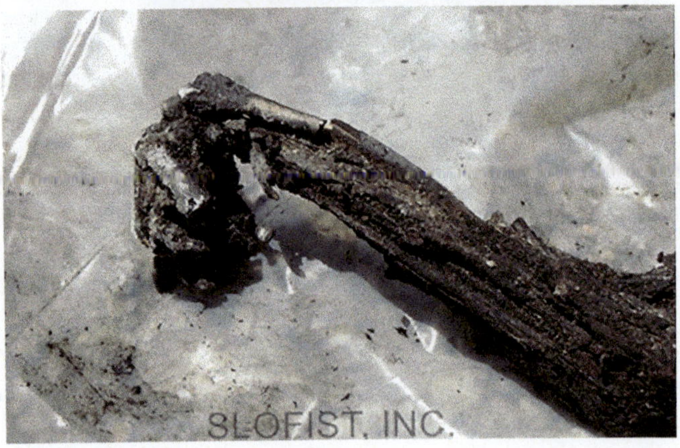

Figure 5.2d Individual #2 in the pugilistic posture, with calcination on right hand.

5.8 Case Study #3

Case study #3 comprises an individual recovered from a structure fire. This individual exhibited widespread (more than 50%) charring and muscle exposure across all regions of the skull, with some bone exposure on the frontal region (see Figures 5.3 and 5.3b). Given, there is some bone exposure present, this individual was scored at a stage five.

When evaluating the trunk, the torso exhibited less than 50% charring across the total surface area, with intestinal exposure (see Figures 5.3 and 5.3b). Given the intestines were exposed, this individual was scored at a stage five.

When evaluating the limbs, the legs exhibited partial (less than 50%) subcutaneous fat exposure and muscle exposure, with bone exposure on the left tibia (see Figure 5.3a). The arms exhibited widespread muscle exposure and charring, but

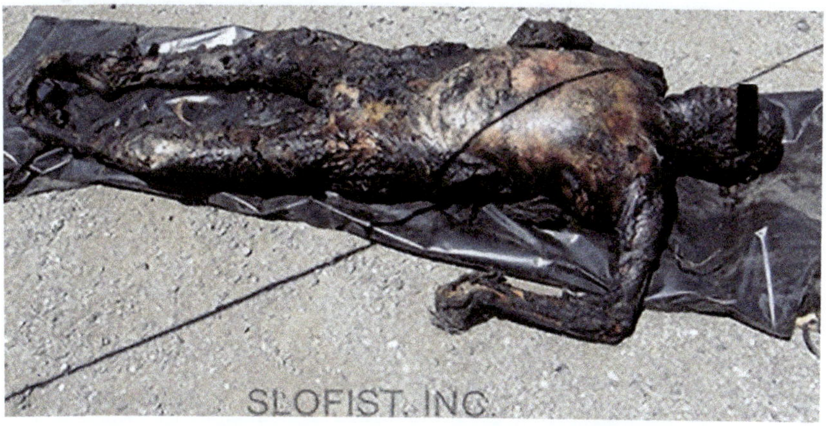

Figure 5.3 Individual #3 with limited (less than 50%) charring to torso.

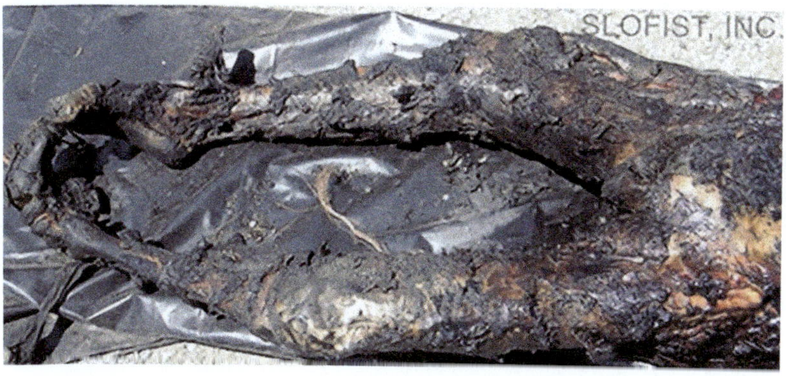

Figure 5.3a Individual #3 with muscle exposure, subcutaneous fat exposure on lower limbs, and bone exposure on feet.

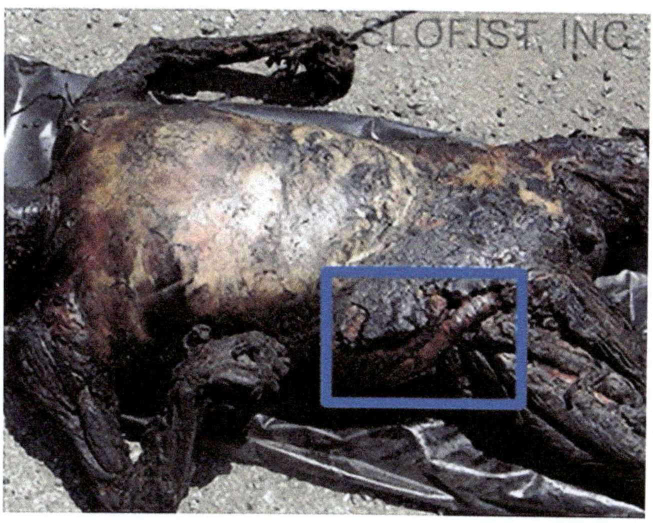

Figure 5.3b Individual #3 exhibiting pugilistic posture in both hands, and intestinal exposure (highlighted in blue box).

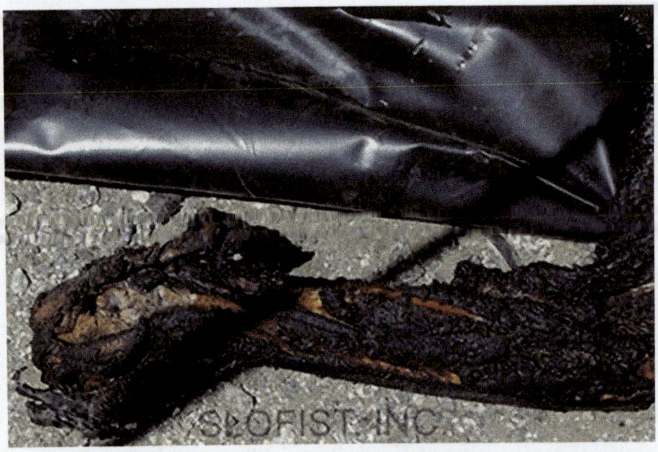

Figure 5.3c Individual #3 with widespread charring and bone exposure.

no bone exposure (see Figures 5.3b and 5.3c). Given there is bone exposure and charring on the left tibia, this individual was scored at a stage seven.

When evaluating the hands and feet, the hands exhibited the pugilistic posture, whereas the feet exhibited bone exposure and charring of bone (see Figures 5.3a and 5.3b). Given there is charring of bone on the feet, this individual was scored at a stage seven. Scores were added together (5 + 5 + 7 + 7), and this individual was given a total body score of 24.

5.9 Case Study #4

Case study #4 comprises an individual recovered from an outdoor context, specifically a trench. The individual had been burned in a trench and then buried. This individual exhibited widespread calcination and fragmentation across all regions of the body (see Figure 5.4). When evaluating the head and neck region, this individual exhibited widespread calcination to the frontal, both parietals, both temporal bones, and the occipital region (see Figures 5.4–5.4b). Given calcination comprised more than 50% of the surface area on the skull and mandible, this individual was scored at a stage seven.

When evaluating the trunk, this individual exhibited partial calcination and fragmentation to the ribs and sternum area of the torso (see Figures 5.4 and 5.4b). Given there was a large portion of muscle still present in this region, the remains were not considered to exhibit widespread calcination and therefore were scored at a stage seven.

When evaluating the long bones, this individual exhibited widespread calcination and fragmentation to both the upper and lower limbs (see Figures 5.4b and 5.4c). The individual exhibited calcination, heat-related fracturing on the humerus,

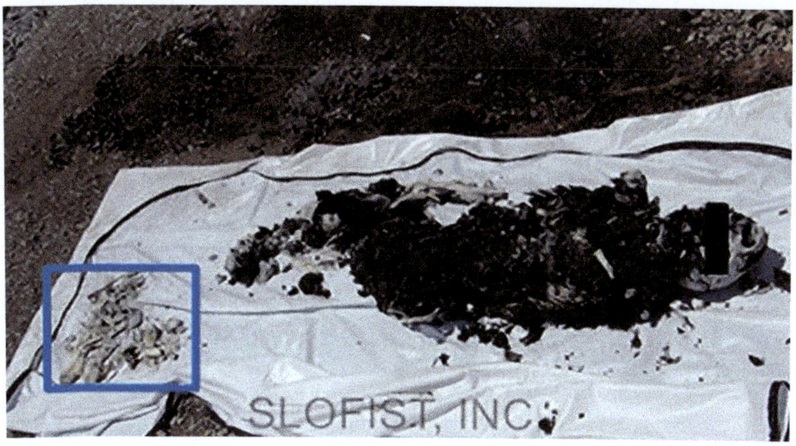

Figure 5.4 Individual #4 with widespread calcination and fragmentation (blue box highlights fragmentary remains of hands and feet).

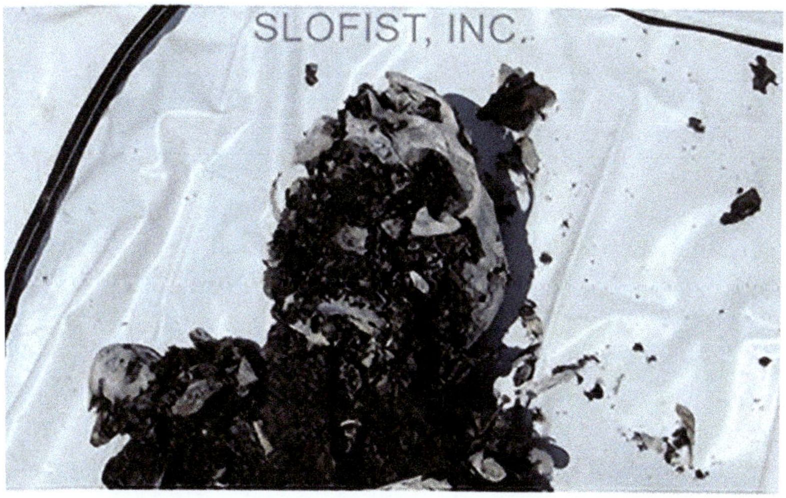

Figure 5.4a Individual #4 with widespread calcination and fragmentation to the frontal, both parietals, temporal, and occipital regions of the skull.

femur, and tibia. Given the remains were in a highly fragmented and calcined state, it was widespread, and therefore the remains were scored at a stage nine.

When evaluating the hands and feet, this individual exhibited widespread calcination and fragmentation (see Figure 5.4). Given the high degree of fragmentation and calcination present, this individual was scored at a stage nine. Scores were added together (7 + 7 + 9 + 9), and this individual was given a total body score of 32.

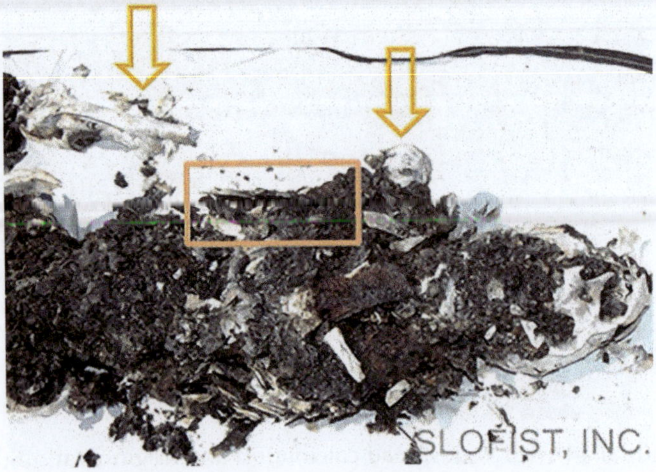

Figure 5.4b Individual #4 with calcined and fragmented ribs (highlighted in orange box above), and a right proximal and distal humerus (yellow arrows above).

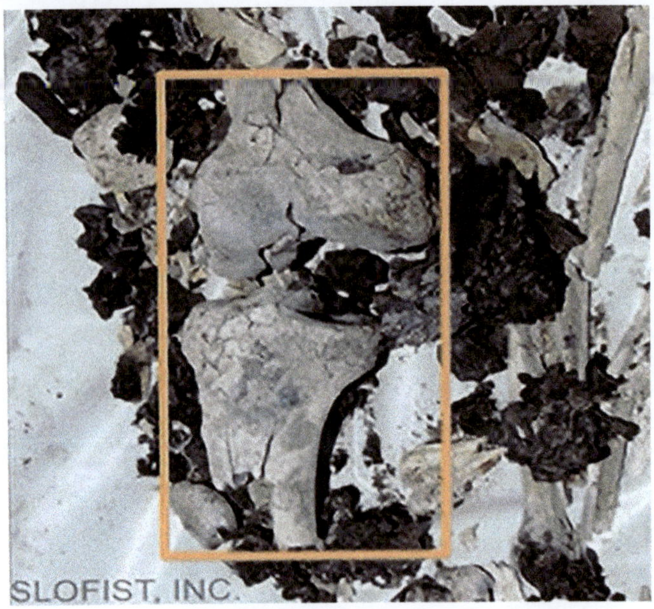

Figure 5.4c Individual #4 with a fragmented and calcined distal femur and proximal tibia (highlighted in orange box above).

5.10 Case Study #5

Case study #5 comprises an individual from a garage fire or structure fire. This individual exhibited widespread muscle exposure on the neck and craniofacial regions, with some bone exposure and charring to the partial bones and mandible (see Figure 5.5). Given there is only partial bone exposure and no calcination present, this individual was scored at a stage five.

When evaluating the trunk, this individual exhibited widespread skin splitting and subcutaneous fat exposure on the torso (see Figure 5.5a). Given there was no partial muscle exposure or bone exposure in this region, this individual was scored at a stage three.

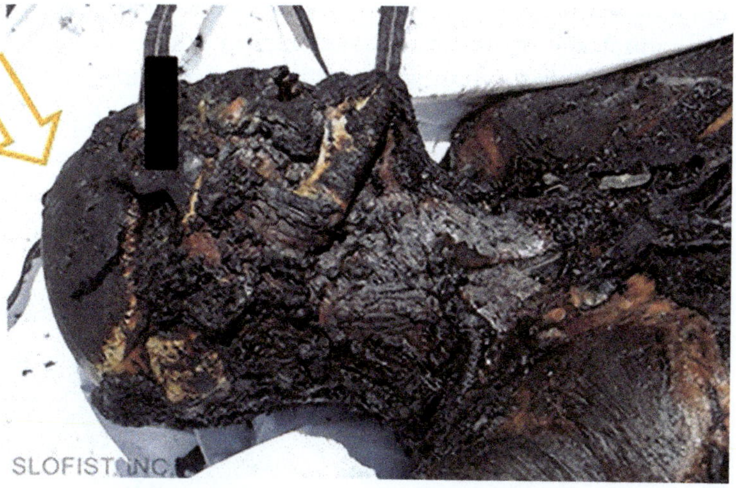

Figure 5.5 Individual #5 with bone exposure on skull (yellow arrow above), and muscle exposure on neck and upper arm regions.

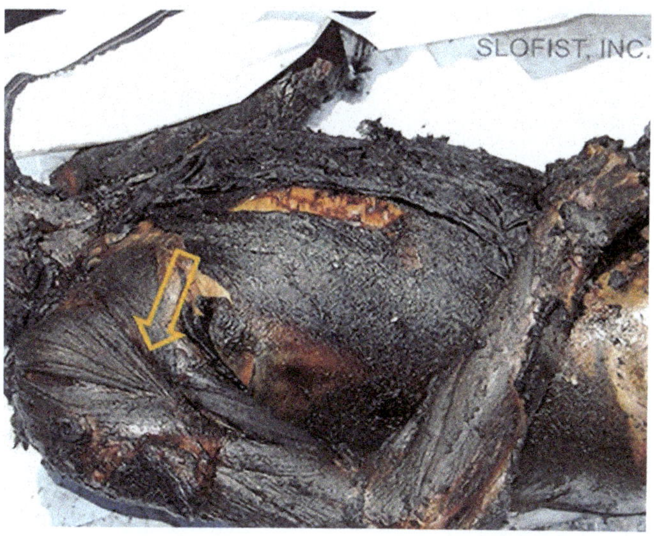

Figure 5.5a Individual #5 with widespread muscle exposure to upper arms (yellow arrow above).

When evaluating the long bones, this individual exhibited widespread muscle exposure on the upper limbs, and partial skin splitting and limited charring to the lower limbs (see Figures 5.5a–5.5c). Given the upper limbs exhibited widespread muscle exposure, the highest score that can be awarded for this individual is a stage five.

When evaluating the hands and feet, this individual exhibited differential charring in these regions. The hands exhibited the pugilistic posture, widespread charring, and muscle exposure, while the feet exhibited partial skin splits with little to no charring (see Figures 5.5a–5.5c). Given the hands exhibited the pugilistic posture, this individual was scored at a stage six. No bone exposure or charring of bone was found in either the hands or feet, so this individual was not scored any higher on this new model. Scores were added together (5 + 3 + 5 + 6), and this individual was given a total body score of 19.

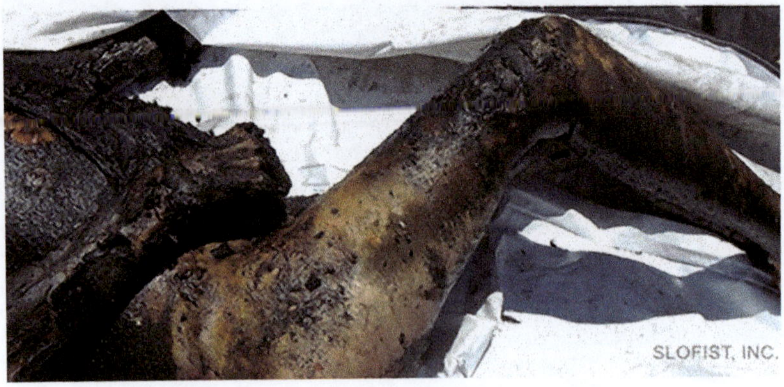

Figure 5.5b Individual #5 with partial charring on lower limbs.

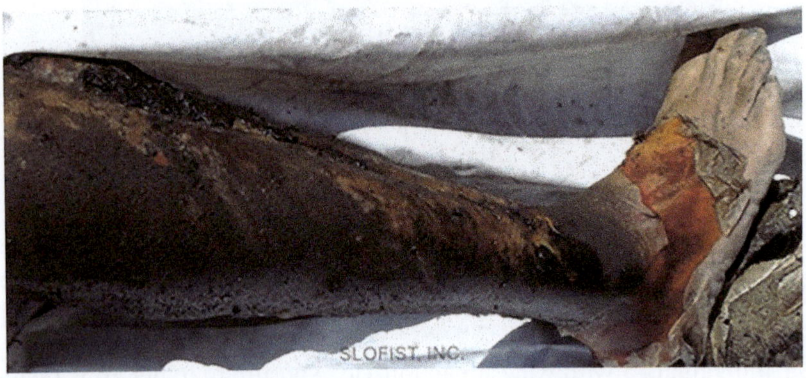

Figure 5.5c Individual #5 with partial skin splitting, and little to no charring on feet.

5.11 Broader Implications

Currently, forensic professionals typically describe the nature and condition of remains, with no attempt to quantify the amount of thermal damage present. This new model provides a way of not only describing thermal alterations but quantifying them using a scale. In contexts where partial remains are present, one can still apply the new model. It is likely that partial remains may be found, especially when remains exhibit the latter stages of burning (like calcination and fragmentation). It is recommended that one visually assesses the remains present per bodily region. If any region cannot be scored, then one would assign a score of zero to that specific area. While it is highly unlikely that all elements from a single bodily region may be missing, it can occur. In the event where partial remains are recovered, it is still possible to use this new model.

This new classification system has laid the foundation for applying quantitative methods to fire environments and provided the first steps in creating models that can be used to estimate *in situ* conditions. Quantitative methods, like the one described in this chapter, can be used to aid investigators in building a legal case and work to minimize misinterpretations of fatal fire scenes.

5.12 Conclusions

This chapter provides an overview of anthropological and medicolegal methods for analyzing burned human remains and highlights the need within the forensic sciences for a new classification system. Previous models provided limited descriptions of thermal alterations, and thus are not widely used today. Previous models (Baby, 1954; Eckert *et al.*, 1988; Glassman and Crow, 1996) progress quickly through the sequence of thermal alterations, often only including a limited amount of soft tissue variables in their descriptions. There is a need within the forensic community for a new classification system that is more broadly applicable to fatal fire cases. A new model was developed based on experimental observations surrounding vehicle, structure, confined space, and outdoor fire contexts. These settings provide a more representative sample of the cases that the medicolegal community are likely to examine. The model developed covers the entire range of thermal alterations from skin blistering to fragmentation. The model also assesses alterations per bodily region and provides a total body score to describe the nature of the remains. This chapter describes how the new classification system was derived and demonstrates how to best apply this new classification system to fatal fire deaths. The case studies mentioned above illustrate how one would go about using this new model to assess thermal alterations. In contexts where alterations may vary between elements (e.g. upper and lower limbs), it is advised that one should use the highest score possible. Once scores are assessed for each region, they are added together to formulate a TBS. TBS scores are then taken and added into a model to predict fire conditions and timing of death events.

This chapter has laid the foundation for a more quantitative approach to be applied within fatal fire research. Primarily, fatal fire research has remained relatively descriptive, with no means to quantify the amount of damage observed. This chapter introduces a new quantifiable method with the hope that more will be developed in the future. Fatal fires often produce some of the most challenging scenes and remains to analyze (Symes *et al.*, 2008; DeHaan, 2012; Lentini, 2013, 2019), and can often lead to misinterpretations that have grave consequences for those wrongly convicted. The ability to use more than one's expertise provides a more solid approach to analyzing and interpreting fatal fire deaths.

Acknowledgments

The experimental research presented in this chapter would not have been possible without the generous support and time of several individuals and organizations. My deepest appreciation goes to the San Luis Obispo Fire Investigation Strike Team (SLOFIST) for generously allowing me to attend their yearly training course and granting me access to data. Thank you for the invaluable training you provide to researchers and the forensic community. A special thanks also goes to the Mountain Desert and Coastal Forensic Anthropologists, the Toelle-Bekken families, and the Bertha Morton Foundation at the University of Montana. The research presented would not have been possible without these organizations and their generous financial contributions.

References

Ahmed, I., Farooq, U., Afzal, W., and Salman, M. (2009) Medicolegal aspect of burn victims: A ten years study. *Pakistan Journal of Medical Sciences*, **25**(5), 797–800.

Arora, A.K., Gupta, P., Kapur, S.S., and Mahajan, S. (2010) An analytical review of burnt bones in Medico-legal Science. *Journal of Punjab Academy of Forensic Medicine and Toxicology*, **10**, 31–36.

Baby, R.S. (1954) Hopewell cremation practices. *The Ohio Historical Society Papers in Archaeology*, **1**, 1–7.

Bass, W.M. (1984) Time interval since death: A difficult decision. In: Human Identification: Case Studies in Forensic Anthropology (eds. T.A. Rathburn and J.E. Buikstra). Charles C. Thomas Publishing, Springfield, IL, pp. 136–147.

Bonhert, M. and Rothschild, M. (2003) Complex suicides by self-incineration. *Forensic Science International*, **131**, 197–201.

Byard, R.W. (2018) The autopsy evaluation of "straightforward" fire deaths. *Forensic Science, Medicine and Pathology*, **14**, 273–275.

Correia, P.M. (1997) Fire modification of bone: A review of the literature. In: Forensic Taphonomy: The Postmortem Fate of Human Remains (eds. W.D. Haglund and M.H. Sorg). CRC Press, Boca Raton, FL, pp. 275–293.

DeHaan, J. (2008) Fire and bodies. In: Analysis of Burned Human Remains (eds. C. Schmidt and S. Steven). Academic Press, London, pp. 1–14.

DeHaan, J. (2012) Sustained combustion of bodies: Some observations. *Journal of Forensic Science*, **10**, 1–6.

DeHaan, J.D., Campbell, S.J., and Nurbakhsh, S. (1999) Combustion of animal fat and its implications for the consumption of human bodies in fires. *Science & Justice*, **39**(1), 27–38.

Dunne, M.J. and McMeekin, R.R. (1977) Medical investigation of fatalities from aircraft-accident burns. *Aviation, Space and Environmental Medicine*, **48**(10), 964–968.

Eckert, W.G., James, S., and Katchis, S. (1988) Investigation of cremations and severely burned bodies. *American Journal of Pathology*, **18**, 163–173.

Fanton, L., Deed, K., Tilhe-Coarlet, S., and Malicier, D. (2006) Criminal burning. *Forensic Science International*, **158**, 87–93.

Fracasso, T., Pfeiffer, H., Pellerin, P., and Karger, B. (2009) The morphology of cutaneous burn injuries and the type of heat application. *Journal of Forensic Science International*, **187**, 81–86.

Galloway, A., Birkby, W.H., Jones, A.M., Henry, T.E., and Parks, B.O. (1989) Decay rates of human remains in an arid environment. *Journal of Forensic Science*, **34**, 607–616.

Giretzlehner, M., Dirnberger, J., Owen, R., Haller, H.L., Lumenta, D.B., and Kamolz, L.-P. (2013) The determination of total burn surface area: How much difference? *Burns*, **39**, 1107–1113.

Glassman, D.M. and Crow, R.M. (1996) Standardization model for describing the extent of burn injury to human remains. *Journal of Forensic Science*, **41**(1), 152–154.

Kashiwagi, M., Hara, K., Takamoto, M., Kageura, M., Masusue, A., Sugimura, T., *et al.* (2009) An autopsy case of suicide by acetylene explosion; a case report. *Medicine, Science, and the Law*, **49**(2), 132–135.

Komar, D.A. (1998) Decay rates in a cold climate region: A review of cases involving advanced decomposition from the Medical Examiner's Office in Edmonton, Alberta. *Journal of Forensic Science*, **43**, 57–61.

Lentini, J. (2013) Scientific Protocols for Fire Investigation. CRC Press, Boca Raton, FL, pp. 1–624.

Lentini, J. (2019) Fire investigation: Historical perspective and recent developments. *Forensic Science Review*, **31**, 37–44.

Martin-de las Heras, S., Valenzuela, A., Villanueva, E., Marques, T., Exposito, N., and Bohoyo, J.M. (1999) Methods for identification of 28 burn victims following a 1996 bus accident in Spain. *Journal of Forensic Science*, **44**(2), 428–431.

Mayne Correia, P.M. (1997) Fire modification of bone: A review of the literature. In: Forensic Taphonomy: The Postmortem Fate of Human Remains (eds. W.D. Haglund and M.H. Sorg). CRC Press, Boca Raton, FL, pp. 275–294.

Megyesi, M., Nawrocki, S., and Haskell, N. (2005) Using accumulated degree-days to estimate the postmortem interval from decomposed human remains. *Journal of Forensic Science*, **50**(3), 618–626.

Moore, R., Waheed, A., and Burns, B. (2019) *Rule of Nine/Wallace Rule of Nines*. National Center for Biotechnology Information, U.S. National Library of Medicine. Stat Pearls Publishing LLC, Baltimore, MD.

Mullins, R.F., Alarm, B., Anwarul Huq Mian, M., Samples, J.M., Friedman, B.C., Shaver, J.R., *et al.* (2009) Burns in mobile home fires-descriptive study at a regional burn center. *Journal of Burn Care and Research*, **30**(4), 694–699.

Parks, J., Noguchi, T., and Klatt, E. (1989) The epidemiology of fatal burn injuries. *Journal of Forensic Science*, **34**(2), 399–406.

Pope, E.J. and Smith, O.C. (2004) Identification of traumatic injury in burned cranial bone: An experimental approach. *Journal of Forensic Science*, **49**(3), 1–10.

Prahlow, J. (2010) Burns and fire related deaths. In: Forensic Pathology for Police, Death Investigators, Attorneys, and Forensic Scientists (ed. J. Prahlow). Springer Press, New York, pp. 481–500.

Symes, S.A., Rainwater, C.W., Chapman, E.N., Gipson, D.R., and Piper, A.L. (2008) Patterned thermal destruction of human remains in a forensic setting. In: The Analysis of Burned Human Remains, 1st edn. (eds. C.W. Schmidt and S.A. Symes). CRC Press, Boca Raton, FL, pp. 15–55.

Thompson, T.J.U. and Chudek, J.A. (2007) A novel approach to the visualization of heat-induced structural change in bone. *Science and Justice*, **47**, 99–104.

Tumer, A., Akcan, R., Karacaoglu, E., Balseven-Odabasi, A., Keten, A., Kanburoglu, C., *et al.* (2012) Postmortem burning of the corpses following homicide. *Journal of Forensic and Legal Medicine*, **19**, 223–228.

Viklund, A., Bjornstig, J., and Larsson, M. (2013) Car crash fatalities associated with fire in Sweden. *Traffic Injury Prevention*, **14**, 823–827.

CHAPTER 6

Burnt Human Remains and Forensic Medicine

Sarah Ellingham[1], PhD; Joe Adserias-Garriga[2], PhD, DDS, D-ABFO and Peter Ellis[3], OAM, MB, FRCPA

[1] *Forensic Coordinator, International Committee of the Red Cross, Switzerland*

[2] *Assistant Professor for Forensic Anthropology and Odontology, Mercyhurst University, USA*

[3] *Forensic Pathologist, Queensland, Australia*

Cases involving burnt remains admitted in a Medical / Coroner's Office can range from superficial burns affecting the soft tissue to calcinated remains where no soft tissue is left and burns affect the hard tissues (bones and teeth).

Determining the manner of death of a body recovered from a fire scene can be very challenging, since the evaluation of the remains will imply pathological, toxicological as well as trauma analysis. This chapter will explore the analysis of burnt remain cases from a medicolegal perspective.

6.1 Fire Death Statistics

A multitude of events can lead to the burning of human remains, be it homicidal, suicidal, accidental, natural disasters, man-made disasters, terror-associated burns, or other. An average of 2800 people in the USA and 330 in the UK die in circumstances involving fire every year, which equates to 10.41 and 6.46 per million population respectively (Woodrow, 2012). While these figures are still staggering, the number of fire deaths has seen a decrease by 66.7% in North America and 64.5% in Western Europe between 1979 and 2007 (US Fire Administration, 2011).

Figure 6.1 depicts the 2017 fire death rate per 100,000 in representatively selected countries, depicting vast discrepancies from 0.2 per 100,000 in Singapore to over 7 in Lesotho (Our World in Data, 2021). While the exact reasons for these divergences are hard to pinpoint, factors such as differences in lifestyle, cultural attitudes towards fire, fire prevention education, and fire safety regulations in infrastructure are likely to play a role. Retrospective analyses of fire fatalities in the USA found 60% of fire deaths to be male, and 40% to be female (Barillo and

Burnt Human Remains: Recovery, Analysis, and Interpretation, First Edition. Edited by Sarah Ellingham, Joe Adserias-Garriga, Sara C. Zapico and Douglas H. Ubelaker.

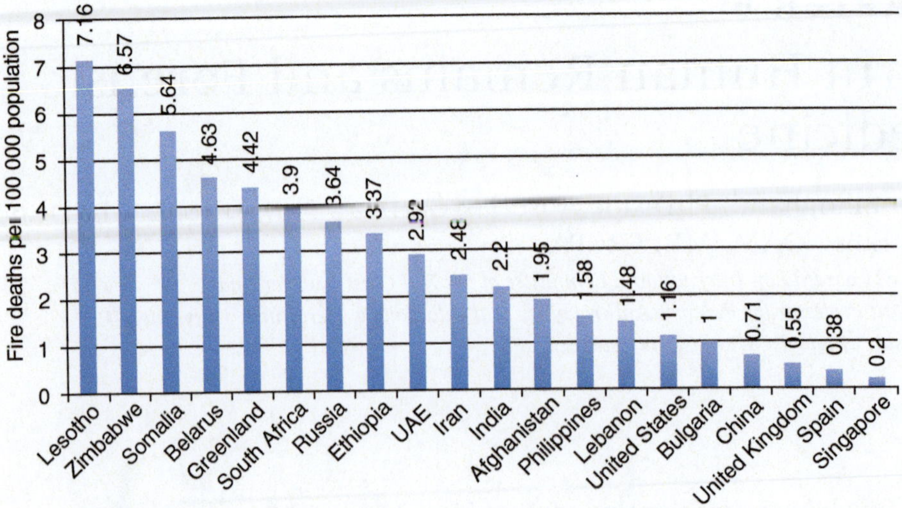

Figure 6.1 Fire deaths per 100,000 population in selected countries.

Goode, 1996). The study further found that 79% of US fires occurred in structure fires, particularly residences. In these cases, 66% of the victims passed away at the scene, 10% were dead on arrival at the hospital, 12.7% lost their lives within six hours following the fire, and 8% were so-called delayed fire deaths, dying over six hours after the event. The average survival for fire deaths recorded in this study was eight days

6.2 Statistics of Manner of Fire-Related Deaths

Manner of death can be divided into five different categories: natural, homicidal, suicidal, accidental, and undetermined. Ascertaining the manner of death from a fire scene can be particularly challenging due to the often severe destruction of the remains and damage to the surrounding structures and may require the consideration of a combination of pathological findings and toxicology, as well as reconstruction of the fire scene and the events and victim activities leading up to the incineration events (DeHaan, 2006). Accidental fire deaths can occur through a variety of scenarios, including building or vehicle fires, natural disasters or terror associated incidents. As mentioned previously, the overall prevalence of fire deaths can be linked to issues such as cultural attitudes to fire or to demographic factors. Particularly numerous fluctuations resulting from cultural or national influences can be found when it comes to the frequency of homicidal and suicidal burns.

6.2.1 Prevalence of Self-Immolation

The prevalence of suicide by self-immolation varies greatly between countries. While in developed countries they account for only 0.06–1% of all suicides, in developing countries this number can reach 40.3% (Copeland, 1985; Ahmadi,

2007). A meta study of 3351 cases of self-immolation worldwide found the highest absolute number of cases and highest fatality rate to be in India, whereas the highest number of per capita cases were found in Sri Lanka (Laloë, 2004). Demographics also varied between countries, with male victims making up the largest proportion of cases in Western countries, and female victims in India and the Middle East. Laloë identified three main groups for self-immolation: psychiatric patients, which is the case mostly in European and Middle Eastern countries (Castellani *et al.*, 1995; Rothschild *et al.*, 2001); people committing suicide by fire for personal reasons, which was mostly the case in India, Sri Lanka, Papua New Guinea, and Zimbabwe; and politically motivated self-immolations, the majority of which can be found in India and South Korea. Asian victims were found to be on average ten years younger than those from Europe, and this discrepancy was most likely to be attributed to the number of women being forced into arranged marriages (Cave Bondi *et al.*, 2001; Laloë, 2004). Faith, however, does not seem to play a significant role, with self-immolations being just as common in Muslim countries as in others.

6.2.2 Prevalence of Criminal Immolation

Similarly to self-immolation, the prevalence of criminal immolation is highly country and culture dependent. In particular, India is experiencing a prevalence of young women dying though immolation due to unfulfilled dowry expectations (Kumar and Tripathi, 2004). Dowry deaths have become such a common phenomenon that they are described in Section 304-B of the Indian penal code as:

> *"the death of a woman… caused by any burns or other bodily injury… within seven years of her marriage, and it is shown that shortly before her death she was subjected to cruelty or harassment by her husband or any relative of her husband's for, or in connection with, any demand for dowry, such deaths will be deemed 'dowry deaths' and her husband or relative will be deemed to have caused her death"*
>
> (Kumar and Tripathi, 2004).

A number of studies have reported 31–55% of fire-related deaths of Indian women to be homicidal, with 90% being young wives between the ages of 16 and 25 (Kumar and Tripathi, 2004; Shaha and Mohanthy, 2006). The majority were dowsed in kerosene before incineration and sustained burns on over 75% of their body surface. The prevalence of women being murdered decreases with increasing education status and it has been found that 72% of homicidal immolation cases in India occurred in rural areas (Shaha and Mohanthy, 2006).

In Brazil, execution through immolation, by placing the victim inside a pile of tires while still alive and then setting it on fire, has become the signature of some drug cartels (Durão *et al.*, 2015). This execution method, known as death in the "microwave oven" is further described in Chapter 19 of this volume.

A ten-year study analyzing all cases of fire fatalities in Lyon, France, from 1993 to 2003, found criminal deaths to make up 31% of incidents, following accidents (52%) and before suicides (16%). Most criminal burns were found to be post-mortem attempts at covering up a crime, whereas immolation homicides only accounted for 25%. These findings echoed previous ones made by Copeland (Copeland, 1985), who looked at cases in the Miami Dade County, USA, from 1977 to 1984, and Büyük and Kocak (Büyük and Koçak, 2009), who evaluated cases in Istanbul, Turkey, between 1998 and 2002.

6.3 Fire Damage to the Body

It is only in a narrow temperature window of 20–44°C that the human body can survive (Knight, 2004). Serious skin damage occurs after only six hours of exposure to 44°C. Between 44°C and 51°C every additional 1°C halves the time it takes for a certain amount of damage to occur (Bohnert, 2004). Uninterrupted prolonged exposure to heat can, depending on temperature and exposure time, ultimately lead to the destruction of a body. It is, however, very rare for a body to combust entirely, and it is more common for a differential preservation of anatomical features to occur. This depends on a multitude of factors, such as the level of temperature and the duration of exposure, the position of the body, and the mode of heat transmission, just to name a few (Bohnert, 2004; DeHaan, 2006). Complete cremation, as associated with the funerary industry, requires constant exposure temperatures of between 900°C and 1100°C for 1–2 hours in a consistently ventilated gas-filled oven (DeHaan, 2006). Even under these conditions, identifiable skeletal elements such as parts of the skull, teeth, or the os coxa remain, so that they are commonly mechanically ground to fine bone dust after cremation.

With prolonged exposure to heat a loss of fluids occurs and this causes a shrinkage of tissue. Externally this is expressed by the skin tightening and splitting and developing a hard, leathery consistency. Also linked to the loss of fluid are the protrusion of the tongue and the appearance of cutaneous petechial hemorrhages in the head and neck area (Lawler, 1993) (Figure 6.2). Continuous high temperatures subsequently cause a vaporization of body fluids as well as a buildup of pressure in closed cavities, and this can cause a rupture of those cavity walls. The fluids which are expressed out of body openings can mimic putrefaction (Bohnert, 2004). Like the skin, internal organs also exhibit fluid loss and shrinkage, turning into small and firm so-called "puppet organs." If the exposure continues, the organ surface takes on a sponge-like residual structure, and eventually, when the tissue is completely desiccated, will disintegrate into ash (Bohnert, 2004). If temperatures exceed 150°C changes to the hair occur. It becomes brittle and its color turns to dark red, brown, or black. From 200°C, gas bubbles can form in the shaft, and at 240°C it becomes frizzy due a melting of the keratin in the hair. From 300°C charring occurs (Bohnert, 2013).

There are multiple factors which can affect the speed of destruction a body undergoes when exposed to fire. Accelerating factors include obesity and clothing. After thorough burning through the skin, the subcutaneous fat is exposed and

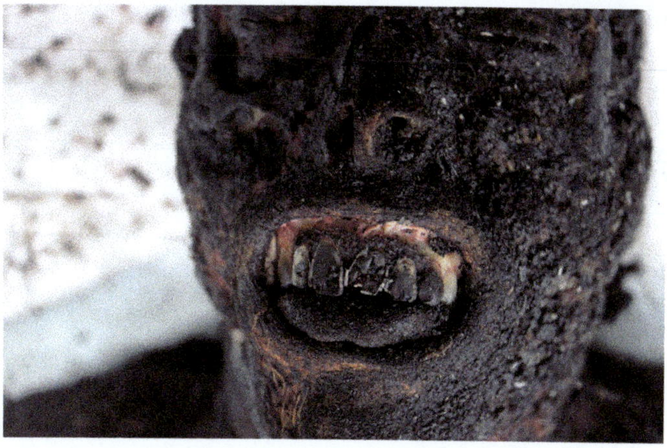

Figure 6.2 Heat induced tightening of the skin around the mouth, protrusion of tongue and fracturing of incisors. (© Institute of Legal Medicine Hamburg).

once ignited it can function as an accelerant, producing flames of 800–900°C (Spitz and Spitz, 2005). In a similar manner, clothing can act as a wick, facilitating a more rapid and more complete combustion process. If exposed to temperatures of over 600°C the muscles shorten and contract due to the dehydration and the denaturing of proteins, and this can lead to the typical "pugilistic stance" which commonly occurs in burn victims after less than ten minutes' exposure (Bohnert *et al.*, 1998). This characteristic stance in which the arms are bent as though presenting the pose of a boxer is caused by the differential size of flexor and extensor muscles on either side of the various shoulder, elbow, wrist, and hand joints. Contractions of the paraspinal muscles can frequently be observed in a notable opisthotonos, the backwards arching of the head, neck, and spine (DeHaan, 2006). Only after considerable exposure time do skeletal structures become exposed. Experimental studies have shown that at an average temperature of 650°C, the rib cage and facial skeleton are exposed after around 20 minutes, and femur and tibia deflesh from around 35 minutes onward. After around one hour tissue destruction proceeds enough for the body to disintegrate (Richards, 1977; Bohnert *et al.*, 1998) (Table 6.1). However, in fire death events, bodies are rarely exposed to constant temperatures resembling the laboratory settings, as fires develop in several stages. It is therefore common for human remains to have differential destruction patterns.

6.4 Classification of the Degree of Fire Damage

Medically, burns are most commonly classified based on the degree of soft tissue destruction, for example with Wilson's three-stage nomenclature (Knight, 2004; Spitz and Spitz, 2005). First degree burns are superficial red discolorations with

Table 6.1 Destruction of the human body in relation to exposure at 670–870°C (Adapted from Bohnert *et al.*, 1998)

Time	Skull	Trunk	Extremities
10 min.	Calvarium free of soft tissue; soft tissue of the face charred	Charring of skin	"Pugilistic stance" of the arms
20 min.	Sparse soft tissue remains in the face; heat fractures of the calvarium	Thorax muscles charred; ribs and sternum exposed	Soft tissue of hands largely combusted, loss of structural integrity, ulna and radius partially exposed; carbonization of leg muscles
30 min.	Tabula externa of the calvarium crumbling	Thoracic and abdominal cavity exposed; organs blackened and shrunken	Hands and distal radius and ulna burned away; tibia and distal femur free of soft tissue and exposed
40 min.	Exposure of the brain; facial bones beginning to disintegrate	Shrunken, charred organs with bumpy surface	Forearms completely combusted and broken away from the body, humerus largely free of soft tissue
50 min.	Facial bones largely combusted, calcined, and disintegrated; base of the skull showing	Organs largely combusted by fire	Arms completely combusted; only calcined stumps of the femur remain

some swelling from edema; however, there is no loss of dermis and usually no blistering. After death, first degree burns may not be recognizable, since gravity causes blood from congested areas to settle into lower parts of the body, leading to fading discoloration and diffusion of swelling into surrounding tissues. In second degree burns, the epidermis is charred and coagulated and large blisters are formed due to subepidermal necrosis. A notable variation to this pattern of second degree burns is white discoloration, swelling, and wrinkling in the palms of hands and soles of feet, which resemble the "washerwoman hands" typically seen in drowning victims. These are caused by fluid filled blisters forming in the stratum germinativum and a clumping of erythrocytes (Bohnert, 2004). For burns to be categorized as third degree, the full thickness of epidermis, dermis, and underlying soft tissue are destroyed. The deep tissue destruction can be of various degrees, ranging from loss of subcutaneous fat and muscle tissue, to charring of bones or even loss of limbs.

In order to describe and specify the extent of burns, the surgical "rule of nines," which divides the body into percentages, is commonly applied (Lawler, 1993; DeHaan, 2006). The head and each of the arms account for 9% of the body, the front and back of the torso as well as front and back of each leg respectively account for 18% and the genitals for 1% of the body surface. If 30–50% of the body surface is affected by heat damage, this is often not compatible with survival (DeHaan, 2006), although this may be dependent on the availability of suitable medical support. Direct thermal damage is not necessary for fire-related deaths to occur; the most common cause of death at a fire scene is smoke inhalation, which can result in a combination of poisoning by carbon monoxide and other inhaled toxic gases, such as cyanide from burning plastics, surfactants being deactivated, as well as other fatal physiological reactions. In addition, delayed deaths due to fluid loss, respiratory failure, or shock a few days after exposure are not uncommon (DiMaio and DiMaio, 2001).

Several approaches to describing the extent of consumption of a body by fire can be found in the literature (Eckert *et al.*, 1988; Glassman and Crow, 1996; Gerling *et al.*, 2001). Until now and from a medicolegal perspective the Crow-Glassman Scale (CGS) has been found to be the most applicable classification for forensic purposes (Bohnert, 2004). It is particularly useful in managing the response to the fire scene and burnt remains recovery. The scale consists of five levels of increasing severity of destruction (Glassman and Crow, 1996). Williams, in Chapter 5 of this volume, argues that the CGS does not include the option to record the full range of possible burn-related features, and that its application can be highly subjective due to it not quantifying the surface percentage of the body affected. Williams therefore proposed an alternative method which allows for separate scoring of the head and neck, trunk, limbs, and hands and feet.

6.5 Medicolegal Determination of Cause of Death

The cause of death, effectively the events that culminate in the death of the victim, is generally established by the medical examiner. A full post-mortem examination should be carried out on all fire-related deaths. While deaths associated with fire are generally divided into early (during fire exposure) or late (a period after the fire exposure), the possibility that the death may have occurred before the outbreak of the fire, must be considered. This may be through natural causes, because of foul play, or following alcohol or drug abuse, just to name a few. The cause of death directly associated with fire most often includes poisoning by carbon monoxide or other toxic gases, cutaneous or mucosal burns, anoxia, hypoxia following respiratory tract mucosal swelling due to the inhalation of hot gasses, hyperthermia, or trauma after falling or being struck by falling objects (DeHaan, 2006). Direct burns, that is, tissue destruction which is accompanied by toxemia (blood poisoning), hypovolemia (low blood volume), hypotension (low blood pressure), hemoconcentration (an increase in accumulated cells in the blood due to plasma loss), hyperkalemia (low potassium levels), and shock, are only rarely the cause of death, and mostly occur in very rapid flash fires (Lawler, 1993). Most burns occur post-mortem. The most common cause of death in fires is toxic gas inhalation. Depending on the nature and composition of the combustible materials involved in the fire, over 300 toxic gases can be produced. These include carbon monoxide (CO), hydrogen cyanide (HCN), nitrogen dioxide (NO_2), nitrogen tetroxide (N_2O_4), benzene (C_6H_6), phosgene ($COCI_2$), ammonia (NH_3), formaldehyde (CH_2O), acrolein (C_3H_4O), hydrogen fluoride (HF), chlorine (CL_2), hydrogen sulphide (H_2S), and other oxides of sulfur (Lawler, 1993).

One of the first steps of the examination is the assessment of vitality, that is to determine whether the individual was alive when the fire started. When possible, toxicological analyses to determine the concentration of carbon monoxide hemoglobin (CO-Hb), methemoglobin (Met-Hb), and cyanide (CN) should be carried out. Concentrations over 10% CO-Hb, and over 0.2 mg l^{-1} are considered lethal (Bohnert, 2013). Positive Met-Hb values are associated with the inhalation of nitrous gases. Other indicators of vitality during fire exposure can be found in the respiratory tract in the form of soot deposits from fire fume inhalation, which can be found on the mucosa of the nose, mouth, pharynx, larynx, trachea, and bronchi, and these may also exhibit bleeding and vesicular detachment (Figure 6.3). The most reliable observations to confirm vital exposure to fire are a combination of CO-Hb concentrations above 10% as well as soot deposits in the respiratory tract, esophagus, and stomach (Bohnert, 2013). Death due to toxic gas poisoning or asphyxiation usually occurs very rapidly, whereas deaths in the days following a fire event are most often associated with shock, fluid loss, or electrolyte imbalance. Deaths occurring with a delay of several weeks tend to be due to organ failure or infections (DeHaan, 2006).

6.6 Medicolegal Determination of Manner of Death

Exposure to fire can make the determination of manner of death a challenging venture. Upon exposure to heat, skin and underlying soft tissue shrinks and contracts, which leads to heat ruptures, which can in some cases exceed 10 cm in length and these can mimic ante-mortem sharp force trauma (Eckert *et al.*, 1988; Lawler, 1993). However, closer examination should find that the heat splits do not exhibit any associated tissue bruising or signs of vital reactions. They further tend to be located near joints and often occur when the rigor mortis is overcome once the muscle begins to heat up.

Also common in fire victims is the formation of a so-called "heat hematoma" of the brain, where blood accumulation resembles a traumatic extradural hemorrhage with a blood volume sometimes exceeding 100 ml. Often occurring bilaterally, the hematoma exhibits a light brown color and a "honeycomb" appearance due to the boiling of fluids (Lawler, 1993; Bohnert *et al.*, 2003) (Figure 6.4). The

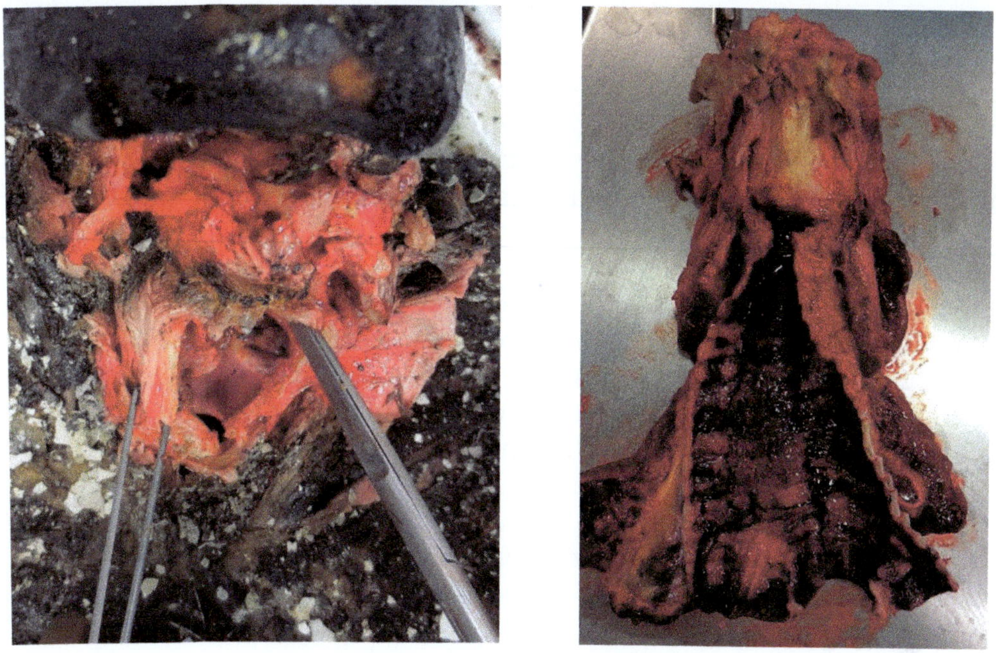

Figure 6.3 Trachea with the absence of soot (a) and the presence of soot in the trachea indicating smoke inhalation (b).

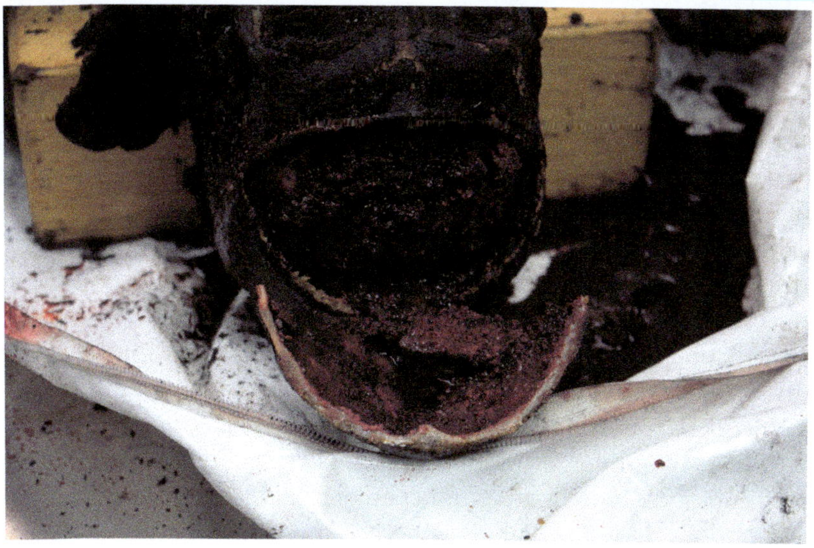

Figure 6.4 Heat hematoma (© Institute of Legal Medicine Hamburg).

hematoma accumulates following the thermal contraction of underlying brain tissue and the filling of the resulting space by blood passively drawn from cranial vessels. Heat hematomas are usually unassociated with any ante-mortem cranial injuries, and their carbon monoxide saturation should be similar to the blood elsewhere in the body. Continuous heat exposure of over half an hour can lead the skull to fracture, which in some instances can lead to difficulties in distinguishing between traumatic injuries and heat fractures (Bohnert *et al.*, 1997). Thermal skull fractures can be divided into two types, one being the result of a rapid increase in intracranial pressure displacing cranial fragments outwards, the other being a consequence of skull desiccation, solely involving the tabula externa, exhibiting stellate, elliptic, or circular fracture lines (Herrmann and Bennett, 1999). It is not uncommon in these types of fractures for the cranial tabula externa to peel off, exposing the underlying diploe; this delamination process produces externally beveled features which can mimic blunt force or ballistic trauma (Pope and Smith, 2004). However, these fractures occur exclusively on the calvarium, never on the base of the skull; fractures on the latter are suggestive of either ante-mortem trauma or post-mortem trauma, which could occur through the impact of falling debris (Bohnert *et al.*, 1997). Other indications of skull fractures having occurred before death are the presence of ante-mortem hematomas (Iwase *et al.*, 1998; Marella *et al.*, 2012). Further, the careful analysis of fracture margins can yield some information on fracture timing. Fractures produced through thermal or mechanical forces produce sharp and well-defined edges, whereas traumatic fractures tend to have blunted, deformed, or warped margins with both the internal and external tables altered due to the prolonged heat exposure, and this becomes most apparent when fractured skulls are reconstructed (Pope and Smith, 2004). Shrinkage induced lacerations to the skin cause some sections of bone to be prematurely exposed to thermal destruction as the skin "degloves."

It can be difficult to distinguish between self-immolation as a means of suicide or immolation homicide, as in both cases the victim is usually doused in flammable liquids, most often gasoline (Rothschild *et al.*, 2001). The determination is further complicated by the above-mentioned heat artifacts which can mimic traumatic ante- or post-mortem injuries. Rothschild *et al.* (2001) evaluated immolation suicides which occurred in Berlin between 1990 and 2000 and made up 0.78% of all registered suicides. They found self-immolations to present themselves with median body surface burns of 78%, mean blood values of 21% CO-Hb and 0.07 µg/m cyanide. Burn shock caused 33% of deaths, while 20% died of a combination of severe burns and smoke intoxication. The CO-Hb values are higher (mean 58%) in individuals who self-immolated in closed spaces such as vehicles (Shkrum and Johnston, 1992). When observing burn patterns it has been found that in self-immolations the soles of the feet are often spared (Makhlouf *et al.*, 2011).

6.7 The Use of Post-Mortem Imaging for the Analysis of Burn Victims

The supplementation of regular autopsies with multi-slice Computer Tomography (MSCT) and/or Magnetic Resonance Imaging (MRI) is becoming a regular practice for the post-mortem examination of burn victims (Figure 6.5). The benefits

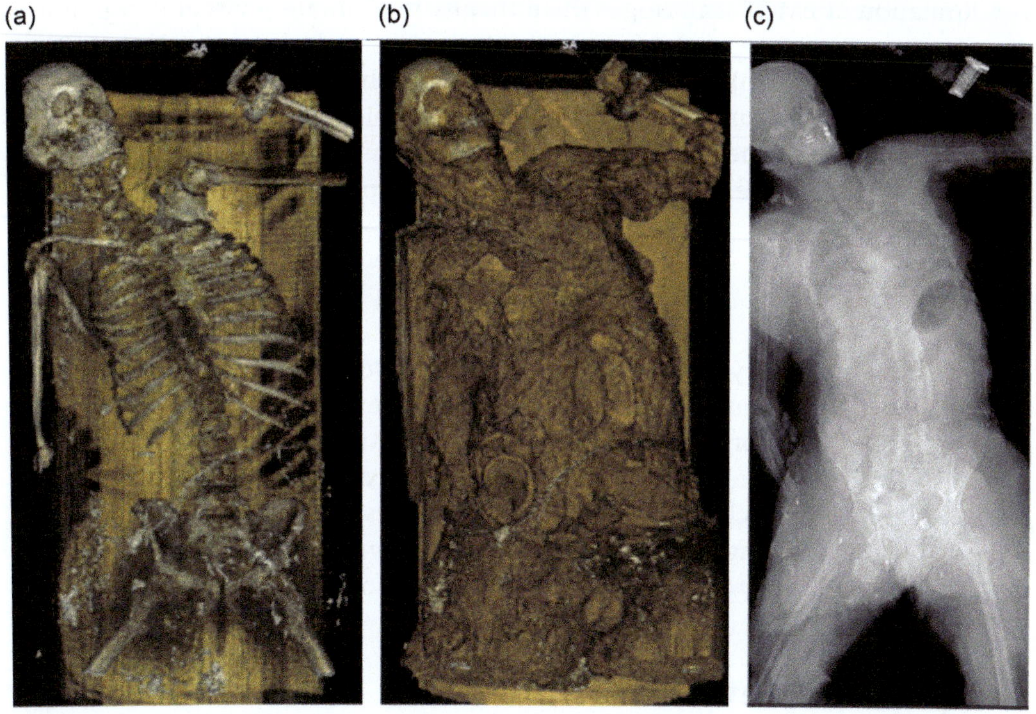

Figure 6.5 a)–c): CT scan of body surface; CT scan threshold set to skeletal view; maximum intensity projection of body (X-ray). Heat induced opisthotonos and pugilistic stance are displayed. (© Institute of Legal Medicine Hamburg).

of post-mortem imaging prior to invasive autopsy are manifold and can reveal a host of information supplementary to traditional post-mortem (Thali *et al.*, 2002). For example, post-mortem CT (PMCT) allows for the examination of body parts not routinely inspected during autopsies, such as the facial skeleton, cervical spine, and limbs. Further studies have found that details of fractures in areas such as the base of the skull, the spine and the pelvis (which may be missed due to the non-routine nature or difficulty of completely dissecting these regions in charred remains) are easily detectable on PMCTs (Levy *et al.*, 2009). It further allows for the documentation of heat-related injuries such as epidural hematoma, gas embolisms, and fractures (Andersen and Boel, 2013). Minimally invasive image-guided biopsies and sampling are also facilitated through post-mortem imaging. The use of PMCT in mass fatality events, often linked to fire-related deaths, has also been discussed in the literature; it can be used as a pre-autopsy triaging tool to locate human remains or hazardous debris in body bags, locating personal effects, medical implants/interventions, or signs of ante-mortem trauma/disease useful for identification, or even facilitate the taking of measurements and data required to fill INTERPOL's DVI forms without the need for invasive autopsies (Brough *et al.*, 2015).

A limitation of PMCT scanning is the difficulty in evaluating visceral organs and vascular structures; augmentations with alternative techniques such as MRI or post-mortem angiographies are better suited to fill these gaps (Levy *et al.*, 2009). Overall, post-mortem imaging techniques, if available, are a low-cost, non-invasive tool to augment the complex process of examining burnt remains, additionally allowing for long-term recording and re-analyzing of images.

6.8 Conclusion

While exhibiting a varying degree of prevalence around the world, fire-related deaths are a global phenomenon. Due to the complexity of fire-induced destruction patterns, post-mortem examination and the determination of cause and manner of death can be very intricate and require experience as well as a variety of examination approaches and analytical techniques. The use of additional technologies such as imaging methods further facilitate and supplement the examinations for more accuracy and long-term storage of information.

Acknowledgments

The authors would like to thank the Institute for Forensic Medicine at the University Medical Center Hamburg-Eppendorf for their permission to publish the images in this chapter.

References

Ahmadi, A. (2007) Suicide by self-immolation: Comprehensive overview, experiences and suggestions. *Journal of Burn Care and Research*, **28**(1), 30–41.

Andersen, A.M. and Boel, L.W.T. (2013) Post Mortem Computed Tomography as an important tool in establishing a cause of death in fire fatalities. *Scandinavian Journal of Forensic Science*, **19**(1), 3–6.

Barillo, D.J. and Goode, R. (1996) Fire fatality study: Demographics of fire victims. *Burns*, **22**(2), 85–88.

Bohnert, M. (2004) Morphological findings in burned bodies. In: *Forensic Pathology Reviews*, Vol. **1**, 1st edn. (ed. M. Tsokos). Humana Press, Totowa, NJ, pp. 3–27.

Bohnert, M. (2013) Burns and scalds. In: *Encyclopedia of Forensic Sciences*, 2nd edn. (eds. J.A. Siegel and P.J. Saukko). Academic Press, Waltham, MA, pp. 11–14.

Bohnert, M., Rost, T., Faller-Marquardt, M., Ropohl, D., and Pollak, S. (1997) Fractures of the base of the skull in charred bodies — Post-mortem heat injuries or signs of mechanical traumatisation? *Forensic Science International*, **87**(1), 55–62.

Bohnert, M., Rost, T., and Pollak, S. (1998) The degree of destruction of human bodies in relation to the duration of the fire. *Forensic Science International*, **95**(1), 11–21.

Bohnert, M., Werner, C.R., and Pollak, S. (2003) Problems associated with the diagnosis of vitality in burned bodies. *Forensic Science International*, **135**(3), 197–205.

Brough, A.L., Morgan, B., and Rutty, G.N. (2015) Postmortem computed tomography (PMCT) and disaster victim identification. *La radiologia medica*, **120**(9), 866–873.

Büyük, Y. and Koçak, U. (2009) Fire-related fatalities in Istanbul, Turkey: Analysis of 320 forensic autopsy cases. *Journal of Forensic and Legal Medicine*, **16**(8), 449–454.

Castellani, G., Beghini, D., Barisoni, D., and Marigo, M. (1995) Suicide attempted by burning: A 10-year study of self-immolation deaths. *Burns*, **21**(8), 607–609.

Cave Bondi, G., Cipolloni, L., Parroni, E., and Cecchi, R. (2001) A review of suicides by burning in Rome between 1947–1997 examined by the Pathology Department of the Institute of Forensic Medicine, University of Rome 'La Sapienza'. *Burns*, **27**(3), 227–231.

Copeland, A. (1985) Suicidal fire deaths revisited. *Zeitschrift Für Rechtsmedizin*, **95**(1), 51–57.

DeHaan, J.D. (2006) Chapter 15: Fire-related deaths and injuries. In: *Kirk's Fire Investigation*, 6th edn. (ed. J.D. DeHaan). Prentice Hall, Upper Saddle River, NJ, pp. 611–654.

DiMaio, V.J. and DiMaio, D. (2001) Chapter 13: Fire deaths. In: *Forensic Pathology*, 2nd edn. (eds. V.J. DiMaio and D. DiMaio). CRC Press, Boca Raton, FL, pp. 367–389.

Durão, C., Machado, M.P., and Daruge Júnior, E. (2015) Death in the "microwave oven": A form of execution by carbonization. *Forensic Science International*, **253**, e1–e3.

Eckert, W.G., James, S., and Katchis, S. (1988) Investigation of cremations and severely burned bodies. *American Journal of Forensic Medicine and Pathology*, **9**(3), 188–200.

Gerling, I., Meissner, C., Reiter, A., and Oehmichen, M. (2001) Death from thermal effects and burns. *Forensic Science International*, **115**(1–2), 33–41.

Glassman, D.M. and Crow, R.M. (1996) Standardization model for describing the extent of burn injury to human remains. *Journal of Forensic Sciences*, **41**(1), 152–154.

Herrmann, N.P. and Bennett, J.L. (1999) The differentiation of traumatic and heat-related fractures in burned bone. *Journal of Forensic Sciences*, **44**(1), 461–469.

Iwase, H., Yamada, Y., Ootani, S., Sasaki, Y., Nagao, M., Iwadate, K., *et al.* (1998) Evidence for an antemortem injury of a burned head dissected from a burned body. *Forensic Science International*, **94**(1–2), 9–14.

Knight, B. (2004) Chapter 11: Burns and scalds. In: *Knight's Forensic Pathology*, 3rd edn. (eds. B. Knight and P. Saukko). CRC Press, Boca Raton, FL, pp. 312–325.

Kumar, V. and Tripathi, C.B. (2004) Burnt wives: A study of homicides. *Medicine, Science and the Law*, **44**(1), 55–60.

Laloë, V. (2004) Patterns of deliberate self-burning in various parts of the world: A review. *Burns*, **30**(3), 207–215.

Lawler, W. (1993) Bodies associated with fires. *Journal of Clinical Pathology*, **46**(10), 886–889.

Levy, A.D., Harcke, H.T., Getz, J.M., and Mallak, C.T. (2009) Multidetector computed tomography findings in deaths with severe burns. *The American Journal of Forensic Medicine and Pathology*, **30**(2), 137–141.

Makhlouf, F., Alvarez, J.-C., and de la Grandmaison, G.L. (2011) Suicidal and criminal immolations: An 18-year study and review of the literature. *Legal Medicine*, **13**(2), 98–102.

Marella, G.L., Perfetti, E., and Arcudi, G. (2012) Differential diagnosis between cranial fractures of traumatic origin and explosion fractures in burned cadavers. *Journal of Forensic and Legal Medicine*, **19**(3), 175–178.

Our World in Data. (2021) *Death Rate from Fires and Burns, 1990 to 2017*. Published online at OurWorldInData.org. https://ourworldindata.org/grapher/fire-death-rates?tab=table.

Pope, E.J. and Smith, O.C. (2004) Identification of traumatic injury in burned cranial bone: An experimental approach. *Journal of Forensic Sciences*, **49**(3), 431–440.

Richards, N.F. (1977) Fire investigation – Destruction of corpses. *Medicine, Science and the Law*, **17**(2), 79–82.

Rothschild, M.A., Raatschen, H., and Schneider, V. (2001) Suicide by self-immolation in Berlin from 1990 to 2000. *Forensic Science International*, **124**(2–3), 163–166.

Shaha, K.K. and Mohanthy, S. (2006) Alleged dowry death: A study of homicidal burns. *Medicine, Science and the Law*, **46**(2), 105–110.

Shkrum, M.J. and Johnston, K.A. (1992) Fire and suicide: A three-year study of self-immolation deaths. *Journal of Forensic Sciences*, **37**(1), 208–221.

Spitz, W.U. and Spitz, D.J. (2005) Chapter XIII: Thermal injuries. In: *Spitz and Fisher's Medicolegal Investigation of Death: Guidelines for the Application of Pathology to Crime Investigation*, 4th edn. Charles C Thomas Publisher Ltd., Springfield, IL, pp. 747–782.

Thali, M.J., Yen, K., Plattner, T., Schweitzer, W., Vock, P., Ozdoba, C., *et al.* (2002) Charred body: Virtual autopsy with multi-slice computed tomography and magnetic resonance imaging. *Journal of Forensic Science*, **47**(6), 1326–1331.

US Fire Administration (2011) Fire death trends: An international perspective. *Topical Fire Report Series*, **12**(8), 1–8.

Woodrow, B. (2012) "Fire as vulnerability": The value added from adopting a vulnerability approach. Geneva: The Geneva Association – Risk and Insurance Economics.

CHAPTER 7

Skeletal Alteration of Burnt Remains through Fire Exposure

Joe Adserias-Garriga, PhD, DDS, D-ABFO
Assisstant Professor, *Department of Applied Forensic Sciences, Mercyhurst University, PA, USA*

Forensic cases involving burnt remains include house fires, mass disasters, motor-vehicle accidents, and criminal burning among others (Bennett and Benedix, 1999; Fanton *et al.*, 2006; Mundorff, 2008). All these scenarios, without exception, are challenging for forensic professionals in the recovery and analysis of the remains.

The proper management of fatal fire scenes and the use of accurate forensic archaeological techniques during recovery are critical to gather the necessary information for the reconstruction of the events (see Chapter 3). The following examination of burnt remains in the lab will be focused on establishing the identity of the deceased and assessing any skeletal trauma. Fatal fire cases frequently involve color, shape, and size altered skeletal elements, which are often heavily fragmented, All these fire induced changes will impact the identification process and skeletal trauma analysis. Due to these limitations, forensic scientists involved in burnt remains analysis should have proper knowledge of the burning process and the alterations that the body undergoes through intense heat exposure.

The comprehension of the burning process and its effects on the body are key for the proper interpretation of the findings at the scene and the following analysis in the lab. The understanding of soft tissue changes is required to properly understand skeletal tissue changes due to fire exposure, since most of burnt remain cases will imply the burning of the hard and soft tissues. As mentioned, forensic professionals analyzing fatal fire remains must have expertise in recognizing the appearance and the burning pattern of the soft and hard tissues to properly interpret the findings in the burnt remains recovery and analysis.

The degree of alteration of the remains will be more significant according to the severity of the burning process. The degree of burning depends on several factors; the most relevant ones are the intensity (or temperature) of the heat and the time of exposure, but also the proximity of the body to the fire, the material being burned, the space where the body is burned, and the kind of heat (fire vs. radiant

Burnt Human Remains: Recovery, Analysis, and Interpretation, First Edition. Edited by Sarah Ellingham, Joe Adserias-Garriga, Sara C. Zapico and Douglas H. Ubelaker.

heat) will play a significant role in the burning process and its effects on the body (Fairgrieve, 2008). All these factors will impact on the condition of the remains, and they will dictate the severity of the alterations in the skeletal elements.

The changes due to heat exposure in the soft and hard tissues occur in a regular fashion, that is, the succession of alterations in the tissues by the fire exposure will present the same order of appearance throughout the burning process. Therefore, the expert's analysis of the conditions of the remains can offer an insight into the burning process that took place on the remains.

This chapter focuses on the changes in the skeletal elements, considering the burning alterations of the soft tissues, and the information that can be obtained from the observation of burnt remains according to their conditions after the fire exposure.

7.1 Assessment of the Severity of the Thermal Damage in the Forensic Context

Different classifications have been proposed to describe the severity of the burning. Their usefulness depends on the context and the role of the professionals that are assessing the burning.

In the clinical context, the classifications of the thermal injuries are based on the depth and the extent of the burning. The classification of burns in degrees, according to their depth, was first introduced in 1634 by Guilhelmus Fabricius Hidanus (Lee *et al.*, 2014), who divided the burn injuries in three degrees. The first degree consisted of erythema and blisters with colorless fluid, the second degree consisted of erythema and blisters with yellow colored fluid, and the third degree consisted in dry dark skin and lack of pain. Fabricius' classification has been modified since then and nowadays the three degrees of burning are divided into: I degree, which consists of erythema, where the epidermis is the only layer affected; IIa degree consists of erythema and blisters, where the epidermis and the most superficial layer of the dermis (papillary dermis) are affected; IIb degree consists of a dry, white appearance of the skin with the loss of epidermal appendages, where the depth of the injury extends to the deeper layer of the dermis (reticular dermis); and III degree consists of a dry leathery consistency of the skin, where epidermis, dermis, and the subcutaneous fat layer of deeper muscle and even bone may be affected (Evers *et al.*, 2010; Lee *et al.*, 2014). While this classification is widely used in the clinical context, it has a very limited use (if any) in the role of treatment required for the patient in the forensic context of fatal fires.

The classification of the thermal injuries according to the extent of the body areas affected corresponds to Wallace's Rule of Nine, where the total body surface area is divided in different body areas: head (9%), anterior and posterior chest (9% each), anterior and posterior abdomen (9% each), upper limb (9% each), anterior and posterior lower limb (9% each), and groin and genitalia (1%)

(Moore *et al.*, 2021). Wallace's Rule of Nine was developed in the clinical contexts, offering a quick assessment of the percentage of the body surface that is burned, assisting in the treatment selection and the prognosis of the patient. Additionally, it is used by the forensic pathologists in the medicolegal context to describe the extent of the thermal injuries in fatal cases.

Subsequently, Eckert's classification was developed to be used in forensic contexts, distinguishing four stages of burning as: *charred*, where internal organs are still preserved; *partial*, where soft tissue is still preserved; *incomplete*, where bone fragments are present; and *complete*, where no distinguishable bone fragments are present (Eckert *et al.*, 1988). Even though this classification was created with the aim of its use in forensic cases, its use is limited nowadays.

The Crow-Glassman Scale was developed as a tool for medical examiners and coroners to get a broad description of the conditions of the bodies in the fire scene. The scale distinguishes five levels of severity. Level 1 is characterized by the presence of blisters and the body has a smoke death appearance, being identifiable by visual recognition. At level 2 the remains are charred. Level 3 represents severe damage in the upper and lower limbs, that can be disarticulated. Severe damage in the skull and small portions of the limbs may be present in level 4. The remains in level 5 of the scale are very fragmentary and there is little or no soft tissue present, making the identifications highly difficult (Glassman and Crow, 1996). Even though the Crow-Glassman Scale does not represent the early stages of burning, it may be of use for managing the scene and the first responders; however, it is of little use in the forensic analysis of the remains by the forensic anthropologists.

In the need of an accurate system to classify the burnt remains in the forensic context that represents the different stages of thermal damage in fatal fire cases, Williams created a scoring model that assesses the different body regions independently (head and neck, trunk, limbs, and hands and feet). This model provides a more realistic and objective classification of burnt bodies that is useful to describe the remains at the scene and for their assessment in the lab (see Chapter 5).

7.2 Soft Tissue Alterations by Fire Exposure

The skin is the largest organ in the human body, covering its entire external surface. Thus, generally, it is the first part of the body to be exposed to heat in the burning process.

The skin consists of three layers of tissue: the epidermis, the dermis, and the subcutaneous tissue, and the thickness of each one varies depending on the body region. The epidermis is the outer, thin, keratinized, and avascular layer of the skin; the adjacent dermis contains blood and lymphatic vessel; and the deepest layer is the subcutaneous tissue (or subcutis), which is highly vascularized and contains adipocytes, highly specialized mesenchymal cells turned into a storage site for fat (Sterry *et al.*, 2006).

The first response of the superficial body tissues to heat exposure is the dilation of the dermal blood vessels. As the heat exposure continues, the circulation in the affected areas ceases and blisters appear that may lead to skin slippage, resulting in the separation of the epidermis from the dermis. As the skin burns, hair is also affected. As the time and temperature of exposure increases, hair experiences alterations, starting with singeing, charring to keratin melting, and complete consumption (Fairgrieve, 2008).

As the heat exposure progresses, the high level of dehydration causes the contraction of the outer layers of the skin, and as a consequence heat ruptures will appear, where the skin will split into what resemble (and should not be confused with) incised wounds (Dolinak *et al.*, 2005). Heat ruptures and the loss of tissue lead to the subcutis exposure and its fat content acts as a fuel, causing an increase in temperature. When this occurs in the thorax area, the internal organs are exposed.

As the fire exposure progresses, the muscles, tendons, and ligaments underlying the subcutaneous tissue shrink and contract, and the body will adopt the pugilistic pose as a result of the overriding effect of the most powerful muscles, tendons, and ligaments. The body in the pugilistic pose shows hyperextension of neck and back, adduction of the shoulders, arms raised above the shoulders with the fingers curled almost in a fist, intense flexion of knees, abduction of the thighs, plantar flexion of the feet, with the toes curled (Fairgrieve, 2008; Symes *et al.*, 2015).

When the body acquires the pugilistic pose during the burning process, some structures are more exposed to the fire flame, such as the forehead and facial structures, the dorsal surface of the hands or the anterior part of the knees; whilst others are more protected from the fire exposure, such as the palmar surface of the hands or the posterior part of the knees.

Symes *et al.* (2008) established a predictable pattern of burning based on the areas that are more exposed and the areas that are more protected from the fire exposure when the body achieves the pugilistic pose. According to this, the superior and anterior part of the neurocranium, the facial structures, sternum, the dorsal surface of the hands, and the anterior part of the knees are the more severely burnt areas in the body, while the anterior part of the vertebrae and sacrum, and the palmar surface of the hands are the less affected areas. Modifications of this pattern should be further investigated, combining the information from the scene with the lab examination of the remains.

7.3 Bone Alteration by Fire Exposure

Bones exposed to fire alter in color, shape, and volume, and fragmentation appears in the skeletal elements. These alterations occur because of changes on the physical and chemical properties that bone experiences when it is exposed to fire (Imaizumi, 2015). As previously mentioned in this chapter, the higher the temperatures and the longer the duration of fire exposure, the more drastic these changes appear.

The understanding of bone structure and composition is key to recognizing the physical and chemical changes that bone will undergo throughout the burning process. In vivo, bone is a dynamic living tissue in constant activity of remodeling and reparation as a response to stress and injury (DeHaan, 2015; Symes *et al.*, 2015). Bone structure is a composite consisting of an organic component (primarily collagen) that is stiffened by a dense inorganic component (primarily hydroxyapatite). While the organic component gives bone elasticity and flexibility, the inorganic component gives bone hardness and rigidity (White *et al.*, 2012; Symes *et al.*, 2015).

When bone is exposed to heat, the organic components suffer evaporation and degradation, and the inorganic components suffer elemental changes; all these alterations significantly impact the bone structure and its properties. The physical and chemical changes that bones undergo in the burning process become macroscopically evident in the gross changes that burnt skeletal remains exhibit. These changes include the aforementioned color alterations, heat-induced fractures, and dimensional changes.

Bone color changes by fire exposure: Bones exposed to fire experience changes in their coloration, progressing from brownish, black, gray-blue, and chalk white, depending on the intensity of the heat and the time of exposure.

Symes *et al.* (2015) proposed a categorization of the color change progression in the bone exposed to heat, defining four color-based categories: the heat line, the border, charring, and calcination.

The heat line is an occasionally occurring feature which is defined as the junction between the unburnt and burnt bone, which is the area of initial transition between the unaltered and heat-altered bone. The border is the area adjacent to the heat line that shows an off-white color; it represents an area protected from direct contact with the flame and it is easily distinguishable as it appears opaque when exposing the bone to backlighting, whereas the unaltered bone appears translucent (Symes *et al.*, 2015). Charred bone corresponds to the black color of carbonization, where some organic material can still be preserved; calcined bone is the chalk white colored bone that has lost all its organic content and moisture (Mayne Correia, 1997; Symes *et al.*, 2015). Calcined bone is extremely brittle and it is often reduced to small fragments (see Figure 7.1).

Heat-induced fractures in bone: Skeletal elements exposed to heat exhibit fractures that experts must recognize, and they should clearly differentiate them from other fractures caused by peri-mortem trauma such as sharp and blunt force trauma. Heat-induced fractures in bones are classified by their morphology, and they include (see Figure 7.2):

Longitudinal fractures are highly frequent heat-related fractures, shown in long bone diaphyses following the longitudinal axis of the skeletal element; they may extend to the bone marrow cavity. They follow a parallel path to the Haversian canals of the bone.

Transverse fractures are another type of highly frequent heat-related fractures, shown perpendicular to the longitudinal axis of the bone. The path of

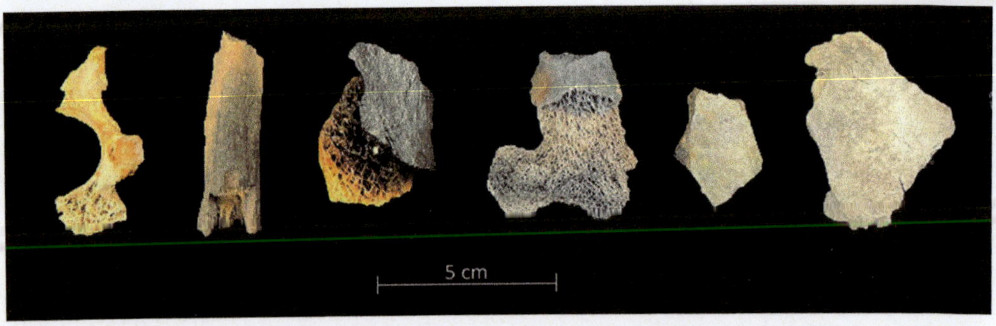

Figure 7.1 Bone color progression in the process of burning from brownish to black, gray and finally chalk white. Black coloration indicates charred and white indicates calcined bone material (Mercyhurst skeletal collection).

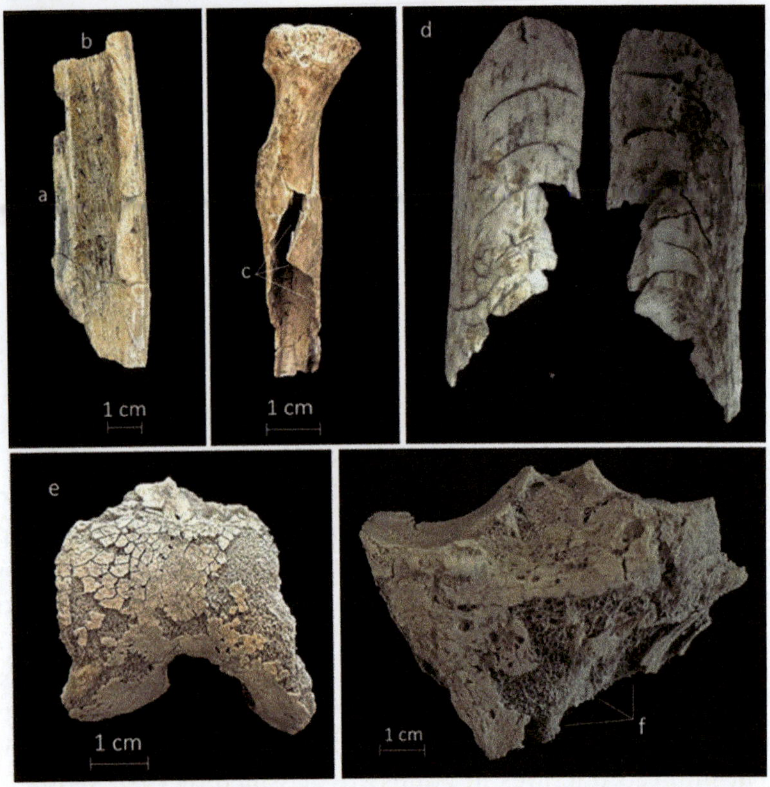

Figure 7.2 Heat-induced fractures in bone. Longitudinal fractures (a) and transversal (b) fractures in a long bone, step fractures in the radius diaphysis (c), curve-transverse fractures in a long bone (d), patina fractures (e) in the articular surface of the distal end of the femur, delamination is noted exposing the trabecular bone (e and f) (Joe Adserias-Garriga research and Mercyhurst skeletal collection).

these fractures transects the Haversian canals. They tend to extend through the marrow cavity, and they can produce a complete cross section of the bone.

Step fractures are created by two longitudinal fractures connected by a transversal fracture. That is, a longitudinal fracture connects in its margin with a transverse fracture, which intersects another longitudinal fracture.

Curve transverse fractures travel around the long bone diaphyses depicting an arch on the circumference of the bone shaft; it is extremely common to present several curve transverse fractures of concentric arches stacked on the diaphysis of the long bones. Fractures in concentric rings, typically shown in fossae, are considered as another form of curve transverse fractures (Symes et al., 2015).

Patina fractures consist of very superficial bone cracks that resemble the patina of an old painting or crazed china (Krogman, 1943). They are commonly seen in flat bones and in long bone epiphyses, especially in the articular surface.

Delamination is characterized by the splinting of the bone layers, resulting in the exposure of the inner layer. This type of fracture is commonly observed in the bones of the cranial vault, where the outer table is separated from the inner table, exposing the trabecular bone of the diploe.

Symes *et al.* (2015) also included the **burn line fractures** in the heat-induced fractures of bone, which occur at the level of the burn borderline, separating the burnt and unburnt parts of the bone.

Several authors have highlighted the role of soft tissue in the creation of patina, delamination, and curve transverse fractures. Krogman (1943) considered the presence of delamination and patina fractures as an indication of soft tissue presence at the time of burning. Symes *et al.* (2015) stated that curve transverse fractures were created by periosteum shrinkage, pulling at the surface of the bone weakened by the heat exposure and forming staked arched fractures on the bone surface. However, the exact production mechanism of these fractures needs further research.

Bone dimensional changes due to heat exposure: Bones experience warping, shrinkage, and deformation when exposed to heat. Bone undergoes four stages of transformation due to the effect of heat: dehydration, decomposition, inversion, and fusion. During the dehydration stage, bone weight is reduced because of water vaporization and the initial combustion of organic materials (Thompson, 2005; Imaizumi, 2015) that will continue in the decomposition stage, where color changes are evident and the bone presents a reduction of its mechanical strength. The inversion stage is characterized by the increase in the crystal size. Finally, in the fusion stage the bone hardens, increasing its mechanical strength due to the fusion of hydroxyapatite crystals (Thompson, 2005).

Bone shrinkage occurs through a combination of losing collagen, chemical changes, and recrystallization of the hydroxyapatite and the subsequent fusion of the crystals (Mayne Correia, 1997; Fairgrieve, 2008; Fredericks *et al.*, 2015). Heat-induced shrinkage of bone has been the topic of research by several authors (Herrmann, 1977; Thompson, 2005; Gonçalves, 2011). Heat-induced shrinkage is a dynamic process that commences during the burning and continues after the cooling down of the remains (Thompson, 2005).

The studies on heat-induced bone shrinkage have carried out the experiments under varied conditions, using human and non-human proxies, fire and radiant heat, and different range of temperatures and times of exposure. These studies have reported bone shrinkage from 1% up to 27% (Herrmann, 1977). The main interest of these studies is to quantify the degree of shrinkage that impairs the metric analysis on the remains. However, no definitive results have been obtained on the quantification of the overall bone volume reduction due to heat exposure; the difficulty in the quantification of the heat-induced shrinkage in bone is to precisely calculate its dimensions when cracks, wrapping, and fragmentation are present.

Shrinkage does not appear uniformly in all areas of the bone. Shrinkage in cortical and trabecular bone presents differently. But the amount of shrinkage shown by the cortical and trabecular bone is still in controversy. Some authors have stated a higher degree of cortical shrinkage in respect to trabecular bone (Gilchrist and Mytum, 1986) and some others have pointed out that trabecular bone experiences a higher degree of shrinking (McKinley, 1994; Fairgrieve, 2008). Therefore, further research is needed to determine the differences between the shrinking mechanisms.

As a result of all these limitations in accurately quantifying the shrinkage in bones exposed to fire, metric analyses should not be applied to burnt remains.

7.4 Teeth Alteration by Fire Exposure

Teeth, like skeletal elements, experience changes in color and dimensions, and show fractures due to heat exposure. However, the changes do not appear uniformly in the tooth structure (Schmidt, 2015); the differential content of organic and inorganic material in the different dental tissues causes them to act differently to the heat exposure. Therefore, the heat-induced changes will appear different in the enamel, cementum, dentine, and pulp.

Enamel is the most external, protective, white layer covering the crown. It consists of a very high percentage (95%) of inorganic, mineralized component (calcium hydroxyapatite) and the remaining 5% of its content corresponds to water and organic matter. Enamel composition makes it the hardest tissue in the human body, but it is also extremely brittle. Cementum is the dull, yellowish external layer covering the root. It is composed of 65% inorganic matter (calcium hydroxyapatite) and 35% water and organic matter, mostly collagen fibers. Cementum is as hard as bone and significantly softer than enamel. Dentin is the hard, yellowish layer underlying the enamel and cementum, which makes up the major bulk of the inner portion of each tooth crown and root. It is composed of 70% calcium hydroxyapatite, 18% organic matter, and 12% water, making it harder than cementum but softer and less brittle than enamel. The pulp cavity is the soft tissue in the cavity underlying the dentin of the crown and root. It has a coronal portion (pulp chamber) and a root portion (root canal). The pulp cavity contains nerves and blood vessels that nourish the tooth (Scheid and Weiss, 2012).

The organic and inorganic content of these dental tissues is one of the main factors to consider in the thermal related changes in the teeth, especially for dimensional changes and fracture pattern.

The dimensional changes in the teeth have been reported to be less intense than those observed in bone. On average, teeth may shrink up to 10–15% of their original dimensions. Enamel is the dental tissue least affected by shrinkage due to its higher levels of organic content (Shipman *et al.*, 1984).

Teeth can exhibit fractures caused by heat exposure, but have a different appearance to the fractures presented in bones. Additionally, the pattern, morphology, and type of heat-induced fractures on teeth differ in the crown and root.

Fractures observed in the root are basically transverse. The crowns tend to fracture along the cusp margins, which is the thinnest part of the enamel layer (Schmidt, 2015; Adserias-Garriga, 2016). Very frequently, fragments of the enamel separate from the inner layers of the tooth, caused by the dentine shrinkage and the brittle status of the enamel.

As mentioned, the different fracture pattern in crowns and roots is due to the differential organic and inorganic components of the enamel, cementum, and dentine.

Color changes in burnt teeth are similar of those presented on bone. The succession of color alteration in teeth starts with a brownish coloration, followed by black, blue-gray, and finally chalk white, that indicates teeth tissue calcination. At this stage water has evaporated, the organic content has been consumed, and only inorganic material is present (Schmidt, 2015). Heat-induced changes in teeth are shown in Figure 7.3.

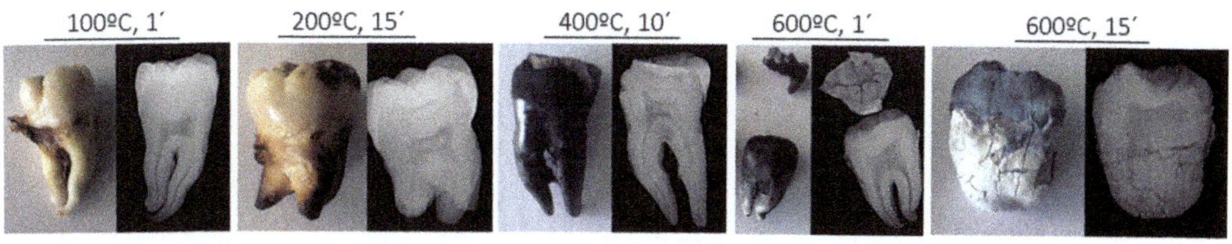

Figure 7.3 Heat-induced changes in teeth and the corresponding radiograph. Color progresses from brown to black (charred), gray and finally chalk white (calcined). Fractures start at the crown and lead to the enamel peel off; root fractures are noted later than those in the crown and basically consist of transversal fractures throughout the root. Fractures can be observed in the radiographs, showing the extension of them into the dental tissues (Joe Adserias-Garriga research).

7.5 Signature Changes in Skeletal Elements after Cremation

Commercial cremation is one of the most intense forms of fire exposure. The process consists of placing the body (within a coffin or carbon box) into the retort where the cremation takes place when a flame is initiated. The cremains resulting from this process are then collected from the retort by a scooping action and the bone fragments are finally pulverized to obtain the powder material commonly referred as ashes (see Figures 7.4 and 7.5).

Commercial cremation offers a realistic and accurate approach to the study of human remains. It allows observation of the gradual tissue changes that take place during the burning process under controlled conditions on human cadavers in direct contact with the fire flame.

The research project conducted by the author consisted in an observational study conducted in Spain including 50 human commercial cremations.

a b c

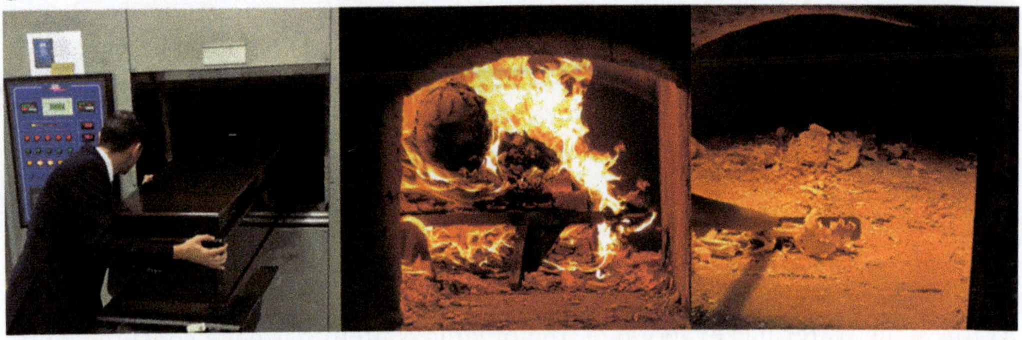

Figure 7.4 Process of commercial cremation: the body is introduced in the retort within the coffin (a), the fire flame is initiated and the body is burning in the retort for three hours (b), the cremains are collected by a scooping action (c) (Joe Adserias-Garriga research).

a b c

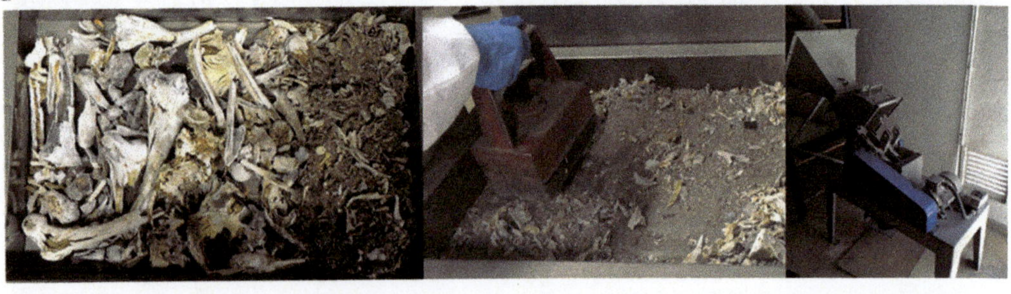

Figure 7.5 Process of commercial cremation (cont.): the cremains obtained from the retort (a), metal material is separated from the cremains by a magnet (b), finally, the cremains are pulverized in the grainer to obtain what is commonly referred to as ashes (c) (Joe Adserias-Garriga research).

The aim of this project was to observe and record the changes in the body (focusing on the skeletal tissues), and to explore how informative this severely burnt material is to reconstruct a biological profile and recognize skeletal signs of trauma and pathology (Adserias-Garriga, 2018).

All cadavers were in a fresh-discoloration stage of decomposition; 24 females and 26 males were included in this study, with the individual's age-at-death ranging from 38 to 95 years. The conditions of the cremation were the same for all the cremations observed: all bodies were placed in the same position in the retort and, the time and temperature of the fire source was the same for all cremations included in the study.

The retort used in this study exhibits one fire source located in the superior part of the cremation space. The bodies were positioned with cranial structures and torso close to the fire flame and the legs and feet in the other end of the retort space (see Figure 7.6). It must be noted that the bodies were placed into the retort within wooden coffins. The fire flame had a constant temperature of 600–700°C, and the maximum temperatures achieved in the retort space ranged 700–1000°C. The time of fire exposure was three hours for all cremations (Adserias-Garriga, 2018).

The pre-cremation examination consisted of recording the individual´s sex, age, ancestry, constitution, cause of death, the presence of amputation or other visible ante-mortem trauma, autopsy performance, shroud or clothes worn, and any other objects included with the body in the cremation retort; additionally, a dental inventory was filled out, including teeth present and absent, dental restorations, crowns and bridges, partial or complete dentures, and dental implants.

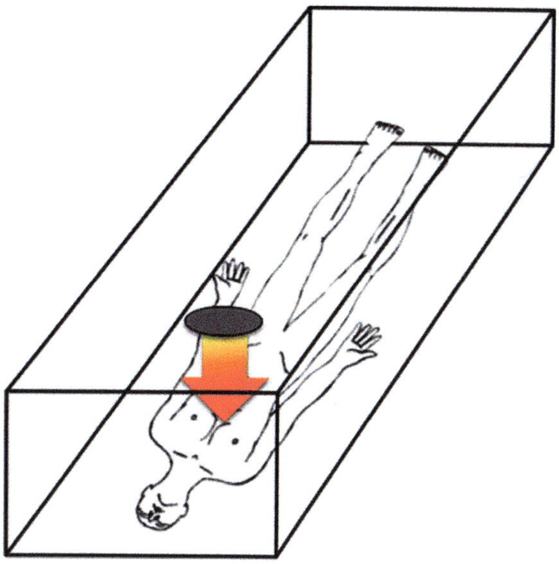

Figure 7.6 Position of the body into the cremation retort, the fire source is indicated with the orange arrow.

The post-cremation observation consisted of recording the coloration, fractures due to fire exposure, deformation or warping, and degree of preservation, which was visually assessed and used to classify the different skeletal elements in less than 25%, between 25 and 50%, between 50 and 75%, and over 75% of the element preserved and distinguishable. Additionally, skeletal indicators of biological profile, trauma, and pathological signs in the cremains were noted, as well as the presence of surgical devices and dental appliances.

The signature findings in color, preservation, fractures, and deformation are discussed according to anatomical regions:

Signature findings after cremation in the skull: The color observed in the cranial remains was mostly chalk white, indicating calcination. In some cases, severely burnt brain tissue fragments were still present, associated with the internal table of the cranium.

Cranial bones fractured often at the sutures, also fracture lines across the bones and patina fractures were observed.

The neurocranium (bones corresponding to the cranial vault) and the viscerocranium, especially bones corresponding to midfacial structures, responded very differently to cremation. The neurocranium presented high preservation and high deformation, while the facial bones presented poor preservation, but deformation was very low in those preserved structures. The high deformation of the neurocranium occurred due to the separation of the outer and the inner layers of the cranial bones exposing the diploe, this phenomenon was observed during the cremation process (see Figure 7.7).

Maxilla and mandible showed an interesting behavior when cremated. Both structures presented a low degree of deformation. With regards to preservation, they showed low preservation in edentulous individuals and high preservation when teeth or dental implants where present in the oral cavity. Thus, the presence

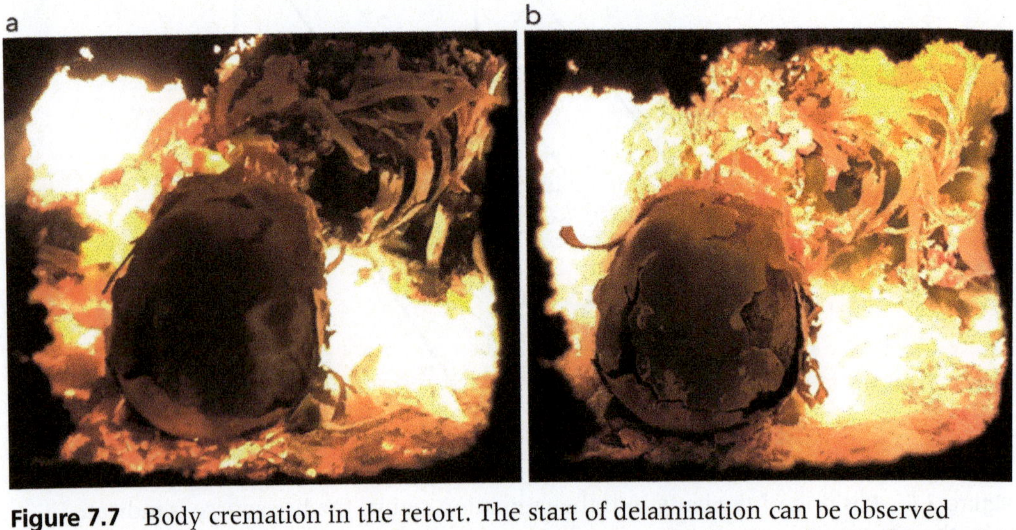

Figure 7.7 Body cremation in the retort. The start of delamination can be observed during the cremation process (a), as cremation progresses the inner and outer layers of the cranium separate and the outer layer curls (b) (Joe Adserias-Garriga research).

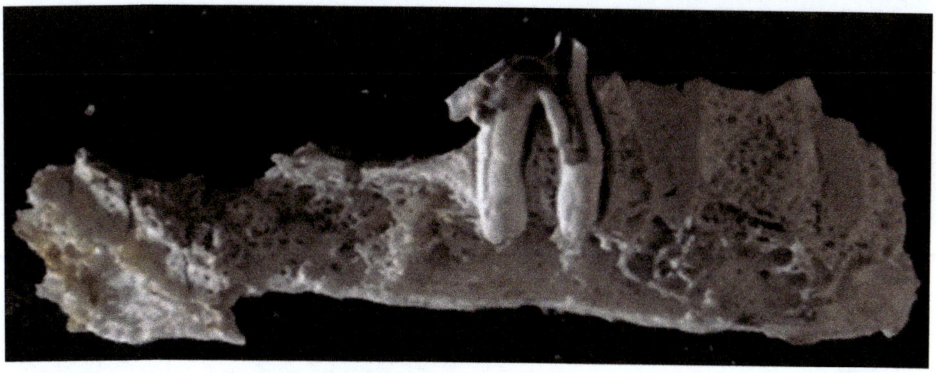

Figure 7.8 Mandible fragment preserving the first molar still in the alveolus, the crown is highly fragmentary and separated from the roots (Joe Adserias-Garriga research).

of teeth (or dental implants) offers a higher resilience of these bones when exposed to fire (see Figure 7.8) (Adserias-Garriga, 2016).

Signature findings after cremation in teeth: Teeth presented chalk white coloration throughout, with some teeth presenting gray areas that corresponded in most cases to the most internal structures surrounding the pulp cavity.

Crowns were in all cases separated from the roots and enamel was very rarely identifiable. Roots were very well preserved. Multirooted teeth roots can fracture near the furcation; however, it is possible to identify the root corresponding to a multirooted tooth by the presence of part of the furcation.

As mentioned above, crowns presented a great fragmentation. Root fractures were mostly transversal fractures, with some vertical fracture lines present, connecting two or more transversal fractures. Most of the time, roots were no longer in their alveolar sockets, and the few cases in which roots were still in the alveoli, corresponded to mandibular molars (see Figure 7.8).

With regards to preservation, all teeth were represented by their roots and crown fragments were present in some cases separated from the roots. No deformation was noted in teeth.

Signature findings after cremation in the thorax and midline structures: Hyoid, sternum, and clavicle showed white coloration throughout. All three skeletal elements showed very low preservation but no deformation. Scapulae presented higher preservation and unlike the other structures, showed high deformation. These low degrees of preservation, especially in clavicle and sternum are the consequence of the body position in the retort with respect the fire source. All these structures were the closest to the fire flame source in the retort where these observations took place. It must be stated that other retorts can present more than one source of fire located in different sites in the cremation space (see Figure 7.6).

Ribs presented white coloration in their external surfaces and light brown coloration could be observed in the inner parts of the rib, where fractures caused trabecular exposure. The fractures observed were mostly transversal (which caused

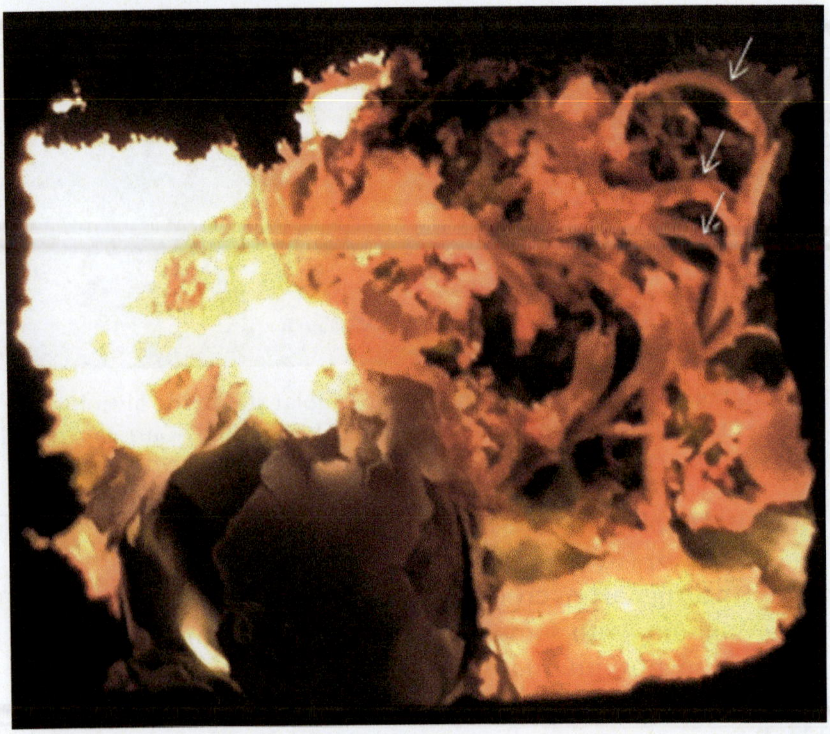

Figure 7.9 Rib fragmentation and deformation (indicated with white arrows) during the cremation process (Joe Adserias-Garriga research).

fragmentation in most of the cases) and longitudinal. High preservation was observed, although high fragmentation and deformation was present (see Figure 7.9).

Vertebrae presented chalk white and very light brown coloration, especially in the trabecular bone exposed. Pedicle fractures were very often observed, causing the separation of the spinous process from the vertebral body. Longitudinal fractures appeared in the spinous process, and patina fractures were noted in the superior and inferior surfaces of the vertebral bodies, as well as in the articular facets. Vertebrae presented high preservation of their structures and very little deformation was noted.

The sacrum presented a similar behavior to vertebrae. White and light brown coloration was noted. Patina fractures were noted in the superior surface of the first sacral element. High preservation, but less fragmentation than vertebrae was present. It must be stated that the posterior part of the sacrum is in contact with the inferior surface of the retort space and in its anterior part it is covered by a significant thick layer of soft tissues (muscle, fat, and internal organs). Therefore, the sacrum is protected by other structures in the process of cremation (see Figure 7.10).

Signature findings after cremation in upper and lower limbs: Upper and lower limb skeletal elements presented chalk white and some sites with light brown coloration, especially in the trabecular bone exposed after fragmentation. This light brown coloration very possibly indicates the most recent fractures and

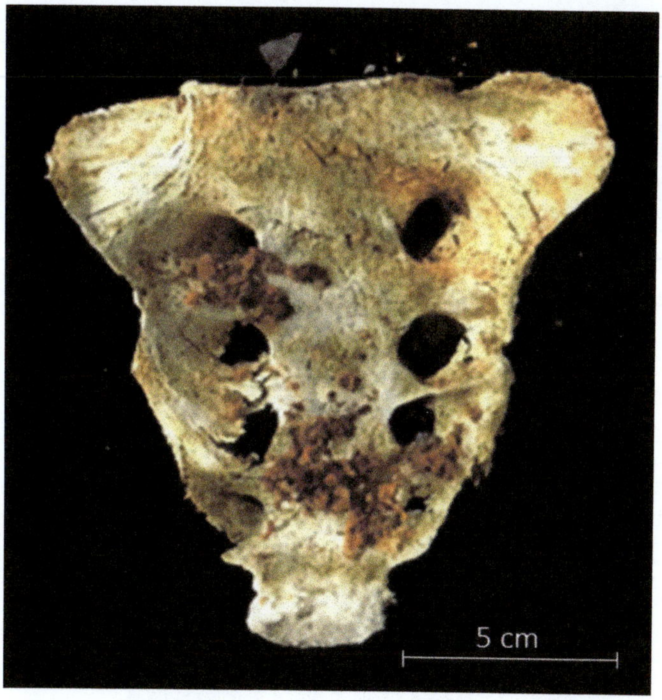

Figure 7.10 Sacrum recovered after the cremation process. Brown matter on the anterior surface corresponds to burnt soft tissue remains (Joe Adserias-Garriga research).

fragmentation sites of the bone, some of them caused by the collection of the remains from the retort.

Long bones resented their epiphyses being separated from the diaphyses. Longitudinal, transversal, step, and curved-transverse fractures were noted in the diaphyses; whilst delamination and patina were observed in the epiphyses.

Curved-transverse fractures have been related to the effect of the superficial cortical bone shrinkage at the same time as the incineration of the soft tissues. However, these hypotheses have not been categorically demonstrated yet. Thus, further research should be invested in determining the role of the soft tissue and the impact of the bone shape in the appearance of curve-transverse fractures.

Delamination was very often found in the femur neck; patina fractures were almost always found in the articulation surfaces of the long bones, as well as on the articular surfaces of the carpal and tarsal elements These articular surfaces are covered by cartilage, which very possibly has a role in their appearance.

Both epiphyses and diaphyses presented high preservation, although diaphyses showed more fragmentation than epiphysis. No deformation was noted in the epiphyses and some was noted in the diaphyses (see Figure 7.11).

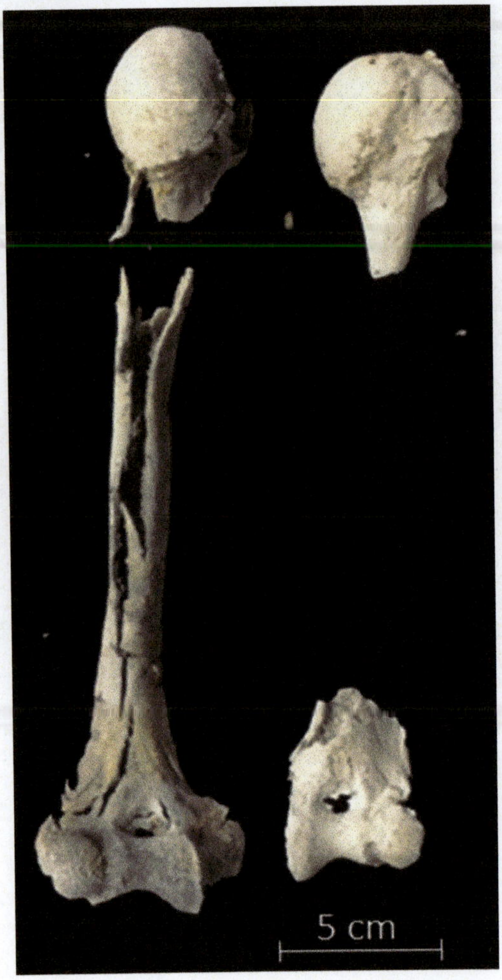

Figure 7.11 Humeri recovered after the cremation process. Calcination is noted throughout, both proximal epiphyses are separated from the diaphyses. Longitudinal fractures are present in the diaphysis, patina fractures are shown in articular surfaces (Joe Adserias-Garriga research).

Biological profile information obtained from the cremains: Informative structures for the reconstruction of the biological profile were preserved and could be used for sex and age assessment.

Fragments of the os coxa and cranial structures such as the mastoid process or the nuchal crest were useful for sex estimation.

Regarding age, dentition was a key element used to classify the individual into adult or juvenile age groups. Vertebral osteophytes or syndesmophytes and bone lipping were indicators of older ages (Adserias-Garriga, 2016, 2018).

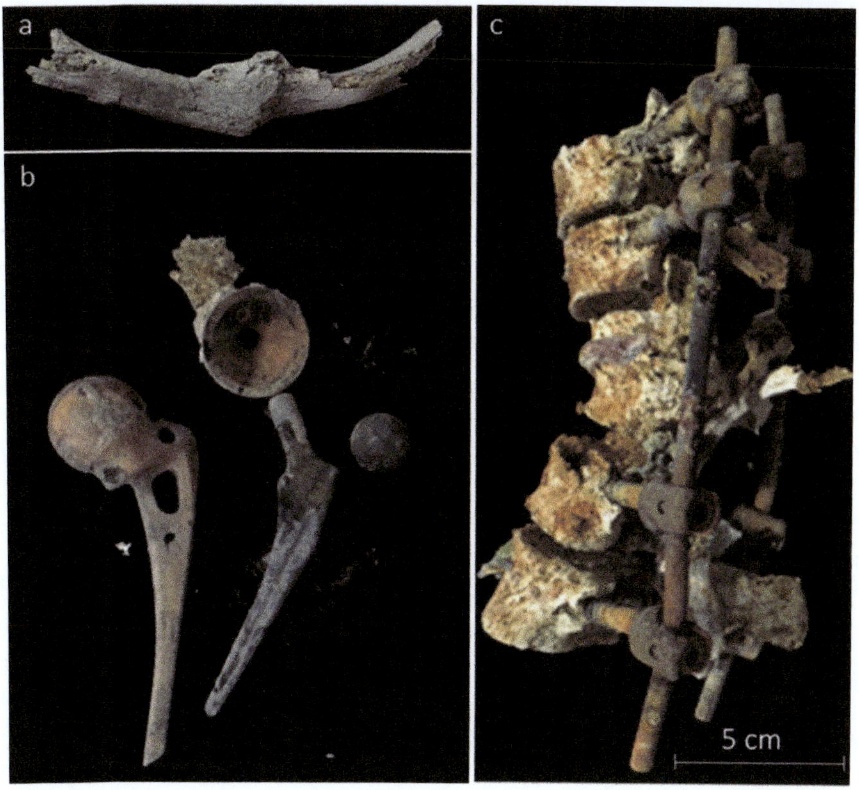

Figure 7.12 Post-cremation findings: Healed fracture in a rib fragment (a), femoral head prosthesis (b), spinal fixation surgical device (c) (Joe Adserias-Garriga research).

Pathology and trauma signs in the cremains: Pathological signs in the cremains were noted in the form of bone lipping, vertebral osteophytes and syndesmophytes, fusion of skeletal elements, as well as the presence of medical devices, such as pacemaker leads (the pulse generator is removed prior to cremation by general protocol, due to the presence of the battery).

Signs of ante-mortem trauma were observed in the form of healed fractures, where a callus could be identified and the presence of surgical devices used to reduce the bone fractures (see Figure 7.12). Ceramic and metal-ceramic dental crowns were intact in their recovery after cremation. Partial dentures were identified by the preservation of their metallic parts, while the resin parts were destroyed by the fire, as were resin complete dentures. All these findings could be of significant assistance in the identification process of the remains.

7.6 Conclusions

The management of fatal fire cases requires an understanding of the burning process and its effects on the anatomical structures, including the soft and hard tissues.

Forensic professionals involved in the recovery and analysis of remains exposed to fire should identify the changes in color and dimension, as well as the heat-induced fractures, and distinguish them from other sources of alteration such as trauma.

Identification and trauma analysis are the main goals in burnt remains investigations. The heat-induced alterations impact on the recovery and analysis of the remains. So fatal fire cases represent a challenging context for forensic scientists.

The amount of information that can be retrieved from burnt remains analysis is indirectly proportional to the severity of burning. That is, the more severely burned the remains are, the more drastic the heat-induced changes are, and the less information can be obtained from the remains analysis.

Commercial cremation represents a very intense body exposure to fire at high temperatures and for a significant amount of time. Therefore the remains resulting from the cremation process show drastic changes from the fire exposure and thus represent an excellent model to observe the fire-induced alterations in the skeletal elements.

The project conducted by the author, consisted of the observational analysis of 50 commercial cremations, with the aim of recording the changes in the cremains and exploring the amount of information that could be obtained from them.

The overall skeletal changes observed after commercial cremation show that the body follows the model of burning pattern proposed by Symes *et al.* (2008). The pugilistic pose could be observed in the cremation observations after most of the coffin was burned in the retort. Bone and teeth color changes are similar, although dimensional changes and heat-induced fracture appearance are different in bones and teeth.

Future research is needed on burnt remains, especially to achieve a better understanding of the mechanism of the generation of certain heat-induced fractures and the dimensional changes (shrinkage and deformation) of bones and teeth exposed to fire.

References

Adserias-Garriga, J. (2016) Fire and teeth. Oral Presentation at the 68th American Academy Forensic Science Annual Meeting, Las Vegas.

Adserias-Garriga, J. (2018) Forensic analysis of incinerated bones and teeth. Some like it hot: Forensic analysis of Burnt Human Remains (Workshop W11) presented at the 70th American Academy of Forensic Sciences Annual Meeting, Seattle.

Bennett, J.L. and Benedix, D.C. (1999) Positive identification of cremains recovered from an automobile based on presence of an internal fixation device. *Journal of Forensic Sciences*, **44**(6), 1296–1298.

DeHaan, J.D. (2015) Fire and bodies. In: *The Analysis of Burned Human Remains*, 2nd edn (eds. C.W. Schmidt and S.A. Symes). Elsevier, Amsterdam, pp. 1–15.

Dolinak, D., Matshes, E., and Lew, E.O. (2005) Environmental injury. In: *Forensic Pathology: Principles and Practice*, 1st edn (eds. D. Dolinak, E. Matshes, and E.O. Lew). Academic Press, Amsterdam and Boston, MA, pp. 240–241.

Eckert, W.G., James, S., and Katchis, S. (1988) Investigation of cremations and severely burned bodies. *American Journal of Forensic Medicine and Pathology*, **18**, 163–173.

Evers, L.H., Bhavsar, D., and Mailänder, P. (September 2010) The biology of burn injury. *Experimental Dermatology*, **19**(9), 777–783. https://doi.org/10.1111/j.1600-0625.2010.01105.x. PMID: 20629737.

Fairgrieve, S. (2008) *Forensic Cremation Recovery and Analysis*. CRC Press, Boca Raton, FL, pp. 37–60.

Fanton, L., Jdeed, K., Tilhet-Coartet, S., and Malicier, D. (2006) Criminal burning. *Forensic Science International*, **158**, 87–93.

Fredericks, J.D., Ringrose, T.J., Dicken, A., Williams, A., and Bennett, P. (2015) A potential new diagnostic tool to aid DNA analysis from heat compromised bone using colorimetry: A preliminary study. *Science & Justice*, **55**, 124–130.

Gilchrist, M. and Mytum, H. (1986) Experimental archaeology and burnt animal bone from archaeological sites. *Circaea*, **4**, 29–38.

Glassman, D.M. and Crow, R.M. (1996) Standardization model for describing the extent of burn injury to human remains. *Journal of Forensic Sciences*, **41**(1), 152–154.

Gonçalves, D. (2011) The reliability of osteometric techniques for the sex determination of burned human skeletal remains. *Homo*, **62**, 351–358.

Herrmann, B. (1977) On histological investigations of cremated human remains. *Journal of Human Evolution*, **6**, 101–103.

Imaizumi, K. (2015) Forensic investigation of burnt human remains. *Research and Reports in Forensic Medical Science*, **5**, 67–74.

Krogman, W.M. (1943) Role of the physical anthropologist in the identification of human skeletal remains, Part I. *FBI Law Enforcement Bulletin*, **12**(4), 17–40.

Lee, K.C., Joory, K., and Moiemen, N.S. (2014) History of burns: The past, present and the future. *Burn Trauma*, **2**, 169–180. https://doi.org/10.4103/2321-3868.143620.

Mayne Correia, P.M. (1997) Fire modification of bone: A review of the literature. In: *Forensic Taphonomy: The Postmortem Fate of Human Remains* (eds. W.D. Haglund and M.H. Sorg). CRC Press, Boca Raton, FL, pp. 275–293.

McKinley, J.I. (1994) *The Anglo-Saxon Cemetery at Spong Hill, North Elmham Part VIII: The Cremations*. East Anglian Archaeology Report No. 69, Norfolk Archaeological Unit, Dereham UK.

Moore, R.A., Waheed, A., and Burns, B. (2021) Rule of Nines. In: *StatPearls* (Internet). StatPearls Publishing, Treasure Island, FL. PMID: 30020659.

Mundorff, A.Z. (2008) Anthropologist-directed triage: Three distinct mass fatality events involving fragmentation of human remains. In: *Recovery, Analysis, and Identification of Commingled Human Remains* (eds. B.J. Adams and J.E. Byrd). Humana Press, Totowa, NJ, pp. 123–144.

Scheid, R.C. and Weiss, G. (2012) *Woelfel's Dental Anatomy*, 8th edn. Wolters Kluwer/Lippincott Williams & Wilkins Health, Philadelphia, PA, pp. 11–14.

Schmidt, C.W. (2015) Burnt human teeth. In: *The Analysis of Burned Human Remains*, 2nd edn (eds. C.W. Schmidt and S.A. Symes). Elsevier, Cambridge, MA, pp. 61–81. ISBN 9780128004517.

Shipman, P., Foster, G., and Schoeninger, M. (1984) Burnt bones and teeth: An experimental study of color, morphology, crystal structure and shrinkage. *Journal of Archaeological Science*, **11**, 307–325.

Sterry, W., Paus, R., and Burgdorf, W. (2006) *Dermatology. Thieme Clinical Companions*. Georg Thieme Verlag, Stuttgart, pp. 1–11.

Symes, S.A., Rainwater, C.W., Chapman, E.N., Gipson, D.R., and Piper, A.L. (2008) Patterned thermal destruction in a forensic setting. In: *The Analysis of Burned Human Remains*, 1st edn (eds. C.W. Schmidt and S.A. Symes). Elsevier, Cambridge, MA, pp. 32–33.

Symes, S.A., Rainwater, C.W., Chapman, E.N., Gipson, D.R., and Piper, A.L. (2015) Patterned thermal destruction in a forensic setting. In: *The Analysis of Burned Human Remains*, 2nd edn (eds. C.W. Schmidt and S.A. Symes). Elsevier, Cambridge, MA, pp. 17–59.

Thompson, T.J.U. (2005) Heat-induced dimensional changes in bone and their consequences for forensic anthropology. *Journal of Forensic Sciences*, **50**(5), 1008–1015. 28.

White, T.D., Black, M.T., and Folkens, P.A. (2012) Bone biology and variation. In. *Human Osteology*, 3rd edn (eds. T.D. White, M.T. Black, and P.A. Folkens). Academic Press, Cambridge, MA, pp. 25–42.

CHAPTER 8

Challenges of Biological Profile Estimation from Burnt Remains

Tim J.U. Thompson, PhD

Dean of School of Health and Life Sciences, Professor of Applied Biological Anthropology, Teesside University

Contexts of death involving the burning of human remains are some of the most challenging for any forensic practitioner to work in. The complexity of the changes that occur to the body because of exposure to fire, combined with the variety of situations in which burnt remains can be found, can be overwhelming for investigative teams. The fact that these continue to be such challenging contexts in which to work, despite having evidence of bodies being burned stretching back thousands of years, is perhaps surprising. Burning then, is a common occurrence.

However, the volume of research activity on this subject has in no way matched the volume of burnt bodies recovered. This is an interesting conundrum and is significant since this lack of engagement with burnt remains over time has implications for modern forensic practice. Historically there has been little interest in studying burnt remains because the perceived understanding was that little information could be gleaned. This is now known not to be true, but even today it can be difficult to convince some forensic and archaeological workers that burnt remains have much to offer an investigation. To some extent this is understandable to those with no experience of this material, since at first sight a burnt and fragmented body can seem destroyed.

Invariably when analyzing burnt human remains, the question of identity emerges. With inhumed or non-burnt forensic casework, the identity of the deceased can be determined using standard identification methods, including the creation of a biological profile if the body is considerably decomposed. Yet the very nature of the heat-induced change we see on the body because of burning will impact every method of identification available to us – both in terms of whether they can be applied to the body and about the accuracy of the output. Thompson (2004) articulated this clearly and little has changed since.

Burnt Human Remains: Recovery, Analysis, and Interpretation, First Edition. Edited by Sarah Ellingham, Joe Adserias-Garriga, Sara C. Zapico and Douglas H. Ubelaker.

8.1 Why Does Burning Affect Methods of Identification?

The key starting point for any forensic investigator to understand is why burning contexts create such difficulties for human identification. Initially this is very simple to answer: burning causes substantial change to the body, and these changes impact standard methods of biological profile estimation. Yet the reality is that these changes are both extreme and subtle, multifactorial, can be simultaneous and progressive, and affect the organic and inorganic component of the hard tissues differently but relatedly.

Heat-induced changes occur first and most intensely closest to the source of the heat. In this regard, it is the skin and soft tissues that are first affected. Burning causes these tissues to dehydrate and contract, causing splitting. This occurs throughout all the soft tissues and recent work has shown that heat will even distort and change coronary artery dimensions and associated luminal diameters in victims (Živković *et al.*, 2020). All these initial changes eventually result in the exposure of the underlying tissues and organs which then go through the same progressive changes. Eventually the shrinkage becomes so extensive that the organs are fully destroyed, and the skeleton is revealed. Bone also undergoes significant change, particularly the loss of organic material and changes to the microstructure of the inorganic material. Numerous publications have described and discussed this change before, for example Schmidt and Symes (2008), Thompson (2015), and Thompson *et al.* (2017) and the reader is directed to these publications for further detail.

Although the full nature of heat-induced skeletal change will not be repeated here, an example will be provided to demonstrate the impact that such changes can have. Heat-induced fragmentation of the skeleton results in multiple challenges for creating biological profiles. For example, anthropological methods are more challenging to apply on small pieces of bone, small bone fragments are harder to recover from the scene, meaning that complete skeletons are less likely to be analyzed, the calculation of MNI is harder, and understanding the taphonomic pathways of the deceased is harder since it can be difficult to know at what point during the context of death, burning, and diagenesis the fragmentation occurred. Archaeological studies and modern forensic case work (such as those by Röst (2017) in Sweden, Godinho *et al.* (2019a) in Portugal, or Ubelaker (2017) in the USA) highlight all of these complexities and the compromises that must be made in the analyses as a result.

One thing which is often forgotten when examining the hard tissues is that there is a very close and intimate relationship between the soft and the hard tissues. In the early stages of the fire and at lower intensities, the soft tissues will act as a buffer, protecting the hard tissues from the effects of the heat. However, as the intensity of the fire increases, the soft tissues become a form of fuel, and therefore damage to the bone can be exacerbated (Ellingham *et al.*, 2015). The reverse is also true, whereby the hard tissues can protect and preserve significant soft tissue structures such as the soft tissues of the oral cavity, which is of interest during forensic pathological investigations of fire-related deaths (Bianchi *et al.*, 2019). Further and at a smaller scale, the collagen bound inside the bones can be preserved. Gonçalves *et al.* (2011) demonstrated the effect of remnants of this soft tissue on the condition of burnt bone, while recent work studying the fate of those who died in Herculaneum following the AD 79 eruption of Vesuvius demonstrated the importance of this close relationship after it was noted that collagen had survived likely as a result of body density in confined spaces (Martyn *et al.*, 2020).

8.2 How Does the Context of Burning Impede the Creation of Biological Profiles?

It is not just the isolated changes to the body that create challenges for human identification, it is the combination of these changes within a complex environmental context. Human remains can become burned in a wide range of situations, the nature of which can also be a key factor in the temperature of the fire, oxygen supply, duration of burning, and the fragmentation of the body. These extrinsic conditions will have an impact on the degree of heat-induced transformation that the skeleton undergoes, and therefore the extent to which such transformations affect methods of identification. Death by fire also has a strong relationship with socio-economic status, with most deaths occurring in low- and middle-income countries (Nayak *et al.*, 2020), creating further challenges due to physical geography and access to forensic facilities.

Burning can also be used as part of a homicide, either as a form of murder or to hide incriminating evidence. Kaur and Byard (2020) give the example of "bride burning" in India. They note that fire is the most common method of so-called dowry deaths and that the female victims usually suffer between 40 and 80% burns, with over three-quarters of victims dying within 24 hours of the attack (Kaur and Byard, 2020). Fire can also be used to hide forensic evidence or to intentionally impede the forensic process. In these cases, accelerants can be used to fuel the fire, which in turn will increase the severity of heat-induced changes to the body. Coulombeix and Schuliar (2017) report just such a case from the Rhône-Alpes region of eastern France, although they concluded that the amount of accelerant used in this instance was not sufficient to completely destroy the bodies of the five victims. This intentional burning may also be accompanied by dismemberment, which increases the surface areas of the body and thus speeds up heat-induced changes.

Yet bodies can be burned in accidental settings too. Indeed, a recent retrospective study of unnatural deaths in Pretoria highlighted that almost 70% of thermal fatalities were accidental (Morobadi *et al.*, 2019). Bodies are routinely recovered from house fires and vehicular accidents. These provide challenges because the collapsing building or surrounding materials can cause additional damage and fragmentation to the remains. In these situations, the scale of the incident may also be a confounding factor regarding biological profiling (de Boer *et al.*, 2020). Further, the burning of materials and fuels, etc. can increase the temperature of the fire and thus the body. Bodies can be burned some time following death due to entirely unrelated factors, but the impact on human identification remains the same. Wegner *et al.* (2020) needed to analyze the remnants of the internal organs to ascertain that the fire occurred days after death, while Garrido-Varas and Intriago-Leiva (2015) used the presence of animal gnawing marks to evidence that burning had happened sometime after decomposition. In Greece, anthropologists used the presence of longitudinal fractures and a lack of warping to determine that decomposition occurred prior to burning (Monetti *et al.*, 2021). Mass fatality incidents can also be associated with highly burnt and fragmented remains which impede identification. For example, there is increasing interest in the recovery and identification of human remains following devastating wildfires (e.g. O'Donnell *et al.*, 2011; Migala and Brown, 2012; Gin *et al.*, 2020) because the speed and intensity of the fires can cause significant bodily damage. Traditional identification methods were only useful in around a quarter of the fatalities resulting from the November 2018 Butte County California wildfire, due to the intensity of the fire (Gin *et al.*, 2020).

There is also work to show that individuals have used fire to commit suicide and self-immolation, which can occur in different environments. Simonit *et al.* (2020) raise the issue of "complicated suicides" whereby the investigation of the original suicide attempt is compounded by additional accidental factors occurring following that suicide attempt. In their case from Italy, a man shot himself in his car, but the car subsequently caught fire destroying much of the evidence. Their challenge was to determine whether the fire was an intentional component of the suicide. The carboxyhemoglobin (COHb) levels in the blood suggested he was alive when the fire began, despite the self-inflicted gunshot wound to the head (Simonit *et al.*, 2020).

It is worth noting that, on occasion, there have been questions of identification after a body has been burned in a modern crematorium. Modern crematoria can heat a body to over 1000°C which will cause the loss of all soft tissues and substantial change to the hard tissues. The use of a cremulator to convert the remains into the more familiar ashes for the bereaved means that traditional methods of biological profiling are not possible. Instead, workers have resorted to the examination of the chemical composition of the powder. In cases with extremely fragmented or highly powdered remains, the analysis of elemental composition has been found to be very helpful for diagnosing conditions of burning and associated biological information (Ellingham *et al.*, 2017; Ubelaker, 2017). Interestingly, some legal systems require a mandatory second post-mortem examination prior to any cremation occurring, which would address these issues. This is just as well since research from Germany noted that 474 cases out of 9981 studied (4.7%) revealed that the first post-mortem had missed some pertinent forensic details (Behrens *et al.*, 2020).

Finally, cremation is also a means of managing large numbers of deceased, particularly when unclaimed or unidentified. It also has a role to play in the wider context of repatriation of the dead, something that Kgatle (2020) discusses in relation to the tensions it creates in the context of traditional funerary practice in Zimbabwe. Moore *et al.* (2020) also discuss the tensions that cremation can create, albeit this time from the perspective of managing large numbers of COVID-19 related dead, noting that the "US inhumane history of enslaved African and African American slaves, Ku Klux Klan cross burnings, burning down of Black homes, churches, and businesses, and the racist burning of Black bodies during the 1919 Red Summer and Jim Crow eras" has resulted in fewer cremations within the Black community compared to other groups. Such tensions surrounding COVID-19 deceased have been noted elsewhere, such as in the Philippines (Go and Doçot, 2021). Soto (2020) describes the use of cremation as part of the process of handling undocumented border crossers in the USA (in this case, at Terrace Park Cemetery, California). Here the cremated remains became part of a political discussion involving the recognition of the deceased as undocumented border crossers. Nonetheless, the challenge in all these examples will be how to undertake biological profile estimation of those who were unidentified yet subsequently cremated.

8.3 Challenges of Biological Profile Estimation of Burnt Remains

Once the human remains have been recovered from the specific burning context, the standard anthropological analysis can be attempted. For the purposes of this chapter, it will be considered that there are two main types of technique that can be used to create a biological profile: morphological and metric methods. Previous work has already explored the relationship between heat-induced changes and osteological methods, and the key conclusions are that heat-induced changes can introduce significant inaccuracies into the results of such methods, but that with patience and perseverance, anthropological methods of identification can nevertheless be performed on burnt skeletons.

8.3.1 Morphological Methods

Morphological methods are those that tend to rely on shape and form for their results. They include the classic approaches to sexual dimorphism and age estimation. Generally, they require the anthropologist to compare the skeletal feature on the body under investigation with a set of standards produced in previous research. They are often comparatively straightforward to apply, but recent discussion within forensic anthropology has highlighted the importance of practitioners' experience in both the application of the methods and the interpretation of the results (Nakhaeizadeh *et al.*, 2020).

As a group of methods, they have popularity with those studying burnt bone. This is because the shape or topographical feature of interest often survives the burning process. The bone may fragment, change color, or recrystallize, but the features can remain. Even shrinkage has a limited effect on these methods. Thus, the sexually dimorphic features of the pelvis and skull, or age-specific changes associated with the epiphyses are still observable. Sex estimation has been successful through the use of the sexually dimorphic regions of the pelvis and skull (e.g. in Piga *et al.*, 2020 or Silva, 2015). Typically, age estimation is performed using epiphyseal fusion or cranial suture closure (such as in Cataroche and Gowland, 2015; Bocquentin *et al.*, 2020; Piga *et al.*, 2020) and as such it can even be argued that age estimation using morphological methods can be applied to very young individuals. Research by Zana *et al.* (2017), for example, demonstrated that foetal bones can survive significant burning events, although bones such as the ethmoid, nasal bones, vomer, lachrymal, maxilla, and deciduous teeth germs do not. Piga *et al.* (2020) reported the use of the temporal bone and neural arches when identifying infant remains from an unusual double burial in Sardinia. Squires *et al.* (2011) combined morphological methods of sex and age estimation with a suite of more advanced analytical methods to explore the relationships between grave goods and demography in an Anglo-Saxon cemetery in England. The same context was later compared to an earlier Roman burial cemetery so that the conditions of burning could be compared and contrasted, including by age and sex as determined through morphological methods (Carroll and Squires, 2020). It is worth noting that although heat-induced changes themselves still allow for morphological methods to be applied, when the impact of external factors, as discussed above, are overlaid, this may be impossible. Price *et al.* (2018) in their archaeological study record high numbers of cremated remains in their Viking sites, yet with such poor preservation that age and sex simply could not be attempted with any real confidence.

On occasion, morphological approaches are required when burnt material must be identified as human or not, such as when they were applied to refute the claim that a set of bony material belonged to Joan of Arc (it was a cat; Charlier *et al.*, 2010). Further, although we often think of morphological methods being applied to broad anatomical surface features, they can also be applied on the microscopic scale. Kutterer *et al.* (2012) recovered small fragments of burnt bone from a Neolithic cave context in the United Arab Emirates. Since the pieces were so fragmented, they applied histological methods to study the shape of the bone microstructure to conclude that the fragments were human and thus were some of the earliest cases of cremation in the region.

8.3.2 Metric Methods

One of the key challenges faced when applying metric methods of biological profiling is that they rely on unmodified bone dimensions for their accuracy. Experimental work has shown how complicated the application of metric methods on burnt bone can be, noting that burning can cause statistically significant dimensional change, that this shrinkage can lead to the misclassification of sex using metric methods, but that to complicate matters even further, burning can also cause an increase in bone dimensions (Thompson, 2002, 2005). We also know from the analysis of micro-CT images that burning causes volumetric shrinkage of bone too (Ellingham and Sandholzer, 2020). Attempts have been made to correct for these heat-induced dimensional changes to take into account likely shrinkage, and while a blanket correction factor may be ineffective (Thompson, 2002; Gonçalves *et al.*, 2020) the application of regression models built from spectroscopic analysis focusing on visible hydroxyl bands within the composition of bone show merit (Gonçalves *et al.*, 2020).

A key tenet of forensic and biological anthropology is that of population specificity. That is, the importance of using population appropriate metric methods on the remains of interest. Using an inappropriate statistical sample will reduce accuracy. Usually when thinking of this, we consider geographical populations, or possibly temporal ones. However, we should also view this in terms of burnt and unburnt populations. Although metric methods are often unreliable when applied to burnt bone, this is because they are derived from unburnt populations. Creation of metric methods specifically for and from burnt remains increases their accuracy. For example, research by Gonçalves *et al.* (2013) achieved correct sex classification rates of over 80% when using appropriately constructed population specific methods, while also proving that sexual dimorphism still exists in burnt bone (and thus should, in theory, still be detectable).

The warping of bone during the burning process, another heat-induced dimensional change, can influence the calculation of metric methods. Although not prevalent in cremation contexts (e.g. Godinho *et al.*, 2019a record it in only 3% of inventoried bone elements), it has been recorded in the bones of both the cranial and post-cranial regions (Godinho *et al.*, 2019a). Research has suggested that the key factor in whether or not warping occurs is the presence of collagen within the bony structure (Vassalo *et al.*, 2019) as opposed to the presence of soft tissue structures *per se* (Gonçalves *et al.*, 2011). In their experimental work, Vassalo *et al.* (2019) were able to show that bone mass is an influencing factor on the degree of warping, with heavier bones displaying more warping in accordance with gravitation pull than lighter bones.

The frustrations experienced when attempting to apply metric methods to burnt bone have led some to explore the potential of the dentition. Tooth crowns are known to be sexually dimorphic and enamel is a robust material that can survive a range of taphonomic factors relatively unscathed. Unfortunately, experimental work has shown that teeth and enamel also experience heat-induced changes (including fragmentation and some dimensional changes) which impact our ability to perform accurate metric analysis (Gouveia *et al.*, 2017; Godinho *et al.*, 2019b). Interestingly, it may be that there is a sex difference in heat-induced shrinkage within the dentition, with females displaying greater shrinkage at temperatures of 900°C (Gouveia *et al.*, 2017).

8.3.3 Other Approaches to Biological Profile Estimation

There is growing interest in the use of imaging on cremated bone to support both morphological and metric analysis. Researchers have applied a range of three-dimensional imaging modalities to burnt bone, which can produce digital images that allow for the visualization and measurement of bone fragments. This is particularly helpful when the burnt remains are within a container of some sort and imaging allows for the safe examination and profiling of the body. Archaeologically, this is often an urn and work has shown that the act of micro-excavating the burnt remains can result in additional fragmentation (Minozzi *et al.*, 2010). Computed tomography (CT) is the preferred modality for this approach and has been shown to be extremely effective for producing images, but also for the subsequent morphological and metric assessments (Minozzi *et al.*, 2010). Anderson and Fell (1995) were probably the first to apply this approach and noted morphological skeletal features within a set of Roman cremation vessels. Harvig *et al.* (2011) were able to take measurements from the CT scans of a series of urns from Bronze Age Denmark, in addition to the identification of morphological features and several heat-induced changes. Thompson and Chudek (2007) were one of the first to attempt to apply magnetic resonance imaging (MRI) to burnt bone with some success, but more recently Cavka *et al.* (2015) were able to analyze bone fragments in Late Bronze Age urns from eastern Croatia / northern Bosnia. In the forensic arena, CT has been used with some considerable success in examining and analyzing burnt human remains, often whilst still contained in their body bags (e.g. Thali *et al.*, 2002; Blau *et al.*, 2008; O'Donnell *et al.*, 2011; de Boer *et al.*, 2020).

Despite the fragmentary nature of much burnt bone and the impact this has on the creation of a biological profile, there has been scant research on the most effective mechanisms for reconstructing, stabilizing, and preserving burnt bone. As Topoleski and Christensen note, "better preservation of skeletal evidence could significantly facilitate forensic anthropological analysis by permitting conclusions and analyses not otherwise possible" (2019:1138). More work is needed in this area since this has the potential to significantly reduce the challenges faced when attempting to create a biological profile from burnt remains; gelatin-based consolidants (Topoleski and Christensen, 2019), acetone solvent (Siegert *et al.*, 2020), and 3D surface scanning (Collings and Brown, 2020) all show promise.

Stable isotopic analysis has long been used on unburnt bone to explore diet and mobility of individuals and is an increasingly common aspect of anthropological profiling. In recent years, these methods have also been applied to forensic casework to provide further information to supplement the traditional anthropological results to great effect. There has always been a concern about applying these to burnt bone, since the process of burning causes significant change to the elemental composition of the bone. In particular, it has been noted that the use of light stable isotopes is not recommended since the carbon and oxygen isotopes can be fractionated by the burning process (Harbeck *et al.*, 2011; Price *et al.*, 2018; Graham and Bethard, 2019), although some work has shown that they are constant up to heating of around 200°C (Harbeck *et al.*, 2011). Interestingly, experimental work has shown that the presence of fuel has an impact on the extent of these changes, with ^{13}C and ^{18}O depleting when fuel is used compared to burning without fuel (Snoeck *et al.*, 2016b).

It has been repeatedly demonstrated that strontium is unaffected by the burning process, and results from burnt bone provide useful bioanthropological information on the last decade or so of an individual's life (Snoeck *et al.*, 2016a). Strontium is effective simply because it is a heavier element and therefore does not exhibit fractionation under heat (Harbeck *et al.*, 2011; Graham and Bethard, 2019). Price *et al.* (2018) undertook strontium isotope analysis from the cremated bone recovered from Viking-era Birka in Sweden. They concluded, perhaps surprisingly for their particular context, that cremation was being performed by both the local and the migratory populations. More recent work has shown that it is possible to combine stable isotope ratios from cremated bone to provide greater interpretative power, as with Grupe *et al.* (2020) who combined strontium and lead analysis of 247 human cremated deposits from the European Alpine region.

Because of its anatomical location, the petrous portion of the temporal bone often survives destructive forces well and this factor, combined with the general robustness of the bone and the lack of remodeling over time, makes it an ideal candidate for successful stable isotope analysis (as well as DNA recovery). In this way, Škvor Jernejčič and Price (2020) were able to use the petrous portion of the temporal bone of cremated human remains in their analysis of mobility in the Bronze to Iron Age transition in Slovenia. Measurement of the $^{87}Sr/^{86}Sr$ ratio demonstrated that the 32 individuals under study were local to the region they were recovered from. This is a useful application of anatomical science to the study of isotopes in burnt bone, but it is also worth noting that once bone has been burned to the point of calcination, it is essentially diagenetically stable and the isotopic composition will not change further (Graham and Bethard, 2019). Regardless, Snoeck *et al.* (2016b) warn of the challenges of using stable isotopes for commenting on the context of burning, since the high levels of variability in conditions around the body during burning result in differing isotopic results in individuals from even the same context.

Finally, a newly developed method of sex determination using tooth enamel peptides is gaining significant interest. The method, developed by Stewart and colleagues (2017), examines sex chromosome-linked isoforms of amelogenin (a protein which forms enamel) and has been demonstrated to have an accuracy of 100% in applications to date. The method is cheaper, quicker, and easier than DNA analysis, and the fact that it is linked to part of the robust hard tissues suggests that it may have some application to burnt human remains, although this has yet to be tested.

8.4 Conclusions

As we can see, there are significant challenges when attempting biological profile estimation from burnt remains. Generally, these stem from the combination of heat-induced changes to the skeleton and the environmental context surrounding the actual burning.

There has been an acknowledgment for many years that our methods of biological profile estimation will be negatively affected by burning, although there are few studies that have attempted to describe the extent of this effect. Recently, Rodrigues *et al.* (2020) recorded that the methods developed for unburnt bones performed better at lower temperatures of burning and that traditional morphological methods were shown to perform poorly at temperatures above 700°C, although some features of the pelvis (including the composite arc) still performed well after burning. Further, the remains of females seem to become "masculinized" when using morphological methods, whereas male remains seem to become "feminized" using metric methods. Ultimately, the authors note that "burns at low to medium temperature intensities are not as innocuous as previously thought regarding the sex estimation of skeletal remains" (Rodrigues *et al.*, 2020).

Burnt human bodies form a significant but challenging aspect of forensic investigation. These are not unmanageable contexts, but they do require burnt body specialists and considerable patience (de Boer *et al.*, 2020). Arguably the discipline has long appreciated the changes that burning causes to the body, yet unfortunately work in this area generally offers few surprises. Therefore continued research on the impact of heat-induced change on the outcomes of our methods of biological profile estimation, the creation of new methods specific to burnt bone, and frameworks for the interpretation of contexts of burning from burnt bone (a *bioarchaeology of cremation*) offer the most fruitful future for mitigating and minimizing the challenges of biological profile estimation from burnt bodies.

References

Anderson, T. and Fell, C. (1995) Analysis of Roman cremation vessels by computerized tomography. *Journal of Archaeological Science*, **22**, 609–617.

Behrens, L.M., Sperhake, J.-P., Püschel, K., and Schröder, A.S. (2020) The postmortem examination prior to cremation: Still a necessary safety measure? *Legal Medicine*, **43**, 101664.

Bianchi, I., Focardi, M., Bugelli, V., Gualco, B., Pradella, F., and Pinchi, V. (2019) The tongue protrusion in post-mortem fire. *Journal of Forensic Odonto-Stomatology*, **37**, 26–31.

Blau, S., Robertson, S., and Johnstone, M. (2008) Disaster victim identification: New applications for postmortem computed tomography. *Journal of Forensic Sciences*, **53**, 956–961.

Bocquentin, F., Anmton, M., Berna, F., Rosen, A., Khalaily, H., Greenberg, H., *et al.* (2020) Emergence of corpse cremation during the Pre-Pottery Neolithic of the Southern Levant: A multidisciplinary study of a pyre-pit burial. *PLoS One*, **15**, e0235386.

Carroll, E.L. and Squires, K.E. (2020) The application of quantitative petrography and macroscopic colour change in a comparative analysis of Roman and Anglo-Saxon cremation practices. *International Journal of Osteoarchaeology*, **30**(6), 882–890.

Cataroche, J. and Gowland, R.L. (2015) Flesh, fire and funerary remains from the Neolithic site of La Varde, Guernsey: Investigations past and present. In: *The Archaeology of Cremation: Burned Human Remains in Funerary Studies* (ed. T.J.U. Thompson). Oxbow Books, Oxford, UK, pp. 19–42.

Cavka, M., Petaros, A., Reiter, G., Nielles-Vallespin, S., Speier, P., Brkljacic, B., *et al.* (2015) MR ultrashort echo time sequence of cremated remains in ancient urns. *Journal of Forensic Radiology and Imaging*, **3**, 117–119.

Charlier, P., Poupon, J., De Mazancourt, P., Gilbert, T., Huynh-Charlier, I., Loublier, Y., *et al.* (2010) The 'relics of Joan of Arc': A forensic multidisciplinary analysis. *Forensic Science International*, **194**, e9–e15.

Collings, A.J. and Brown, K. (2020) Reconstruction and physical fit analysis of fragmented skeletal remains using 3D imaging and printing. *Forensic Science International: Reports*, **2**, 100114.

Coulombeix, A. and Schuliar, Y. (2017) Analysis and interpretation of burned human remains from a homicide. In: *Taphonomy of Human Remains: Forensic Analysis of the Dead and the Depositional Environment* (eds. E.M.J. Schotsman, N. Márquez-Grant, and S.L. Forbes). Wiley, Chichester, UK, pp. 438–444.

De Boer, H.H., Roberts, J., Delabarde, T., Mundorff, A.Z., and Blau, S. (2020) Disaster victim identification operations with fragmented, burnt, or commingled remains: Experience-based recommendations. *Forensic Sciences Research*, **5**, 191–201.

Ellingham, S.T.D. and Sandholzer, M.A. (2020) Determining volumetric shrinkage trends of burnt bone using micro-CT. *Journal of Forensic Sciences*, **65**, 196–199.

Ellingham, S.T.D., Thompson, T.J.U., and Islam, M. (2015) The effect of soft tissue on temperature estimation from burnt bone using Fourier Transform Infrared Spectroscopy. *Journal of Forensic Sciences*, **61**, 153–159.

Ellingham, S.T.D., Thompson, T.J.U., and Islam, M. (2017) Scanning Electron Microscopy-Energy-Dispersive X-Ray (SEM/EDX): A rapid diagnostic tool to aid the identification of burnt bone and contested cremains. *Journal of Forensic Sciences*, **63**(2), 504–510.

Garrido-Varas, C. and Intriago-Leiva, M. (2015) The interpretation and reconstruction of the post-mortem events in a case of scattered burned remains in Chile. In: *The Archaeology of Cremation: Burned Human Remains in Funerary Studies* (ed. T.J.U. Thompson). Oxbow Books, Oxford, UK, pp. 227–242.

Gin, K., Tovar, J., Bertelink, E.J., Kendell, A., Milligan, C., Willey, P., *et al.* (2020) The 2018 California wildfires: Integration of rapid DNA to dramatically accelerate victim identification. *Journal of Forensic Sciences*, **65**. https://doi.org/10.1111/1556-4029.14284.

Go, M.C. and Docot, D. (2021) Fire and fear: Rapid cremations in the Philippines amidst COVID-19. *Forensic Science International: Synergy*, **3**, 100132.

Godinho, R.M., Gonçalves, D., and Valera, A.C. (2019a) The preburning condition of Chalcolithic cremated human remains from the Perdigões enclosures (Portugal). *International Journal of Osteology*, **29**, 706–717.

Godinho, R.M., Oliveria-Santos, I., Pereira, M.F.C., Maurício, A., Valera, A., and Gonçalves, D. (2019b) Is enamel the only reliable hard tissue for sex metric estimation of burned skeletal remains in biological anthropology? *Journal of Archaeological Science: Reports*, **26**, 101876.

Gonçalves, D., Thompson, T.J.U., and Cunha, E. (2011) Implications of heat-induced changes in bone on the interpretation of funerary behaviour and practice. *Journal of Archaeological Science*, **38**, 1308–1313.

Gonçalves, D., Thompson, T.J.U., and Cunha, E. (2013) Osteometric sex determination of burned human skeletal remains. *Journal of Forensic and Legal Medicine*, **20**, 906–911.

Gonçalves, D., Vassalo, A.R., Makhoul, C., Piga, G., Mamede, A.P., Parker, S.F., *et al.* (2020) Chemosteometric regression models of heat exposed human bones to determine their pre-burnt metric dimensions. *American Journal of Physical Anthropology*, **173**(4), 734–747.

Gouveia, M.F., Oliveira Santos, I., Santos, A.L., and Gonçalves, D. (2017) Sample-specific odontometric sex estimation: A method with potential application to burned remains. *Science & Justice*, **57**, 262–269.

Graham, D.D. and Bethard, J.D. (2019) Reconstructing the origins of the Perrins Ledge cremains using strontium isotope analysis. *Journal of Archaeological Science: Reports*, **24**, 350–362.

Grupe, G., Klaut, D., Otto, L., Mauder, M., Lohrer, J., Kröger, P., *et al.* (2020) The genesis and spread of the early Fritzens-Sanzeno culture (5th/4th cent. BCE) – Stable isotope analysis of cremated and uncremated skeletal finds. *Journal of Archaeological Science: Reports*, **29**, 102121.

Harbeck, M., Schleuder, R., Schneider, J., Wiechmann, I., Schmahl, W.W., and Grupe, G. (2011) Research potential and limitation of trace analyses of cremated remains. *Forensic Science International*, **204**, 191–200.

Harvig, L., Lynnerup, N., and Amsgaard Ebsen, J. (2011) Computed tomography and computed radiography of late Bronze Age cremation urns from Denmark: An interdisciplinary attempt to develop methods applied in bioarchaeological cremation research. *Archaeometry*, **54**, 369–387.

Kaur, N. and Byard, R.W. (2020) Bride burning: A unique and ongoing form of gender-based violence. *Journal of Forensic and Legal Medicine*, **75**. https://doi.org/10.1016/j.jflm.2020.102035.

Kgatle, M.S. (2020) Dealing with the cultural and financial challenges during death of a loved one and repatriation of the remains: A mission to the wounded. *HTS Teologiese Studies/Theological Studies*, **76**(4), 1–8.

Kutterer, A.U., Doppler, S., Uerpmann, M., and Uerpmann, H.-P. (2012) Neolithic cremation in south-east Arabia: Archaeological and anthropological observations at FAY-NE10 in the Emirate of Sharjah (UAE). *Arabian Archaeology and Epigraphy*, **23**, 125–144.

Martyn, R., Craig, O.E., Ellingham, S.T.E., Islam, M., Fattore, L., Sperduti, A., *et al.* (2020) A re-evaluation of manner of death at Roman Herculaneum following the AD 79 eruption of Vesuvius. *Antiquity*, **94**, 76–91.

Migala, A.F. and Brown, S.E. (2012) Use of human remains detection dogs for wide area search after wildfire: A new experience for Texas task force 1 search and rescue resources. *Wilderness & Environmental Medicine*, **23**, 337–342.

Minozzi, S., Giuffra, V., Bagnoli, J., Paribeni, E., Giustini, D., Caramella, D., *et al.* (2010) An investigation of Etruscan cremations by Computed Tomography (CT). *Antiquity*, **84**, 195–201.

Monetti, L., Voulgari, M., Karagiorgou, I., and Moraitis, K. (2021) Macroscopic determination of the pre-burning conditions of human remains recovered from an unusual forensic context: A case report. *Journal of Forensic and Legal Medicine*, **78**, 102115.

Moore, S.E., Jones-Eversley, S.D., Tolliver, W.F., Wilson, B.L., and Jones, C.A. (2020) Six feet apart of six feet under: The impact of COVID-19 on the Black community. *Death Studies*, 1–11.

Morobadi, K., Blumenthal, R., and Saayman, G. (2019) Thermal fatalities in Pretoria: A 5-year retrospective review. *Burns*, **45**, 1707–1714.

Nakhaeizadeh, S., Morgan, R.M., Olsson, V., Arvidsson, M., and Thompson, T.J.U. (2020) The value of eye-tracking technology in the analysis and interpretations of skeletal remains: A pilot study. *Science & Justice*, **60**, 36–42.

Nayak, M., Merchant, S., and Shah, K. (2020) Trends & pattern in unnatural female death cases due to burn: A one year retrospective study. *Indian Journal of Forensic Medicine and Toxicology*, **14**, 19–23.

O'Donnell, C., Iino, M., Mansharan, K., Leditscke, J., and Woodford, N. (2011) Contribution of postmortem multidetector CT scanning to identification of the deceased in a mass disaster: Experience gained from the 2009 Victorian bushfires. *Forensic Science International*, **205**, 15–28.

Piga, G., Orquín, R.P., Guirguis, M., Gonçalves, D., Pimenta, C., Tereso, J.P., *et al.* (2020) Woman and child: The singular testimony of a Punic tomb in the necropolis of Monte Sirai (Carbonia-Sardinia, Italy). *Journal of Archaeological Science: Reports*, **29**, 102095.

Price, T.D., Arcini, C., Gustin, I., Drenzel, L., and Kalmring, S. (2018) Isotopes and human burials at Viking Age Birka and the Mälaren region, east central Sweden. *Journal of Anthropological Archaeology*, **49**, 19–38.

Rodrigues, C.O., Ferreira, M.T., Matos, V., and Gonçalves, D. (2020) "Sex change" in skeletal remains: Assessing how heat-induced changes interfere with sex estimation. *Science & Justice*, **61**(1), 26–36.

Röst, A. (2017) Building by stone and bone: Handling cremated remains in Late Bronze Age Sweden. In: *Cremation and the Archaeology of Death* (eds. J.I. Cerezo-Román, A. Wessman, and H. Williams). Oxford University Press, Oxford, UK, pp. 130–147.

Schmidt, C.W. and Symes, S.A. (2008) *The Analysis of Burned Human Remains*. Academic Press, San Diego, CA.

Siegert, C.C., Hamilton, M.D., Erhart, E.M., and Devlin, J.B. (2020) A comparative assessment of consolidation materials applied to burned bone, *Forensic Science International*, **310**, 110224.

Silva, F.C. (2015) The funerary practice of cremation at Augusta Emerita (Mérida, Spain) during High Empire: Contributions from the anthropological analysis of burned human bone. In: *The Archaeology of Cremation: Burned Human Remains in Funerary Studies* (ed. T.J.U. Thompson). Oxbow Books, Oxford, UK, pp. 123–150.

Simonit, F., Da Broi, U., Furioso, C., and Desinan, L. (2020) A burned body with a gunshot wound in the mouth and a suicide note: A complex or complicated suicide? *Journal of Forensic and Legal Medicine*, **72**. https://doi.org/10.1016/j.jflm.2020.101958.

Škvor Jernejčič, B. and Price, T.D. (2020) Isotopic investigations of human cremations from the Late Bronze Age/Early Iron Age cemetery of Ljubljana – Dvorišče SAZU, Slovenia. *Journal of Archaeological Science: Reports*, **34**, 102594.

Snoeck, C., Pouncett, J., Ramsey, G., Meighan, I.G., Mattielli, N., Goderis, S., *et al.* (2016a) Mobility during the Neolithic and Bronze Age in northern Ireland explored using strontium isotope analysis of cremated human bone. *American Journal of Physical Anthropology*, **160**, 397–413.

Snoeck, C., Schulting, R.J., Lee-Thorp, J.A., Lebon, M., and Zazzo, A. (2016b) Impact of heating conditions on the carbon and oxygen isotope composition of calcined bone. *Journal of Archaeological Science*, **65**, 32–43.

Soto, G. (2020) Absent and present: Biopolitics and the materiality of body counts on the US-Mexico border. *Journal of Material Culture*, **26**(1), 43–63.

Squires, K.E., Thompson, T.J.U., Islam, M., and Chamberlain, A. (2011) The application of histomorphometry and Fourier Transform Infrared Spectroscopy to the analysis of early Anglo-Saxon burned bone. *Journal of Archaeological Science*, **38**, 2399–2409.

Stewart, N.A., Gerlach, R.F., Gowland, R.L., Gron, K.J., and Montgomery, J. (2017) Sex determination of human remains from peptides in tooth enamel. *PNAS*, **114**, 13649–13654.

Thali, M.J., Yen, K., Plattner, T., Schweitzer, W., Vock, P., Ozdoba, C., *et al.* (2002) Charred body: Virtual autopsy with multi-slice computed tomography and magnetic resonance imaging. *Journal of Forensic Sciences*, **47**, 1326–1331.

Thompson, T.J.U. (2002) The assessment of sex in cremated individuals: Some cautionary notes. *Canadian Society of Forensic Sciences Journal*, **35**, 49–56.

Thompson, T.J.U. (2004) Recent advances in the study of burned bone and their implications for forensic anthropology. *Forensic Science International*, **146S**, S203–S205.

Thompson, T.J.U. (2005) Heat-induced dimensional changes in bone and their consequences for forensic anthropology. *Journal of Forensic Sciences*, **50**, 1008–1015.

Thompson, T.J.U. (2015) Fire and the body; fire and the people. In: The Archaeology of Cremation: Burned Human Remains in Funerary Studies (ed. T.J.U. Thompson). Oxbow Books, Oxford, UK, pp. 1–17.

Thompson, T.J.U. and Chudek, J.A. (2007) A novel approach to the visualisation of heat-induced structural change in bone. *Science & Justice*, **47**, 99–104.

Thompson, T.J.U., Gonçalves, D., Squires, K., and Ulguim, P. (2017) Thermal alternation to the body. In: Taphonomy of Human Remains: Forensic Analysis of the Dead and the Depositional Environment (eds. E.M.J. Schotsman, N. Márquez-Grant, and S.L. Forbes). Wiley, Chichester, UK, pp. 318–334.

Topoleski, J.J. and Christensen, A.M. (2019) Use of a gelatin-based consolidant to preserve thermally-altered skeletal remains. *Journal of Forensic Sciences*, **64**, 1135–1138.

Ubelaker, D.H. (2017) Interpretation of burned remains: Lessons from modern forensic cases. In: Cremation and the Archaeology of Death (eds. J.I. Cerezo-Román, A. Wessman, and H. Williams). Oxford University Press, Oxford, UK, pp. 104–113.

Vassalo, A.R., Mamede, A.P., Ferreira, M.T., Cunha, E., and Gonçalves, D. (2019) The G-force awakens: The influence of gravity in bone heat-induced warping and its implications for the estimation of the pre-burning condition of human remains. *Australian Journal of Forensic Sciences*, **51**, 201–208.

Wegner, A., Doberentz, E., and Madea, B. (2020) Fire exposure after lethal hypothermia. *Forensic Science, Medicine, and Pathology*. https://doi.org/10.1007/s12024-020-00286-5.

Zana, M., Magli, F., Mazzucchi, A., Castoldi, E., Gibelli, D., Caccia, G., *et al.* (2017) Effects of cremation on fetal bones. *Journal of Forensic Sciences*, **62**, 1140–1144.

Živković, V., Cvetković, D., Zaletel, I., Byard, R., and Nikolić, S. (2020) The effects of elevated temperature on coronary artery dimensions. *Forensic Science International*, **314**. https://doi.org/10.1016/j.forsciint.2020.110390.

CHAPTER 9

Victim Identification: The Role of Incinerated Dental Materials

Peter J. Bush[1], BS; Mary A. Bush[2], DDS and Raymond Miller[3], DDS

[1] *Director of the South Campus Instrument Center at the State University of New York School of Dental Medicine, USA*

[2] *Associate Professor and Associate Dean for Students, Community, and Professional Initiatives at SUNY at Buffalo School of Dental Medicine, USA*

[3] *Clinical Associate Professor at the University at Buffalo School of Dental Medicine; forensic dental consultant to the Office of the Erie County Medical Examiner in Buffalo, NY, USA*

9.1 Introduction

In victim identification of incinerated remains, every clue is utilized to establish a connection to ante-mortem (AM) identity. While it has been long established that surgically implanted materials such as prostheses can be of particular interest (Ubelaker and Jacobs, 1995; Berketa *et al.*, 2015), more recently it has been shown that dental materials and their method of placement can provide useful information (Bush *et al.*, 2006, 2008; Bonavilla *et al.*, 2008). Dental materials can consist of a very wide array of substances such as restorative materials, those used in endodontic, orthodontic, and other procedures. Dental prostheses can include bridges, crowns, dentures, wires, brackets, posts and implants, resins, sealers, and cements. The manufacturers of these products have either by design or default included components that are unique in chemical and physical structure. They might, for example, produce contrast in a dental radiograph, resulting from inclusion of materials that have an atomic number higher than the surrounding tooth structure. The higher atomic number causes absorption of X-rays, thus showing as bright areas in a radiograph, revealing the presence of the material (Chesne *et al.*, 1999).

Recognition of these procedures and their resulting placement has augmented the basis of traditional dental identification of non-incinerated victims in which AM dental X-rays are visually compared with post-mortem (PM). Restorations using dental materials can be very helpful in victim ID. With additional knowledge

Burnt Human Remains: Recovery, Analysis, and Interpretation, First Edition. Edited by Sarah Ellingham, Joe Adserias-Garriga, Sara C. Zapico and Douglas H. Ubelaker.

of analytical methods, chemistry, and microstructure, there is the potential for positive identification based on proven scientific methods, going beyond a simple visual comparison.

Under exposure to high temperature, the multitude of dental materials will undergo different chemical and structural evolutions, depending on the exposed temperature. As is well known, organic materials (composed principally of hydrogen, oxygen, and carbon) will decompose up to around 400°C, leaving the elements higher in the periodic table as residuals.

Enamel crowns may separate from the tooth roots, resulting in loss of restorative materials and disruption of the physical integrity of the teeth. In this case, comparing shape and arrangement of tooth and jaw structure is more difficult, but there may remain valuable information to aid in identification. This involves knowledge of the physical and chemical properties of the materials used in dentistry and of the methods and circumstances in which they are used.

9.2 Microstructural Changes in Teeth after Incineration

There have been a number of studies documenting the macroscopic structural and color changes in teeth exposed to ranges of temperatures (Harsanyi, 1975; Muller *et al.*, 1998). Here, focus will be laid on the microstructural changes. The structure of teeth comprises three main components, enamel, dentin, and cementum. These are composite materials consisting of hydroxyapatite mineral and organic phases. Enamel and dentin have distinct microstructures which can be recognized both before and after incineration. Cementum, however, has an amorphous structure. Fresh enamel has a u-shaped prism structure around 4–5 microns in diameter. Each prism is composed of acicular (needle-like) crystals of hydroxyapatite with a cross-sectional dimension of 100 nm. Dentin has a tubular structure, with the peritubular dentin similarly composed of acicular mineral crystals (Summitt *et al.*, 2001). Following high temperature incineration, the acicular crystals in both enamel and dentin melt, recrystallize, and are no longer recognizable. However, the enamel prism structure and, remarkably, the dentin tubules are both still recognizable and can be used to confirm the nature of a specimen. The use of a scanning electron microscope (SEM) is necessary to visualize these structures. Except where noted, the following images are taken with high resolution field emission SEMs (see Figures 9.1–9.5).

The pictures in this section represent extremes: fresh specimens versus those exposed to high temperatures, typically 1000°C for at least 30 minutes. At temperatures in between these extremes, there is a gradation of structural changes.

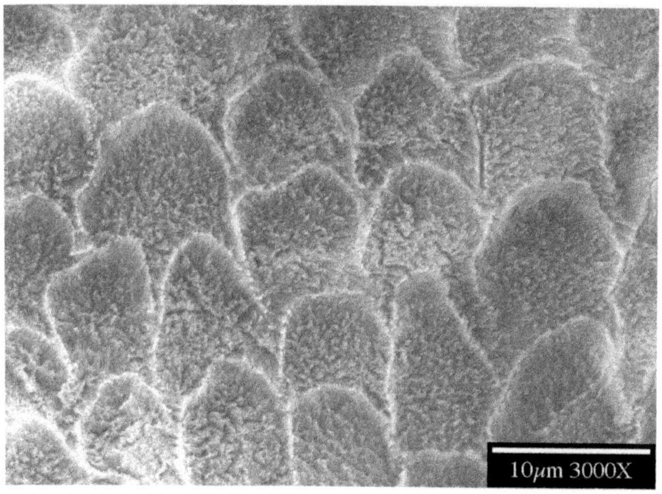

Figure 9.1 Fresh enamel, etched to reveal the inverted u-shaped prism structure. Here the prisms are viewed perpendicular to the prism long dimension.

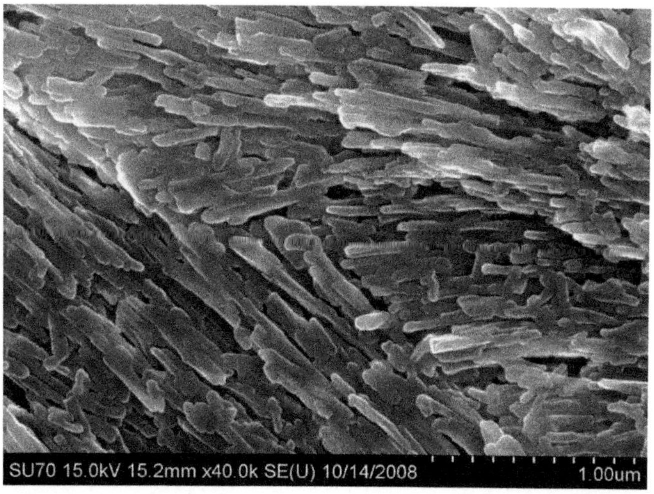

Figure 9.2 High magnification image of fresh enamel micro-crystallites, 40,000x. The needle diameter averages around 100 nm. A prism boundary can be seen extending from top left towards bottom right. At temperatures of 600–800°C, these crystals melt, fuse, and form larger crystal agglomerates.

9.3 Structural Changes Due to Restorative Procedures

During restorative procedures such as placing a filling or preparing a crown, the tooth structure is altered by the clinician. Such changes can be recognized after incineration and may indicate which procedure was performed on the tooth, even though the restorative material itself may not be present or retrieved.

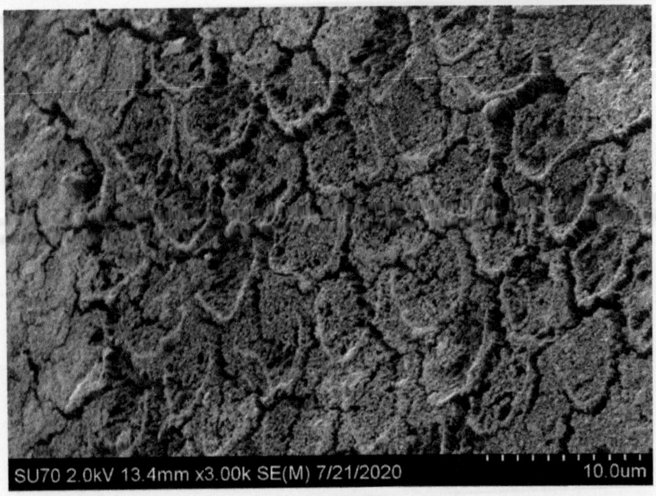

Figure 9.3 Incinerated enamel surface (1000°C 1 hour). The prism structure is still recognizable after recrystallization (compare Figure 9.1). Cracking principally occurs at the prism boundaries.

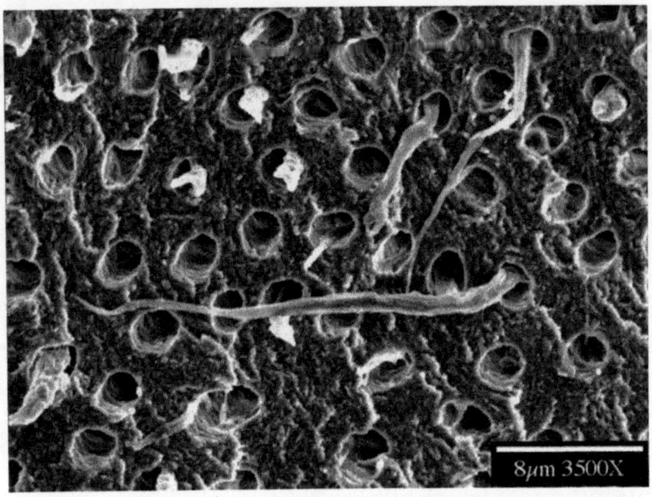

Figure 9.4a Fresh dentin. Some cellular processes can be seen protruding from the tubules. Tubule dimension approximately 2 microns.

The information retrieved from the example given in Figures 9.6–9.8 may provide the investigator with a piece of evidence that may otherwise go undetected, namely that this individual had a tooth colored filling in this tooth, even though the material itself was not evident. In this case, the AM record confirmed this conclusion.

Rather than detail the chemical and structural changes after incineration of the hundreds of dental materials, some case studies will be presented to illustrate how this information may be used in victim identification.

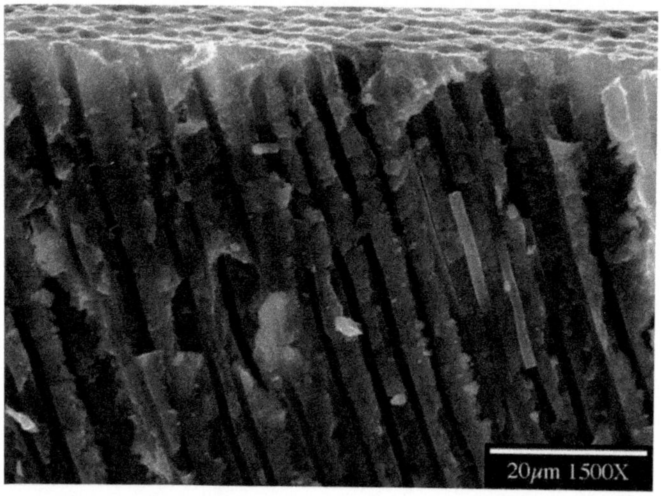

Figure 9.4b View parallel to the tubules.

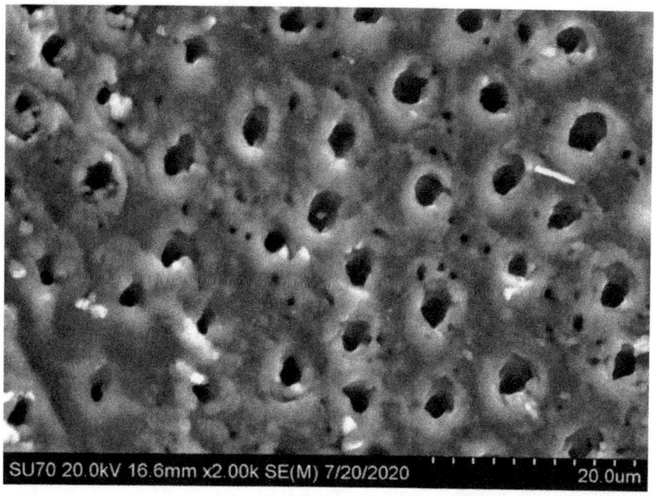

Figure 9.5a Incinerated dentin (1000°C, 1 hour). The peritubular dentin has recrystallized to form larger apatite crystals.

9.4 Case Reports

9.4.1 Case Report 1: Airline Crash

Airline crashes are usually multi-fatality incidents encompassing the destructive forces of trauma and fire, leading to fragmentation of human remains, including the dentition. Although the dentition inherently has been shown to survive such insults, the combinations of these forces will inflict damage and complicate the identification process.

A transportation accident in north-east USA exemplified the results of such incidents whereby application of advanced analytical technologies assisted in the

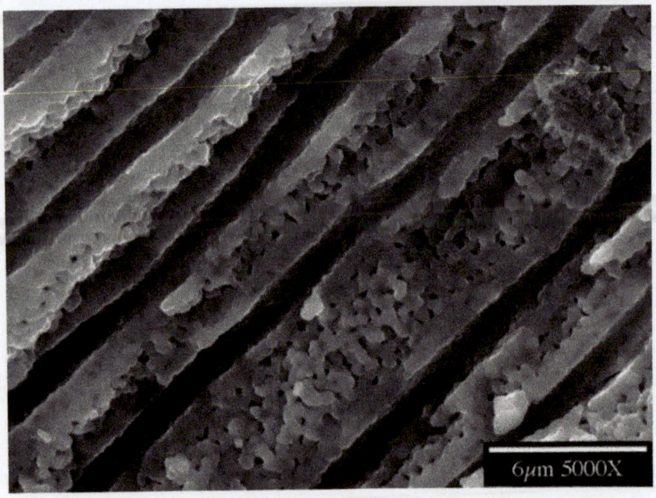

Figure 9.5b View parallel to the tubules. Larger crystallites are evident in the peritubular dentin. The tubular structure is still obvious after incineration.

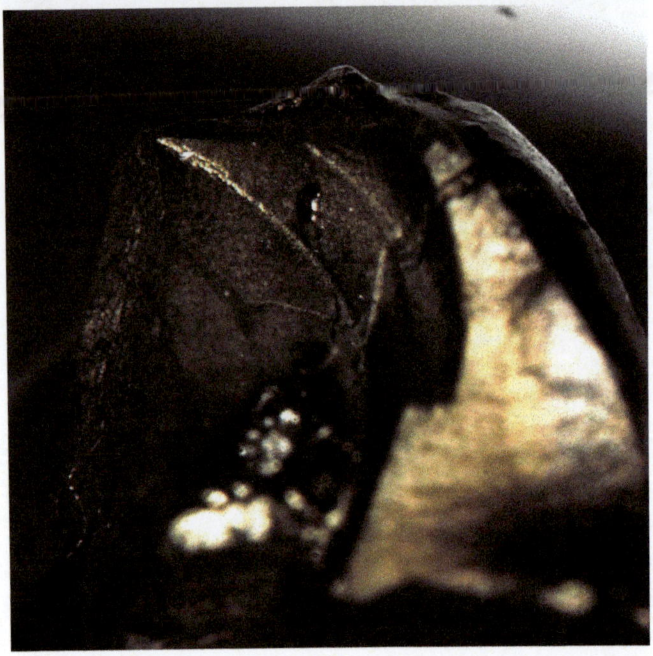

Figure 9.6 Optical image of a cremated tooth fragment. Note darkened color.

victim identification process. This incident involved the previously mentioned forces of initial physical trauma, the impact of the aircraft free-falling into a home in a residential neighborhood. This was followed by significant thermal trauma. The physical trauma caused fractures of the skull and associated structures such as the maxilla, mandible, and individual teeth. This impact trauma further exposed these structures, leading to direct thermal trauma. This thermal damage was

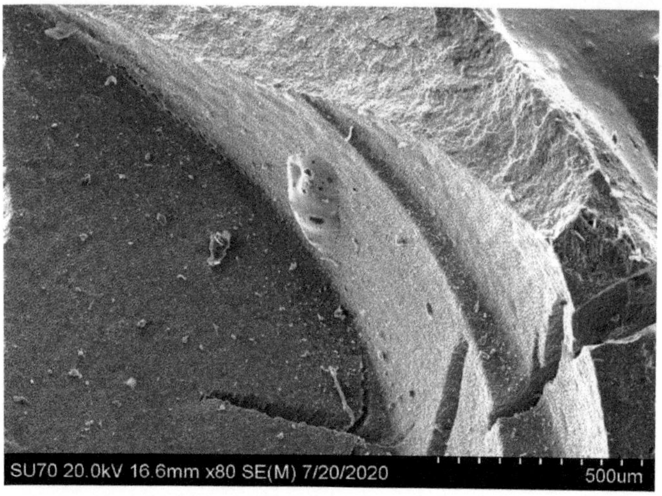

Figure 9.7 SEM image of tooth fragment as shown in Figure 9.6. Curving and flat features are clearly evident. These are the structures that resulted from the use of a dental bur during preparation for placing a filling.

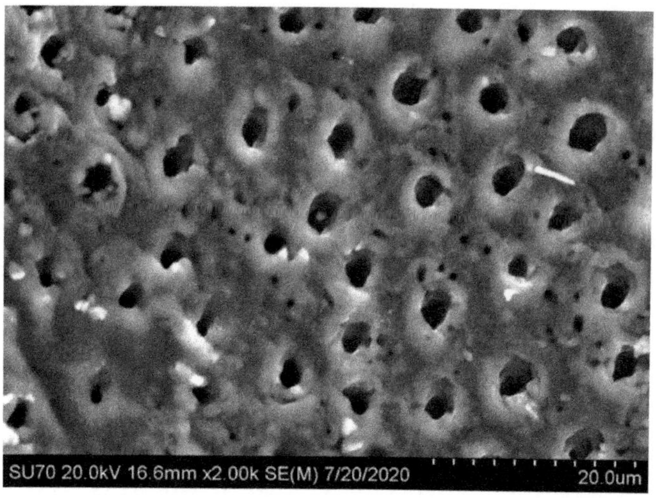

Figure 9.8a Image taken from fractured dentin at right in Figure 9.7.

increased in areas directly associated with the home's gas line and location of fuel cells of the aircraft. This was documented by body location as mapped out from recovery logs. Basically, proximity to thermal intensity adversely affected body condition and increased the difficulty in establishing identity.

The physical and thermal trauma also make the recovery process difficult. Careful and thorough anthropological and archaeological techniques need be employed. Layers of aircraft, house, and other debris are carefully removed to uncover evidence of human remains. Upon identifying the location of victims, protocols are in place to recover all human tissue for further analysis, keeping in

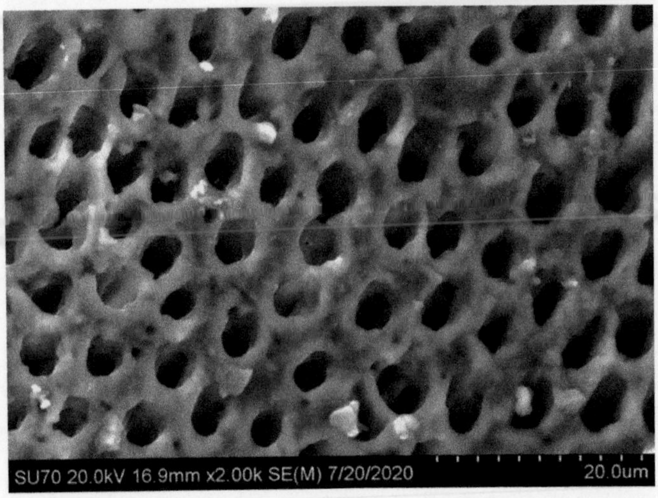

Figure 9.8b Image from the flat area at left in Figure 9.7. The dentin tubules are more open, indicating that the dentist used a phosphoric acid etch prior to placing a tooth-colored filling.

mind the possibility for fragmentation and commingling. Individual teeth, restorations, and prostheses are part of this process and can provide very critical information in the identification process.

A knowledgeable and well-trained recovery team, usually composed of anthropologists, will locate significant human tissues for pathological, biological, anthropological, and odontological analysis. Odontologists and other disciplines can also be involved in the recovery, based on their unique ability to recognize specific materials for association and identification. Items such as a single tooth or jaw fragments can provide enough information to establish identity when thoroughly and comprehensively analyzed.

Examples of advanced analytical techniques and dental victim identification in the above mass fatality transportation incident will be presented in the next few paragraphs.

The first example is the recovery of a single tooth. This recovered tooth presented with evidence of AM treatments involving root canal therapy, prefabricated post, and placement of a composite resin core. The AM radiographs presented a compilation of these treatments. One exhibits the coronal portion with the core and post evident in a bitewing (Figure 9.9). The other, a periapical (Figure 9.10), demonstrates the root with the completed root canal without the core or post. Pattern comparison of the size, shape, location, and unique attributes of the root, post, and core, when compared with the recovered PM tooth and associated radiograph (Figure 9.11) should be sufficient to establish dental identity. Since this identity involves single tooth identification, advanced analytics utilizing X-ray fluorescence (XRF) analysis would have provided additional evidential confirmation.

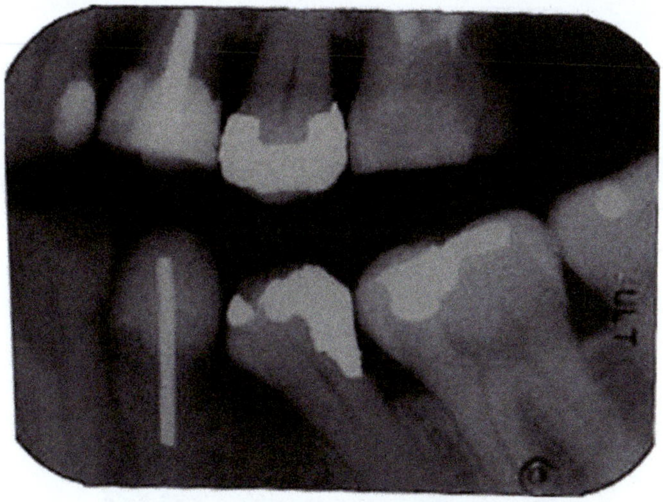

Figure 9.9 AM Bitewing.

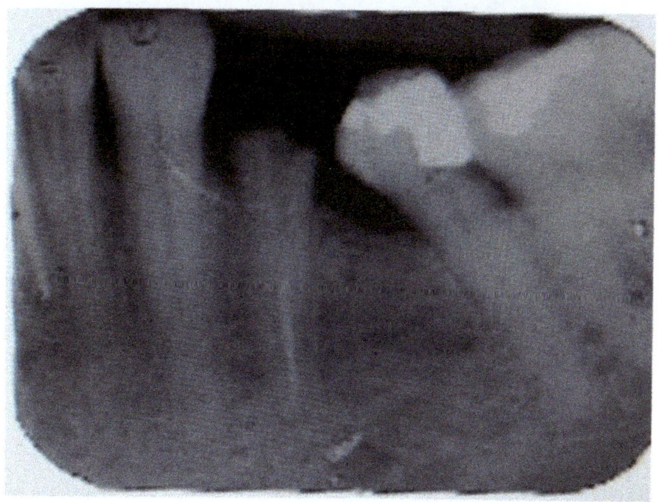

Figure 9.10 AM Periapical.

The information from the XRF provided the elemental composition of the core material and based on research at the State University of New York at Buffalo's School of Dental Medicine's South Campus Instrument Center and their compiled database of commercially available composite resins, the recovered restoration was identified as to brand name. The core was determined to be Heliomolar (Ivoclar-Vivadent)) as seen on the display from the XRF (Figure 9.12). This comparison is dependent on the provider accurately documenting material identity in the dental record (Figure 9.13) regarding tooth #21 (Universal), the lower left second premolar. This information provided additional comparative data to confirm identity.

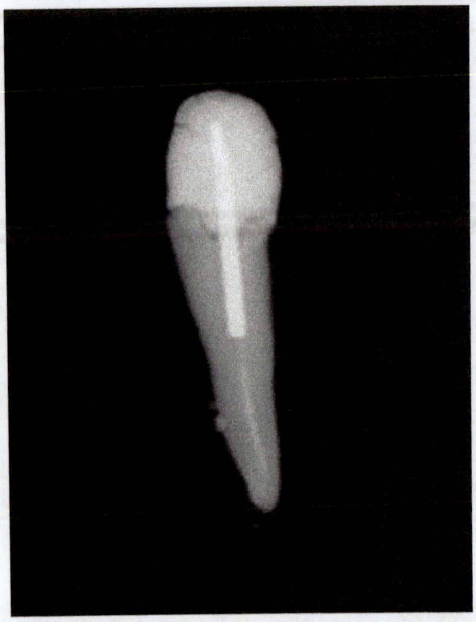

Figure 9.11 PM Radiograph.

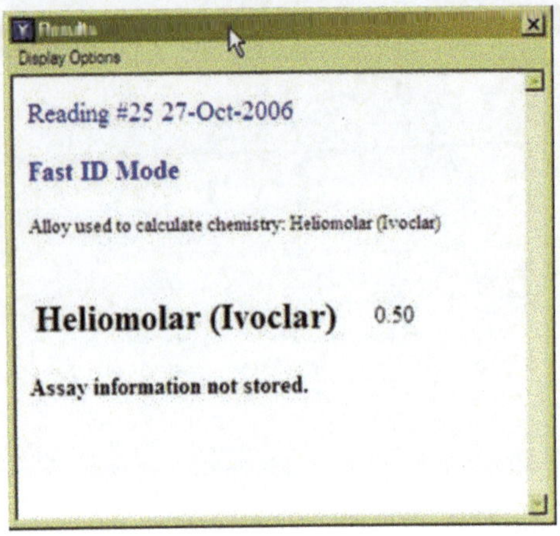

Figure 9.12 XRF display identifying composite brand as Heliomolar.

The second example from this incident involves a recovered mandibular fragment containing the roots of two teeth determined to be teeth #30 and #31(FDI) the lower right first and second molar (Figure 9.14). Radiographic analysis of the PM fragment revealed root canal therapy #30 and missing #32 (Universal) (Figure 9.15). No other restorative treatments were clinically or radiographically evident.

Using further analytical techniques of stereomicroscopy (Figures 9.16 and 9.17) and SEM (Figures 9.18 and 9.19) with energy dispersive spectroscopy (EDS) (Figure 9.20) the root canal therapy was confirmed. The elemental composition of the root canal sealer was determined using an established database of root canal

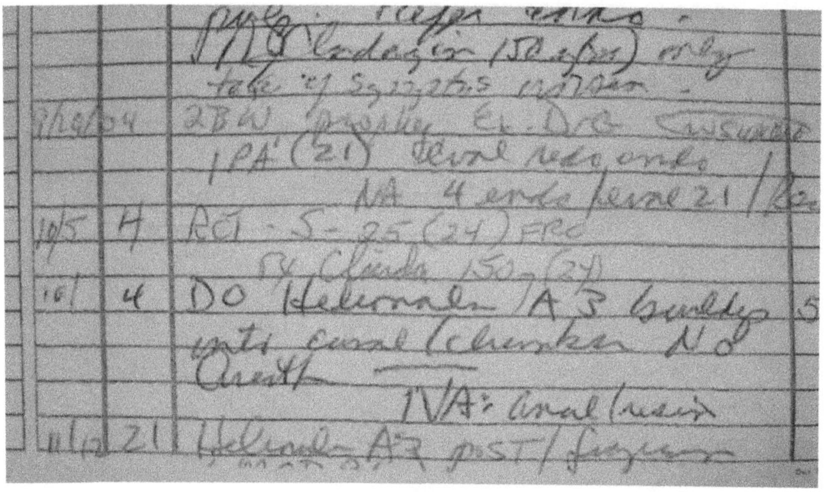

Figure 9.13 Dental chart entry indicating Heliolmolar used as restorative material in tooth #21.

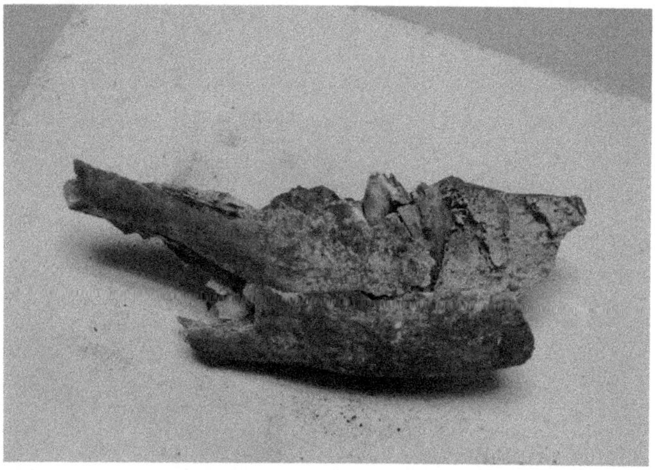

Figure 9.14 Recovered right mandibular fragment in debris field of airline crash.

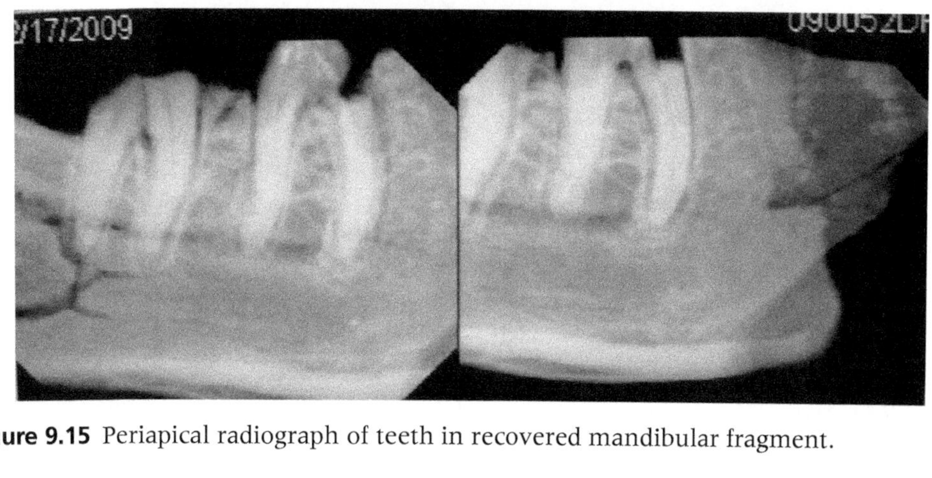

Figure 9.15 Periapical radiograph of teeth in recovered mandibular fragment.

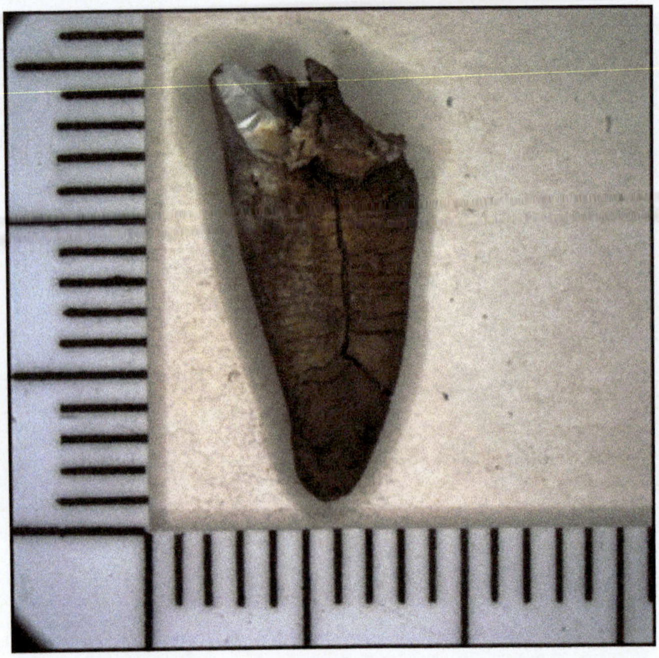

Figure 9.16 Distal root tooth #30 (Universal) with thermal damage.

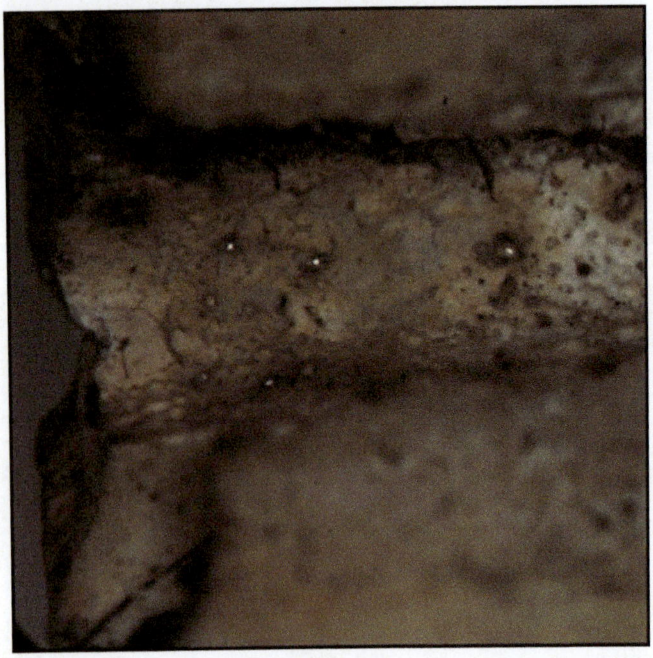

Figure 9.17 Stereomicroscope view of canal of #30 (Universal) root with evidence of silver from root canal sealer.

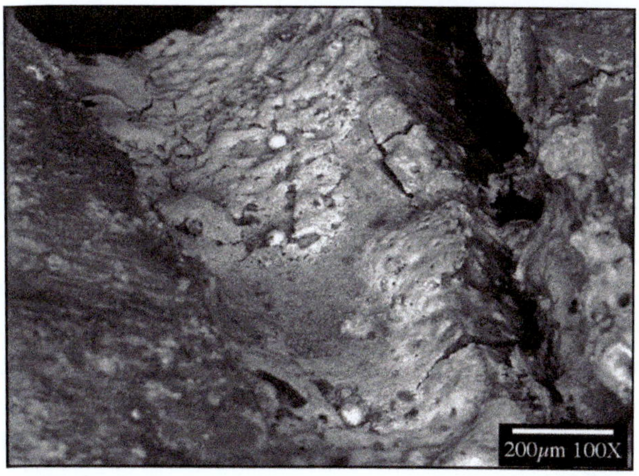

Figure 9.18 200x SEM view of canal of #30 (Universal) root with evidence of silver and paste from root canal sealer.

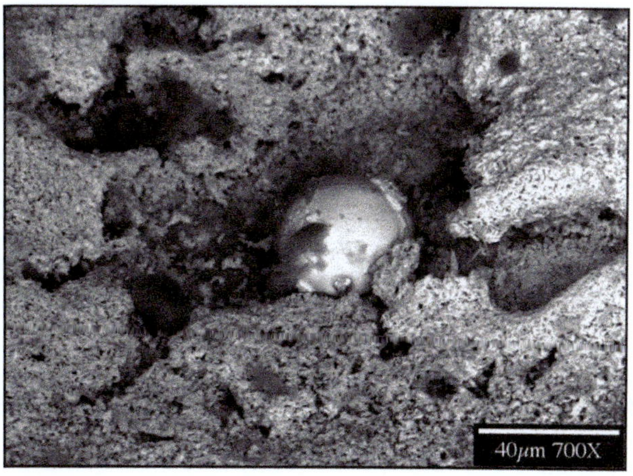

Figure 9.19 700X view of canal of #30 (Universal) root with evidence of silver and paste from root canal sealer.

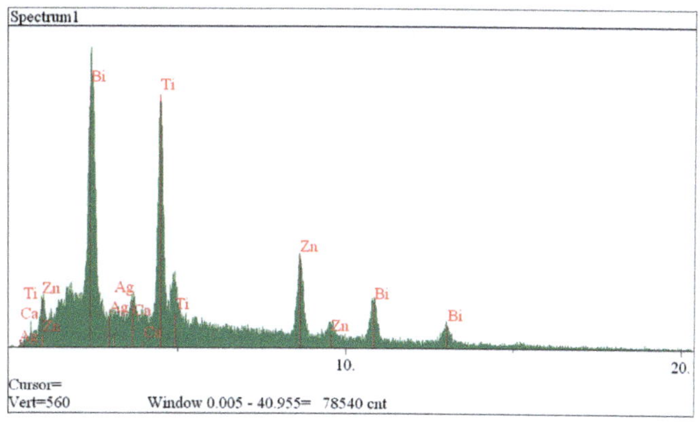

Figure 9.20 Energy Dispersive Spectrogram of root canal sealer from recovered root #30 (Universal).

sealers and the material was associated as to brand. The sealer was identified as AH26 (Dentsply) and the use of this specific sealer was documented in the dental record (Figure 9.21).

Following established disaster victim identification protocols, a thorough database of dental treatments for the presumed victims had been created. This database included only two potential victims with the profile #30 root canal therapy, #31 present, #32 missing (Universal). The AM radiographs (Victim A: Figure 9.22 and Victim B: Figure 9.23) when compared to the PM image (Figure 9.15) based on root anatomy, bone trabeculation, and treatments is more consistent with Victim A; however, it is not conclusive. The additional conformational information of the specific root canal sealer used in the treatment of Victim A provided another level of material evidence to establish a positive identity of this PM fragment being associated with this victim.

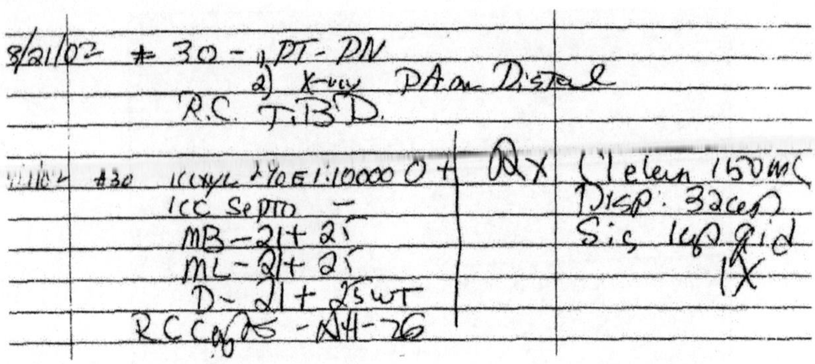
8/21/02 #30 - 1) PT - DN
2) X-ray PA on Distal
R.C. T.B.D.
#30 1:100000
1cc Septo
MB-21+25
ML-21+25
D-21+25WT
RC ... -AH-26
Rx Cleocin 150mg
Disp: 32caps
Sig 1cap qid

Figure 9.21 Presumed victim dental chart note indicating use of AH26 as sealer in tooth #30 (Universal).

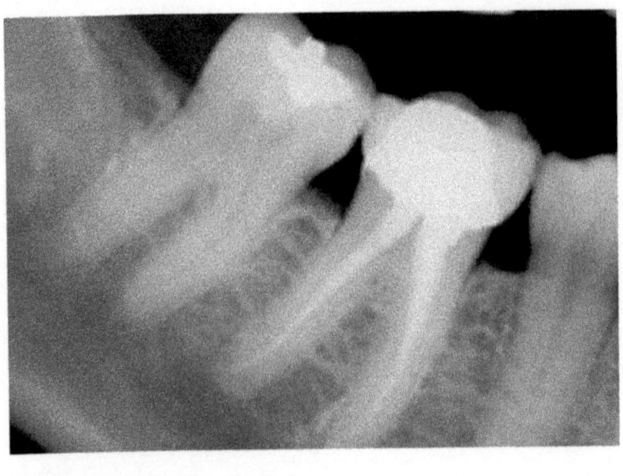

Figure 9.22 Victim A.

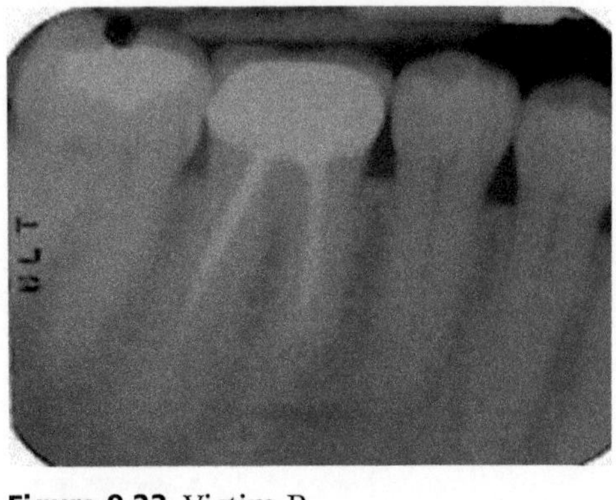

Figure 9.23 Victim B.

9.4.2 Case Report 2: Double Homicide

In the summer of 2011, the incinerated remains of two individuals were discovered on an estate in north-eastern USA. A thorough anthropological recovery uncovered burnt bone fragments, teeth, and dental restorations that were believed to be porcelain laminate veneers (PLVs) of teeth #8 and 9 (Universal) (Figure 9.24). The identification of the two individuals was presumed to be the male and female residents of the home. Skull fragments of each individual revealed beveled, circular injuries consistent with bullet wounds. Homicide was the suspected manner of death.

The female was identified through dental records. There was difficulty in identifying the male victim since the recovered remains were incinerated and unable to yield DNA for analysis. Individual teeth were located but again physical and thermal trauma and lack of adequate dental identifiers did not provide a dental profile sufficient for comparison to AM records.

The recovered PLVs were considered a key to identification, but with no associated tooth structure and the fact that neither individual had these types of restorations it appeared that a conclusive dental identification of the male was not likely. This inability to identify the male caused a suspect's defense attorney to request dismissal of charges for lack of evidence. They proposed the counter theory that the male resident was the actual murderer and the discovered male was another individual. Further analysis of the PLVs was requested. First, the restorations were analyzed by SEM-EDS. This analysis revealed that the restorations contained alumina consistent with alumina-oxide ceramic restorations. Second, stereomicroscopy analysis of the

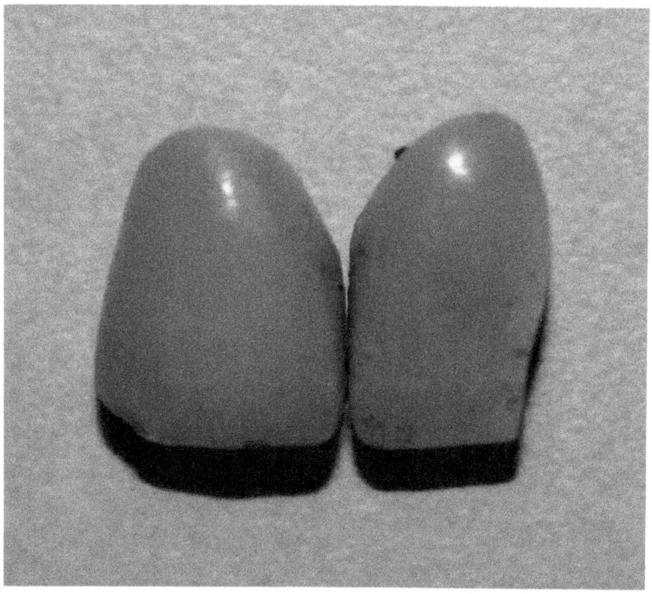

Figure 9.24 Recovered fractured crowns #8, 9 (Universal), labial view.

restoration showed margins consistent with fractures. This, along with shape and size determined that these were actual fractured full coverage crowns and not PLVs. The suspected male victim's AM profile did include full coverage alumina-oxide ceramic crowns #7–10 (FDI) (Figures 9.25 and 9.26). Although material, shape, and size were consistent the data was not sufficient to confirm a positive dental identification.

Fortunately, digital records of the suspected male's prepared teeth were available. These 3D records allowed for the dies to be reproduced. The recovered fractured crowns were adapted to the dental dies of teeth #8 (Universal) (Figures 9.27 and 9.28) and #9 (Universal) (Figures 9.29 and 9.30), exact duplicates of the male victim's prepared teeth, and the marginal and internal adaptation of crowns to

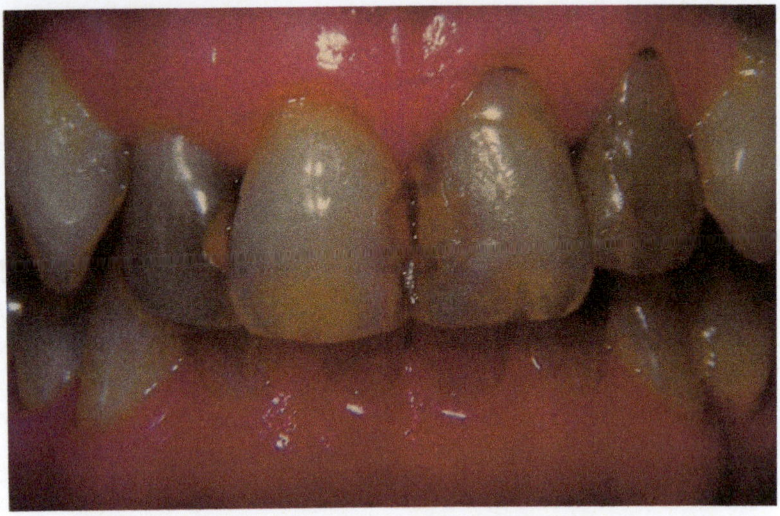

Figure 9.25 Pre-treatment image of presumed homicide victim.

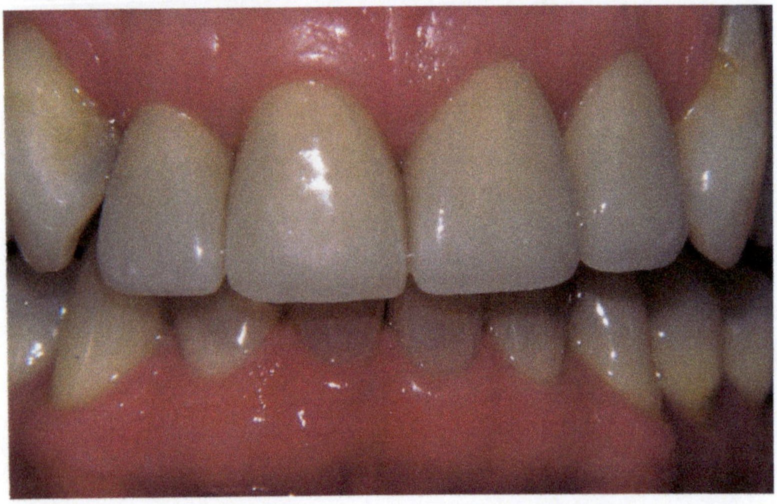

Figure 9.26 Post-treatment Procera® crowns teeth #7, 8, 9, 10 (Universal).

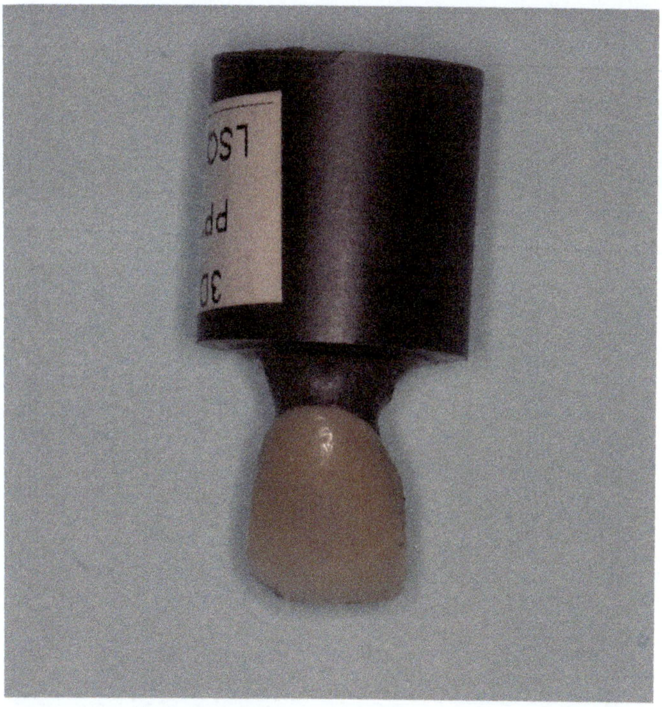

Figure 9.27 Labial view of analogue die of presumptive victim with recovered fractured crown #8 (Universal) seated in place.

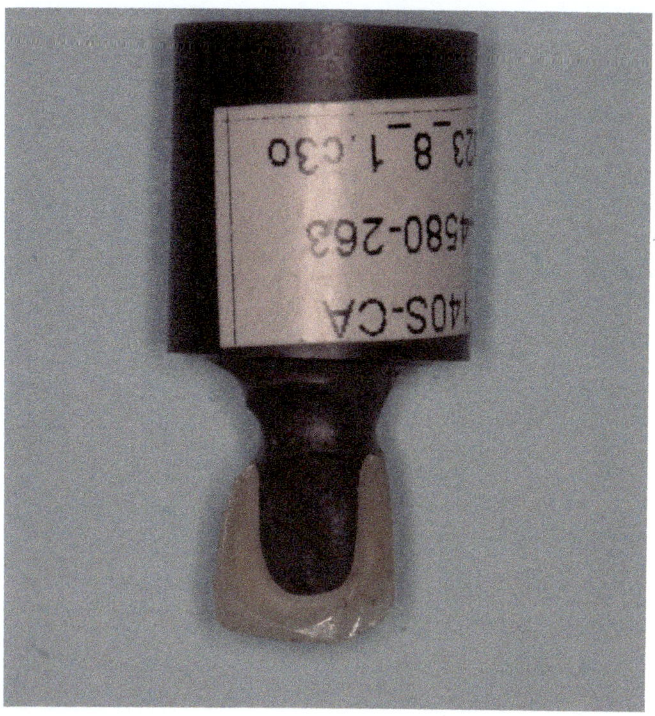

Figure 9.28 Palatal view of analogue die of presumptive victim with recovered fractured crown #8 (Universal) seated in place.

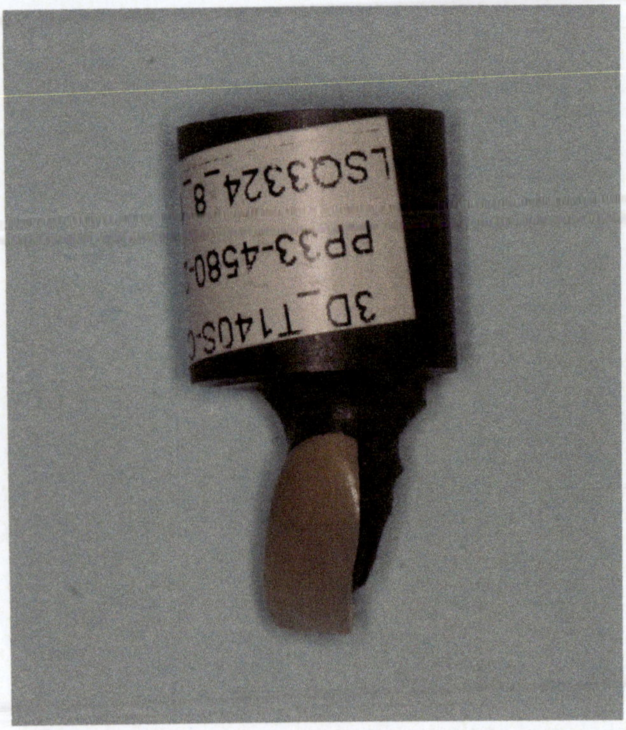

Figure 9.29 Labial view of analogue die of presumptive victim with recovered fractured crown #9 (Universal) seated in place.

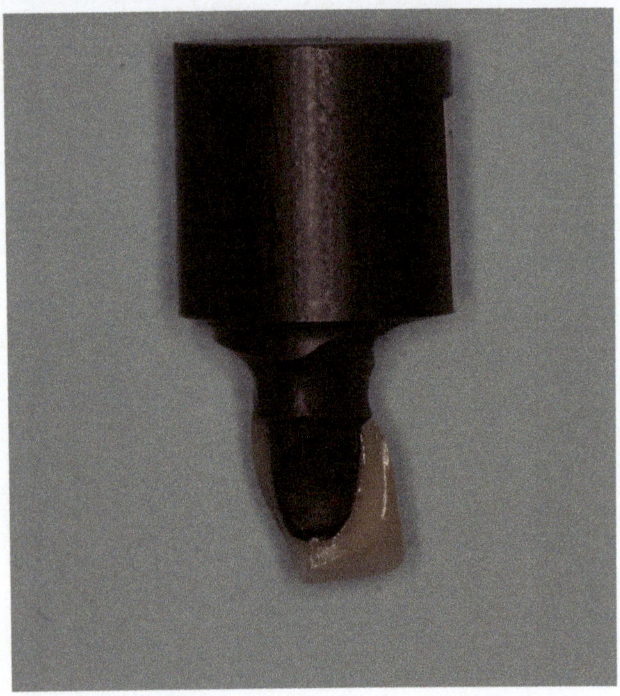

Figure 9.30 Palatal view of analogue die of presumptive victim with recovered fractured crown #9 (Universal) seated in place.

dies was precise and correct. The crowns were determined to be associated with the resident male victim. The material consistency, type of restoration, and exact adaptation of crown to die confirmed a positive dental identification of the male. This identification allowed prosecution of the suspect to proceed, leading to a plea deal and a long prison term.

The incineration and thermal trauma fractured the crowns but did not alter the size or elemental composition of the crowns. This allowed them to be analyzed to determine type of ceramic crown and verify the individuality of the restoration to the presumed victim. The adaption revealed no gaps or marginal discrepancies. The fracturing of the crowns provided a view of internal adaptation of the crown, beyond marginal integrity, to the prepared tooth. This is not normally visualized when determining the fit of a crown to a tooth in clinical practice and further proof of the relationship of the recovered crowns to the presumed male victim. This was despite the suspect's attempts to destroy evidence of the victims through physical and thermal trauma.

9.5 Conclusions

Historically, dental evidence that was severely degraded by incineration or thermal damage rendered data or information that was not of forensic significance. The thermal damage eliminated the DNA or organic evidence. It also altered the clinical and radiographic morphology of the teeth and their restorations. These alterations did not allow for the normal process of radiographic pattern comparison between the AM and PM images. Radiographic comparison has long been the standard for victim identification. When the PM evidence is severely damaged this odontological analysis is eliminated from the identification process.

Now, technology, using SEM/EDS, has discovered that significant information persists despite significant incineration of the dentition. Alterations in tooth morphology and structure, along with tool marks, can be viewed under SEM magnification. Remnants of restorative materials are also discoverable, and through EDS their elemental composition can be determined. This information, which persists through the thermal process, can potentially lead to specific brands of restorative materials being identified. This identification of specific brands, if adequately notated in the dental record, may provide another level of certainty and confirmation in the victim identification process.

Thermally damaged dental evidence significantly degraded by incineration was once thought to be of limited value in victim identification. Research has shown that significant information and PM data can be collected when appropriate technological analysis is applied.

References

Berketa, J.W., Simpson, E., Graves, S., O'Donohue, G., and Liu, Y.L. (2015) The utilization of incinerated hip and knee prostheses for identification. *Forensic Science, Medicine, and Pathology*, **11**(3), 432–437.

Bonavilla, J.D., Bush, M.A., Bush, P.J., and Pantera, E.A. (2008) Identification of incinerated root canal filling materials after exposure to high heat incineration. *Journal of Forensic Sciences*, **53**(2), 412–418.

Bush, M.A., Bush, P.J., and Miller, R.G. (2006) Detection and classification of composite resins in incinerated teeth for forensic purposes. *Journal of Forensic Sciences*, **51**(3), 636–642.

Bush, M.A., Miller, R.G., Norrlander, A.L., and Bush, P.J. (2008) Analytical survey of restorative resins by SEM/EDS and XRF: Databases for forensic purposes. *Journal of Forensic Sciences*, **53**(2), 419–425.

Chesne, A.D., Benthaus, S., and Brinkmann, B. (1999) Forensic identification value of roentgen images in determining tooth-colored dental filling materials. *Archiv fur Kriminologie*, **203**(3–4), 86–90.

Harsanyi, L. (1975) Scanning electron microscopic investigation of thermal damage of the teeth. *Acta Morphologica Academiae Scientiarum Hungaricae*, **23**(4), 271–281.

Muller, M., Berytrand, M.F., Quatrehomme, G., Bolla, M., and Rocca, J.P. (1998) Macroscopic and microscopic aspects of incinerated teeth. *The Journal of Forensic Odonto-stomatology*, **16**(1), 1–7.

Summitt, J.B., Robbins, J.W., and Schwartz, R.S. (2001) *Fundamentals of Operative Dentistry: A Contemporary Approach*. 2nd edn. Quintessence Publishing Company, Batavia, IL.

Ubelaker, D.H. and Jacobs, C.H. (1995) Identification of orthopedic device manufacturer. *Journal of Forensic Science*, **40**(2), 168–170.

CHAPTER 10

Techniques for the Differentiation of Blunt Force, Sharp Force, and Gunshot Traumas from Heat Fractures in Burnt Remains

Hanna Friedlander[1], MA; Megan Moore[2], PhD, D-ABFA and Pamela Mayne Correia[3], MA

[1] *Missing Persons Coordination Unit, Michigan State Police*

[2] *Department of Sociology, Anthropology, and Criminology, Eastern Michigan University*

[3] *Department of Anthropology, University of Alberta*

10.1 Introduction

One of the most consequential roles of the forensic anthropologist is to determine the type and timing of trauma to human bone for medicolegal investigations. This task becomes more complicated when thermal damage (i.e. burning) is involved. Although forces that cause perimortem bone fractures fall along a continuum based on the velocity of the force and the area of the impact (Kroman, 2007; Kroman and Symes, 2013), the forensic anthropologist must endeavor to distinguish between the sometimes subtle trauma signatures of blunt force, sharp force, and high velocity projectiles. The forensic anthropologist must differentiate these trauma signatures on bone in addition to distinguishing whether the timing of the trauma occurred antemortem (exhibiting evidence of healing), perimortem (and possibly relevant to the cause of death), or postmortem (presenting with more brittle fracture characteristics). Ultimately, the bone fractures provide the crucial evidence of this timing, as the biomechanical properties of bone change, based on whether the bone is fresh/wet or dry/burnt when the fracture occurs; however,

Burnt Human Remains: Recovery, Analysis, and Interpretation, First Edition. Edited by Sarah Ellingham, Joe Adserias-Garriga, Sara C. Zapico and Douglas H. Ubelaker.

characteristics of fresh bone fractures can persist well into the postmortem interval. Postmortem thermal damage may mask some of the characteristics of perimortem trauma, but it will not erase the evidence completely. This chapter reviews the biomechanics and characteristics of different types of bone trauma with additional thermal damage to help the practitioner better interpret the type and timing of trauma with thermal damage, and to provide an overview of new techniques, as well as case study examples.

10.2 Bone Fracture Biomechanics: Fresh Bone

The biomechanics of bone fractures are dependent upon the mass and velocity of impact, the bone shape, and the bone material properties. The condition of the bone as either fresh/wet or dry/burnt can alter the material properties and change how fractures propagate through the bone. Living bone is made up of inorganic hydroxyapatite and organic collagen (and other proteins), amorphous polysaccharides, and water, making it both stiff and viscoelastic (Galloway, 1999). As a viscoelastic material, bone material properties will vary between a liquid and a solid state, based on the mass and velocity of impacts (Berryman and Symes, 1998; Symes *et al.*, 2012a; Berryman *et al.*, 2018). This elastic property of fresh bone includes the ability to return to its original shape once a force is removed (Galloway, 1999; Berryman *et al.*, 2012, 2018; Symes *et al.*, 2012a; Moore, 2013; Green and Schultz, 2017). This material strength of bone can be measured in terms of stress (applied force divided by cross-sectional area) and strain (the actual change or deformation in shape) (Frankel and Nordin, 1980). The stiffness of the bone helps fresh bone resist forces of compression, and the ductility and elasticity allow bone to resist forces of tension (Galloway, 1999). When forces are applied to fresh bone beyond the yield point (based on Young's modulus of elasticity), permanent plastic deformation occurs, changing the shape of the bone. As strain causes alterations beyond the failure point, the bone can no longer withstand the forces and will ultimately fracture, failing under the strain (Frankel and Nordin, 1980; Galloway, 1999; Kroman, 2007; Passalacqua and Fenton, 2012; Symes *et al.*, 2012a; Kroman and Symes, 2013; Moore, 2013).

The macroscopic and microscopic shape of bone make it anisotropic, and so it responds differently to forces in different directions. Bone is stronger in compression. It fails first in tension, which is an important consideration for the interpretation of fracture patterns (Berryman and Symes, 1998; Galloway, 1999; Symes *et al.*, 2012a). Macroscopically, long bones are composed of mostly compact cortical bone surrounding a medullary canal, with the epiphyses composed of mostly trabecular bone. Microscopically, this compact bone is composed of Haversian systems (i.e., osteons), which consist of bone matrix cylinders of concentric and circumferential lamellae, with blood vessels along the central canal and interspersed with osteocytes that are connected via fluid-filled networks of canaliculi (Berryman and Haun, 1996; White *et al.*, 2012; Wedel and Galloway, 2014)(see also Chapter 14 of this book). Long bones and irregular bones differ from one another in that cortical bone is the main component of long bones. The heft of cortical bone provides structure and integrity to the skeletal system; the strength stems from the lamellar bone oriented around Haversian canals in alternate directions (Weiner *et al.*, 1999; Vaughan *et al.*, 2012). As bone is remodeled, the primary osteons are replaced by secondary osteons, and the lamellar structure is once again reorganized. This reorganization gives the bone rigidity (Vaughan *et al.*, 2012) that allows bone to respond to forces from various directions, and not to succumb to heavy loads (Berryman and Haun, 1996). The trabecular portion of long bones, which is predominantly longitudinally orientated (Vaughan *et al.*, 2012), is constantly remodeled as well. This lightweight inner portion of bone allows for flexibility and impact resistance from many different angles (Wedel and Galloway, 2014). Cranial bones consist of two layers of cortical bone around a diploic, spongy center. Irregular bones are particularly lightweight and highly vascularized, with one thin cortical layer and dense trabecular centers (White *et al.*, 2012). These variations in bone structure directly impact how force, compression, and deformation occur.

The energy of extrinsic forces of trauma propagate through bone and follow the path of least resistance (Berryman and Symes, 1998; Symes *et al.*, 2012a). As forces build and move across the surface of a bone, stressors rise beyond the failure point and ultimately cause primary fractures. These primary fractures in fresh bone occur at more oblique angles or in a radial pattern, with smooth, sharp edges of the fracture margins (Wheatley, 2008; Cattaneo *et al.*, 2017). An example of a primary fracture in bone is the circular defect of the entrance wound that results from a high-velocity projectile. Secondary fractures radiate from the impact site, and follow the path of least resistance; they circumnavigate Haversian canals and rebound off interstitial fluids and cilia, creating radiating and then tertiary concentric fractures, if the force is great enough (Fairgrieve, 2008; Berryman *et al.*, 2018). As bone loses moisture after death, the viscoelastic quality decreases and the brittleness of bone increases, losing the ability to absorb and dissipate forces (Fairgrieve, 2008; Symes *et al.*, 2012a; Green and Schultz, 2017). The stressors can proceed through the bone directly, with no osteocytic response, or interstitial fluids to dissipate forces to prevent further damage (Moraitis and Spiliopoulou, 2006; Fairgrieve, 2008; Chen *et al.*, 2010). Similarly, organic components and water decrease in bone because of burning, which causes the bone to lose its viscoelastic properties and become more rigid and fragile, no longer able to absorb and dissipate the forces. It responds mechanically as a brittle material.

10.3 Bone Fracture Biomechanics: Stages of Thermal Damage

With thermal damage, the loss of moisture happens rapidly and can alter the bone in shape and chemistry. Thermal damage due to heat exposure occurs in four stages: dehydration, decomposition, inversion, and then fusion (Shipman *et al.*, 1984; Mayne Correia, 1997). Heat-induced changes are typically assessed via color patterns and overall bone degradation, starting with the onset of dehydration and the decomposition of the remains. First, dehydration (i.e. water loss) allows for the propagation of heat fractures and determines the extent of the heat-related damage. The pugilistic pose is the most frequently observed product of dehydration. Muscles, tissues, and ligaments shrink and pull on the skeletal system, especially in the stronger flexor muscles. The pugilistic pose generates fractures on surrounding bones, as arms, legs, hands, and feet, become adducted and flexed (see Figure 10.1). The pulling of the tendons, ligaments, and muscles causes the dehydrated bone to snap under pressure, as the organic matrix of the bone weakens under thermal alteration (Wedel and Galloway, 2014; Symes *et al.*, 2015). Next, decomposition (i.e., removal of organic components from bone witnessed by carbonization) permits direct fracturing, as dehydrated bone has no viscoelasticity to dissipate forces; thus the fractures propagate with less resistance. Then inversion (the loss of all carbonates and the end of the carbonization process) creates shrinking, warping, and general degradation of the bones exposed to heat. Finally, fusion, or the melting of bone crystals, is the last stage, when the structures of bone disintegrate, and the fragility of the new structures is evident in the extensive damage that follows (Dzierzykray-Rogalski, 1967; Herrmann, 1977; Mayne

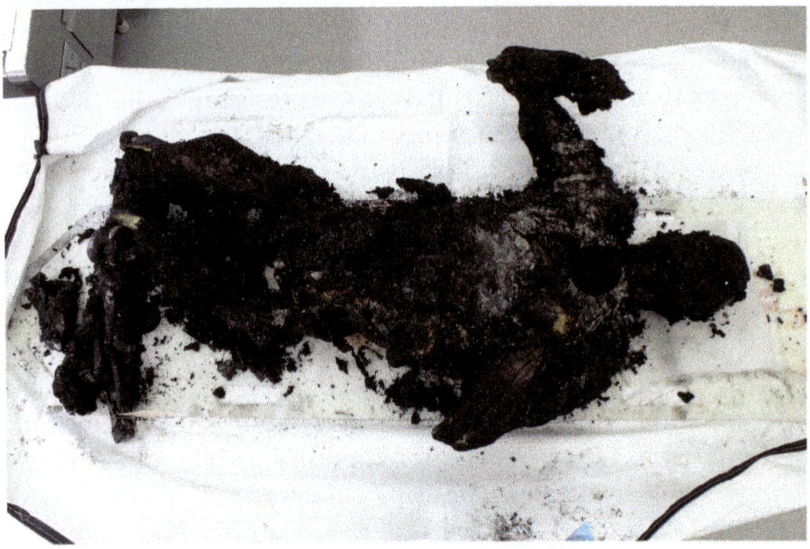

Figure 10.1 Pugilistic pose with heat-related fractures to lower limbs.

Correia, 1997). When inversion and fusion occur, this causes distortion and color changes to bone. Thompson and colleagues (2017) note the importance of the duration that bone is exposed to heat, the amount of oxygen fueling the fire, and whether and how much of an accelerant was used; this can gravely impact the extent of the heat damage.

10.4 Heat Fractures

As organic components dissipate from bone during heating, heat fractures begin to propagate. The dehydration of the bone causes bones to crack, sending rifts through the cortical and trabecular bone layers (Dzierzykray-Rogalski, 1967; Herrmann, 1977; Mayne Correia, 1997; Pope and Smith, 2004). Heat fractures are in essence predictable in their formation – lack of collagen, fluids, and bony response allow heat fractures to develop straight, sharp margins that are crisp and clean (Marella *et al.*, 2012). These fractures do not always propagate across bone entirely and can be superficial or deep depending on the bone type. Irregular bones, for example, have thinner cortical layers, which makes them more susceptible to heat-related breakage. Long bones, on the other hand, are thicker, and take more time to dehydrate and allow heat fractures to form on the surface of the bone. Herrmann and Bennett (1999) point out that the fracture mechanics differ substantially between dry/burnt and wet/unburnt bone; therefore, the fractures should be structurally different. In essence, differentiation of trauma from heat fractures is straightforward depending on the severity of heat exposure.

The general, breakdown of bones that have been exposed to heat is predictable in nature. Long bones, for example, break down systematically (Chamay and Tschantz, 1972). There is noted fracturing, splintering, and warping along the diaphysis of long bones, breaching the cortical bone, and eventually disintegrating the cortical bone (Binford, 1963). Long bones frequently exhibit longitudinal fractures, stepped or transverse fractures, delamination, and curvilinear (or curved transverse) fractures (Symes *et al.*, 2015; Galtés and Scheirs, 2019). The study of this breakdown of long bones is broad and it includes the study of variances in heat exposure, temperatures reached, and musculature present or absent. On the other hand, irregular bones, such as crania, pelves, ribs, and vertebrae are less studied. Irregular bones are predicted to show linear fractures, patina breakage, sharp margins, shrinkage, and warping, as heat fractures dissipate through the bones (Pope and Smith, 2004). Their bony structure is different from their long bone counterparts, which causes differences in their breakdown when exposed to heat. The thinned cortical layers of these bones add to a quicker carbonization process. The exception is with fully fleshed remains, where the pelves, ribs, and vertebrae are protected by thickened musculature (Bohnert *et al.*, 1997). Tissue shielding initially protects some cranial bones under thicker muscles, as with the temporal bones and the cranial base (Baby, 1954; Symes *et al.*, 2015). This does

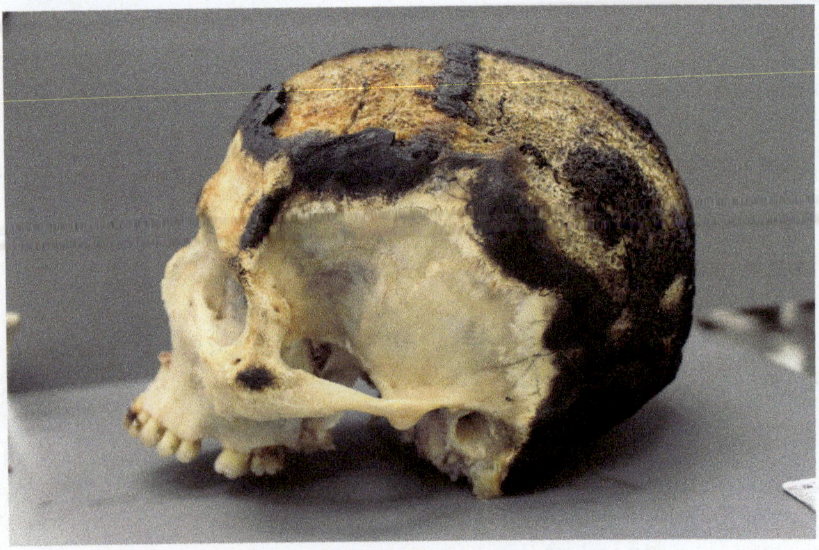

Figure 10.2 Heat-related fractures to cranium exposing diploë.

not, however, stop delamination fractures from occurring across the superficial cranium, as cortical layers flake off in chunks, exposing the diploic interior (see Figure 10.2). Understanding how bones break down when exposed to heat provides direct indicators for the differentiation of various perimortem traumas from heat fractures, as burnt bone can still show remnants of blunt force, sharp force, and gunshot traumas. In most traumas, especially when tissues are present prior to burning, longitudinal and transverse fractures appear typically at a distance from the edge of a wound; this is likely due to soft tissue shrinkage (Collini *et al.*, 2015).

10.5 Blunt Force Trauma in Burnt Remains

Blunt force trauma (BFT) is the result of relatively slow loading forces (e.g., resulting from a fall, interpersonal violence, or from a vehicle accident). BFT typically has a clear impact site and is categorized as abrasions, contusions, lacerations, and depressions caused by the impact of a blunt object (Moraitis and Spiliopoulou, 2006; Symes *et al.*, 2012a). If the force is great enough, BFT causes fracture propagation to occur gradually across the bone, with secondary radiating linear fractures and then tertiary circular concentric fractures (Hart, 2005; Kroman and Symes, 2013). The concentric fractures of the skull will exhibit internally beveled concentric fractures compared to the externally beveled concentric fractures observed in gunshot trauma (GST) (Hart, 2005). BFT in the long bones is characterized by butterfly, avulsion, angulation, or crushing fractures (Galloway, 1999; Symes *et al.*, 2012a). The surface area of contact between a blunt force object and bone causes interstitial fluids to disperse to counteract the damage as the bone is crushed and begins to collapse. Of course, the intrinsic and extrinsic factors of a blunt object and the impact on bone play a crucial role on what trauma is seen. The damage to bone relies largely on the object used (size, shape), the force deployed, and the overall health of the bone (Symes *et al.*, 2012a).

BFT is not seen as a "straight line" wound, like sharp force trauma (SFT) markers. The low velocity impact can have radiating, concentric, and compression fractures that include delamination of bone, internal beveling of concentric fractures, and elastic and plastic deformation (Symes *et al.*, 2012a). Due to the slower velocity in BFT, the microstructure of the fracture surface will not be as smooth as with high velocity projectiles because the bone is able to withstand some of the energy and behave more elastically. As a result, the surface may appear microscopically slightly rough and billowed, with macroscopic evidence of a breakaway spur (Symes *et al.*, 2012a). Passalacqua and Fenton (2012) described the type of trauma in BFT as quasistatic and the roughened surface the result of tortuous fracturing, as the bone resists the stress. The characteristics of the BFT fracture pattern (e.g. contusions, radiating fractures, depressions, internal beveling) and surface features of the fracture margin will still be visible after burning and the application of fractography of the fracture margin may help determine whether the fractures are the result of BFT, thermal damage, or otherwise.

When burned, BFT tends to show extensive charring around the impact site due to exposure of trabecular bone to heat. The transverse, longitudinal, curvilinear, and radiating fractures that stem from the impact site may be partially eroded due to charring. Other times, these fractures can be masked by heat fractures, which will spread through bone until impacted by another fracture line (Galtés and Scheirs, 2019). Scheirs *et al.* (2017) point out that BFT causing compression of bones will leave significant markers, beginning with chipped layers of cortical bone, "waves" (rounded, jagged edges) along long fracture edges, scaling near fracture margins, crushed bone on the cortical surface, and flaking. When BFT is recognized in burnt bone, Galtés and Scheirs (2019) note similar characteristics can still be seen, based on the severity of the heat exposure. Longitudinal fractures, created by both BFT and heat exposure, can be misconstrued if not carefully observed. With an understanding of bone biomechanics, though, it can be concluded that fracture walls which are smooth tend to be traumatic in nature, whereas those which are sharp and abrupt are heat fractures (Herrmann and Bennett, 1999). BFT markers will lose their sharpness, becoming rough and uneven as exposure to heat increases (Macoveciuc *et al.*, 2017). This is a sharp contrast to heat fracture morphology. When assessing BFT in burnt remains, it has been noted that, specifically in depressed fractures, traumas appear larger post-carbonization (Collini *et al.*, 2015). This is due to surface area exposure of the wound.

Koch and Lambert (2017) utilized radiographs and macroscopic examination of SFT, BFT, and GST. The BFT experiment consisted of two pig carcasses that were hit with a sledgehammer on the torso and limbs. Each carcass was then radiographed to document the trauma markers. One pig was subsequently burned for eight minutes, reaching a peak of about 600°C; the second was burned for about 22.5 minutes, reaching a high temperature of about 1000°C. Prior to the burns, it was noted that each pig's limbs were held together largely by scarce skin and tissue, the bones were highly fragmented. Due to the skin/tissue rupture from the sledgehammer, the fire was able to break down the tissues and impact the bone, leaving minimal remains for post-burn analysis. What remained showed extensive heat fractures and longitudinally splintered bones. The torso blows, impacting the ribs, were able to be assessed, unlike the limbs, as the skin was not broken prior to the burn. The protective tissues and skin of the torso kept the ribs largely untouched by the fire (Koch and Lambert, 2017).

Fractography may provide the necessary lexicon for differentiating perimortem BFT from postmortem thermal damage, although it has not yet been validated in burnt bones. Fractography is the study of fracture surfaces as it relates to fracture propagation and is typically used to analyze material failure, first used for the study of glass and ceramics (Christensen *et al.*, 2018). Christensen and colleagues (2018) apply this analytical technique to the analysis of BFT of long bone shafts. This is similar to the method of analyzing the fracture surface topography proposed by Symes *et al.* (2012a) and Galloway and Zephro (2005), who describe the blunt force fracture surfaces as billowy or jagged. Passalacqua and Fenton (2012) described the roughened surface of blunt force fractures as tortuous, resulting from the fresh bone resisting the lower velocity forces before ultimately fracturing. BFT, as interpreted through fractography, starts with a "mirror zone," or relatively smooth area, that turns into a roughened area (identified as "bone hackle") and as the force moves away from the point of impact, the fracture surface becomes more jagged (an area described as "wake features" with discontinuous "arresting ridges") (Christensen *et al.*, 2018) (see Figure 10.3). One benefit of this approach to practitioners is that these features are relatively visible with a naked eye, but can be enhanced with standard light microscopy. Contrast can be increased quickly and inexpensively with fingerprint powder (Christensen *et al.*, 2018). All fracture surfaces should be analyzed and photographed prior to any attempts at reconstruction to verify the presence of these features to determine the impact site and direction of force. Future research should verify whether these features persist after thermal damage and whether they can be differentiated from fractures due to thermal damage, although previous research by Galtés and Scheirs (2019) suggests that the roughened BFT fracture surface characteristics are discernible in burnt bone. It is equally important to determine that heat-related fractures do not mimic these BFT characteristics in fresh bone.

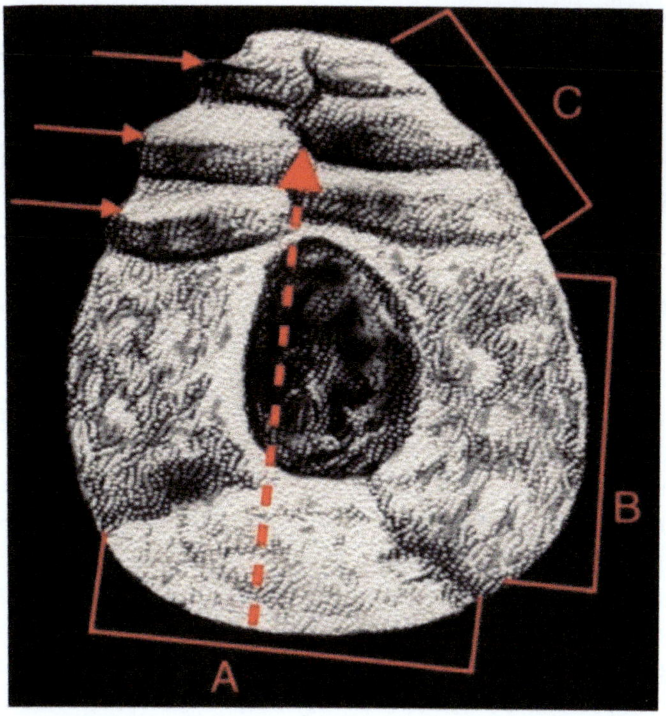

Figure 10.3 Illustration of femoral cross section with characteristics described using fractography. The letter characterizations are as follows: A. Mirror zone, B. Bone Hackle, C. Wake features. The solid arrows represent arrest ridges, while the dotted arrow shows the fracture initiation direction, which is opposite of the direction of force.

10.6 Sharp Force Trauma in Burnt Remains

SFT is essentially BFT with a sharp object (Symes *et al.*, 2002; Kroman and Symes, 2013). SFT can be categorized by weapon class and the characteristics of the weapon to cut, incise, puncture, chop, dent, or crush bone (Kimmerle and Baraybar, 2008). The impact of SFT on bones can cause compression, create a kerf indicative of the implement, and cause raised or curled edges (Symes *et al.*, 2002; Klepinger, 2006; Kimmerle and Baraybar, 2008). Cortical and trabecular bone tissue will respond to SFT differently. Thicker bone will hold the fracture markers better, as the density of the bone will allow for a deep wound to show in depth and length. A thinner bone will crack, splinter, and break as a sharp object pierces it (Wedel and Galloway, 2014). SFT markers are well defined by Symes *et al.* (2012a), indicating that these markers derive from stabbing, cutting, and sawing of bone from a slow velocity. The impact site can be surrounded by radiating, concentric, and compression fractures. These wounds are typically straight in nature and puncture the bone directly. The wound impressions and direct mutilation from the sharp force weapon (Cattaneo and Porta, 2009) produce fracture walls and floors that are distinct, based on weapon type; there are some limitations, however, to the assessment of these wounds (Symes *et al.*, 2012a; Crowder *et al.*, 2013).

In fleshed, burnt remains, the incised flesh can promote heat exposure to the bone and more rapid burning (Waltenberger and Schutkowski, 2017). Kerf floors and walls show significant destruction in that cut marks are skewed and macroscopic analysis cannot always detect SFT markers based on the level of calcination (Waltenberger and Schutkowski, 2017). Marciniak (2009) noted that various saw marks will be seen post-cremation depending on exposure to fire, heat, and bony response. The striae patterns can be seen post-cremation, though distorted, and lead to definitive identification of trauma from heat fractures (Marciniak, 2009; Symes *et al.*, 2012b; Tutor *et al.*, 2020). But, when the fire damage is overwhelming and cortical bone is lost, fracture information can deteriorate and severely decrease the visibility of SFT markers (Kooi and Fairgrieve, 2012). The survivability of SFT markers in burnt bones will vary depending on the weapon utilized. More shallow etchings are more likely to deteriorate or be intertwined with heat fractures due to the superficial nature of the wound (Herrmann and Bennett, 1999), although Emanovsky and colleagues were able to discern shallow SFT in calcined deer bone (Emanovsky *et al.*, 2002).

The most common technology used to assess SFT in burnt remains is stereomicroscopic analysis (SM) technology. Scanning electron microscopy (SEM) technology highlights the signature markers left from SFT traumas, including kerf walls and tool mark striations. SM works to magnify and enhance visualization of SFT marker length and depth in burnt remains. Based on the literature available, high resolution digital microscopy, or SEM assessment of SFT, when combined with SM technology are the primary techniques used to assess SFT markers in burnt bone (Amadasi *et al.*, 2012; Gibelli *et al.*, 2012; Kooi and Fairgrieve, 2012; Robbins *et al.*, 2014; Alunni *et al.*, 2018).

Alunni *et al.* (2018) assessed whether SM technology could accurately identify hacking traumas after burning. They utilized four femurs from eight-month-old piglets, which had been deceased for four days, and fully macerated before thirty lesions were produced via a piston calibrated device. The femora were placed on wooden pyres for ten minutes, until completely carbonized, then cooled for one hour. SEM measurements were taken prior to and after carbonization. Alunni and colleagues (2018) noted that SEM worked well for SFT in both burnt and unburnt bone, revealing specific alterations such as the edge "upraisings." There were no visible vertical striae before or after burning; however, the linear and V-shaped lesions, as well as lateral push back, were easily identifiable. The study concluded that in all cases V-shaped kerfs and "lateral pushing back" were observable after burning via SEM (Alunni *et al.*, 2018).

Kooi and Fairgrieve (2012) used five racks of pig ribs, with the subcutaneous fat removed, and produced two cut marks on each rib: one vertebral and one sternal. The racks were then cut in half to control burning. Approximately 100 SFT markers were created, with 40 being observed post-burning. The ribs were burned in a fish basket for about one hour, until the tissue had completely burned off. The SFT marks were then coated in gold and mounted for SEM analysis. Additionally,

SM analysis was utilized to look for "a linear cut with a V-shaped cross section, the presence or absence of mounding of tissue on either side of the defect, associated fractures arising from the trauma, striations, and wastage." By using SEM, in combination with a stereomicroscope, the authors were able to more readily identify SFT markers, such as V-shaped kerf floors, hinge fractures next to the toolmark, and differentiation of those markers from transverse and longitudinal heat fractures. Though the SFT characteristics decreased post-carbonization, critical features were still viewable via SEM.

10.7 Gunshot Trauma in Burnt Remains

Unlike SFT and BFT, GST is derived from high velocity impact. The high velocity at impact causes the viscoelastic material properties of bone to behave as a brittle material and shatter (Berryman *et al.*, 2012). The rapid propagation of bullets, or items from blast/explosives, can cause plug-and-spall bone fragments to break away from the whole bone, and radiating and concentric fractures move outward from the site of impact. The elasticity, age, and general bone health, in combination with the caliber, weapon type, distance, and positioning of the shooter to victim all play a crucial role in bone reaction to GST. The amount of tissue surrounding the impact site is directly responsible for how secondary fracture propagation will occur (Kimmerle and Baraybar, 2008; Collini *et al.*, 2015; Berryman, 2019). GST is known for its internal and external beveling, seen around the point of impact, where the bone deforms and reacts by bending and breaking, creating clear entrance and exit wounds (Symes *et al.*, 2012a). Common indicators of GST on the cranium are circular defects, keyhole-shaped defects, and gutter-shaped defects that cause displaced bone fragments and beveling, and extensive fragmentation (Berryman, 2019). The overall design of the projectile, including size, determines the impact site damage based on bullet mass and velocity from gun propulsion (Berryman, 2019). GST can cause single or multiple lesions depending on whether a handgun, rifle, or shotgun was used. Directionality of the lesions can be determined by originating fractures from the wound, the keyhole defect (cranial), and beveling (Cattaneo and Porta, 2009).

Macroscopically, tissue thickness and heat exposure ultimately impact what remains from GST in cases of cremation. In a controlled experiment by Collini and colleagues (2015), bovine ribs that were calcined showed round and beveled lesions even after temperatures reached 800°C. Like BFT and SFT, GST will develop heat fractures around the edges of the wound impact site, as well as off the longitudinal and transverse fractures stemming from the GST (Collini *et al.*, 2015). As carbonization shrinks the bone, the GST features can become skewed or even lost. When soft tissues are present, they can pull and conceal morphological GST characteristics (Poppa *et al.*, 2011; Fais *et al.*, 2012). The use of X-ray can help locate bullet(s) and additional fragments. Where the bullet previously caused chipping, flaking, or depressed markers around the entrance/exit wounds, much like BFT, these margins will shrink (therefore enlarging the trauma site), burn, and shatter with advanced heating (Collini *et al.*, 2015). In some instances, where remains are not completely calcined, perimortem fractures stemming from GST show extensive color changes. Symes and colleagues (2015) theorized that this occurs in crania as fluids and tissues push out of the fragmented vault, cooling and slowing the carbonization in these areas. If this is the case, analysis of GST and the surrounding impact site could lead to variances and differentiation of perimortem fractures from heat fractures.

Fais and colleagues (2012) utilized micro-computed tomography (micro-CT) scans to attempt to identify firing distance and differentiation in entrance and exit wounds from GST in burnt bone. Twenty-four sections of human calf, measuring 6 cm each, were shot perpendicular to the skin surface from various distances (5, 15, and 30 cm). The segments were then burned in a wood burning stove for four minutes at 600°C. Once cool, each segment was embedded in resin, cut into 5-micron thick sections and subjected to micro-CT scanning. The authors concluded that the entrance wounds from all distances appeared similar, most likely due to the charring and splitting of soft tissues post-carbonization. Macroscopically, the GST exit wounds mimicked SFT. Micro-CT analysis around the wounds revealed radiopaque material (with a density higher than 1000 HU) visible around the entrance, with no metal particles observed near the exit wound (Fais *et al.*, 2012).

Unfortunately, most of the articles surrounding GST identification in carbonized remains are focused on the detection of gunshot residues (GSR), not identification of the trauma itself. Even beyond that, there are limited studies on GST and GSR evaluations post-cremation. Amadasi and colleagues (2012) were the first to look at SEM/EDX (scanning electron microscope/energy dispersive X-ray spectrometry) for detecting GSR after remains had been burned. The authors worked with 16 adult bovine ribs, cut to approximately 20–27 cm in length and 2–5 cm thick. Eight of the ribs were left covered with muscle; the other eight were macerated. Both unjacketed and full metal-jacketed bullets were used to test projectile type differentiation after cremation. The ribs were burned and cooled over a 24-hour period, with the first 12 hours heating to 800°C, and the last 12 hours left for cooling. All ribs were assessed with SEM/EDX before and after calcination. Upon examination, Amadasi *et al.* (2012) discovered the unjacketed bullets had different entrance wound shapes from full metal-jacketed bullets, but both bullet types left metal residues on and around the entrance wound; however, the unjacketed bullets left more residue particles. Copper (Cu) and Zinc (Zn) are the main components of GST, and lead (Pb), barium (Ba), and antimony (Sb) are the main components of GSR noted in previous SEM/EDX studies (Bai *et al.*, 2007; Amadasi *et al.*, 2012; Fais *et al.*, 2012; Vermeij *et al.*, 2012; Berryman, 2019). Therefore the identification of these particles in this study, after calcination, could allow for the differentiation of ante- and postmortem trauma, or GST identification, in remains where tissues and lesions cannot be macroscopically assessed.

10.8 Case Study: 3D Modelling of Traumatic and Heat Fractures in Cranial and Irregular Bone

Formalin, due to its high combustion rate, was specifically looked at in the study by Friedlander (2018) to determine the applicability of utilizing embalmed human remains as animal substitutes in forensic reconstructions. Two femur samples were used and burned differentially to determine how formalin impacted osteonal structuring, collagen structure, and heat fracture prevalence. By burning samples at various temperatures (see Friedlander, 2018), this study provided results closely aligned with ideas brought about by Mason and O'Leary (1991), stating that formalin has minimal effects on the structure of burnt bone. Gustavson (1947) and Thavarajah *et al.* (2012) came to similar conclusions, claiming formalin does not impact the collagen structure within bones, but instead embeds in the peptides of the collagen, therefore, not constricting or expanding Haversian systems.

The fact that formalin minimally impacts bone structure (and that the combustion of formalin does not dramatically alter burn rates and times) provides validation for formalin fixed bone in additional research on thermally altered bone. Five formalin fixed human calottes and five human hemipelves were used in a second study focused on differentiating heat fractures from BFTs and SFTs in burnt irregular bones (Friedlander, 2018). Prior to carbonization, one of each bone type was

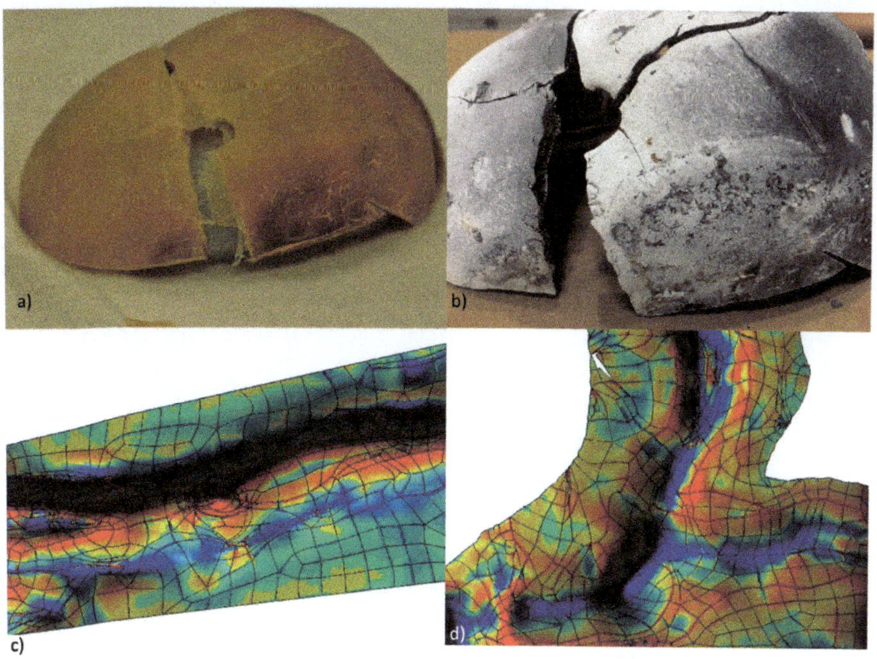

Figure 10.4 A and B show BFT impact pre- and post-carbonization. C highlights the double reverse curvature, seen at points of impact, where the CCM changes from red to dark blue, with a color scale in between, then flips back to red. Conversely, D represents a heat fracture, with minimal color change from red to blue.

set aside as a control, two of each were inflicted with trauma via a tire iron demonstrating BFT (see Figure 10.4a), and two of each with a kitchen knife demonstrating SFT (see Figure 10.5a). All fractures were counted and photographed. The calottes and hemipelves both burned for just over six minutes, with temperatures spanning 350–650°C (see Figures 10.4b and 10.5b). After burning, 180 fractures were counted, with a mix of both traumatic and heat fractures (Friedlander, 2018).

A Keyence VHX-2000 microscope was used for depth analysis photography, magnified between 20x and 50x depending on the visibility of the fracture markers. 3D depth analysis was generated from the bottom of each fracture to the top; this was automatically done by the computer software associated with the Keyence VHX-2000. Exporting each .csv point cloud file from the Keyence and importing it into Geomagic Studio 2014 software allowed for the production of computer-aided design (CAD) models that were saved as .stl files. These files were uploaded into Geomagic Design X 2016, where each polygon underwent non-uniform rational basis spline (NURBS) surfacing. For a more detailed explanation of the methods, please refer to Friedlander (2018). The Accuracy Analyzer™ tool was then utilized to generate curvature color maps (CCMs), which gave visual representation of fracture boundary lines, slopes, and variances in traumatic and heat fracture walls (Friedlander, 2018).

Microscopically, it was evident that traumatic fractures and heat fractures were characteristically different. Traumatic fractures showed variances in the CCMs

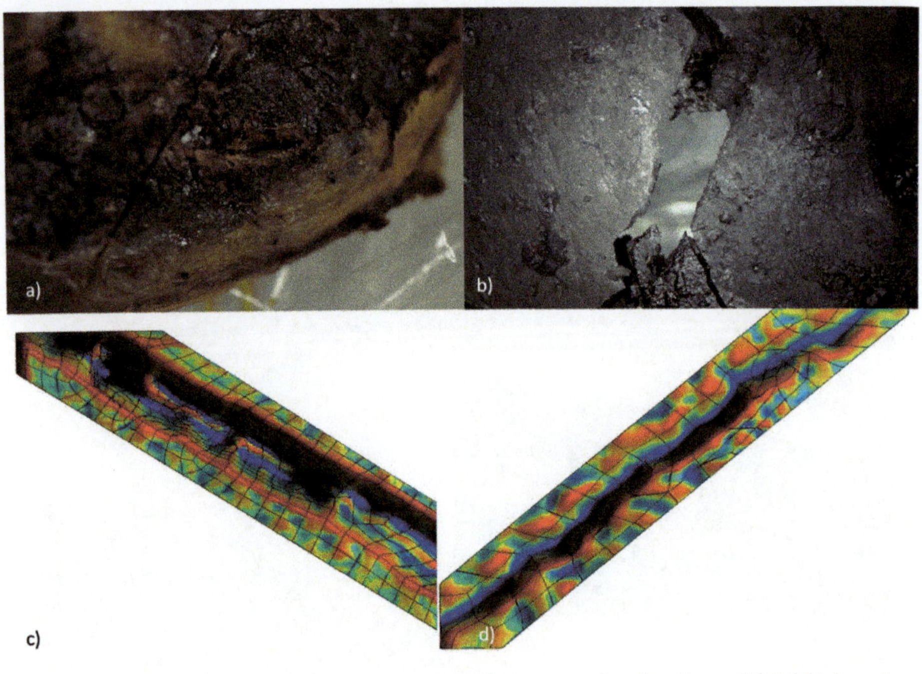

Figure 10.5 A and B show SFT impact, pre- and post- carbonization. C highlights the double reverse curvature, with island features, seen at points of impact, where the CCM changes from red to dark blue, with a color scale in between, then flips back to red. Conversely, D represents a heat fracture, with minimal color change from red to blue.

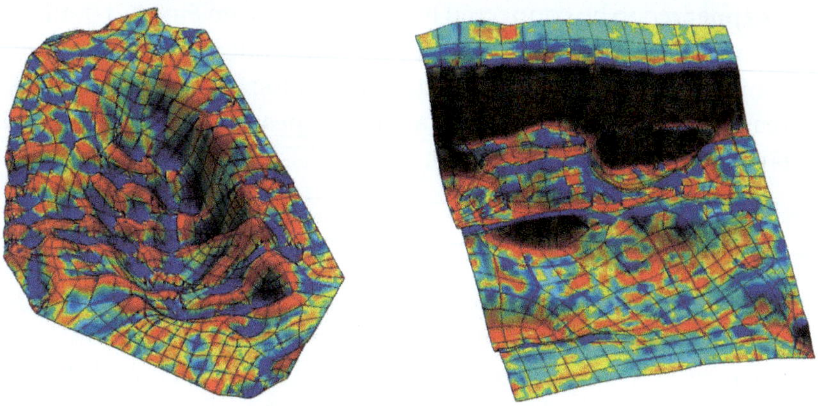

Figure 10.6 Bubble wrap texture of color from shallow SFT.

depending on whether they were from the point of impact, or secondary fractures (Friedlander, 2018). Points of impact showed a double reverse curvature, where the CCM changed from red to dark blue, with a color scale in between, then flipped back to red (see Figures 10.4c and 10.5c). This pattern repeated between the fracture walls. In shallow SFT, the double reverse curvature appeared almost like bubble wrap, with the colors transitioning from red to blue and back again (see Figure 10.6). In BFT and SFT, there are noted "islands" of color as well, where a small double reverse curvature can be seen between the fracture walls (see Figures 10.5c and 10.7) . This is most commonly seen in secondary fractures. There is a large gradient from red to dark blue, where each color in between can be seen. Conversely, heat fractures tended to drastically change from red to dark blue, with minimal variation in between (see Figures 10.4d and 10.5d). Some heat fractures showed a pinching pattern at the base of the fracture walls, where the two

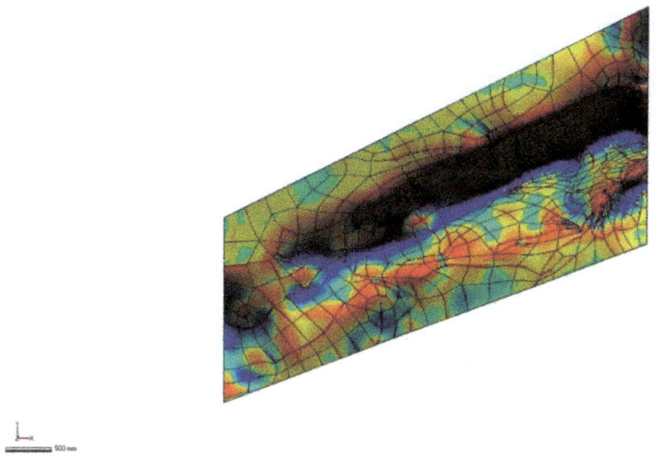

Figure 10.7 "Islands" of color with a small double reverse curvature can be seen between the trauma related fracture walls.

fracture walls appeared to be connected by a line of red (see Figure 10.4d). Successful qualitative analysis was documented in this experiment; however, quantitative analysis attempts failed, possibly due to the technology used and possibly due to a need for greater examination of the fracture slopes, patterns, and general morphology seen on the CCMs (Friedlander, 2018).

10.9 Discussion

A variety of technologies/methodologies used to differentiate traumatic fractures from heat fractures exist (fractography, SM, SEM, micro-CT, and 3D modeling); however, the most used methodology appears to be a combination of SM and SEM technology. Although SM and SEM allows for greater fracture detail and visualization, they are destructive processes that inhibit further examination afterwards and are cost prohibitive to most practitioners. In cases of SFT, SM technology can highlight traumatic markers in kerf walls, kerf floors, and striations, as well as show tooth markers from saw blades. SEM, on the other hand, has revealed various metallic residues in SFT wounds, as shown by Gibelli and colleagues (2012), in which sharp tools left metal particles in the walls of the fractures as tools were inserted into and pulled out of bones. The authors theorize the location of these particles could even lead to a possibility of weapon class identification (Gibelli *et al.*, 2012).

In GST studies, SEM/EDX has been proven in cases of cremation to illuminate GSR. Amadasi and colleagues (2012) showed that even as the temperature rose to 800°C, and bones became calcified, GSR was still able to be detected. This means, regardless of macroscopic assessment of GST, if SEM/EDX can pick up on metal particles known to be associated largely with bullets, GST may be present. The limitation of this is the possibility of contamination to the samples analyzed. The particle size, shape, and morphology found around the entrance wounds in this study could be used to locate entrance wounds in otherwise unrecognizable GST samples. Unfortunately, for the purposes of this review, there is a lack of literature on SEM and SEM/EDX technology utilized on burnt remains impacted by BFT.

Of course, SEM and SEM/EDX have limitations, primarily surrounding the cleaning of remains and samples, the recognition of particles in the machinery, and contamination of metal residues from outside sources. The microtraces of samples caused from SFT, BFT, and GST show gray in color, whereas bone particles and organic materials appear black when set to standards developed by Vermeij and colleagues (2012). Any cleaning done to remains, prior to SEM or SEM/EDX processing, including maceration, chemicals, and insects for cleaning can erode particles and residues from the fragment edge(s). Likewise, understanding the particle composition, size, shape, and color is critical to completing SEM and SEM/EDX analysis. Vermeij and colleagues (2012) state that even bone dust particles, if not assessed properly, can mimic aluminum particles. Finally, the contamination of fragments from other metals, while cleaning or excavating remains, can leave secondary transfer particles on the remains' surface. This can skew results and analysis of SEM and SEM/EDX (Vermeij *et al.*, 2012).

Micro-CT scans are non-destructive and allow for detailed assessment of bone surfaces. Imaizumi (2015) was able to use micro-CT scans to assess the Haversian and lamellar patterns of burnt bone to study how heat impacts bone on a histological level. Alunni and colleagues (2018) tested SFT and micro-CT analysis, proving in some instances that SFT markers can still be seen post-cremation. Thermal damage does not seem to impact the ability of micro-CT scans to aid in the identification of SFT. Micro-CT, in this study, highlighted new fossae formations around the inner cortical layer of bone where the trauma markers were located. Alunni and colleagues (2018) stated in their study that V-shaped kerf walls and lateral push back of bone were visible in all their carbonization and calcination samples. However, Waltenberger and Schutkowski (2017) caution that the floor angles of knife marks have not been well documented or studied under thermal alteration, and irregularities in their alteration may be evident. There are no current correlations between floor angle alteration and carbonization, due to limited studies in this area. The literature falls short in the assessment of BFT with micro-CT analysis of burnt remains. Fractography shows promise for this area of research, by identifying the area of impact from the fracture margin and identifying the "mirror zone," "bone hackle," and "wake features" that indicate the direction of force, but this analytical method must be demonstrated to be observable after post-mortem thermal damage.

Fais and colleagues (2012) determined micro-CT analysis can estimate firing range and aid in the identification of entrance and exit wounds from GST. Even when the bullet track was not detected, metallic residues were located. Those portions of bone where residues were found were conclusively identified as the entrance wound, where the exit wound and tested stab wounds showed no metallic residues. Poppa *et al.* (2011) used neutron activation analysis (NAA) to aid in quantifying the metallic particles left in gunshot wounds. This was combined with high-heat environments to see if thermal damage would alter the GSR. The authors were able to successfully identify and quantify the traces of particles in the carbonized samples. Compared to SEM technology, when micro-CT was tested to see if metallic residues could be identified from both SFT and GST, there were no noted particles found according to Galtés and Scheirs (2019). So, although in-depth and non-destructive, micro-CT is expensive, time consuming, and presents limitations in the ability to recognize metallic residues that are important in trauma analysis.

A new solution, which is non-destructive and easy to replicate, is presented in the Friedlander (2018) case study. The 3D models allow for a colorful, in-depth analysis of fracture walls in blunt force, sharp force, and heat-related fractures. Variances in the CCM models were evaluated and show differences in the way trauma and heat fractures are visualized. In particular types of trauma, such as a stab wound where a double reverse curvature mimicking bubble wrap is seen, or a BFT fracture in which the trauma penetrates through the bone completely, leaving only a waterfall of color, trauma fractures can look similar to one another, with minute differences in how the CCM is presented. This can be problematic when trying to discern the type of trauma fracture seen; however, the method still provides a way for the differentiation of trauma from heat fractures. Heat fractures are noted to have common characteristics not seen on traumatic fractures, such as a quick digression from red to dark blue on the CCM. There are outliers found in this study, which need to be acknowledged, as in some instances, deeper heat fractures looked very similar to traumatic fractures. As this is the only current use of 3D CAD modelling of traumatic and heat fractures in bone, there are some notable limitations; however, this study opens new avenues of research for future fracture differentiation studies.

Perhaps the largest limitation surrounding trauma differentiation from heat fractures relies on the trauma itself. In some cases of SFT and BFT, the weapon simply does not damage the bone, only the soft tissues; therefore, SFT, BFT, and GST will not be evident if the impact only damages soft tissues. This concealment is unavoidable, but inevitably skews the anthropological assessment of the remains (Tutor *et al.*, 2020) and is a reminder that the absence of evidence is not the evidence of absence (Wright, 1888).

10.10 Conclusions

Thermal alteration of bone is a highly studied topic within forensic anthropology, especially in terms of how the biomechanical material properties of bone change with heat. Thermal damage from heat causes bone to dehydrate, decompose, shrink and warp, change color, and eventually melt the crystalline structure. These changes in the material properties weaken the ability of bone to resist forces, leading to additional heat-related fractures. These heat-related fractures can confound the analysis of perimortem trauma and the research presented here suggests that a variety of technologies are available to discern the type and timing of fractures in burnt bone, with some limitations for each of these methods. It is evident that tested methods, such as SEM, SEM/EDX, micro-CT scans, and 3D modelling can be useful in identifying trauma. Though, in some instances, these methodologies have not been tested on various trauma types, combined with carbonization. For example, the current technologies heavily rely on particle identification from weapon types, especially in SFTs and GSTs. These methodologies are not tested on BFT, which begs the question of whether BFT is too unique to be mistaken for anything other than what it is, or does the thermal damage alter the bone too much to properly study BFT under SEM, SEM/EDX, micro-CT, and 3D CAD modelling?

New methods and techniques need to be established to better aid forensic anthropologists on the determination of trauma from heat fractures in cases of cremation. While burn patterns are useful to overall circumstances of death, especially in determining the cause of death (Bytheway *et al.*, 2014), burn patterns are not enough to definitively aid in the discrimination of trauma and heat fractures. Based on the literature, it can be argued that various traumas, or markers for those traumas such as gunshot residue, survive high-burn temperatures. It is clear that tissues protect deep traumas as well, in cases of incomplete cremation. By incorporating technology into the assessment of burnt human remains, particularly those which are skeletonized, the forensic anthropologist has a wider tool kit at their disposal to better study, identify, and classify trauma types, traumatic fractures, and heat fractures in cases of cremation.

Acknowledgments

A special recognition to the individuals from the cases described herein and to the many missing and unidentified individuals and their families. Dr. Jeffrey Jentzen and Dr. Carl Schmidt of the UM Department of Pathology, MI, and all the pathologists, autopsy technicians, and the medical examiner investigators who provided their assistance and expertise in the analysis of these cases. To the work and dedication of the Michigan State Police towards solving their missing and unidentified persons cases and aiding local law enforcement agencies in this effort as well. A debt of gratitude is owed to Jason Papirny, the Anatomical Gift Program (AGP) coordinator for the University of Alberta, and the professors who aided in the highlighted case study of this chapter from the Department of Anthropology, Civil Engineering, and Division of Anatomy. Finally, thank you very much to our family and friends for all their help and support. We appreciate all you do.

Permissions

Permission for the use of the images in this chapter were granted by donors and/or medical examiner personnel, amidst anonymization of the individuals.

References

Alunni, V., Nogueira, L., and Quatrehomme, G. (2018) Macroscopic and stereomicroscopic comparison of hacking trauma of bones before and after carbonization. *International Journal of Legal Medicine*, **132**(2), 643–648. https://doi.org/10.1007/s00414-017-1649-8.

Amadasi, A., Brandone, A., Rizzi, A., Mazzarelli, D., and Cattaneo, C. (2012) The survival of metallic residues from gunshot wounds in cremated bone: A SEM–EDX study. *International Journal of Legal Medicine*, **126**(4), 525–531. https://doi.org/10.1007/s00414-011-0661-7.

Baby, R.S. (1954) Hopewell cremation practices. *Ohio Historical Society Papers in Archaeology*, **1**, 1–8.

Bai, R., Wan, L., Li, H., Zhang, Z., and Ma, Z. (2007) Identify the injury implements by SEM/EDX and ICP-AES. *Forensic Science International*, **166**(1), 8–13. https://doi.org/10.1016/j.forsciint.2006.03.008.

Berryman, H.E. (2019) A systematic approach to the interpretation of gunshot wound trauma to the cranium. *Forensic Science International*. https://doi.org/10.1016/j.forsciint.2019.05.019.

Berryman, H.E. and Haun, S.J. (1996) Applying forensic techniques to interpret cranial fracture patterns in an archaeological specimen. *International Journal of Osteoarchaeology*, **6**(1), 2–9.

Berryman, H.E. and Symes, S.A. (1998) Recognizing gunshot and blunt cranial trauma through fracture interpretation. In: *Forensic Osteology: Advances in the Identification of Human Remains*, 2nd edn. (ed. K.J. Reichs). Charles C. Thomas, Springfield, IL, pp. 333–352.

Berryman, H.E., Lanfear, A.K., and Shirley, N.R. (2012) The biomechanics of gunshot trauma to bone: Research considerations within the present judicial climate. In: *A Companion to Forensic Anthropology* (ed. D.C. Dirkmaat). Wiley-Blackwell, Chichester, UK, pp. 390–399.

Berryman, H.E., Berryman, J.F., and Saul, T.B. (2018) Bone trauma analysis in a forensic setting. *Forensic Anthropology*, 213–234. https://doi.org/10.1002/9781119226529.ch11.

Binford, L.R. (1963) An analysis of cremations from three Michigan sites. *Wisconsin Archaeology*, **44**(2), 98–110.

Bohnert, M., Rost, T., Faller-Marquardt, M., Ropohl, D., and Pollak, S. (1997) Fractures of the base of the skull in charred bodies – Post-mortem heat injuries or signs of mechanical traumatisation? *Forensic Science International*, **87**(1), 55–62.

Bytheway, J.A., Larison, N.C., and Ross, A.H. (2014) Recognition of atypical burn patterns and pre-cremation blunt force trauma observed on human remains in two forensic cases in the United States. *Anthropology*, **2**(5), 136. https://doi.org/10.4172/2332-0915.1000136.

Cattaneo, C., Cappella, A., and Cunha, E. (2017) Post mortem anthropology and trauma analysis. In: *P5 Medicine and Justice: Innovation, Unitariness and Evidence* (ed. S.D. Ferrara). Springer, Switzerland, pp. 166–179.

Cattaneo, C. and Porta, D. (2009) Trauma analysis of skeletal remains. *Wiley Encyclopedia of Forensic Science*. https://doi.org/10.1002/9780470061589.fsa461.

Chamay, A. and Tschantz, P. (1972) Mechanical influences in bone remodeling. Experimental research on Wolff's law. *Journal of Biomechanics*, **5**(2), 173–180.

Chen, J., Liu, C., You, L., and Simmons, C.A. (2010) Boning up on Wolff's Law: Mechanical regulation of the cells that make and maintain bone. *Journal of Biomechanics*, **43**(1), 108–118.

Christensen, A.M., Hefner, J.T., Smith, M.A., Webb, J.B., Bottrell, M.C., and Fenton, T.W. (2018) Forensic fractography of bone: A new approach to skeletal trauma analysis. *Forensic Anthropology*, **1**(1), 32–51.

Collini, F., Amadasi, A., Mazzucchi, A., Porta, D., Regazzola, V.L., Garofalo, P., *et al.* (2015) The erratic behavior of lesions in burnt bone. *Journal of Forensic Sciences*, **60**(5), 1290–1294.

Crowder, C., Rainwater, C.W., and Fridie, J.S. (2013) Microscopic analysis of sharp force trauma in bone and cartilage: A validation study. *Journal of Forensic Sciences*, **58**, 1119–1126.

Dzierzykray-Rogalski, T. (1967) New methods of investigation of bone remains from cremation graves. *Anthropologie*, **4**(3), 41–45.

Emanovsky, P.D., Hefner, J.T., and Dirkmaat, D.C. (2002) *Identification of Sharp Force Trauma in burned remains utilizing Odocoileus virginianus as a Valid Research Tool*. Poster presented at American Academy of Forensic Science 54th Annual Meeting. American Academy of Forensic Sciences, Atlanta, Georgia.

Fairgrieve, S.I. (2008) *Forensic Cremation: Recovery and Analysis*. CRC Press, Boca Raton, FL.

Fais, P., Giraudo, C., Boscolo-Berto, R., Amagliani, A., Miotto, D., Feltrin, G., *et al.* (2012) Micro-CT features of intermediate gunshot wounds severely damaged by fire. *International Journal of Legal Medicine*, **127**(2), 419–425. https://doi.org/10.1007/s00414-012-0775-6.

Frankel, V.H. and Nordin, M. (eds.). (1980) *Basic Biomechanics of the Skeletal System*. Lea and Febiger, Philadelphia, PA.

Friedlander, H. (2018) Differentiation of perimortem trauma from heat fractures in cranial and irregular bones in cases of cremation. Master thesis. University of Alberta.

Galloway, A. (ed.). (1999) *Broken Bones: Anthropological Analysis of Blunt Force Trauma*. Charles C. Thomas, Springfield, IL.

Galloway, A. and Zephro, L. (2005) Skeletal trauma analysis of the lower extremity. In: *Forensic Medicine of the Lower Extremity: Human Identification and Trauma Analysis of the Thigh, Leg and Foot* (eds. J. Rich, D.E. Dean, and R.H. Powers). Humana Press Inc., Totowa, pp. 253–277.

Galtés, I. and Scheirs, S. (2019) Differentiation between perimortem trauma and heat-induced damage: The use of perimortem traits on burnt long bones. *Forensic Science, Medicine & Pathology*, **15**(3), 453–457. https://doi.org/10.1007/s12024-019-00118-1.

Gibelli, D., Mazzarelli, D., Porta, D., Rizzi, A., and Cattaneo, C. (2012) Detection of metal residues on bone using SEM-EDS – Part II: Sharp force injury. *Forensic Science International*, **223**(1–3), 91–96. https://doi.org/10.1016/j.forsciint.2012.08.008.

Green, A.E. and Schultz, J.J. (2017) An examination of the transition of fracture characteristics in long bones from fresh to dry in central Florida: Evaluating the timing of injury. *Journal of Forensic Sciences*, **62**(2), 282–291.

Gustavson, K.H. (1947) Note on the reaction of formaldehyde with collagen. *Journal of Biological Chemistry*, **169**(3), 531–537.

Hart, G.O. (2005) Fracture pattern interpretation in the skull: Differentiating blunt force from ballistics trauma using concentric fractures. *Journal of Forensic Sciences*, **50**(6), 1276–1281.

Herrmann, B. (1977) On histological investigations of cremated human remains. *Journal of Human Evolution*, **6**(2), 101–103.

Herrmann, N.P. and Bennett, J.L. (1999) The differentiation of traumatic and heat-related fractures in burned bones. *Journal of Forensic Sciences*, **44**(3), 461–469.

Imaizumi, K. (2015) Forensic investigation of burnt human remains. *Research and Reports in Forensic Medical Science*, **5**, 67–74.

Kimmerle, E.H. and Baraybar, J.P. (eds.). (2008) *Skeletal Trauma: Identification of Injuries Resulting from Human Rights Abuse and Armed Conflict*. Taylor & Francis, Boca Raton, FL.

Klepinger, L.L. (2006) Trauma. In: *Fundamentals of Forensic Anthropology* (eds. M. Cartmill and K. Brown). Wiley-Liss, Hoboken, NJ, pp. 101–116.

Koch, S. and Lambert, J. (2017) Detection of skeletal trauma on whole pigs subjected to a fire environment. *Journal of Anthropology Reports*, **2**(1), 113.

Kooi, R.J. and Fairgrieve, S.I. (2012) SEM and stereomicroscopic analysis of cut marks in fresh and burned bone. *Journal of Forensic Sciences*, **58**(2), 452–458. https://doi.org/10.1111/1556-4029.12050.

Kroman, A. (2007) Fracture biomechanics of the human skeleton. Doctoral dissertation, University of Tennessee, Knoxville, TN.

Kroman, A.M. and Symes, S.A. (2013) Investigation of skeletal trauma. In: *Research Methods in Human Skeletal Biology* (eds. E.A. DiGangi and M.K. Moore). Academic Press, San Diego, CA, pp. 219–239.

Macoveciuc, I., Márquez-Grant, N., Horsfall, I., and Zioupos, P. (2017) Sharp and blunt force trauma concealment by thermal alteration in homicides: An in-vitro experiment for methodology and protocol development in forensic anthropological analysis of burnt bones. *Forensic Science International,* **275**, 260–271. https://doi.org/10.1016/j.forsciint.2017.03.014.

Marciniak, S. (2009) A preliminary assessment of the identification of saw marks on burned bone. *Journal of Forensic Sciences,* **54**(4), 779–785.

Marella, G.L., Perfetti, E., and Arcudi, G. (2012) Differential diagnosis between cranial fractures of traumatic origin and explosion fractures in burned cadavers. *Journal of Forensic and Legal Medicine,* **19**(3), 175–178.

Mason, J.T. and O'Leary, T.J. (1991) Effects of formaldehyde fixation on protein secondary structure: A calorimetric and infrared spectroscopic investigation. *Journal of Histochemistry & Cytochemistry,* **39**(2), 225–229.

Mayne Correia, P. (1997) Fire modification of bone: A review of the literature. In: *Forensic Taphonomy: The Postmortem Fate of Human Remains* (eds. W.D. Haglund and M.H. Sorg). CRC Press, Boca Raton, FL, pp. 275–293.

Moore, M.K. (2013) Functional morphology and medical imaging. In: *Research Methods in Human Skeletal Biology* (eds. E.A. DiGangi and M.K. Moore). Academic Press, San Diego, CA, pp. 397–424.

Moraitis, K. and Spiliopoulou, C. (2006) Identification and differential diagnosis of perimortem blunt force trauma in tubular long bones. *Forensic Science, Medicine & Pathology,* **2**(4), 221–230. https://doi.org/10.1385/fsmp:2:4:221.

Passalacqua, N.V. and Fenton, T.W. (2012) Developments in skeletal trauma: Blunt-force trauma. In: *A Companion to Forensic Anthropology* (ed. D.C. Dirkmaat). Wiley-Blackwell, Chichester, UK, pp. 400–411.

Pope, E.J. and Smith, O.C. (2004) Identification of traumatic injury in burned cranial bone: An experimental approach. *Journal of Forensic Sciences,* **49**(3), 1–10.

Poppa, P., Porta, D., Gibelli, D., Mazzucchi, A., Brandone, A., Grandi, M., *et al.* (2011) Detection of blunt, sharp force and gunshot lesions on burnt remains: A cautionary note. *The American Journal of Forensic Medicine and Pathology,* **32**(3), 275–279. https://doi.org/10.1097/PAF.0b013e3182198761.

Robbins, S., Fairgrieve, S., and Oost, T. (2014) Interpreting the effects of burning on pre-incineration saw marks in bone. *Journal of Forensic Sciences,* **60**(Suppl 1), S182–S187. https://doi.org/10.1111/1556-4029.12580.

Scheirs, S., Malgosa, A., Sanchez-Molina, D., Ortega-Sánchez, M., Velázquez-Ameijide, J., Arregui-Dalmases, C., *et al.* (2017) New insights in the analysis of blunt force trauma in human bones. Preliminary results. *International Journal Legal Medicine,* **131**(3), 867–875.

Shipman, P., Foster, G., and Schoeninger, M. (1984) Burnt bones and teeth: An experimental study of color, morphology, crystal structure and shrinkage. *Journal of Archaeological Science,* **11**, 307–325.

Symes, S.A., L'Abbé, E.N., Chapman, E.N., Wolff, I., and Dirkmaat, D.C. (2012a) Interpreting traumatic injury from bone in medicolegal investigations. In: *A Companion to Forensic Anthropology* (ed. D.C. Dirkmaat). Wiley-Blackwell, Chichester, UK, pp. 340–389.

Symes, S.A., Dirkmaat, D.C., Ousley, S., Chapman, E., and Cabo, L. (2012b) Recovery and interpretation of burned human remains. Final technical report. National Institute of Justice Award Number #2008-DN-BX-K131.

Symes, S.A., Rainwater, C.W., Chapman, E.N., Gipson, D.R., and Piper, A.L. (2015) Patterned thermal destruction in a forensic setting. In: *The Analysis of Burned Human Remains* (eds. C.W. Schmidt and S.A. Symes). Academic Press, London, UK, pp. 17–59. https://doi.org/10.1016/b978-0-12-800451-7.00002-4.

Symes, S.A., Williams, J.A., Murray, E.A., Hoffman, J.M., Holland, T.D., Saul, J.M., *et al.* (2002) Taphonomic context of sharp-force trauma in suspected cases of human mutilation and dismemberment. In: *Advances in Forensic Taphonomy: Method, Theory, and Archaeological Perspectives* (eds. W.D. Haglund and M.H. Sorg). CRC Press, Boca Raton, FL, pp. 403–434.

Thavarajah, R., Mudimbaimannar, V., Elizabeth, J., Rao, U., and Ranganathan, K. (2012) Chemical and physical basics of routine formaldehyde fixation. *Journal of Oral and Maxillofacial Pathology*, **16**(3), 400–405.

Thompson, T.J., Gonçalves, D., Squires, K., and Ulguim, P. (eds.). (2017) Thermal alteration to the body. In: *Taphonomy of Human Remains: Forensic Analysis of the Dead and the Depositional Environment* (eds. E.M.J. Schotsmans, N. Márquez-Grant, and S.L. Forbes). Wiley, Chichester, UK, pp. 318–334. https://doi.org/10.1002/9781118953358.ch21.

Tutor, P.M., Márquez-Grant, N., Rojas, C.V., García, A.M., Guzmán, I.P., and Sánchez, M.B. (2020) Through fire and flames: Post-burning survival and detection of dismemberment-related toolmarks in cremated cadavers. *International Journal of Legal Medicine*, **135**, 1–15.

Vaughan, T., McCarthy, C., and McNamara, L. (2012) A three-scale finite element investigation into the effects of tissue mineralisation and lamellar organisation in human cortical and trabecular bone. *Journal of the Mechanical Behavior of Biomedical Materials*, **12**, 50–62.

Vermeij, E.J., Zoon, P.D., Chang, S.B.C.G., Keereweer, I., Pieterman, R., and Gerretsen, R.R.R. (2012) Analysis of microtraces in invasive traumas using SEM/EDS. *Forensic Science International*, **214**(1–3), 96–104. https://doi.org/10.1016/j.forsciint.2011.07.025.

Waltenberger, L. and Schutkowski, H. (2017) Effects of heat on cut mark characteristics. *Forensic Science International*, **271**, 49–58.

Wedel, V.L. and Galloway, A. (eds.). (2014) *Broken Bones: Anthropological Analysis of Blunt Force Trauma*. Charles C. Thomas, Springfield, IL.

Weiner, S., Traub, W., and Wagner, H. (1999) Lamellar bone: Structure–function relations. *Journal of Structural Biology*, **126**(3), 241–255.

Wheatley, B.P. (2008) Perimortem or postmortem bone fractures? An experimental study of fracture patterns in deer femora. *Journal of Forensic Sciences*, **53**(1), 69–72.

White, T.D., Black, M.T., and Folkens, P.A. (2012) *Human Osteology*, 3rd edn. Academic Press, San Diego, CA.

Wright, Rev. W. (1888) The Empire of the Hittites. In: *Journal of the Transactions of the Victoria Institute, or Philosophical Society of Great Britain*, 21, Meeting January 3, 1887, (Paper read at the meeting by the author). The Victoria Institute, London, p. 59.

PART 3
Analytical Approaches to the Analysis of Burnt Bone

CHAPTER 11
Biochemical Alterations of Bone Subjected to Fire

Sarah Ellingham[1], PhD and Sara C. Zapico[2], PhD, ABC-MB

[1] *Forensic Coordinator, International Committee of the Red Cross, Geneva, Switzerland*

[2] *Assistant Professor, Department of Chemistry and Environmental Science, New Jersey Institute for Technology, NJ, USA*

11.1 The Biological and Chemical Makeup of Fresh Bone

11.1.1 Introduction

In order to understand the changes undergone by bone once it is subjected to fire, one must first understand its makeup in vivo. Around 90% of bone volume is accounted for by its extracellular matrix, which is a two-phase composite material comprised of a mineral phase (65 wt.%), an organic phase (25 wt.%) and water (10 wt.%) (Chen *et al.*, 2011). The organic phase's primary component is type I collagen, which consists of fibrils made up of three chains with a sequence of (Gly-Xxx-Yyy)n, which are wound together into a left-handed so-called polyproline II helix. Three of these helices in turn form a right-handed triple helix, stabilized by hydrogen bonds which connect the amino group of glycine (Gly) to the carboxyl group of the Xxx residue in an adjacent chain (Bächinger and Davis, 1991; Downey and Siegel, 2006). The triple helices forming the structural features of collagen I, are around 300 nm in length and 1.4 nm wide, consisting of about 1000 amino acid residues per chain, with a highly homogenous sequence. Fibrils are aligned to form larger structures, the collagen fibers. Non-collagenous proteins, such as glycoproteins, proteoglycans, and Y-glutamic acid containing proteins, form the secondary organic components of bone. These play a role in regulating the indurating mineral matrix's crystal size, orientation, and habit; in fact these non-collagenous proteins act as nucleators, without which collagen would be unable to nucleate hydroxyapatite deposits itself (Rho *et al.*, 1998; Olszta *et al.*, 2007; Robey, 2008).

The mineral phase of bone consists of dahllite, a poorly crystalline non-stochiometric form of hydroxyapatite ($Ca_{10}(PO_4)_6(OH)_2$). Dahllite can incorporate several

Burnt Human Remains: Recovery, Analysis, and Interpretation, First Edition. Edited by Sarah Ellingham, Joe Adserias-Garriga, Sara C. Zapico and Douglas H. Ubelaker.

elemental substitutions; calcium (Ca) ions can be replaced by a plethora of elements, the most common being magnesium (Mg), zinc (Zn) chromium (Cr), copper (Cu), and manganese (Mn), which are all used in the growing process (Zimmerman *et al.*, 2015). The phosphate group (PO_4^{3-}) has been found to be substituted by citrate, phosphate esters, pyrophosphates, diphosphonates, and amino acids, whereas the hydroxyl group (OH^-) can be replaced by chlorine (Cl) or fluoride (F) (Zimmerman *et al.*, 2015). However, the most common substitution is carbonate (3–8 wt. %), which, depending on the position of its crystals, can either be classified as "Type A" (OH^-) or "Type B" (PO_4^{3-}) substitution, with the latter being more commonly found in human bone (Klepinger, 1984; Castro *et al.*, 2010; Figueiredo *et al.*, 2010; Wang *et al.*, 2010). This is relevant to the analysis of taphonomic factors, as lattice substitutions through carbonate decrease bone's crystallinity and accelerate its biodegradation rate (Figueiredo *et al.*, 2010). The mineral salts of the bone account for 99% of the body's calcium, 85% of its phosphorous, and 40–60% of its sodium and magnesium (Downey and Siegel, 2006). This in organic matrix maintains the extracellular fluid-ion concentrations needed for physiological functions such as nerve conduction and muscle contractions. Water in the bone is found bound to minerals and collagen or loose in the vascular-lunar-canalicular cavities. It is crucial for the bone's viscoelasticity (Nyman *et al.*, 2006). Depending on the skeletal element or factors such as age, disease, pathologies, or species, the geometrical spatial arrangements, as well as the composition of bone may vary (Quelch *et al.*, 1983; Aerssens *et al.*, 1998).

The remaining 10% of bone volume is accounted for by cellular elements, such as osteocytes, osteoblasts, osteoclasts, and bone lining cells. Osteoblasts are formed from undifferentiated mesenchymal cells during both endochondral and intramembranous bone formation and are densely stacked along the bone's surface lining. Active osteoblasts are oval in shape, have a nucleus in the middle and contain large quantities of rough endoplasmic reticula (RER), mitochondria, and Golgi apparatus. They are responsible for the synthesis of the organic matrix as well as depositing minerals into this matrix. Once osteoblasts cease to be active, they either turn into osteocytes surrounded by matrix, or become thin, elongated bone lining cells which cover the surface in adult skeletons (Downey and Siegel, 2006). These bone lining cells build a lining between osteoblasts and osteoclasts and the bone marrow. They further digest spare bone matrix which has not been completely absorbed by osteoclasts and deposit thin layers of collagen into clean resorption pits to initiate new bone formation (Parfitt, 2001; Everts *et al.*, 2002). Osteocytes comprise around 90% of bone cells in adults. While still immature, osteocytes look similar to the osteoblasts they used to be, still retaining large amounts of RER, Golgi apparatus, and mitochondria. However, during the maturation process they lose their cytoplasm and become smaller and deeply embedded into the bone tissue. Mature osteocytes are positioned in the lacunae, and feature elongated cytoplasmic processes that project through the matrix' canaliculi and connect with adjacent cell processes. This is important as it allows for nutrition flow within the mineral matrix, as well as facilitating cell communication. The final type of bone cells are the osteoclasts, which facilitate bone resorption. Osteoclasts are multi-nucleated and significantly larger than the other cells of bone. They are generally found on the bone surface and are very mobile, moving from site to site.

In terms of bone structure, there are several different variants, which differ in their arrangement of fibril patterns. These include parallel fibrils (common in fish and amphibian bones), woven fibers (common in amphibians and reptiles, but also found in mammalian embryos and areas of new bone formation), radial fibril arrays (found in dentine), and lamellar bone, which is the most common type in human bones. In this type of bone the lamellae are typically folded into a cylinder shape, the so-called Haversian systems or osteons (Rho *et al.*, 1998; Weiner and Wagner, 1998). During the constantly ongoing internal remodeling process of the bone, osteoclasts form tunnels into the bone; these are refilled by osteoblasts that deposit a thin layer of cement on the tunnel surface, which is followed by a new layer of lamellae. Only a narrow channel is left at the center, which acts as a blood vessel. These structures are the Haversian canals, orthogonally to which smaller capillary-like tunnels called Volkmann's canals connect Haversian canals with each other as well as with the periosteum (Olszta *et al.*, 2007).

On a macroscopic level, lamellar bone can be separated into two types, compact bone and trabecular bone (also referred to as spongy or cancellous bone). Trabecular bone, which is found in the interior of many bones, is highly porous and very metabolically active. It remodels itself more frequently than compact bone, which is very dense and found on the surface, or cortex, of all bones (Rho *et al.*, 1998; Ritchie *et al.*, 2009).

11.2 Bone Transformation When Subjected to Heat

The in vivo bone structure and makeup undergoes several changes via diagenetic processes post-mortem. These changes are accelerated and more severe when the bone is subjected to heating. There are four main stages that bone undergoes when subjected to high temperatures: 1) dehydration, which is characterized by the breaking of the hydroxyl bonds as well as the loss of the water loosely bound to the mineral bone matrix; 2) decomposition, which is the stage in which the bone's organic components are lost through pyrolysis; 3) inversion, marked through the loss of carbonate; 4) fusion, the final stage in the process, in which the bone's crystal matrix sinters and coalesces (Mayne Correia, 1997; Thompson, 2004; Ellingham *et al.*, 2015a). These phases are attended by a multitude of structural alterations which can be observed in changes to the bone's color, microstructure, morphology, mechanical strength, and crystallinity.

There is a plethora of analytical approaches to observe and measure the changes undergone by bone when subject to heating, a selection of which will be introduced in the next sections.

11.3 Analytical Approaches to Observing Bone Transformation

11.3.1 Colorimetry

One of the earliest approaches to distinguish and quantify heat-induced alterations to bone was through the classification of color changes. While going through the different phases associated with heat exposure, bone undergoes distinct color changes; fresh bone exhibits a light ivory color, which darkens through dehydration, changing over brown into black because of carbonization in the decomposition phase through the incineration of organic materials. This gives way to a gray shading starting with the inversion phase, which finally turns into white, signalling the complete loss of all organic compounds and fusion of the bone minerals.

Since the 1980s visual comparisons with the Munsell Soil Color Charts were used as a means of standardizing observations of bone color changes (Shipman *et al.*, 1984). The obvious drawbacks of this method being its proneness to bias and inter and intra observer error (Ellingham *et al.*, 2015b). Nowadays colors are most often electronically recorded by spectrophotometers, which do not only minimize observer errors, but allow for the mathematical modelling and 3-D plotting of colors in an Euclidean space (Trujillo *et al.*, 1996; Schafer, 2001; Devlin and Herrmann, 2008). The most commonly used system to record bone color data is the CIE L*a*b* (CIELAB) uniform color space, which is based on a tristimulus value (Devlin and Herrmann, 2008; Ellingham *et al.*, 2015b). The L* axis depicts the lightness ranked from 0 (black) to 100 (white), the a* axis reflects red / green colors (red being positive, green negative values) and the b* axis yellow / blue colors (yellow being positive, blue negative). Other color schemes, such as RGB (measuring red, green, and blue components), HSL (measuring Hue, Saturation and Lightness) or the Windows used WinHSL240, to name a few, work in analogue ways and can also be applied (Ellingham *et al.*, 2015b). The spectrophotometer records color values by producing a light beam which passes though the sample; each sample component absorbs or transmits light over a specific wavelength. Colorimetry is discussed more in depth in Chapter 13.

It is important to note, however, that bone color changes are dependent on many factors other than just burn temperature, such as moisture, the oxygen levels of the environment, etc., and therefore correlations between bone color and exposure time/temperature should be drawn with caution.

11.3.2 SEM-EDX

Scanning electron microscopes (SEM) enable the surface analysis of heterogeneous organic and inorganic materials by using a focused electron beam that reacts with the sample to be analyzed and produces a topological image (Goldstein *et al.*, 2012; Mutalibov *et al.*, 2017). When it contacts the sample, the electron beam produces secondary electrons (SE), backscatter electrons (BSE), and characteristic X-rays, which can be detected with the according detectors and displayed on a monitor

(Mutalib *et al.*, 2017). The SEM image is formed based on the interaction between the emitted beam of electrons and the sample. These interactions can be elastic, or inelastic. In the latter, the sample emits low-energy SEs after bombardment from the electron beam and the energy is transferred to the sample atoms. In elastic interactions the primary electron beam is deflected when encountering the sample atomic nucleus or electrons of similar energy. Elements with higher atomic numbers deflect more electrons as their nucleus has more positive ions (Mutalib *et al.*, 2017). BSE electrons contain a lot of information on the structure below the sample surface. For SE, which is the most common signal type used for SEM, detection only occurs to a few nanometers of the sample surface. Its strength lies in the depiction of topological contrast of the sample, such as surface texture. The contrast of an image is generated depending on the signal intensity of the beam-specimen interaction that is measured point to point across the sample surface, which is scanned in a raster. The image magnification is equivalent to the ratio between the linear size of the raster on the specimen and the linear size of the viewing screen (Goldstein *et al.*, 2012). A 100 µm wide raster on a sample, for example, would appear 1000× magnified when displayed on a 10 cm wide viewing screen.

Energy dispersive X-ray spectroscopy (EDX) is involved in detecting samples' elemental composition by using SEM. EDX works by picking up sample characteristic X-rays after the collision of electron beam with a sample in the regular SEM process. The X-ray is the result of the interaction between the primary electron beam and the sample's atom nucleus. As no two elements have the same X-ray emission spectrum, they can be differentiated and their concentration measured (Goldstein *et al.*, 2012). The advantage of the SEM-EDX combination is that information on gross elemental sample distribution can be directly linked to a sample image (Turner-Walker and Syversen, 2002). SEM-EDX further lends itself to the analysis of bone, as it has a superior resolution of three-dimensional structures compared to conventional light spectroscopy and achieves a much higher magnification (Shipman, 1981).

SEM analyses of burnt bone depict soft tissue remnants being present adhering to the bone surface up until temperatures of 300°C. From around 400°C bones are soft and tissue free, with some retained tissue appearing as bubbly char. The combustion of soft tissue around 400°C coincides with the observation of thumbnail fracturing on the bone. Cracking becomes more frequent as temperatures pass 500°C. Fracturing is a sign of structural failure of a material, and in the case of burnt bone is a direct result of the loss of collagen, which in vivo provides tensile strength to the bone. From around 600°C, near the end of the decomposition phase and loss of organic material, bone porosity is seen to increase throughout the inversion phase up until circa 900°C, where the bone surface starts to exhibit a marked granularity. Exposure temperatures of over 1000°C leave the bone with a "melted" smooth surface, a product of the fusion process (Ellingham *et al.*, 2018). Ellingham and colleagues' (2018) analysis of burnt bones using EDX found that while there are some fluctuations in the atomic percentage of elements depending on the transformation stage, the overall elemental composition of bone does not change significantly regardless of temperature, allowing for the detection of an osseous "fingerprint," enabling the differentiation of bone from other material in cases of contested cremains.

11.3.3 Fourier Transform Infrared-Spectroscopy

A commonly used analytical technique for the analysis and characterization of biomaterials, Fourier transform infrared-spectroscopy (FTIR) lends itself to the analysis of burnt bone, as it is a rapid technique that allows for a simultaneous examination of organic and inorganic tissue components (Thompson *et al.*, 2009; Howes *et al.*, 2012; Ellingham *et al.*, 2015b, 2016). Molecular spectroscopy, such as FTIR and Raman spectroscopy, builds on the fact that photons experience absorption, emission, or scattering by a molecule if a change in energy of the molecule occurs. Infrared spectroscopy probes molecular bond vibrations when infrared radiation passes through a sample (Kourkoumelis *et al.*, 2019). The peaks in the FTIR spectrum correspond to the frequency of molecular bond vibrations, which are localized to specific functional groups. The position of absorption bands (measured in wavenumber units, cm^{-1}) depends on the type of molecular bonds, vibrating masses, the intra- and intermolecular environment, and their electron donating or withdrawing effects, as well as coupling with other vibrations (Barth, 2007; Kourkoumelis *et al.*, 2019).

The FTIR spectra of bone can be roughly separated into two distinct blocks, where the organic and inorganic components exhibit specific peaks. In the FTIR spectra the area between 1200 cm^{-1} and 1800 cm^{-1} is representative for the bone's organic components and therefore allows for the observation of changes to the collagen structure. The band around 1654 cm^{-1} depicts the so-called amide-I band, the peptide C = O stretching vibration, which in vivo is responsible for the visco-elasticity of the fibrillar collagen matrix (Chadefaux *et al.*, 2009; Paschalis, 2009). The band at 1544 cm^{-1} depicts the amide-II band, a combination of the C-N and N-H vibration.

The strong absorption band at 900–1200 cm^{-1} is linked to the $_{v1}$ and $_{v3}$ normal mode of the phosphate ion of the hydroxyapatite and is the result of symmetric ($_{v1}$) and asymmetric ($_{v3}$) P-O stretching vibrations (Lebon *et al.*, 2010). Anti-symmetrically bending $_{v4}$ phosphate ions appear as well-defined double peaks at 563 and 604 cm^{-1}. This split peak has traditionally been used to determine the so-called crystallinity index (CI). A carbonate $_{v3}CO_3^{2-}$ band at around 1456 cm^{-1} overlaps with the absorption bands of the organic material (Kourkoumelis *et al.*, 2019) and a $_{v2}CO_3^{2-}$ band is present at 871 cm^{-1} (Table 11.1).

When analyzing burnt bone with the FTIR it becomes apparent that the amide II structure is the first to be compromised from temperatures of around 300°C onwards, closely followed by the amide I and amide II structures. The carbonate peak at 871 cm^{-1} declines in height proportionally to increasing temperature, and is only rudimentarily present at temperatures above 900°C. Similarly, the $_{v3}CO_3^{2-}$ carbonate band declines until its disappearance from 700°C exposure temperatures onwards. At temperatures above 650°C the $_{v4}PO_4$ band exhibits an additional splitting, the so-called phosphate high temperature (PHT) peak (Figures 11.1a–c).

Table 11.1 FTIR band assignments for bone

Peak position (cm^{-1})	Component assignment
563 and 604 cm^{-1}	$PO_4^{-3}v_4$
871 cm^{-1}	$_{v2}CO_3^{-2}$
900–1200 (1028) cm^{-1}	$PO_4^{-3}v_1$
900–1200 (1028) cm^{-1}	$PO_4^{-3}\boldsymbol{v}_3$
1456 cm^{-1}	$_{v3}CO_3^{-2}$
1242 cm^{-1}	amide III
1544 cm^{-1}	amide II
1654 cm^{-1}	amide I

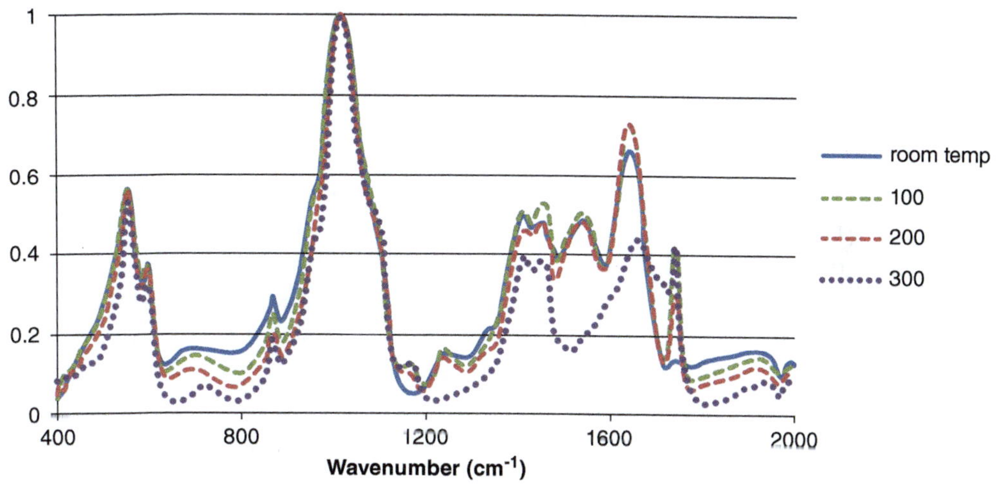

Figure 11.1a FTIR spectra of bone burnt at low temperatures (100–300°C).

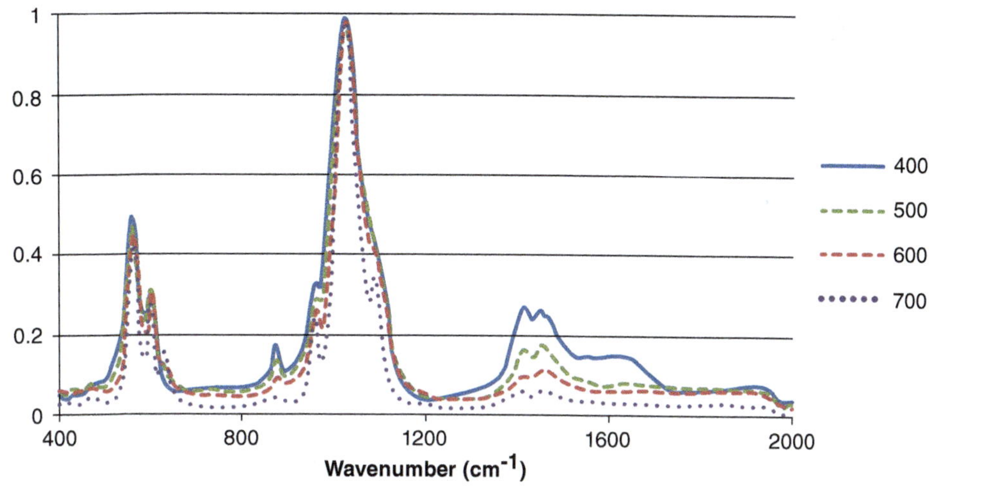

Figure 11.1b FTIR spectra of bone burnt at medium temperatures (400–700°C).

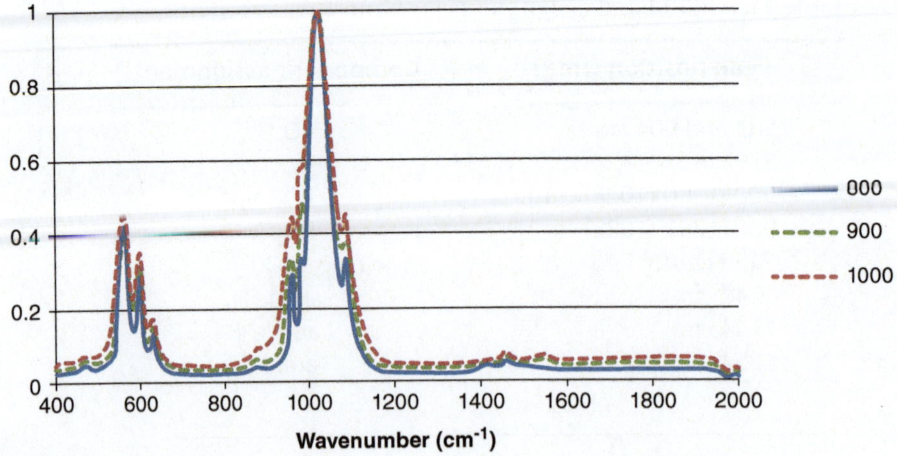

Figure 11.1c FTIR spectra of bone burnt at high temperatures (800–1000°C).

Several studies have utilized peak ratios to quantify these heat-induced changes in order to retrospectively determine the temperatures that bone has been exposed to (Thompson *et al.*, 2013; Ellingham *et al.*, 2015b). Ellingham *et al.* (2016) found that while the burning exposure time does not have a significant impact on the degradation stage of the bone, the presence or absence of soft tissue, however, does significantly alter the process. At low temperatures (under 400°C) soft tissue functions as a buffer, shielding the bone from the effects of the heat, whereas at temperatures above 700°C it acts as an accelerator, amplifying the process (Ellingham *et al.*, 2016).

11.3.4 Raman Spectroscopy

Raman spectroscopy is complementary to infrared spectroscopy, functioning on the basis of vibrational bands being different; while in infrared spectroscopy light absorption is being measured, Raman spectroscopy measures inelastic light scattering. Some vibrational modes may be detectable in one of the two techniques, but not the other (Mamede *et al.*, 2018). In Raman spectroscopy, samples are irradiated by monochromatic radiation from a laser source, which can be in the ultraviolet, visible, or near-infrared spectral region (785–1064 nm) (Larkin, 2011). When the radiation interacts with a molecule, its electron cloud will be temporarily perturbed, producing an oscillating electric moment where electrons couple with the photons and lead to scattering (Mamede *et al.*, 2018). This scattering can either be elastic (Rayleigh scattering), meaning the scattered light is the same frequency as the incident one (ν_0), or inelastic (Raman scattering), which means the scattered light is either higher ($\nu_0 + \nu_{vib}$) or lower ($\nu_0 - \nu_{vib}$) than the incident radiation. It is mainly the higher inelastic scatter, which is picked up by the Raman

Table 11.2 Ramen band assignments for bone.

Peak position (cm^{-1})	Component assignment
422–454	$PO_4^{-3}v_2$
568–617	$PO_4^{-3}v_4$
815–921	C-C stretching
957–962	$PO_4^{-3}v_1$
1006–1055	$PO_4^{-3}v_3$
1065–1071	CO_3^{-2}
1243–1269	amide III
1595–1720	amide I

spectroscopy, making it a fairly weak process since it only picks up a fraction of the inelastic scattering (Mamede *et al.*, 2018).

Like the FTIR, Raman spectroscopy provides simultaneous quantitative and qualitative information on both the mineral and organic portions of bone, and the same components can be analyzed. The typical Raman band assignment for bone can be found in Table 11.2 (Khan *et al.*, 2013). In the literature Ramen spectroscopy has been performed on bone mainly in medical settings and not on diagenetically altered or burnt samples; nonetheless if applied to burnt bone, findings are expected to be in conformity with observations conducted with FTIR.

11.3.5 X-Ray Diffraction

X-ray diffraction (XRD) has been a popular tool for the determination of change to the bone matrix since the 1980s (Shipman *et al.*, 1984). In material science it is widely used to perform qualitative and quantitative analyses of crystalline materials. It works because of structural interference produced with monochromatic X-rays with a crystal sample. The X-ray beams are scattered by the electrons associated with the atoms of any crystal and experience interference, depending on the differential arrangement of atoms and crystal symmetry. The measurement of direction of the outgoing beams allows for the determination of the properties of the crystalline structure, such as its symmetry and unit cell (Smith, 2019). In powder diffraction, three types of information can be found in the diffraction pattern: geometrical, represented by the angular position of the diffraction peak; structural, embodied in the intensity of the diffraction peak; and the physical state, represented in the peak profile (Smith, 2019). This three-dimensional diffraction information is condensed into one direction in diffraction space. The angle between the ingoing and outgoing beam is called 2θ. The position of the diffraction peak is controlled by Bragg's Law ($n\lambda = 2d \sin \theta$), where λ is the beam wavelength, d is the space between the diffracting crystal planes, and θ the incident angle (Rogers and Daniels, 2002; Rogers *et al.*, 2010).

In the analysis of osseous material with XRD, the CI is the most observed feature (Bartsiokas and Middleton, 1992). The CI is the intensity ratio of the (300)/(200) line profile of the apatite when using Cu Kα radiation and an angular range of 15–120° in 2θ (Piga *et al.*, 2008; Ellingham *et al.*, 2015b). Changes in the crystal structure are observable from 600°C onwards and manifest themselves as increasing separations of the diffraction peaks and an increase in XRD-CI, which continues up to 900°C (van Hoesel *et al.*, 2019). From 700°C, Piga *et al.* (2009) further observed the appearance of a calcium oxide peak at 37.5°C and disappearance of the calcide peak at 36°C in 2θ from around 775°C onwards. These observations make XRD a useful technique for the determination of high burning temperatures over 600°C, but less effective to determine lower burn exposure temperatures.

11.3.6 Thermogravimetric Analysis (TGA) and Differential Scanning Calorimetry (DSC)

Thermogravimetric analysis (TGA) and differential scanning calorimetry (DSC) are well established in material science to determine the properties of natural and synthetic hydroxyapatites for tissue engineering (Figueiredo *et al.* 2010). The techniques depict heat effects occurring when the material phase transitions and chemical reactions when exposed to changing temperatures. TGA measures a sample's mass during heating or cooling, whereas DSC measures the absorbed or released energy of the sample (Mkukuma *et al.*, 2004; Ellingham *et al.*, 2015a).

Experimental research using TGA clearly showed bone exhibiting three main weight loss phases. The first, peaking around 100–150°C is attributed to the evaporation of water in an endothermic event. The most severe weight loss is linked to the exothermic process of collagen combustion and the recrystallization commencing at around 300–350°C, interrupted by a brief endothermic event linked to the decomposition of carbonate around 450°C, continuing in the exothermic process until the complete combustion of all organic components, peaking at around 500°C and continuing until the commencement of mineral sintering in an endothermic process from 750°C onwards (Ellingham *et al.*, 2015a). It was found that an increase in exposure time to a certain temperature increases mass loss; however, in order for specific phase changes to occur, a certain "activation temperature" needs to be reached, a mere time increase is not sufficient (Ellingham *et al.*, 2015a) (Figures 11.2a–c).

11.3.7 Amino Acid Racemization

A method ideal for determining the thermal stability of collagen is amino acid racemization (AAR). With the exception of glycine, all 20 amino acids found in proteins have asymmetric chiral carbon atoms and can exist as L or D-amino acid stereoisomers. These typically start out as L-amino acids but convert to D-amino acids over time. The process of reaching an equilibrium between L and D forms is time and temperature dependent and known as racemization (Collins *et al.*, 1999). When systematically conducting AAR on bone which had been experimentally heated to different temperatures, Ellingham (2015) found the concentration of

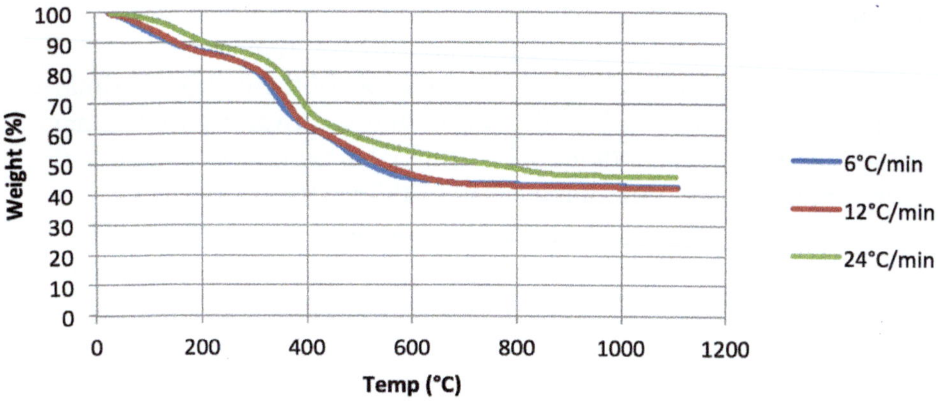

Figure 11.2a Average TGA curves of bones subjected to differing heating regimes.

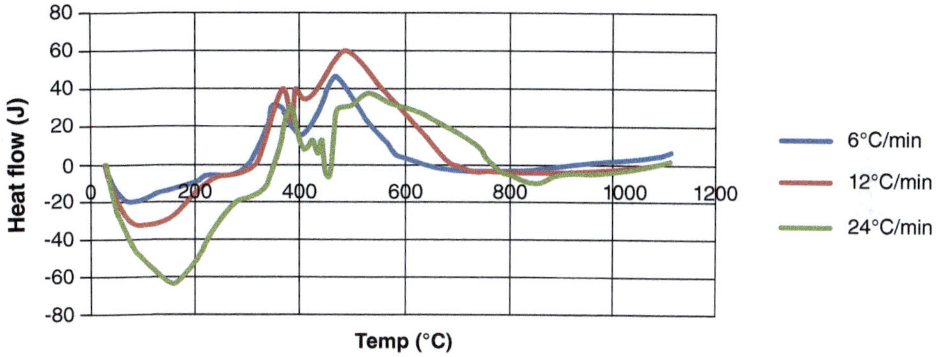

Figure 11.2b Average DSC curves of bones subjected to different heating regimes.

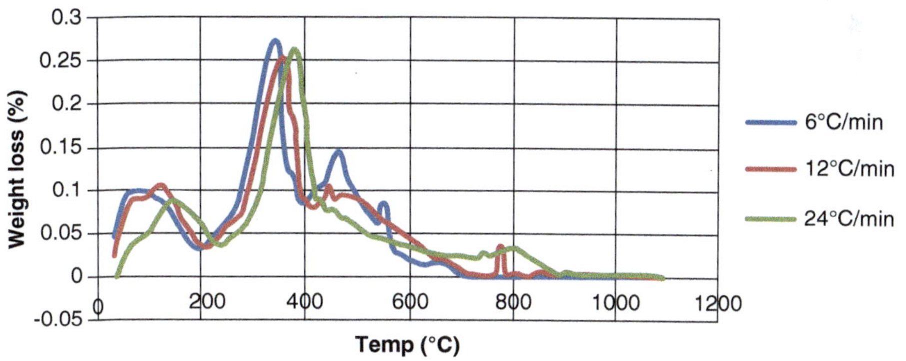

Figure 11.2c Average TGA first derivative curves from bones subjected to different heating regimes.

amino acids in bone collagen to rapidly decrease from 250°C onwards, with concentrations dropping below detection level from 400°C. Up to 250°C aspartic acid (Asx), the derivative of asparagine (Asg) and glutamine, is the only amino acid to racemize, reaching a D/L ratio of 0.3 at 250°C. This is not surprising given Asx is one of the only amino acids which can racemize while still internally bound (Collins *et al.*, 1999), and has the highest racemization rate, in general. It is simultaneously strongly suggestive of the fact that most of the collagen primary structure is still intact (Collins *et al.*, 2009). From 300°C onwards glutamic acid (Glx), serine (Ser), alanine (Ala), valine (Val), phenylalanine (Phe), leucine (Leu), tyrosine (Tyr), arginine (Arg), threonine (Thr), histidine (His), and isoleucine (Ile) also commence racemization. The composition of amino acids is dominated by collagen up until 400°C. Collagen begins to locally unravel its triple helical structure when heated. This process is reversible to temperatures of up to 58 +/– 10°C, after which irreversible denaturing of collagen occurs (Kronick and Cooke, 1996; Bozec and Odlyha, 2011). Once the denaturing sets in, the breaking of hydrogen cross-links causes severe conformational changes to the collagen fibrils. The release of collagen stabilizing H-bonded water leads to the gradual collapse of the triple helical structure, a process which occurs from 150°C onwards. An observed sudden drop in the total amino acid racemization and the commencing of racemization of all other amino acids between 250 and 300°C coincides with the complete conformational change from triple helix to random coil, the cleavage of individual amino acids and the shift from an endothermic to exothermic combustion process (Bozec and Odlyha, 2011; Ellingham *et al.*, 2015a). The now free amino acids continue to racemize until their complete combustion around 400°C (Figures 11.3a–b).

11.4 DNA

There are only a few studies analyzing the specific effects of fire on DNA. The majority aim to assess the recovery of a full nuclear DNA profile with identification purposes. To serve this objective, bones and/or teeth were subjected to different temperatures and times to evaluate DNA yield, amplification, and profiling. The study of Alvarez

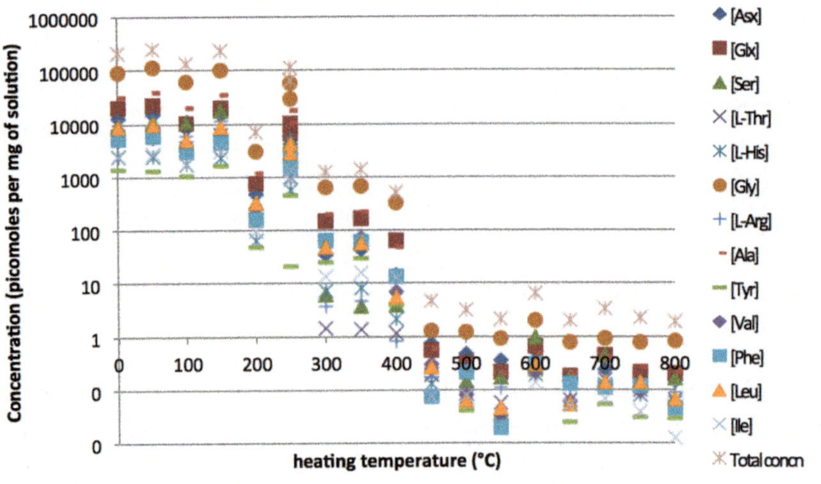

Figure 11.3a Total amino acid concentration.

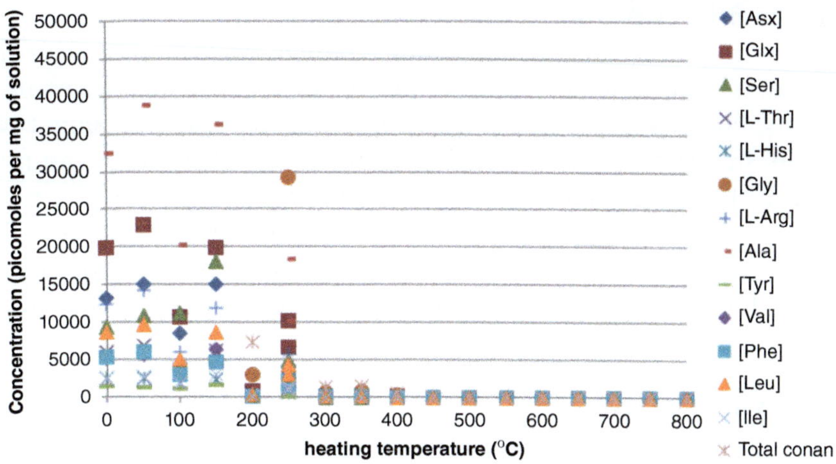

Figure 11.3b Amino acid concentration on a logarithmic scale.

Garcia *et al.* (1996) on tooth samples found that at lower temperatures of 4°C, 20°C, and 40°C, amplification of nuclear DNA was possible, whereas in contrast higher temperatures of around 500°C with an exposure time of two minutes did not allow for any amplification. This is in concordance with the study of Adserias-Garriga *et al.* (2016), which also used teeth, and which found the amplification of STRs to decrease from 300°C and 1–5 minutes of exposure time, although this depended on the STR. In bone samples, Harbeck *et al.* (2011) demonstrated the amplification of mitochondrial DNA up to 700°C and one and a half hours of exposure time. In contrast, Imaizumi *et al.* (2014) using metacarpal bones only found positive amplification of mitochondrial DNA up to 200°C exposed to 15 minutes. The study of Maciejewska *et al.* (2015) analyzed both the retrieval of STR profiles and mtDNA amplification. Full STR profiles were obtained from teeth after 100°C, five and ten minutes' exposure time. At higher temperatures and prolonged exposure the number of retrieved alleles decreased. However, they found it was possible to sequence mtDNA up until exposure to 500°C for five minutes. With respect to bone samples, it was possible to obtain a full DNA profile up to 800°C with five minutes' exposure time, and mtDNA sequence up to 900°C exposed for the same duration. mtDNA performed better than nDNA as there are several mtDNAs in each mitochondrion, and several mitochondria in each cell; thus, it is more likely, in extreme conditions to obtain mtDNA. Additional studies were carried out based on forensic cases. An extensive review of this topic can be found in Chapter 12.

11.5 Changes to the Bone at Different Temperatures

11.5.1 100°C Exposure

At exposure to temperatures of 100°C macroscopically bone remains relatively unchanged, exhibiting a neutral white to yellow white color. Microscopically, osseous cells and organic tissue are still clearly determinable. Collagen fibers begin to take on a cord-like structure and start to denature. This can be seen through the process of amino acid racemization, the change of L-amino acids to their D-stereoisomers. The first amino acids to racemize at temperatures of around 100°C are Asp and Asn, which can be recorded as a combined signal Asx. The triple helical structure of the collagen is still retained at these temperatures (Ellingham, 2015). The bone experiences a first weight loss phase, peaking at temperature ranges between 100°C and 150°C, which can be attributed to the breakage of hydroxyl bonds and evaporation of water which was loosely mechanically bound to the bone matrix (Herrmann, 1972). This is known as the dehydration phase (Thompson, 2005).

11.5.2 200°C Exposure

The dehydration phase, including evaporation and weight loss, continues up to temperatures of around 250°C. Macroscopically, bone takes on a brown yellowish color and exhibits a "glassy," slightly greasy, albeit granular looking surface (Shipman *et al.*, 1984). Microscopically, crystals are in a polyhedral formation. While the infrared spectra of bones exposed to 200°C are virtually indistinguishable from fresh bone, amino acid racemization shows a continued unraveling of the collagen superhelix and its reduction to random coils at around 250°C, from which point the racemization of other amino acids commences and the overall amino acid concentration drops (Ellingham, 2015).

11.5.3 300°C Exposure

Exposure to temperatures of 300°C marks the onset of the decomposition phase, which is characterized by the removal of the bone's organic components by pyrolysis, causing the onset of the most severe weight loss phase, simultaneously introducing the exothermic process of hydroxyapatite re-crystallization from polyhedral to cubic shaped crystals. On FTIR spectra this is reflected in the plateauing of the CO/P value and a sudden increase in the CO/CO_3 and C/C ratios. The combustion of organic components can also be visualized through FTIR spectra, which show a compromising of the amide II peak from 300°C onwards, closely followed by amide I and amide III peak, which are almost completely degraded by 350°C (Ellingham *et al.*, 2015b). The collagen continues to denature and separates into cord-like structures which microscopically become more compact and exhibit an irregular structure. The free amino acids continue racemization, while the overall amino acid concentration drastically drops (Ellingham, 2015). The granular bone surface is covered in a peeling, bubbling layer of char, which manifests itself as a spike in the atomic percentage of carbon when analyzed with the EDX, and visually can be identified in the entirely black color of the bone.

Bone still covered in soft tissue shows less heat-induced damage at 300°C than defleshed bones, as the soft tissue acts as a de facto shield which creates a buffer effect and a boiling rather than burning environment on the bone surface (Ellingham *et al.*, 2015b).

11.5.4 400°C Exposure

At 400°C the combustion of the bone's organic components continues. The amino acid concentration plummets drastically, until from 450°C onwards no collagen can be detected in the bone anymore. This collagen combustion process goes hand in hand with the commencement of a strong exothermic phase, which follows a short endothermic event from the decomposition of carbonate. On the FTIR spectra a decrease in height of the amide peaks leading to a total disappearance at 500°C can be seen (Ellingham *et al.*, 2016). These occurrences are accompanied by a sudden and dramatic weight loss and volumetric shrinkage of the bone. The shrinkage, in combination with the loss of elasticity that goes inherent with the loss of collagen, causes structural failure and thus cracking on the osseous surface which manifests as thumbnail fractures. The re-crystallization of minerals continues at these temperatures. Soft tissue remnants still adherent to the bone take on a bubbly charred appearance and the bone exhibits a jet black color (Ellingham *et al.*, 2015b).

11.5.5 500°C Exposure

At 500°C the strong exothermic phase accompanies the bone's collagen combustion and the re-crystallization of minerals peaks. Bone crystals have a cubic shape. The thumbnail fractures turn into branched micro cracks and their number increases. Some residual charred soft tissue remains on the bone surface, which takes on a light brownish gray color (Castillo *et al.*, 2013; Ellingham *et al.*, 2015b).

11.5.6 600°C Exposure

Exposure to 600°C sees the exothermic phase of organic tissue combustion and recrystallization of the mineral phase continue. The most notable change on the FTIR spectrum occurs at around 650°C, with the appearance of a so-called "phosphate high temperature" peak, which is an additional splitting of the ${}_{v4}PO_4$ phosphate peak. Any remaining soft tissue will combust in this temperature range (Ellingham *et al.*, 2015b). Microscopically the bone becomes more porous, which is linked to the voids in the mineral grid of the bone left behind by the combusted organic phase. Cubic crystals give way to more irregular crystal structures (Castillo *et al.*, 2013). Visually, bone exposed to temperatures of around 600°C exhibits a whitish gray color.

11.5.7 700°C Exposure

The exothermic incineration process continues until at around 750°C all organic components have been completely combusted. While at this temperature no more mass is lost, the bone undergoes shrinkage, which has the consequence of increasing surface fractures and porosity (Ellingham *et al.*, 2015a). The bone crystals are taking on a more rounded shape (Castillo *et al.*, 2013). At temperatures exceeding 700°C, any fat and muscle tissue immediately ignite, acting as a form of fuel or accelerant, causing temperatures reaching the bone to spike and consequently increasing the bone recrystallization, which resembles a sintering process.

Exposed to temperatures of 700°C, bone takes on a completely white color, signalling the complete absence of organic material.

11.5.8 800°C Exposure

From around 800°C onwards the bone minerals begin to sinter and carbonate is lost in an endothermic event (Ellingham *et al.*, 2015a). These phenomena become evident through the bone's FTIR spectra, depicting a sudden drop in the CI simultaneous to an increase in CO_3/P and C/P ratios (Ellingham *et al.*, 2016). Bone shrinkage processes are accelerated through the re-crystallization and sintering of the bone matrix. Individual crystals coalesce into larger ones with crystal size reaching its maximum. There is an observable increase in micro-porosity on the bone's surface (Ellingham *et al.*, 2018).

11.5.9 900°C Exposure

Temperatures of around 900°C mark the onset of the fusion phase. This entails the continued sintering of the mineral matrix and a loss of carbonate. The bone experiences a dramatic increase in volumetric shrinkage (Ellingham and Sandholzer, 2020). Microscopically, the bone surface exhibits decreasing porosity and a more granular appearance, as crystals sinter into significantly smaller, rounded granular structures. Bones exposed to this temperature range have been observed to exhibit a white color, with occasional orange/pink staining which has been attributed to any copper present in the bone oxidizing (Dunlop, 1978; Ellingham *et al.*, 2015b).

11.5.10 1000°C Exposure

At temperatures of around 1000°C the fusion phase is in full swing. The mineral matrix continues to sinter and coalesce, micropores are being filled in and newly formed micro crystals form a compact surface, giving the bone a smooth appearance (Ellingham *et al.*, 2018). The re-crystallization of hydroxyapatite leads to the formation of ß-tricalcium phosphate. The bone exhibits a white or white/pink color due to the oxidizing copper.

11.6 Conclusion

The analysis of burnt bone is a rapidly growing sub-field of forensic anthropology. Like its mother discipline its core objectives are the reconstruction of an individual's life, circumstances of death, and post-depositional history. However, due to the extreme modification bone undergoes because of heat exposure, the analyses become increasingly complex and may require the application of different analytical techniques to unlock the information stored in the bone. Methods described in this chapter are by no means exhaustive and the research is ever evolving; nonetheless they give a glimpse into the most commonly available techniques and what information can be gleaned about the bone.

Acknowledgment

The authors would like to thank Dr. Kirsty Penkman, University of York, for performing the amino acid racemization and providing the graphs.

References

Aerssens, J., Boonen, S., Lowet, G., and Dequeker, J. (1998) Interspecies differences in bone composition, density, and quality: Potential implications for in vivo bone research. *Endocrinology*, **139**(2), 663–670.

Adserias-Garriga, J., Ubelaker, D.H., and Zapico, S.C. (2016) Evaluation of macroscopic changes and the efficiency of DNA profiling from burnt teeth. *Science & Justice: Journal of the Forensic Science Society*, **56**(6), 437–442.

Alvarez Garcia, A., Munoz, I., Pestoni, C., Lareu, M.V., Rodriguez-Calvo, M.S., and Carracedo, A. (1996) Effect of environmental factors on PCR-DNA analysis from dental pulp. *International Journal of Legal Medicine*, **109**(3), 125–129.

Bächinger, H.P. and Davis, J.M. (1991) Sequence specific thermal stability of the collagen triple helix. *International Journal of Biological Macromolecules*, **13**(3), 152–156.

Barth, A. (2007) Infrared spectroscopy of proteins. *Biochimica et Biophysica Acta (BBA)-Bioenergetics*, **1767**(9), 1073–1101.

Bartsiokas, A. and Middleton, A.P. (1992) Characterization and dating of recent and fossil bone by X-ray diffraction. *Journal of Archaeological Science*, **19**(1), 63–72.

Bozec, L. and Odlyha, M. (2011) Thermal denaturation studies of collagen by microthermal analysis and atomic force microscopy. *Biophysical Journal*, **101**(1), 228–236.

Castillo, R.F., Ubelaker, D.H., Acosta, J.A.L., and de la Fuente, G.A.C. (2013) Effects of temperature on bone tissue. Histological study of the changes in the bone matrix. *Forensic Science International*, **226**(1–3), 33–37.

Castro, W., Hoogewerff, J., Latkoczy, C., and Almirall, J.R. (2010) Application of laser ablation (LA-ICP-SF-MS) for the elemental analysis of bone and teeth samples for discrimination purposes. *Forensic Science International*, **195**(1–3), 17–27.

Chadefaux, C., Le Hô, A., Bellot-Gurlet, L., and Reiche, I. (2009) Curve-fitting micro-ATRFTIR studies of the amine I and II bands of type I collagen in archaeological bone materials. *E-Preservation Science*, **6**(1), 129–137.

Chen, P., Toroian, D., Price, P.A., and McKittrick, J. (2011) Minerals form a continuum phase in mature cancellous bone. *Calcified Tissue International*, **88**(5), 351–361.

Collins, M.J., Waite, E.R., and Van Duin, A.C.T. (1999) Predicting protein decomposition: The case of aspartic-acid racemization kinetics. *Philosophical Transactions of the Royal Society B: Biological Sciences*, **354**(1379), 51–64.

Collins, M.J., Penkman, K.E., Rohland, N., Shapiro, B., Dobberstein, R.C., Ritz-Timme, S., *et al.* (2009) Is amino acid racemization a useful tool for screening for ancient DNA in bone? *Proceedings of the Royal Society of London B: Biological Sciences*, **276**(1), 2971–2977.

Devlin, J.B. and Herrmann, N.P. (2008) Bone color as an interpretive tool of the depositional history of archaeological cremains. In: *The Analysis of Burned Human Remains* (eds. C.W. Schmidt and S.A. Symes). Academic Press, Boston, MA, pp. 109–138.

Downey, P.A. and Siegel, M.I. (2006) Bone biology and the clinical implications for osteoporosis. *Physical Therapy*, **86**(1), 77–91.

Dunlop, J.M. (1978) Traffic light discoloration in cremated bones. *Medicine, Science and the Law*, **18**(3), 163–173.

Ellingham, S.T.D. (2015) Advanced analytical analysis and interpretation of biochemical and structural changes in burnt bone from forensic and archaeological contexts. PhD. Thesis. Teesside University, Middlesbrough.

Ellingham, S. and Sandholzer, M. (2020) Determining volumetric shrinkage trends of burnt bone using micro-CT. *Journal of Forensic Sciences*, **65**(1), 196–199.

Ellingham, S.T.D., Thompson, T.J.U., and Islam, M. (2015a) Thermogravimetric analysis of property changes and weight loss in incinerated bone. *Palaeogeography, Palaeoclimatology, Palaeoecology*, **438**, 239–244.

Ellingham, S.T.D., Thompson, T.J., Islam, M., and Taylor, G. (2015b) Estimating temperature exposure of burnt bone – A methodological review. *Science & Justice*, **55**(3), 181–188.

Ellingham, S.T.D., Thompson, T.J., and Islam, M. (2016) The effect of soft tissue on temperature estimation from burnt bone using Fourier transform infrared spectroscopy. *Journal of Forensic Sciences*, **61**(1), 153–159.

Ellingham, S.T.D., Thompson, T.J., and Islam, M. (2018) Scanning Electron Microscopy–Energy-Dispersive X-Ray (SEM/EDX): A rapid diagnostic tool to aid the identification of burnt bone and contested cremains. *Journal of Forensic Sciences*, **63**(2), 504–510.

Everts, V., Delaissié, J.M., Korper, W., Jansen, D.C., Tigchelaar-Gutter, W., Saftig, P., *et al.* (2002) The bone lining cell: Its role in cleaning Howship's lacunae and initiating bone formation. *Journal of Bone and Mineral Research*, **17**(1), 77–90.

Figueiredo, M., Fernando, A., Martins, G., Freitas, J., Judas, F., and Figueiredo, H. (2010) Effect of the calcination temperature on the composition and microstructure of hydroxyapatite derived from human and animal bone. *Ceramics International*, **36**(8), 2383–2393.

Goldstein, J.I., Newbury, D.E., Echlin, P., Joy, D.C., Roming, A.D., Jr, Lyman, C.E., *et al.* (eds.) (2012) *Scanning Electron Microscopy and X-ray Microanalysis: A Text for Biologists, Materials Scientists, and Geologists*, 1st edn. Springer Science & Business Media.

Harbeck, M., Schleuder, R., Schneider, J., Wiechmann, I., Schmahl, W.W., and Grupe, G. (2011) Research potential and limitations of trace analyses of cremated remains. *Forensic Science International*, **204**(1–3), 191–200.

Herrmann, B. (1972) Zur Beurteilung von Kohlenstoffverfärbungen bei Leichenbränden. *Ausgrabungen Und Funde*, **17**(1), 275–277.

Howes, J.M., Stuart, B.H., Thomas, P.S., Raja, S., and O'Brien, C. (2012) An investigation of model forensic bone in soil environments studied using infrared spectroscopy. *Journal of Forensic Sciences*, **57**(5), 1161–1167.

Imaizumi, K., Taniguchi, K., and Ogawa, Y. (2014) DNA survival and physical and histological properties of heat-induced alterations in burnt bones. *International Journal of Legal Medicine*, **128**(3), 439–446.

Khan, A.F., Awais, M., Khan, A.S., Tabassum, S., Chaudhry, A.A., and Rehman, I.U. (2013) Raman spectroscopy of natural bone and synthetic apatites. *Applied Spectroscopy Reviews*, **48**(4), 329–355.

Klepinger, L.L. (1984) Nutritional assessment from bone. *Annual Review of Anthropology*, **13**(1), 75–96.

Kourkoumelis, N., Zhang, X., Lin, Z., and Wang, J. (2019) Fourier transform infrared spectroscopy of bone tissue: Bone quality assessment in preclinical and clinical applications of osteoporosis and fragility fracture. *Clinical Reviews in Bone and Mineral Metabolism*, **17**(1), 24–39.

Kronick, P.L. and Cooke, P. (1996) Thermal stabilization of collagen fibers by calcification. *Connective Tissue Research*, **33**(4), 275–282.

Larkin, P. (2011) Chapter 2 Basic principles. In: *Infrared and Raman Spectroscopy* (ed. P. Larkin). Elsevier, Oxford, pp. 7–25.

Lebon, M., Reiche, I., Bahain, J., Chadefaux, C., Moigne, A., Fröhlich, F., *et al.* (2010) New parameters for the characterization of diagenetic alterations and heat-induced changes of fossil bone mineral using Fourier transform infrared spectrometry. *Journal of Archaeological Science*, **37**(1), 2265–2267.

Maciejewska, A., Wlodarczyk, R., and Pawlowski, R. (2015) The influence of high temperature on the possibility of DNA typing in various human tissues. *Folia histochemica et cytobiologica*, **53**(4), 322–332.

Mamede, A.P., Gonçalves, D., Marques, M.P.M., and Batista de Carvalho, L.A. (2018) Burned bones tell their own stories: A review of methodological approaches to assess heat-induced diagenesis. *Applied Spectroscopy Reviews*, **53**(8), 603–635.

Mayne Correia, P.M. (1997) Fire modification of bone: A review of the literature. In: *Forensic Taphonomy: The Postmortem Fate of Human Remains* (eds. W.D. Haglund and M.H. Sorg). CRC Press, Boca Raton, FL, pp. 275–294.

Mkukuma, L.D., Skakle, J.M.S., Gibson, I.R., Imrie, C.T., Aspden, R.M., and Hukins, D.W.L. (2004) Effect of the proportion of organic material in bone on thermal decomposition of bone mineral: An investigation of a variety of bones from different species using thermogravimetric analysis coupled to mass spectrometry, high-temperature X-ray diffraction, and Fourier transform infrared spectroscopy. *Calcified Tissue International*, **75**(4), 321–328.

Mutalib, M., Rahman, M.A., Othman, M.H.D., Ismail, A.F., and Jaafar, J. (2017) Scanning electron microscopy (SEM) and energy-dispersive X-ray (EDX) spectroscopy. In: *Membrane Characterization* (eds. N. Hilal, A.F. Ismail, T. Matsuura, and D. Oatley-Radcliffe). Elsevier, Amsterdam. pp. 161–179.

Nyman, J.S., Roy, A., Shen, X., Acuna, R.L., Tyler, J.H., and Wang, X. (2006) The influence of water removal on the strength and toughness of cortical bone. *Journal of Biomechanics*, **39**(5), 931–938.

Olszta, M.J., Cheng, X., Jee, S.S., Kumar, R., Kim, Y., Kaufman, M.J., *et al.* (2007) Bone structure and formation: A new perspective. *Materials Science and Engineering R: Reports*, **58**(3–5), 77–116.

Parfitt, A.M. (2001) The bone remodeling compartment: A circulatory function for bone lining cells. *Journal of Bone and Mineral Research*, **16**(9), 1583–1585.

Paschalis, E.P. (2009) Fourier transform infrared analysis of bone. *Osteoporosis International*, **20**(1), 1043–1047.

Piga, G., Malgosa, A., Thompson, T.J.U., and Enzo, S. (2008) A new calibration of the XRD technique for the study of archaeological burned human remains. *Journal of Archaeological Science*, **35**(8), 2171–2178.

Piga, G., Thompson, T.J.U., Malgosa, A., and Enzo, S. (2009) The potential of X-ray diffraction in the analysis of burned remains from forensic contexts. *Journal of Forensic Sciences*, **54**(3), 534–539.

Quelch, K.J., Melick, R.A., Bingham, P.J., and Mercuri, S.M. (1983) Chemical composition of human bone. *Archives of Oral Biology*, **28**(8), 665–674.

Rho, J., Kuhn-Spearing, L., and Zioupos, P. (1998) Mechanical properties and the hierarchical structure of bone. *Medical Engineering and Physics*, **20**(2), 92–102.

Ritchie, R.O., Buehler, M.J., and Hansma, P. (2009) Plasticity and touchiness in bone. *Physics Today* **6**(1), 41–47.

Robey, P.G. (2008) Noncollagenous bone matrix proteins. In: *Principles of Bone Biology*, Vol. **1**, 3rd edn. (eds. J.P. Bilezikian, L.G. Raisz, and T.J. Martin). Elsevier Academic Press, San Diego, CA, pp. 335–349.

Rogers, K., Beckett, S., Kuhn, S., Chamberlain, A., and Clement, J. (2010) Contrasting the crystallinity indicators of heated and diagenetically altered bone mineral. *Paleogeography, Palaeoclimatology, Palaeoecology*, **296**(1–2), 125–129.

Rogers, K.D. and Daniels, P. (2002) An X-ray diffraction study of the effects of heat treatment on bone mineral microstructure. *Biomaterials*, **23**(12), 2577–2585.

Schafer, A.T. (2001) The colour of the human skull. *Forensic Science International*, **117**(1–2), 53–56.

Shipman, P. (1981) Applications of scanning electron microscopy to taphonomic problems. *Annals of the New York Academy of Sciences*, **376**(1), 357–385.

Shipman, P., Foster, G., and Schoeninger, M. (1984) Burnt bones and teeth: An experimental study of color, morphology, crystal structure and shrinkage. *Journal of Archaeological Science*, **11**(4), 307–325.

Smith, F. (ed.). (2019) *Industrial Applications of X-ray Diffraction*. CRC Press, Boca Raton, FL.

Thompson, T.J.U. (2004) Recent advances in the study of burned bone and their implications for forensic anthropology. *Forensic Science International*, **146**(SUPPL.), S203–S205.

Thompson, T.J.U. (2005) Heat-induced dimensional changes in bone and their consequences for forensic anthropology. *Journal of Forensic Sciences*, **50**(5), 1–8.

Thompson, T.J.U., Gauthier, M., and Islam, M. (2009) The application of a new method of Fourier Transform Infrared Spectroscopy to the analysis of burned bone. *Journal of Archaeological Science*, **36**(3), 910–914.

Thompson, T.J.U., Islam, M., and Bonniere, M. (2013) A new statistical approach for determining the crystallinity of heat-altered bone mineral from FTIR spectra. *Journal of Archaeological Science*, **40**(1), 416–422.

Trujillo, O., Vanezis, P., and Cermignani, M. (1996) Photometric assessment of skin colour and lightness using a tristimulus colorimeter: Reliability of inter and intra-investigator observations in healthy adult volunteers. *Forensic Science International*, **81**(1), 1–10.

Turner-Walker, G. and Syversen, U. (2002) Quantifying histological changes in archaeological bones using BSE-SEM image analysis. *Archaeometry*, **44**(3), 461–468.

van Hoesel, A., Reidsma, F.H., van Os, B.J., Megens, L., and Braadbaart, F. (2019) Combusted bone: Physical and chemical changes of bone during laboratory simulated heating under oxidising conditions and their relevance for the study of ancient fire use. *Journal of Archaeological Science: Reports*, **28**, 102033.

Wang, X., Zuo, Y., Huang, D., Hou, X., and Li, Y. (2010) Comparative study on inorganic composition and crystallographic properties of cortical and cancellous bone. *Biomedical and Environmental Sciences*, **23**(1), 473–480.

Weiner, S. and Wagner, H.D. (1998) The material bone: Structure-mechanical function relations. *Annual Review of Materials Science*, **28**(1), 271–298.

Zimmerman, H.A., Meizel-Lambert, C.J., Schultz, J.J., and Sigman, M.E. (2015) Chemical differentiation of osseous, dental, and non-skeletal materials in forensic anthropology using elemental analysis. *Science & Justice*, **55**(2), 131–138.

CHAPTER 12

DNA Profiling from Burnt Remains

Sara C. Zapico[1,2], PhD, ABC-MB and Rebecca Stone-Gordon[3], MSc

[1] *Assistant Professor, New Jersey Institute for Technology, Department of Chemistry and Environmental Science, Newark, NJ, USA*

[2] *Smithsonian Institution, National Museum of Natural History, Washington, DC*

[3] *American University, Washington, DC*

12.1 Introduction

The identification of burnt remains constitutes one of the most challenging tasks of a forensic scientist. These situations comprise different scenarios: natural, accidental, arson fires, and mass disasters. These contexts prompt a multidisciplinary approach towards the identification of the remains based on fingerprint analysis, dental and medical records' comparison, and DNA analysis. At the same time, particularly in mass disaster settings, there are challenges associated with the analysis of the remains, such as determination of the number of victims, mechanisms of body destruction, extent of body fragmentation, and body accessibility (Alonso *et al.*, 2005).

Bone and teeth represent reliable sources of DNA, even in adverse environmental conditions (Watherston *et al.*, 2018). Different skeletal elements retrieve different DNA yields (Montelius and Lindblom, 2012). Based on the identification efforts of the World Trade Center (9/11) disaster in 2001, it was determined that skeletal samples from the femur and metatarsal bones offered the most amount of DNA (Mundorff *et al.*, 2009). In fact, current recommendations suggest the collection of femoral shaft samples (Watherston *et al.*, 2018). Teeth and their location in the jawbone provide protection from environmental and physical conditions. However, DNA quality and quantity retrieved from teeth depends on the type of tooth and tissue (Zapico and Ubelaker, 2013).

Even though bone and teeth are the preferred sources of DNA from remains subjected to fire, different factors (temperature, time of exposure, among others) could affect the appropriate recovery of DNA, and as a result hamper the correct identification of the victims.

Burnt Human Remains: Recovery, Analysis, and Interpretation, First Edition. Edited by Sarah Ellingham, Joe Adserias-Garriga, Sara C. Zapico and Douglas H. Ubelaker.

The present chapter will provide an overview of the studies related to DNA extraction and profiling from burnt remains, the challenges encountered in these processes, as well as current and new methodologies developed to overcome these problems.

12.2 Research Studies on Burnt Remains

An early study of Álvarez García *et al.* (Alvarez Garcia *et al.*, 1996) described the impact of different temperatures and times on the retrieval and analysis of DNA from dental pulp. In this work, teeth were kept at 4°C, 20°C, and 40°C for periods ranging from 2 weeks to 36 months. Additionally, 168 teeth were subjected to incineration for one and two minutes at 75°C, 100°C, 200°C, 300°C, 400°C, and 500°C. Likewise, teeth were exposed to 100°C and 200°C for five and ten minutes. After isolating the pulp, the method chosen for DNA extraction was chelating resin. The assessed markers were HLA DQA1, D1S80, HUMTH01, HUMFES/FPS, and the amelogenin gene. At lower temperatures (4°C, 20°C, and 40°C) positive amplification results were obtained in most of the samples during the different time periods. On teeth subjected to incineration, negative amplification results were obtained at 500°C at two minutes, except for amelogenin. Other temperatures and times retrieved positive amplification from most of the samples. Exposure to 100°C for ten minutes gave positive amplification results; however, when the temperature was increased (200°C) for the same time interval, the results became poorer. Additionally, this study retrieved DNA from three unidentified cremated bodies. All the markers used gave positive results. Since these were actual forensic cases, the teeth were protected by muscular and skeletal structures, as well as dental structures such as enamel and cementum, providing the ideal environment to protect pulp DNA.

Harbeck *et al.* (Harbeck *et al.*, 2011) developed a combined study to determine the maximum degree of bone cremation that can be reached at which robust, original signals from DNA and stable isotope analysis can still be retrieved. They used tibiae of modern cattle and subjected them to temperatures ranging from 100°C to 1000°C in increments of 100°C for one and a half hours and four hours. DNA was extracted through two methods: silica-based columns and InViSorb Forensic Kit (InViTek). The target gene was the mitochondrial hypervariable region one (HVS1) (129 bp), which was sequenced. From the samples subjected to fire for one and a half hours, it was possible to retrieve and amplify DNA up to 700°C applying the silica-based column extraction method. In contrast, the same samples extracted through InViSorb kit only yielded amplifiable DNA at temperatures of 100°C, 200°C, 300°C, and 700°C. For samples exposed for four hours, applying the InViSorb extraction kit, it was possible to obtain reproducible results up to a temperature of 600°C. This work also referred to a previous study (von Wurmb-Schwark *et al.*, 2005), where the authors tried to obtain a DNA profile from samples from a modern crematory. However, they only found non-authentic DNA profiles in the cremated remains, based on the disparities between the DNA profile obtained from the bone vs. DNA profile obtained from buccal swabs. The authors hypothesized that the reason for these inconsistencies is the contamination of the remains during their treatment in the crematorium.

Schwark *et al.* (Schwark *et al.*, 2011) conducted a systematic study to analyze the possibility of retrieving authentic DNA profiles from forensic cases. They collected 71 bone fragments from 13 human bodies during autopsy, dividing them into five groups based on thermal impact: "well preserved"; "semi-burnt"; "black burnt"; "blue-grey burnt"; "blue-grey-white burnt." Authentic genetic profiles were obtained from blood. DNA was extracted from 400–500 mg bone powder using Invisorb Forensic Kit I (Invitek, Germany). Samples were not previously decalcified. The quality of DNA was tested using a multiplex PCR, including amelogenin gene and two Y-STRs; two autosomal markers, vWA and TH01; and two mitochondrial fragments from the hypervariable region I (HVI), as described in a previous work (von Wurmb-Schwark *et al.*, 2009). STR analysis was performed using AmpFISTR Identifiler (Thermo Fisher Scientific). Additionally, amplification of two regions of the Hypervariable region I (HVI) of mitochondrial DNA was carried out. In terms of quality and quantity of DNA, the first two groups ("well preserved" and "semi-burnt") gave a full profile. The "well preserved" group retrieved higher DNA concentration than the "semi-burnt" group. "Black burnt" bones showed a variable profile pattern and lower DNA concentrations. The last two groups retrieved negative results in terms of DNA profile retrieval and the lowest DNA concentrations. AmpFISTR Identifiler was used on the samples which had retrieved a full profile on the previous phase. Full profiles were obtained from "well preserved" samples. From "semi-burnt" samples, 83.3% of the samples showed profiles with 14–15 STRs or 10–13 STRs. Again, "black burnt" bones presented a variable profile pattern. From the last two groups it was only possible to amplify five loci in one case. With respect to mtDNA amplification and sequencing, "well preserved" and "semi-burnt" bones exhibited enough quantities of both HVI fragments for subsequent sequencing analysis. However, six samples of this group retrieved lower amounts of mtDNA products, and the authors referred to a potential inhibitor present (collagen I). The problem was solved by reducing the amount of the DNA used for the PCR (1 µl instead of 5 µl). "Black burnt" bones again retrieved heterogeneous results in mtDNA analysis. The authors suggested that an inhibitor could be playing a role in this case. From the last two groups it was only possible to amplify the smaller HVI fragment. This was expected based on the previous results as well as the temperatures to which these remains were subjected (Cattaneo *et al.*, 1999). This study pointed to the possibility of obtaining reliable and reproducible DNA profiles from "well preserved" and "semi-burnt" bones.

Imaizumi *et al.* (Imaizumi *et al.*, 2014) conducted another temperature/time study using bovine metacarpal bones. They analyzed physical changes on the bone as well as the retrieval of DNA. The DNA specimens were exposed to temperatures from 150°C to 300°C in 50°C increments and burnt over short time intervals (15, 30, 45, 60, 120, and 180 minutes). The samples were decalcified and posteriorly extracted applying phenol-chloroform protocol, concentrating the extracts with a filter device. PCR was performed on 419-bp product within the bovine mtDNA D-loop region, and a 128-bp product within a 16S ribosomal RNA coding region of bovine mtDNA. Negative amplification was found in all specimens burnt at temperatures above 250°C. In contrast, it was possible to amplify both mtDNA fragments in samples burnt for 180 minutes at 150°C. At 200°C, only bone specimens burnt for 15 minutes showed amplification for both products. These results were consistent with a previous study from another group (Cattaneo *et al.*, 1999).

Maciejewska *et al.* (Maciejewska *et al.*, 2015) assessed the possibility of retrieved DNA profiles from different human tissues at different temperatures and times. They selected thigh skeletal muscle, liver, cardiac muscle, adipose tissue, long bones (fibula), and teeth. These tissues were exposed to 100°C, 300°C, 500°C, 700°C, 800°C, 900°C, and 1000°C for five or ten minutes. Hair and nails were subjected to temperatures of 100°C, 300°C, 500°C, 700°C, or 800°C for five minutes. DNA was isolated applying phenol-chloroform protocol followed by purification and concentration on Microcon 100 columns (Merck Millipore). AmpFISTR SGM Plus and AmpFISTR MiniFiler (Thermo Fisher Scientific) were used to obtain DNA profiles. HVI of mtDNA was sequenced using the HVI F15971 R16410 primers and the BigDye Terminator Cycle Sequencing Kit (Thermo Fisher Scientific). No amplification of autosomal STRs or mtDNA was obtained for hair and nail samples subjected to temperatures ranging from 100°C to 800°C. In teeth, the three tested markers (SGMPlus, MiniFiler and mtDNA) retrieved profiles after exposure to 100°C for five and ten minutes. For the SGMPlus, teeth exposure to 300°C for five and ten minutes, 63% and 31% of the alleles, respectively, gave a positive signal. Teeth exposed to 300°C for five and ten minutes provided full MiniFiler profiles. Temperatures of 500°C and beyond did not allow for retrieval of SGMPlus or MiniFiler profiles. In contrast, complete sequences of HVI mtDNA were obtained from teeth samples exposed to 100°C, 300°C, and 500°C for five minutes. Fibula fragments subjected to temperatures of 100°C, 300°C, 500°C, 700°C, and 800°C for five minutes retrieved full MiniFiler and SGMPlus profiles. At 900°C and five minutes' exposure, nuclear DNA was degraded and only the amelogenin gene in two samples was amplified, and four out of six samples gave a reliable HVI sequence. With respect to the other two samples, the Primer-Extension Preamplification (PEP) method was applied (Maciejewska *et al.*, 2013). It was possible to obtain a complete and reliable HVI mtDNA sequence for one of the samples. Temperatures above 900°C caused incineration of all the tested tissues, and it was not possible to retrieve nuclear or mitochondrial DNA. SGMPlus, MiniFiler, and mtDNA profiles could be obtained from adipose tissues exposed to

100–500°C for five minutes. Beyond these temperatures amplifiable DNA was not retrieved. In contrast, it was possible to obtain partial SGMPlus profiles at 700°C with five minutes' exposure time from other soft tissues. Above this temperature, no amplification products were obtained. However, MiniFiler and mtDNA profiles could be retrieved at temperatures of 100–800°C with five minutes' exposure. No profiles were obtained beyond 800°C. An increase of exposure time reduced the ability to obtain full profiles at 100–300°C. From adipose tissue, exposure to higher temperatures (500°C) did not yield amplification in any of the markers. However, the other soft tissue samples retrieved partial SGMPlus profiles and full MiniFiler and mtDNA profiles. Temperatures of 800–1000°C resulted in the lack of DNA amplification in all the analyzed systems. This study indicates that DNA stability and retrieval in tissues exposed to high temperatures depends on tissue type, temperature, and time of exposure.

The study of Adserias-Garriga *et al.* (Adserias-Garriga *et al.*, 2016) analyzed the efficiency of DNA profiling on human teeth subjected to temperatures of 100–700°C in 100°C increments and exposure times of 1, 5, 10, and 15 minutes. DNA was extracted from the whole tooth, applying a silica-based column methodology without a previous decalcification step (Zapico and Ubelaker, 2013). The amelogenin gene was amplified by conventional PCR, and the efficiency of STR profiling was estimated using real-time PCR by analysis of different STRs: D7S820, D13S317, D5S818, CSF1PO, TPOX, TH01, vWA, D16S539, AND FES/FPS. Based on the DNA quantification by fluorometry, it was possible to obtain DNA from almost all samples, except 400°C at 10 and 15 minutes; 500°C at 15 minutes; 600°C at 5 and 15 minutes; 700°C at 5, 10, and 15 minutes gave quantification values below the detection limit of the assay. STR amplification similar to the controls was possible to obtain in the first temperatures and times intervals (100°C and 200°C at one and five minutes). In the majority of STRs, the amplification was very low, from 300°C and one or five minutes. At this temperature the color of the teeth was grey, which agrees with previous described studies (Schwark *et al.*, 2011). Similar results were obtained with the amelogenin gene. Amplification was possible up to 300°C with 15 minute exposure, although at this temperature and time it was still possible to see slight amplification bands. Based on these results the authors pointed to a differential amplification between STRs located on the p arm vs. the q arm. The latter showed higher amplification even at temperatures and times where it was not possible to get amplification, which may indicate that these genes are better protected than the p arm. GAPDH, a housekeeping gene for the real-time PCR, was also amplified. This gene retrieved positive signals for all combination of temperatures and times, although the amplification was inversely proportional to the increase of temperatures and times. The amplification of this gene opened the possibility of being able to amplify other DNA regions in these cases, like SNPs. The authors included an important limitation of this study: the teeth used in this work were isolated extracted teeth. In vivo, teeth are surrounded and protected by maxillary and mandibular bones as well as facial soft tissues. This protection would increase the resistance of teeth to fire. This must be considered in a forensic case.

In this line of research, Ramlal *et al.* (Ramlal *et al.*, 2017) used teeth samples exposed to 700°C for 15–20 minutes and later deposited in soil for six and twelve months to analyze DNA retrieval under environmental conditions. The method chosen for DNA extraction was phenol-chloroform, later concentrated with Centricon-100. mtDNA was obtained from eight out ten samples from the six-month group, and six out of ten samples from the twelve-month group. The concentration of DNA was variable among samples from the same group, ranging at 0.43–0.84 µg/ml in the six-month group; and 0.45–0.8 µg/ml in the twelve-month group. The authors did not find any statistically significant differences between these two groups in terms of DNA retrieval.

Samsuwan *et al.* (Samsuwan *et al.*, 2018) used porcine teeth and bone to analyze DNA retrieval under different conditions. Among them, they burnt bone and teeth samples with rubber for three hours. DNA was extracted applying the phenol-chloroform protocol. Porcine nuclear ACTB gene was amplified by PCR. HVI and HV2 regions of mtDNA were also amplified by PCR. Only teeth samples showed a positive amplification of both ACTB and mtDNA. This study suggested that teeth could be a better source for DNA retrieval and profiling from burnt remains than bone.

This section has given an overview of some of the studies dedicated to analyzing the possibility of DNA retrieval from burnt remains, providing potential methodologies to improve the DNA yield.

12.3 Forensic Cases

Forensic cases constitute a good source of the strategic approaches that forensic scientists develop to be able to recover identifiable DNA from human remains.

The study of Holland *et al.* (Holland *et al.*, 2003) proposed different strategies to improve the DNA profiling of the remains from the 9/11 victims. The first one was a modified protocol to increase the DNA recovered from the bones containing both EDTA and collagen to remove the potential inhibitors of the samples. The other strategy was the development of two mini-STR multiplexes to improve the DNA profiling. Both approaches improved the outcome of obtaining DNA profiles; however, the condition of the remains is still an issue to successfully achieve the identification goal.

Staiti *et al.* (Staiti *et al.*, 2004) explained the workflow they used in identification of three bodies from different forensic cases. From the third body, which was burnt, they decided to use endochondral bone. Prior to DNA extraction, the bones were decalcified for three days, and later a modified Promega IQ protocol was applied for DNA recovery. This protocol was compared with the traditional phenol-chloroform protocol. Using AmpFLSTR Identifiler, the authors were able to obtain a full DNA profile from the three bodies, with the modified IQ protocol performing better in terms of DNA yield and purity than the traditional phenol-chloroform.

The usefulness of mitochondrial DNA analysis in cold cases was demonstrated by Nelson *et al.* (Nelson and Melton, 2007). They recovered 116 bone/teeth samples from cases submitted to their laboratory between February 1999 and May 2005. There were two different aims for these analyses: some samples were used for body identifications submitted by law enforcement; other samples were submitted to answer historical or familiar identity questions. The method chosen for DNA extraction was silica-based columns. HV1 and HV2 regions of mtDNA were sequenced. In terms of type of samples, 92% of femurs and 90% of teeth provided full or partial profiles. Despite these results, the authors concluded that burnt samples were not successful in retrieving profiles (11 out of 16 burnt samples failed to lead to identification). Additionally, amplifying DNA from cremains (the remains obtained after a cremation) was uniformly unsuccessful, which is consistent with previous studies (Cattaneo *et al.*, 1999).

Ohira *et al.* (Ohira *et al.*, 2009) described the identification process of two bodies recovered after a house fire in Yokohama City, Japan. The remains were supposedly a father and a son. They were identified based on ante-mortem and post-mortem X-ray films and dental records. In addition to these analyses, the authors used teeth samples from the remains to determine the DNA profile and compare it to reference samples from the father's brother and daughter (son's sister). Teeth were decalcified prior to DNA extraction, which was achieved through the phenol-chloroform protocol. The AmpFISTR Identifiler Kit was used for nuclear DNA profiling. Additionally, sequencing of the HV1 of mtDNA was performed. The results of STR analysis confirmed the relationship between the father and his brother. The STR and mtDNA sequence analysis established the parent-child relationship among father-son-daughter. Thus, it is important to consider both nuclear and mitochondrial markers for correctly assigning kinship associations.

Hartman *et al.* (Hartman *et al.*, 2011) described the laboratory workflow for the identification of the remains of the Victoria bushfires disaster. Depending on the condition of the remains, they collected blood, tissue, and bone samples. Bones were collected when the remains were severely burned and it was not possible to obtain blood or tissue. All samples were extracted using the Qiagen DNA Investigator Kit. DNA profiling was performed using the AmpFISTR Profiler Plus. In contrast to previously referred studies, 100% of the bone samples yielded full DNA profiles, as well as 91% of tissue samples; the lowest percentage of full profiles was obtained from blood specimens (77%). Overall, DNA analysis assisted in the identification of 67 of the 163 victims, 12 from direct matches, using Guthrie cards or pathology specimen, and 55 from kinship matches. 32 out of 67 cases used DNA as primary identifier, while 35 applied additional scientific information, such as forensic odontology. This forensic scenario highlights the importance of the recovery of ante-mortem samples, an appropriate triage of post-mortem samples, and a multidisciplinary approach for disaster victim identification.

Continuing with disaster victim identification scenarios, Ricci *et al.* (Ricci *et al.*, 2015) describe the identification efforts of seven corpses recovered after a fire in a textile factory in Florence, Italy, where Chinese workers were illegally employed. Since the bodies were completely charred, different samples were collected: from the pterygoid muscles and the posterior part of the tongue; small fragments of brain; two feet and a hand bone. Reference samples were collected from the relatives: two brothers; two sisters; one daughter; one son; and one mother. DNA was extracted by EZ1 Advanced using the EZ1 Tissue Kit (Qiagen). The AmpFlSTR NGM PCR Amplification Kit (Thermo Fisher Scientific) and the PowerPlex Y23 System (Promega) were used for male samples. The amelogenin gene showed that there were five males and two females. Direct comparison was made between the autosomal profile of the mother's sample, as well as one daughter and one son, identifying their relatives. Y-STR profiles were used to compare the two brothers' profiles, which were fully matched with their respective relatives. However, in these two cases and the cases of the two sisters, likelihood ratios and probabilities were calculated to determine the kinship match. In this case, the authors did not discuss the efficiency of the different samples for DNA analyses; however, they recommended using tissue fragments taken from parts protected from the fire.

Zgonjanin *et al.* (Zgonjanin *et al.*, 2015) depict the identification of a taxi driver who was found burnt in the trunk of his car. They used a bone sample of the body and additionally assessed five DNA extracts from different femoral samples, corresponding to five different burnt body identification cases. For DNA extraction, they used the phenol-chloroform protocol without previous decalcification, and posteriorly purified by ultra-filtration on Centricon-100. AmpFlSTR Identifiler Plus; AmpFlSTR NGM; and AmpFlSTR Yfiler (Thermo Fisher Scientific) were used to obtain the DNA profiles and the Y-STR profiles. The taxi driver case provided successful amplification with the three kits, identifying the victim based on the reference sample from his son, comparing both STRs and Y-STRs. With respect to the other cases, full STR profiles were obtained in four cases. In the fifth case 10/16 loci were amplified with Identifiler and 13/16 with NGM. Two victims were identified by comparison to daughters; two victims were identified by comparison to sons. In these cases, only STRs were compared. The last victim was matched to his father, where both STRs and Y-STRs were compared. Based on these results the authors suggested not to generalize the expectation of potential success of sample analysis based on their appearance, that is, the remains of the taxi driver were severely burned yet identifiable DNA profiles were retrieved.

Ferreira *et al.* (Ferreira *et al.*, 2015) discussed the efficiency of DNA profiling among different tissues in three severely burnt bodies due to a car crash in Brazil. From each of the three bodies they collected deep red muscle and cartilage from the hip joint (head of the femur), and a swab from inside the urinary bladder. The method chosen for DNA extraction was phenol-chloroform. PowerPlex Fusion Kit was used to obtain the DNA profiles. All the samples retrieved DNA yields higher than 1 ng/μl. In two bodies, cartilage samples had DNA yields higher than muscle and the swab from the urinary bladder. Full profiles were obtained from all samples of cartilage, deep red muscle, and swabs from the urinary bladder. This demonstrated the usefulness of these samples as a source of DNA typing of severely burnt bodies in disaster victim identification.

This section described technical approaches carried out by forensic scientists to retrieve DNA profiles towards the identification of human remains in forensic cases.

12.4 Alternative Approaches and New Technologies

12.4.1 Assessment of DNA Damage

Fredericks *et al.* (Fredericks *et al.*, 2012) studied the possibility of using Fourier transform infrared (FTIR) spectroscopy to assess DNA integrity. They used bovine femur bone fragments subjected to temperatures of 50–1000°C for two or four hours. DNA extraction was carried out with a previous demineralization step and applying the All-tissue DNA-extraction kit (Gen-ial Gmbh). They amplified three DNA fragments of different sizes to represent the amplification of full STRs, miniSTRs, and single nucleotide polymorphisms. As expected, DNA degradation was a function of the temperature and duration of heat treatment. DNA was relatively stable at temperatures below 150°C. This correlated with the analysis of the amide I to phosphate ratio, measured by FTIR, which represents a semi-quantitative method for collagen content of bone. Based on this measure, between 150°C and 600°C collagen molecules undergo degradation. Beyond these temperatures, no amide I bands were detected, which is consistent with previous studies that pointed out that bone heated at temperatures above 600°C loses its organic component. This study suggested that the degradation of collagen and DNA occur at a similar temperature. Additionally, the authors reported changes on mineral components of the bone, which could also be correlated with the success of DNA amplification. Thus, the authors proposed the use of FTIR spectroscopy as a "screening" tool prior to attempting DNA extraction and analysis.

The previous group (Fredericks *et al.*, 2015) developed a subsequent study analyzing the correlation between color changes and changes in collagen, mineral, and DNA integrity, using a colorimeter. The procedure of bone heating and DNA extraction was similar to the previous work (Fredericks *et al.*, 2012). In addition, they used the StockMarks for Cattle Bovine Genotyping Kit (Thermo Fisher Scientific) for amplification and analysis of 11 unlinked microsatellite loci. No DNA targets were successfully amplified at 210°C or above, with a pallet code of the Munsell color chart 9Y9/6. However, this color chart alone was not enough to distinguish the subtle changes in color to correlate with DNA integrity. Additionally, this is very subjective. Despite these limitations, and based on their results, the authors agreed that with further development, this technique could be useful as a diagnostic tool to aid DNA analysis.

Ginart *et al.* (Ginart *et al.*, 2019) developed a methodology to assess DNA degradation based on quantitative-PCR followed by high-resolution melting. Moreover, it determines the sex of the DNA donor. Three amplicons were evaluated: a Y-linked gene; a large-target sequence; and a small-target sequence. An imbalance between the small and long target melting peak heights permitted the estimation of the extent of DNA degradation. They tested this methodology in experimental DNA samples heated to 95°C for different times (0–40 minutes), and, in forensic casework samples, both yielding full profiles and partial profiles. In experimental samples, it was possible to assess the degradation of DNA. In forensic samples, the results were compared to Plexor HY on full profiles and PowerQuant on partial profiles. In the former, the new technique was able to detect the Y-melting peaks more efficiently than the kit. In the latter, it was possible to determine the degradation of the samples and detection of the male DNA. Thus, in general this methodology could be a useful tool to detect DNA degradation before the STR analysis.

12.4.2 Alternatives for DNA Extraction

Researchers have looked for alternative tissues to recover DNA from burnt remains. Theodore Harcke *et al.* (Theodore Harcke *et al.*, 2009) documented the recovery of DNA from the spinal cord or surrounding dura mater in 11 cases of severely burnt human remains, aided by digital radiographs (DR) and multidetector computer tomography (MDCT). DNA was extracted using Chelex, and the chosen STR kit was the PowerPlex 15 Amplification kit (Promega). In comparison to the routine sample results, spinal cord and surrounding tissues were comparable with other organ tissue as a source of nuclear DNA. Additionally, the processing time was shorter than bone samples. The authors referred to limitations of this study: spinal cord samples were from the lower thoracic and upper lumbar spine, so it is not possible to assume that samples from other areas (like cervical) can be used in burnt cases.

As described previously in this chapter, Owen *et al.* (Owen *et al.*, 2013) also evaluated the possibility of using bladder samples for DNA analysis. The authors recovered bladder swabs from 28 forensic cases exposed to fire. DNA was extracted using the QIAamp DNA investigator kit with a slightly modification of the protocol. DNA profile was obtained using the AmpFISTR Identifiler Plus STR (Thermo Fisher Scientific). In comparison with other samples, bladder swabs retrieved greater nuclear DNA yields (muscle and blood), and lower when the other sample was a bone. All but one of the bladder samples gave full DNA profiles, the other gave a partial profile. Additionally, the quality of the profiles from bladder samples was similar or better when compared to the conventional samples. Thus, this study ratified the usefulness of bladder swabs as an alternative source of DNA for the identification of burnt remains.

De Lourdes Chávez-Briones *et al.* (de Lourdes Chávez-Briones *et al.*, 2013) were able to obtain the DNA profile of burnt remains from maggots colonizing the body. Three maggots were collected; from each one they removed the crop, a diverticulum of the cephalic end of the gut. DNA extraction was performed using phenol-chloroform. STR analysis was performed using AmpFISTR Identifiler kit (Thermo Fisher Scientific). As a reference sample, DNA from the father of a missing person was used. The genetic profiles were similar from the three different maggots. It was possible to determine the sex based on amelogenin gene, and 12 loci were amplified, sharing at least one allele with the alleged father, leading to the identification of the victim. This study described the value of collecting maggots at the crime scene, not only to determine the post-mortem interval, also, for identification purposes.

In an article of Emery *et al.* (Emery *et al.*, 2020), two different DNA extraction methods were assessed to improve the possibility of obtaining full DNA profiles from burnt remains. Bone and teeth were recovered from 23 forensic cases exposed to fire at different temperatures (based on teeth/bone color). Two different extraction protocols were assessed: Loreille extraction protocol, and a modified version of Dabney protocol, extensively used for ancient DNA extraction (aDNA) (Loreille *et al.*, 2007, 2010; Dabney *et al.*, 2013). STR amplification was carried out with PowerPlex ESX 17 Fast Systems kit (Promega). With both methods, there was an inverse correlation between average DNA yields and increasing temperatures. In terms of STR profile, higher quality full and partial profiles using the Dabney protocol were generated in comparison with the Loreille protocol. The authors suggested applying this modified version of the Dabney protocol to improve DNA profiling from burnt remains.

12.4.3 New Technologies

The introduction of Next Generation Sequencing (NGS) technologies, as well as forensic DNA phenotyping and ancestry determination seem to be the next step to improve DNA analysis from burnt remains.

Hollard *et al.* (Hollard *et al.*, 2017) used Ancestry Informative Markers (AIMs) to aid the identification of a carbonized body found in a city dump near Paris, France. A tooth and a piece of muscle were the chosen samples. The authors analyzed the HVI of mtDNA and determined the Y-STR profile based on the Yfiler Plus PCR Amplification kit. Eye color prediction was based on the IrisPlex system. The method chosen for AIMs was the HID-Ion AmpliSeq Ancestry Panel (Thermo Fisher Scientific) on the Ion PGM system (Thermo Fisher Scientific), composed by 165 autosomal SNPs. The mtDNA haplotype obtained was HV0, found in West Eurasian populations. The Y-chromosome haplogroup was E1b1, which according to the literature, matched two Tunisian haplogroups. Applying two SNP panels, one concluded that the sample could be of Southwest Asian origin (85%) (Kidd panel) and the other European origin (60%) (Seldin). The IrisPlex system predicted brown eyes. Thus, according to these results, the individual had brown eyes and his probable origin was in the Mediterranean Basin or South-west Asia. This information could be useful to include on the unidentified body report to increase the chances for identification.

Wai *et al.* (Wai *et al.*, 2018) evaluated the performance of the Early Access AmpliSeq Mitochondrial Panel (Thermo Fisher Scientific) on experimentally degraded samples using the Ion Torrent platform (Thermo Fisher Scientific). DNA from saliva samples was extracted applying the QIAamp DNA Mini Kit (Qiagen). This DNA was heated at 125°C for 30, 60, 120, and 240 minutes. As expected, the quality of DNA decreased with heat treatment for as little as 30 minutes. Despite these results, when applying the mitochondrial panel, it was possible to obtain complete sequences in all samples and resolved kinship and haplogroup assignments. This panel could be helpful towards the identification of highly degraded samples.

Following this previous line of research, Elwick *et al.* (Elwick *et al.*, 2019) evaluated the efficiency of two NGS kits and two NGS platforms for DNA profiling of challenged human remains. Bone and teeth were recovered from human remains and subjected to different treatments: bones were cremated in an oven at 900°C for 2.5 hours; teeth were thermally degraded in an oven at 232°C for 45 minutes; remains were ignited with gasoline in a house (mock arson scene) and burnt until they self-extinguished. Bone and tooth DNA were extracted using the Loreille total demineralization protocol (Loreille *et al.*, 2010). Regular STR analysis by Capillary Electrophoresis (CE) was performed using GlobalFiler (Thermo Fisher Scientific). For NGS, AmpliSeq STR and iiSNP panel on the Ion S5 System was used; and the ForenSeq DNA Signature Prep Kit on the MiSeq FGx system. In general, both NGS systems performed better than the CE system, as it was possible to recover more information from the degraded samples, including SNPs; providing more information aided the identification of the remains.

Sharma *et al.* (Sharma *et al.*, 2020) ratified the usefulness of the ForenSeq DNA Signature Kit in experimentally degraded DNA samples in comparison with regular CE (PowerPlex Fusion). Extracted DNA was heated at 95°C for 0, 5, 10, 15, 20, and 30 minutes (first experiment) and 40, 50, 60 minutes (second experiment). Additionally mock case-type samples were used to test the system. The results of this study pointed to an outperformance of the ForenSeq DNA Signature Prep kit with respect to the PowerPlex Fusion kit. As described in the previous paragraph, the analysis of SNPs and other non-traditional markers could be useful for the identification of the remains.

Gaudio *et al.* (Gaudio *et al.*, 2019) described the usefulness of retrieved DNA from petrous bones, and applying Dabney extraction method, in combination with NGS towards the determination of the sex and geographic origin. As previously mentioned, this additional information could be helpful towards the identification of the remains.

One of the growing fields on forensic genetics is the application of Rapid DNA for identification. Gin *et al.* (Gin *et al.*, 2020) described the utility of this new methodology in a disaster victim identification scenario, the 2018 California Wildfires. Different samples were collected from the bodies: blood, organs, muscle, and bone fragments. Furthermore, ante-mortem specimens and buccal swabs from the relatives were collected. ANDE Rapid DNA identification system was used. This system is based on the automation and integration of four laboratory processes: purification of genomic DNA from a sample; rapid multiplexed amplification of 27 STR loci (including amelogenin, and three Y-STR loci);

separation of the fragments; locus and allele assignation. Thanks to the application of this technology, approximately 90% of the samples submitted to Rapid DNA generated STR profiles, which was the primary identification modality in this scenario, leading to the identification of 58 victims. Thus, based on the simplicity and quick results, Rapid DNA technology should be considered as a potential tool to aid with identification in disaster contexts.

This section gave an overview of the current strategies for improving the identification of burnt remains at different levels: assessment of DNA damage; alternatives for DNA extraction; and new cutting-edge technologies.

12.5 Conclusions

This chapter covered the different approaches that forensic scientists apply for the identification of burnt remains based on DNA analysis. Figure 12.1 summarizes these approaches. The conditions the remains are exposed to (temperature and time of exposure) constitute the first hallmark towards the retrieval of identifiable DNA. As described, using alternative tissues instead of bone and teeth, like bladder swabs, seems to improve this goal. Likewise, modification of DNA extraction techniques could also help to get complete DNA profiles. New methodologies, like NGS, performed better when compared to traditional STR analysis. In addition, NGS kits for identification include additional STRs and SNPs analyses, which increase the information retrieved from the remains, improving the chances of identification. The election of one methodology over another, or the integration of them on the identification workflow will depend on the availability and conditions of the remains.

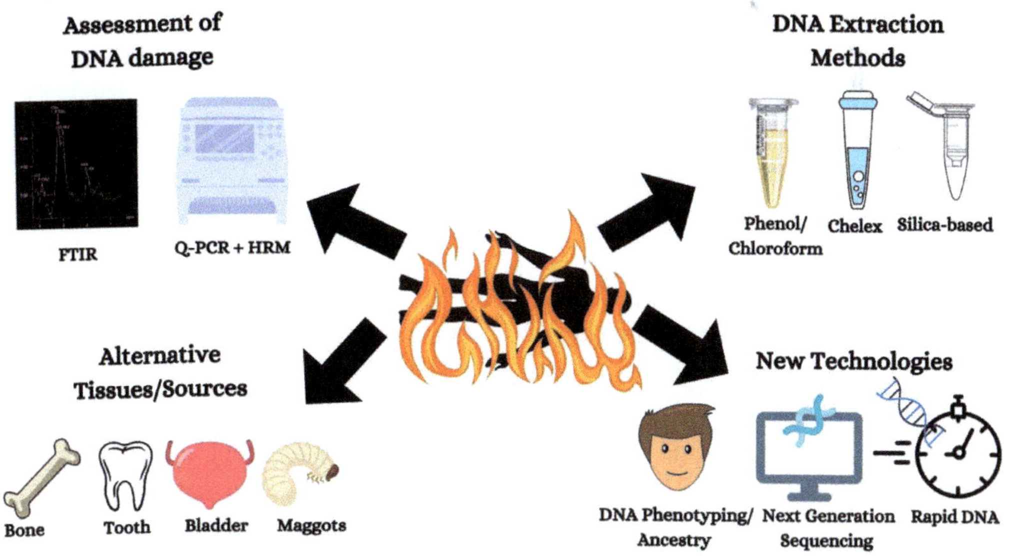

Figure 12.1 Summary of the approaches to improve DNA profiling from burnt remains. FTIR, Fourier Transformation Infrared; Q-PCR + HRM, Quantitative PCR + High Resolution Melting.

References

Adserias-Garriga, J., Ubelaker, D.H., and Zapico, S.C. (2016) Evaluation of macroscopic changes and the efficiency of DNA profiling from burnt teeth. *Science & Justice*, **56**(6), 437–442. https://doi.org/10.1016/j.scijus.2016.06.006

Alonso, A., Martin, P., Albarran, C., Garcia, P., Fernandez de Simon, L., Jesus Iturralde, M., *et al.* (2005) Challenges of DNA profiling in mass disaster investigations. *Croatian Medical Journal*, **46**(4), 540–548. https://www.ncbi.nlm.nih.gov/pubmed/16100756

Alvarez Garcia, A., Munoz, I., Pestoni, C., Lareu, M.V., Rodriguez-Calvo, M.S., and Carracedo, A. (1996) Effect of environmental factors on PCR-DNA analysis from dental pulp (Research Support, Non-U.S. Gov't). *International Journal of Legal Medicine*, **109**(3), 125–129. http://www.ncbi.nlm.nih.gov/pubmed/8956985

Cattaneo, C., DiMartino, S., Scali, S., Craig, O.E., Grandi, M., and Sokol, R.J. (1999) Determining the human origin of fragments of burnt bone: A comparative study of histological, immunological and DNA techniques (Comparative Study). *Forensic Science International*, **102**(2–3), 181–191. http://www.ncbi.nlm.nih.gov/pubmed/10464934

Dabney, J., Knapp, M., Glocke, I., Gansauge, M.T., Weihmann, A., Nickel, B., *et al.* (2013) Complete mitochondrial genome sequence of a Middle Pleistocene cave bear reconstructed from ultrashort DNA fragments. *Proceedings of the National Academy of Sciences of the United States of America*, **110**(39), 15758–15763. https://doi.org/10.1073/pnas.1314445110

de Lourdes Chávez-Briones, M., Hernández-Cortés, R., Díaz-Torres, P., Niderhauser-García, A., Ancer-Rodríguez, J., Jaramillo-Rangel, G., *et al.* (2013) Identification of human remains by DNA analysis of the gastrointestinal contents of fly larvae. *Journal of Forensic Sciences*, **58**(1), 248–250. https://doi.org/10.1111/j.1556-4029.2012.02279.x

Elwick, K., Bus, M.M., King, J.L., Chang, J., Hughes-Stamm, S., and Budowle, B. (2019) Utility of the Ion S5™ and MiSeq FGx™ sequencing platforms to characterize challenging human remains. *Legal Medicine (Tokyo)*, **41**, 101623. https://doi.org/10.1016/j.legalmed.2019.08.001

Emery, M.V., Bolhofner, K., Winingear, S., Oldt, R., Montes, M., Kanthaswamy, S., *et al.* (2020) Reconstructing full and partial STR profiles from severely burned human remains using comparative ancient and forensic DNA extraction techniques. *Forensic Science International: Genetics*, **46**, 102272. https://doi.org/10.1016/j.fsigen.2020.102272

Ferreira, S.T.G., Paula, K.A., Nogueira, R.F., Oliveira, E.S., and Moraes, A.V. (2015) A comparative study between muscle, cartilage, and swab from inside the urinary bladder samples for DNA typing of severely burnt bodies in disaster victim identification (DVI). *Forensic Science International: Genetics Supplement Series*, e617–e618. https://doi.org/10.1016/j.fsigss.2015.09.243

Fredericks, J.D., Bennett, P., Williams, A., and Rogers, K.D. (2012) FTIR spectroscopy: A new diagnostic tool to aid DNA analysis from heated bone. *Forensic Science International: Genetics*, **6**(3), 375–380. https://doi.org/10.1016/j.fsigen.2011.07.014

Fredericks, J.D., Ringrose, T.J., Dicken, A., Williams, A., and Bennett, P. (2015) A potential new diagnostic tool to aid DNA analysis from heat compromised bone using colorimetry: A preliminary study. *Science & Justice*, **55**(2), 124–130. https://doi.org/10.1016/j.scijus.2014.10.005

Gaudio, D., Fernandes, D.M., Schmidt, R., Cheronet, O., Mazzarelli, D., Mattia, M., *et al.* (2019) Genome-wide DNA from degraded petrous bones and the assessment of sex and probable geographic origins of forensic cases. *Scientific Reports*, **9**(1), 8226. https://doi.org/10.1038/s41598-019-44638-w

Gin, K., Tovar, J., Bartelink, E.J., Kendell, A., Milligan, C., Willey, P., *et al.* (2020) The 2018 California Wildfires: Integration of rapid DNA to dramatically accelerate victim identification. *Journal of Forensic Sciences*, **65**(3), 791–799. https://doi.org/10.1111/1556-4029.14284

Ginart, S., Caputo, M., Corach, D., and Sala, A. (2019) Human DNA degradation assessment and male DNA detection by quantitative-PCR followed by high-resolution melting analysis. *Forensic Science International*, **295**, 1–7. https://doi.org/10.1016/j.forsciint.2018.11.013

Harbeck, M., Schleuder, R., Schneider, J., Wiechmann, I., Schmahl, W.W., and Grupe, G. (2011) Research potential and limitations of trace analyses of cremated remains. *Forensic Science International*, **204**(1–3), 191–200. https://doi.org/10.1016/j.forsciint.2010.06.004

Hartman, D., Drummer, O., Eckhoff, C., Scheffer, J.W., and Stringer, P. (2011) The contribution of DNA to the disaster victim identification (DVI) effort. *Forensic Science International*, **205**(1–3), 52–58. https://doi.org/10.1016/j.forsciint.2010.09.024

Holland, M.M., Cave, C.A., Holland, C.A., and Bille, T.W. (2003) Development of a quality, high throughput DNA analysis procedure for skeletal samples to assist with the identification of victims from the World Trade Center attacks. *Croatian Medical Journal*, **44**(3), 264–272.

Hollard, C., Keyser, C., Delabarde, T., Gonzalez, A., Vilela Lamego, C., Zvénigorosky, V., *et al.* (2017) Case report: On the use of the HID-Ion AmpliSeq™ Ancestry Panel in a real forensic case. *International Journal of Legal Medicine*, **131**(2), 351–358. https://doi.org/10.1007/s00414-016-1425-1

Imaizumi, K., Taniguchi, K., and Ogawa, Y. (2014) DNA survival and physical and histological properties of heat-induced alterations in burnt bones. *International Journal of Legal Medicine*, **128**(3), 439–446. https://doi.org/10.1007/s00414-014-0988-y

Loreille, O.M., Diegoli, T.M., Irwin, J.A., Coble, M.D., and Parsons, T.J. (2007) High efficiency DNA extraction from bone by total demineralization. *Forensic Science International: Genetics*, **1**(2), 191–195. https://doi.org/10.1016/j.fsigen.2007.02.006

Loreille, O.M., Parr, R.L., McGregor, K.A., Fitzpatrick, C.M., Lyon, C., Yang, D.Y., *et al.* (2010) Integrated DNA and fingerprint analyses in the identification of 60-year-old mummified human remains discovered in an Alaskan glacier. *Journal of Forensic Sciences*, **55**(3), 813–818. https://doi.org/10.1111/j.1556-4029.2010.01356.x

Maciejewska, A., Jakubowska, J., and Pawlowski, R. (2013) Whole genome amplification of degraded and nondegraded DNA for forensic purposes. *International Journal of Legal Medicine*, **127**(2), 309–319. https://doi.org/10.1007/s00414-012-0764-9

Maciejewska, A., Wlodarczyk, R., and Pawlowski, R. (2015) The influence of high temperature on the possibility of DNA typing in various human tissues. *Folia Histochemica et Cytobiologica*, **53**(4), 322–332. https://doi.org/10.5603/fhc.a2015.0029

Montelius, K. and Lindblom, B. (2012) DNA analysis in disaster victim identification. *Forensic Science, Medicine and Pathology*, **8**(2), 140–147. https://doi.org/10.1007/s12024-011-9276-z

Mundorff, A.Z., Bartelink, E.J., and Mar-Cash, E. (2009) DNA preservation in skeletal elements from the World Trade Center disaster: Recommendations for mass fatality management. *Journal of Forensic Sciences*, **54**(4), 739–745. https://doi.org/10.1111/j.1556-4029.2009.01045.x

Nelson, K. and Melton, T. (2007) Forensic mitochondrial DNA analysis of 116 casework skeletal samples. *Journal of Forensic Sciences*, **52**(3), 557–561. https://doi.org/10.1111/j.1556-4029.2007.00407.x

Ohira, H., Yamamuro, Y., Kitagawa, Y., Nakagawa, K., Yamamoto, I., and Yamada, Y. (2009) Effective appropriate use of dental remains and forensic DNA testing for personal identity confirmation. *Legal Medicine (Tokyo)*, **11**(Suppl 1), S560–562. https://doi.org/10.1016/j.legalmed.2009.01.085

Owen, R., Bedford, P., Leditschke, J., Schlenker, A., and Hartman, D. (2013) Post mortem sampling of the bladder for the identification of victims of fire related deaths. *Forensic Science International*, **233**(1–3), 14–20. https://doi.org/10.1016/j.forsciint.2013.07.018

Ramlal, G., Vevaraju, D., Vemula, A.Y., Swapna, T., and Bindu, P.H. (2017) Extrication of DNA from burnt teeth exposed to environment. *Journal of Clinical and Diagnostic Research*, **11**(8), Zc120–zc122. https://doi.org/10.7860/jcdr/2017/26911.10525

Ricci, U., Carboni, I., Iozzi, S., Nutini, A.L., Contini, E., Torricelli, F., *et al.* (2015) Genetic identification of burned corpses as a part of disaster victim identification effort. *Forensic Science International: Genetics Supplement Series,* e447–e448. https://doi.org/10.1016/j.fsigss.2015.09.177

Samsuwan, J., Somboonchokepisal, T., Akaraputtiporn, T., Srimuang, T., Phuengsukdaeng, P., Suwannarat, A., *et al.* (2018) A method for extracting DNA from hard tissues for use in forensic identification. *Biomedical Reports,* **9**(5), 433–438. https://doi.org/10.3892/br.2018.1148

Schwark, T., Heinrich, A., Preusse-Prange, A., and von Wurmb-schwark, N. (2011) Reliable genetic identification of burnt human remains. *Forensic Science International: Genetics,* **5**(5), 393–399. https://doi.org/10.1016/j.fsigen.2010.08.008

Sharma, V., van der Plaat, D.A., Liu, Y., and Wurmbach, E. (2020) Analyzing degraded DNA and challenging samples using the ForenSeq™ DNA Signature Prep kit. *Science & Justice,* **60**(3), 243–252. https://doi.org/10.1016/j.scijus.2019.11.004

Staiti, N., Di Martino, D., and Saravo, L. (2004) A novel approach in personal identification from tissue samples undergone different processes through STR typing. *Forensic Science International,* **146**(Suppl), S171–173. https://doi.org/10.1016/j.forsciint.2004.09.052

Theodore Harcke, H., Monaghan, T., Yee, N., and Finelli, L. (2009) Forensic imaging-guided recovery of nuclear DNA from the spinal cord. *Journal of Forensic Sciences,* **54**(5), 1123–1126. https://doi.org/10.1111/j.1556-4029.2009.01114.x

von Wurmb-Schwark, N., Ringleb, A., Gebuhr, M., and Simeoni, E. (2005) Genetic analysis of modern and historical burned human remains. *Anthropologischer Anzeiger,* **63**(1), 1–12. https://www.ncbi.nlm.nih.gov/pubmed/15830583

von Wurmb-Schwark, N., Preusse-Prange, A., Heinrich, A., Simeoni, E., Bosch, T., and Schwark, T. (2009) A new multiplex-PCR comprising autosomal and y-specific STRs and mitochondrial DNA to analyze highly degraded material. *Forensic Science International: Genetics,* **3**(2), 96–103. https://doi.org/10.1016/j.fsigen.2008.11.007

Wai, K.T., Barash, M., and Gunn, P. (2018) Performance of the Early Access AmpliSeq™ Mitochondrial Panel with degraded DNA samples using the Ion Torrent™ platform. *Electrophoresis,* **39**(21), 2776–2784. https://doi.org/10.1002/elps.201700371

Watherston, J., McNevin, D., Gahan, M.E., Bruce, D., and Ward, J. (2018) Current and emerging tools for the recovery of genetic information from post mortem samples: New directions for disaster victim identification. *Forensic Science International: Genetics,* **37**, 270–282. https://doi.org/10.1016/j.fsigen.2018.08.016

Zapico, S.C. and Ubelaker, D.H. (2013) Sex determination from dentin and pulp in a medicolegal context. *Journal of the American Dental Association,* **144**(12), 1379–1385. http://www.ncbi.nlm.nih.gov/pubmed/24282268

Zgonjanin, D., Petković, S., Maletin, M., Vukovic, R., and Draskovic, D. (2015) Case report: DNA identification of burned skeletal remains. *Forensic Science International: Genetics Supplement Series,* e444–e446. https://doi.org/10.1016/j.fsigss.2015.09.176

CHAPTER 13

Applying Colorimetry to the Study of Low Temperature Thermal Changes in Bone

Christopher W. Schmidt[1], PhD and Alexandria McDaniel[2], MS
[1] *Professor of Anthropology, University of Indianapolis, Indianapolis, IL, USA*
[2] *Medicolegal Investigator, Office of the Chief Medical Examiner, New York City, NY, USA*

13.1 Introduction

Archaeologists and forensic anthropologists have documented in detail the changes bone experiences when exposed to temperatures high enough to ignite it (e.g. Shipman *et al.*, 1984; Buikstra and Swegle, 1989; Mayne Correia, 1997; Bohnert *et al.*, 1998; McKinley and Bond, 2001; Walker *et al.*, 2008; Symes *et al.*, 2014, 2015; DeHaan, 2015; Keough *et al.*, 2015; Thompson, 2015). As bone heats up, it dehydrates, losing water bound to its matrix. Next, it loses its collagen and other organic components in a process called decomposition. This is followed by inversion, where it loses its carbonate. Lastly, bone crystals melt and eventually coalesce (Thompson, 2004, 2005, 2015; Ellingham *et al.*, 2014:182).

Bone dehydration begins around 100°C and its loss of collagen starts around 300°C. Around 600°C, the fusion of its crystals begins. As bone temperature exceeds 300°C, it changes from its natural color to a brown, then a charred black as tissues carbonize. As collagen exits, the bone takes on a bluish gray hue before taking on a stark white, or calcined state, where little more than mineral remains. As these color changes take place, bone also fractures, shrinks, and warps (e.g. Ellingham *et al.*, 2014; Symes *et al.*, 2015).

Burnt bones, therefore, have diagnostic color and morphological signatures that distinguish them from bones affected by other taphonomic agents. However, the color changes bones experience when heated to temperatures below their ignition point are not so well understood, especially when compared to the colors experienced by burnt bones. In archaeological contexts, such heated but unburnt conditions can occur when people cook vertebrate animals; when funerary fires are near to, but not directly in contact with a body; and when people are buried

Burnt Human Remains: Recovery, Analysis, and Interpretation, First Edition. Edited by Sarah Ellingham, Joe Adserias-Garriga, Sara C. Zapico and Douglas H. Ubelaker.

by volcanic ash (e.g. Bennett, 1999; Oestigaard, 2000; Roberts *et al.*, 2002; Koon *et al.*, 2003; Walker *et al.*, 2008; Asmussen, 2009; Irish *et al.*, 2015; Schmidt *et al.*, 2015; Solario *et al.*, 2015; Weitzel and McKenzie, 2015; Greenfield and Beattie, 2017). Unburnt, but heated, bones occur in forensic contexts when brief duration heating events, such as a rapidly moving brush fires, elevate bone temperatures but do not burn them because the fire exits the area before a person's soft tissues are consumed (Symes *et al.*, 2014).

There are many ways to detect thermal changes in bone, particularly at microscopic scales (e.g. Herrman, 1977; Nelson, 1992; Hiller *et al.*, 2003; Koon *et al.*, 2003; Mkukuma *et al.*, 2004; Thompson, 2004, 2005, 2015; Etok *et al.*, 2007; Hanson and Cain, 2007; Figueiredo *et al.*, 2010; Gonçalves *et al.*, 2011; Gonçalves, 2012; Ellingham *et al.*, 2014; Mahoney and Miszkiewicz, 2015). Perhaps the oldest approach has been to observe macroscopic changes in bone surface color because they tend to be distinct and intuitive to document (e.g. Webb and Snow, 1945; Baby, 1954; Wells, 1960; Binford, 1963; Walker *et al.*, 2008; Symes *et al.*, 2014, 2015; Keough *et al.*, 2015; Ullinger and Sheridan, 2015; Williams, 2015). Systems for documenting bone color are wide ranging, from using the human eye to using automated color detection devices like colorimeters. This chapter focuses on documenting bone color, in part, because inspecting bone colors is readily accomplished and does not require bone sectioning. Specifically, this chapter discusses colorimetry because it collects data in a way that is intuitive and highly replicable (e.g. Krap *et al.*, 2019).

13.2 Colorimetry

Colorimetry is the measurement of color based primarily on wavelength detection (Fairchild, 2005:53). Differences in color relate to their hue, value, and chroma, which vary because of combinations of chromatic and achromatic content. Hue refers to the pure color; it is the range of colors depicted on a color wheel or viewed once white light has passed through a prism. Value (also called lightness or luminance) is the brightness of a color. Value is not a color on its own, rather it is a color's relative lightness or darkness. Chroma is the purity of a color. If one adds gray to navy blue to tone down the starkness of its appearance, the added color makes the blue less pure and changes its chroma. Saturation is a term that at times is used synonymously with chroma, but technically chroma and saturation are different aspects of a similar phenomenon. Where chroma refers to the deviation of a color from its pure state, saturation is how strong or weak a color appears (Commission Internationale de L'Eclairage (CIE), 2019).

Chromatic colors are those with hue, such as red, orange, yellow, green, blue, violet, etc. In contrast, white, gray, and black are achromatic because they lack hue (Fairchild, 2005). There are multiple means of organizing color, such as the RGB (red-green-blue) and CMYK (cyan-magenta-yellow-black) systems. When color models link to a color map, they make up a color space; one such color space is CIELAB (León *et al.*, 2006). CIELAB gives scores for three components: L* for lightness from black (0) to white (100), a* for green (below zero) to red (above zero), and b* for blue (below zero) to yellow (above zero) (see Figure 13.1). CIELAB (developed by the International Commission on Illumination) detects colors in a manner that is similar to the ways humans perceive them and it conceivably includes billions of colors (McLaren, 1976). It also provides quantitative output suitable for empirical study (López *et al.*, 2005; Devlin and Herrmann 2015). For these reasons, CIELAB color space (henceforth L*a*b*) is commonly employed to document colors expressed on thermally altered bone (e.g. Devlin and Hermann, 2015).

Colorimetry has several advantages over other means of detecting color in heated bones. The primary advantage is that once calibrated, the colorimeter repeatedly produces consistent color data for a given area of bone. The output is very precise, which means there may be minor differences for one or more of the L*, a*, and b* values from one collection event to the next, which is why it is common practice to take consecutive measurements and to use the average of those. The colorimeter employed in the case study discussed in section 13.4 had a default of taking four measurements. In addition to being reliable, the colorimeter produces valid data, that is, data that produces colors that are identical to the color of the object being studied.

Testing the colorimeter before collecting osteological data on white and black surfaces, as well as red, yellow, and blue surfaces provides an intuitive way to assess colorimetry output. A black surface produces an L* of 0 and a white surface, an L* of 100. Reds produce positive a* values, and blues produce negative b* values. Analysts can also use a color converter to assess colorimeter output. Several are available as web-based programs where one enters the L*a*b* data

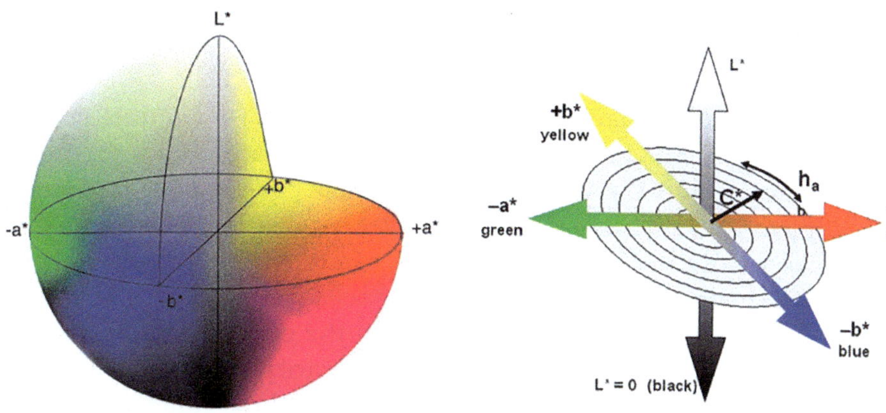

Figure 13.1 Depiction of CIELAB color space. L* marks the axis that ranges from white to black, a* is green to red, and b* is blue to yellow.

and the color it represents is presented on screen. Of course screen resolution can affect color quality, but in general the converters produce an image suitable for assessment. If, for example, a red surface appears green or brown, it is likely the colorimeter is not set up properly, or it has light bleeding into the collector during data collection.

Colorimetry is more precise than visual color identification. Visual color identification places bone colors into color categories, that is, brown, black, blue, gray, white. The colorimeter, on the other hand, records specific numeric values based on the wavelengths it detects. Where the visually based color system records six colors or so, colorimeters can detect a plethora of variations within each of the visually based color categories. Such precision may not be useful in every circumstance, but it certainly gives analysts more to work with as they investigate thermal changes in detail.

One way to improve visual inspection is to use a Munsell color reference to standardize color determination. This involves matching bone color to standard color plates organized by hue, value, and chroma. Employing Munsell references can be beneficial, but it is best employed by analysts having a sound knowledge of color organization and the roles value and chroma play in color determination. Again, the colorimeter collects color data automatically, regardless of the analysts' ability to match colors. Thus, using a colorimeter in most osteological cases is a superior option to the use of a Munsell standard for collecting color data.

Another advantage of colorimetry is that it produces interval-scale data suitable for parametric analyses. The range for L^* is 0–100, and the ranges for a^* and b^* are usually truncated between -128 and 127; each component can be explored individually or collectively. In contrast, visual inspection methods tend to place colors into ordinal ranks that do not account for color components individually. Using ranked data has its advantages in certain instances (see section 13.3) but it gives fewer options for study.

13.3 Challenges of Colorimetry

Despite its precision, accuracy, and intuitive output, using a colorimeter presents certain challenges. The first is that colorimeters collect data from specific areas of a surface; handheld units may collect color data from an area no greater than one or two centimeters across. This means it may take several data collection events to record a representative sample of a given bone. Moreover, its precision means that it may indicate subtle color differences along a region of bone that to the naked eye is basically the same color. It is plausible that the color nuances are so varied that the color data are too complex to compare to previously collected data acquired by less precise means. On the other hand, these nuanced data better reflect surface variations and will help analysts consider ranges of color rather than discrete color categories.

A particularly germane challenge to using colorimetry on bones is that colorimeters work best on flat surfaces; the color detector should not have stray light hitting it. It should only collect light reflecting directly off the specimen being studied. Bones tend to be round, which means ambient light easily enters the detector. To overcome this, it is advised that the ambient light be turned off and the data collection take place in a dark room. Using a color converter is a convenient way to detect evidence of ambient light contamination in the L*a*b* output.

Despite the value of colorimetry, it does not obviate other means of bone color data collection in every case. Specific instances where visual inspection suffices are likely many, but generally visual inspection may be preferred when there are thousands of bones to score, or when access to the remains is limited, particularly when the decedent is recently deceased. In these circumstances, a trained analyst will find the visually produced color data are suitable to answer questions such as what aspects and what percentage of individual skeletons had thermal alterations, how many people had thermal alterations, and what condition of thermal alteration (i.e. blackened or calcined) characterized the individual or the group. In cases where colorimetry is at first impractical, it may be possible to photograph bones and to collect colorimetry data from the photographs at a later date (e.g. Hermanns and Piérard, 2006).

13.4 Case Study

An example of employing a colorimeter and the L*a*b* color space for the study of thermally altered bones comes from McDaniel (2020). In this study, experimentally heated pig femora were used as proxies for human bones to determine if bone changes color when exposed to low thermal energies, that is, temperatures above room temperature but below bone ignition point. Defleshed pig bones were used because they are common substitutes for human bones (Li *et al.*, 2015). Complete pig femora were heated in a laboratory oven but not allowed to burn. Peak temperatures were kept at 125°C. The goal of the study was to document changes in bone color related to temperatures around the boiling point of water (100°C).

The colorimeter used was a handheld PCE Instruments CSM 2 set to collect color data using the L*a*b* color space. There are numerous colorimeters available; the advantage of this model was its ease of use, precision, ability to collect L*a*b* data, and price. The study collected bone color data before and after each heating event. It also controlled for temperature, duration, and weight.

The colorimetry results indicated that bone midshaft colors changed in a consistent and predictable way as bone temperatures increased, which in some ways mirrored the process seen in burnt bones. The low temperature color changes, however, were nowhere near as dramatic as those seen in burnt bones. In essence, the bones became browner, presumably as fluids, including blood, moved through

Haversian systems. The L* also indicated that they became lighter in color. Prior to heating they were darker, less red, and less yellow. Metaphyseal color changes were more pronounced than those at the midshafts, but overall the range of color changes was similar at both bone locations (Figure 13.2).

Duration and temperature affected bone color; the L* and a* components had linear relationships with both. But, of the two, temperature had a more dramatic effect. This is similar to results found in studies of experimental burning where temperature had a greater impact on bone color (e.g. Walker *et al.*, 2008; Beach *et al.*, 2015). Thirty minutes at 75°C was sufficient to initiate bone color changes, but these were more vivid as bones approached 100°C, regardless of duration. Importantly, corresponding L*a*b* color values before and after heating did not correlate, meaning the colors at which a bone started the study did not affect their colors after the heating events. The heat-related color changes were enough that a discriminant function properly distinguished heated and non-heated L*a*b* values for 26 of 27 bones. The lone misclassification was for the bone that reached the lowest temperature after heating (38.9°C).

This case study underscores the importance of colorimetry in the determination of thermal changes in bone. In this study, the color changes were at times subtle. The color changes were not homogenous; rather, the bone had what is termed a "mottled" appearance (e.g. Schmidt *et al.*, 2015). In fact, a mottled condition may characterize bone that is heated but not yet burned, like that found among the people of Herculaneum who died via a pyroclastic event, or in instances of cooking where burning is intentionally mitigated, but the bone reaches temperatures of at

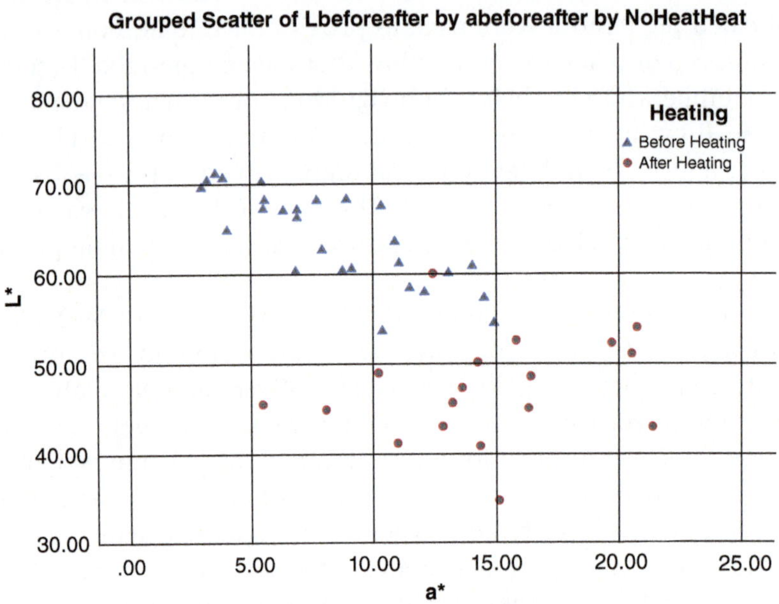

Figure 13.2 Metaphysis L* and a* values for bones before heating and after.

least 75°C for a sustained period. In such cases, the bone bears several colors in a small area, likely as fluids move through but fail to completely exit it (Figure 13.3). Mottling is a color category, like brown or black. It is not something that shows up in L*a*b* data. The various colors of mottled surfaces collectively take on a beige hue once color converted. Thus, mottling should be limited to qualitative descriptions of bone along with "charred" and "calcined." It is a useful descriptor but not indicative of any particular region of the L*a*b* color space.

That the metaphyses changed more dramatically than the midshafts may be due to metaphyseal cortical bone being thinner than midshaft cortices and so may reflect color changes more readily. When bones are burned the metaphyses are often more friable than midshafts. This may be due to the rapid loss of metaphyseal fluids prior to burning, as well as the spongy bone dominated metaphyseal architecture (e.g. Symes *et al.*, 2015). If this is the case, the color changes that take place prior to burning are indicating that the stage is being set for an environment ripe for combustion should temperatures get high enough.

Interestingly, the experimentally heated bones did not reach water's boiling point, yet they experienced color changes. The heated bone L*a*b* values became distinguished from their unheated colors at around 40°C. Moreover, every bone in the study lost some fluid, even those heated for only 30 minutes at the lowest temperature, and the longer a bone was in the oven, the more fluid it lost. One bone lost 26% of its total weight, another lost 19%. On average, bones lost around 12% of their weight. Clearly fluid loss affects color, yet the relationship is not fully understood. One possible application of the understanding of low temperature

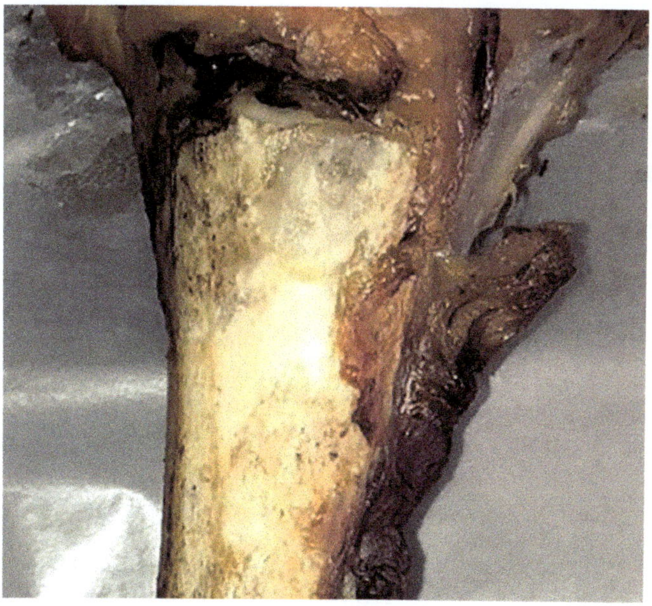

Figure 13.3 Mottled metaphyseal bone heated to below 90°C.

changes beyond the study of human bones concerns bones found in archaeological settings. The case study above may help archaeologists understand the colors of bone thought to have been cooked. It is conceivable that one could estimate cooking temperatures based on the L*a*b* color space data provided by McDaniel (2020), although such an application would benefit from verification efforts on other species of animals. Since the L*a*b* values before heating did not correlate with their values after heating, McDaniel's study should be repeatable no matter the original colors, weights, and temperatures of the bones used in future experiments.

13.5 Conclusion

In the end, this chapter's focus on colorimetry provides another example of colorimetry's efficacy in the study of heated bones. Analysts have used colorimetry in osteology for decades (see Devlin and Herrmann, 2015) and its use continues to expand (e.g. Fredericks *et al.*, 2015; McDaniel, 2020). Coupling colorimetry with the study of bone colors is another step in the ongoing improvements analysts are making in osteology. It is important to bear in mind that the techniques discussed here, particularly those regarding colorimetry, are not the extent of the frontier it offers; instead it is a brief glimpse into a realm of study with a great deal of potential. With technology prices moderating, an increase in available web-based support resources, and an ever-improving literature, now is an excellent time for osteologists to consider colorimetry and related means of analysis, for the study of thermally altered remains. There is a need for more experimental burning studies in controlled environments using technology that produced precise data and reproducible results.

References

Asmussen, B. (2009) Intentional or incidental thermal modification? Analysing site occupation via burned bone. *Journal of Archaeological Science*, **36**, 528–536.

Baby, R.S. (1954) Hopewell cremation practices. *Ohio Historical Society Paper Archaeology*, **1**, 1–17.

Beach, J., Passalacqua, N.V., and Chapman, E.N. (2015) Heat-related changes in tooth color. In: *The Analysis of Burned Human Remains*, 2nd edn. (eds. C.W. Schmidt and S.A. Symes). Academic Press, Amsterdam, pp. 139–148.

Bennett, J. (1999) Thermal alteration of burned bone. *Journal of Archaeological Science*, **26**, 1–8.

Binford, L.R. (1963) An analysis of cremations from three Michigan sites. *Wisconsin Archaeology*, **44**, 98–110.

Bohnert, M., Rost, T., and Pollak, S. (1998) The degree of destruction of human bodies in relation to the duration of the fire. *Forensic Science International*, **95**, 11–21.

Buikstra, J.E. and Swegle, M. (1989) Bone modification due to burning: Experimental evidence. In: *Bone Modification* (eds. R. Bonnichsen and M. Sorg). University of Maine, Orono, ME, pp. 247–258.

Commission Internationale de L'Eclairage. (2019) *ISO/CIE 11664-3:2019 Colorimetry – Part 3: CIE tristimulus values*. CIE, Vienna.

DeHaan, J.D. (2015) Fire and bodies. In: *The Analysis of Burned Human Remains*, 2nd edn. (eds. C.W. Schmidt and S.A. Symes). Academic Press, Amsterdam, pp. 1–15.

Devlin, J.B. and Hermann, N.P. (2015) Bone color. In: *The Analysis of Burned Human Remains*, 2nd edn. (eds. C.W. Schmidt and S.A. Symes). Academic Press, Amsterdam, pp. 119–137.

Ellingham, S.T.D., Thompson, T.J.U., Islam, M., and Taylor, G. (2014) Estimating temperature exposure of burnt bone – A methodological review. *Science and Justice*, **55**, 181–188.

Etok, S.E., Valsami-Jones, E., Wess, T.J., Miller, J.C., Maxwell, C.A., Keith, D., *et al.* (2007) Structural and chemical changes of thermally treated bone apatite. *Journal of Materials Science*, **42**, 9807–9816.

Fairchild, M.D. (2005) *Color Appearance Models*, 2nd edn. John Wiley and Sons Ltd, Chichester, West Sussex.

Figueiredo, M., Fernando, A., Martins, G., Freitas, J., Judas, F., and Figueiredo, H. (2010) Effect of the calcination temperature on the composition and microstructure of hydroxyapatite derived from human and animal bone. *Ceramic International*, **36**, 2383–2393.

Fredericks, J.D., Ringrose, T.J., Dicken, A., Williams, A., and Bennett, P. (2015) A potential new diagnostic tool to aid DNA analysis from heat compromised bone using colorimetry: A preliminary study. *Science & Justice*, **55**, 124–130.

Gonçalves, D. (2012) The micro-analysis of human burned bones: Some remarks. *Cadernos do GEEvH*, **1**, 32–40.

Gonçalves, D., Thompson, T.J.U., and Cunha, E. (2011) Implications of heat-induced changes in bone on the interpretation of funerary behaviour and practice. *Journal of Archaeological Science*, **38**, 1308–1313.

Greenfield, H.J. and Beattie, A. (2017) A practical macroscopic approach for distinguishing burned and boiled bones in zooarchaeological assemblages. In: *The Wide Lens in Archaeology: Honoring Brian Hesse's Contributions to Anthropological Archaeology* (eds. J. Lev-Tov, P. Hesse, and A. Gilbert). Lockwood Press, Atlanta, GA, pp. 43–87.

Hanson, M. and Cain, C.R. (2007) Examining histology to identify burned bone. *Journal of Archaeological Science*, **34**, 1902–1913.

Hermanns, J.-F. and Piérard, G.E. (2006) High-resolution epiluminescence colorimetry of striae distensae. *Journal of the European Academy of Dermatology and Venereology*, **20**(3), 282–287.

Herrman, B. (1977) On histological investigations of cremated human remains. *Journal of Human Evolution*, **6**, 101–103.

Hiller, J.C., Thompson, T.J.U., Evison, M.P., Chamberlain, A.T., and Wess, T.J. (2003) Bone mineral change during experimental heating: An X-ray scattering investigation. *Biomaterials*, **24**, 5091–5097.

Irish, J.D., Potter, B.A., and Reuther, J.D. (2015) An 11,500-year-old human cremation from eastern Beringia (central Alaska). In: *The Analysis of Burned Human Remains*, 2nd edn. (eds. C.W. Schmidt and S.A. Symes). Academic Press, Amsterdam, pp. 295–306.

Keough, N., L'Abbé, E.N., Steyn, M., and Pretorius, S. (2015) Assessment of skeletal changes after post-mortem exposure to fire as an indicator of decomposition stage. *Forensic Science International*, **246**, 17–24.

Koon, H.E.C., Nicholson, R.A., and Collins, M.J. (2003) A practical approach to the identification of low temperature heated bone using TEM. *Journal of Archaeological Science*, **30**, 1393–1399.

León, K., Mery, D., Pedreschi, F., and León, G. (2006) Color measurement of L*a*b* units from RGB digital images. *Food Research International*, **39**, 1084–1091.

Li, Y., Chen, S.-K., Li, L., Qin, L., Wang, X.-L., and Lai, Y.-X. (2015) Bone defect animal models for testing efficacy of bone substitute biomaterials. *Journal of Orthopedic Translation*, **3**, 95–104.

López, F., Valiente, J.M., Baldrich, R., and Vanrell, M. (2005) Fast surface grading using color statistics in the CIE Lab Space. *Iberian Conference on Pattern Recognition and Image Analysis*, **2**, 666–673.

Mahoney, P. and Miszkiewicz, J. (2015) Formation times in thermally altered enamel. In: *The Analysis of Burned Human Remains*, 2nd edn. (eds. C.W. Schmidt and S.A. Symes). Academic Press, Amsterdam, pp. 355–363.

Mayne Correia, P.M. (1997) Fire modification of bone: A review of the literature. In: *Forensic Taphonomy: The Postmortem Fate of Human Remains* (eds. W.D. Haglund and M.H. Sorg). CRC Press, Boca Raton, FL, pp. 275–293.

McDaniel, A. (2020) Low temperature thermal changes in bone. M.S. Thesis. University of Indianapolis, Indianapolis, IN.

McKinley, J.I. and Bond, J.M. (2001) Cremated bone. In: *Handbook of Archaeological Sciences* (eds. D.R. Brothwell and A.M. Pollard). Wiley, Chichester, pp. 281–290.

McLaren, K. (1976) The development of the CIE 1976 (L* a* b*) uniform colour space and colour-difference formula. *Coloration Technology*, **92**, 338–341.

Mkukuma, L.D., Skakle, J.S., Gibson, I.R., Imrie, C.T., Aspden, R.M., and Hukins, D.W.L. (2004) Effect of the proportion of organic material in bone on thermal decomposition of bone mineral: An investigation of a variety of bones from different species using thermogravimetric analysis coupled to mass spectrometry, high-temperature X-ray diffraction, and Fourier transform infrared spectroscopy. *Calcified Tissue International*, **75**, 321–328.

Nelson, R. (1992) A microscopic comparison of fresh and burned bone. *Journal of Forensic Science*, **37**, 1055–1060.

Oestigaard, T. (2000) Sacrifices of raw, cooked, and burnt humans. *Norwegian Archaeological Review*, **33**, 41–58.

Roberts, S.J., Smith, C.I., Millard, A., and Collins, M.J. (2002) The taphonomy of cooked bone: Characterizing boiling and its physico-chemical effects. *Archaeometry*, **44**, 485–494.

Schmidt, C.W., Oakley, E., D'Anastasio, R., Brower, R., Remy, A.J., and Viciano, J. (2015) Herculaneum. In: *The Analysis of Burned Human Remains*, 2nd edn. (eds. C.W. Schmidt and S.A. Symes). Academic Press, Amsterdam, pp. 149–162.

Shipman, P., Foster, G., and Schoeninger, M. (1984) Burnt bone and teeth: An experimental study of color, morphology, crystal structure, and shrinkage. *Journal of Archaeological Science*, **11**, 307–325.

Solario, A., Olivera, D., Gordillo, I., Bosch, P., Fetter, G., Lara, V.H., *et al.* (2015) Cooked bones? Method and practice for identifying bones treated at low temperatures. *International Journal of Osteoarchaeology*, **25**, 426–440.

Symes, S.A., L'abbé, E.N., Pokines, J.T., Yuzwa, T., Messer, D., Stromquist, A., *et al.* (2014) Thermal alteration to bone. In: *The Manual of Forensic Taphonomy* (eds. J.T. Pokines and S.A. Symes). CRC Press, Boca Raton, FL, pp. 367–402.

Symes, S.A., Rainwater, C.W., Chapman, E.N., Gipson, D.R., and Piper, A.L. (2015) Patterned thermal destruction in a forensic setting. In: *The Analysis of Burned Human Remains*, 2nd edn. (eds. C.W. Schmidt and S.A. Symes). Academic Press, Amsterdam, pp. 17–56.

Thompson, T.J.U. (2004) Recent advances in the study of burned bone and the implications for forensic anthropology. *Forensic Science International*, **146**, 203–205.

Thompson, T.J.U. (2005) Heat-induced dimensional changes in bone and their consequences for forensic anthropology. *Journal of Forensic Science*, **50**, 1008–1015.

Thompson, T.J.U. (2015) The analysis of heat-induced crystallinity change in bone. In: *The Analysis of Burned Human Remains*, 2nd edn. (eds. C.W. Schmidt and S.A. Symes). Academic Press, Amsterdam, pp. 323–334.

Tristan Krap, T., Ruijter, J.M., Nota, K., Karel, J., Lieke Burgers, A., Aalders, M.C.G., Oostra, R.J., and Duijst, W. (2019) Colourimetric analysis of thermally altered human bone samples. *Nature Scientific Reports*, **9**, 8923. https://doi.org/10.1038/s41598-019-45420-8.

Ullinger, J. and Sheridan, S.G. (2015) Bone color changes in a burned burial structure from early Bronze Age Bab adh-Dhra', Jordan. In: *The Analysis of Burned Human Remains*, 2nd edn. (eds. C.W. Schmidt and S.A. Symes). Academic Press, Amsterdam, pp. 403–414.

Walker, P.L., Miller, K.W.P., and Richman, R. (2008) Time, temperature, and oxygen availability: An experimental study of the effects of environmental conditions on the color and organic content of cremated bones. In: *The Analysis of Burned Human Remains* (eds. C.W. Schmidt and S.A. Symes). Academic Press, Amsterdam, pp. 129–136.

Webb, W.S. and Snow, C.E. (1945) The Adena People No. 2. The University of Kentucky Reports in Anthropology and Archaeology #6. University of Kentucky Press, Lexington, KY.

Weitzel, M.A. and McKenzie, H.G. (2015) Fire as a cultural taphonomic agent. In: *The Analysis of Burned Human Remains*, 2nd edn. (eds. C.W. Schmidt and S.A. Symes). Academic Press, Amsterdam, pp. 203–216.

Wells, C.A. (1960) A study of cremation. *Antiquity*, **342**, 9–37.

Williams, H. (2015) Towards an archaeology of cremation. In: *The Analysis of Burned Human Remains*, 2nd edn. (eds. C.W. Schmidt and S.A. Symes). Academic Press, Amsterdam, pp. 259–287.

CHAPTER 14

The Use of Histology to Distinguish Animal from Human Burnt Bone with Reference to Some Limitations

Pamela Mayne Correia[1], MA; Kalyna Horocholyn[2], MA and Kassandra Pointer[3], BA, B.Ed

[1] *Curator and Forensic Anthropologist, Department of Anthropology, University of Alberta, Edmonton, Alberta, Canada*

[2] *Department of Anthropology (formerly), University of Alberta, Edmonton, Alberta, Canada*

[3] *Department of Anthropology (formerly), University of Alberta, Edmonton, Alberta, Canada*

14.1 Introduction

Histological analysis of human bone tissue within the field of biological anthropology has had a long tradition for interpreting the bones origin and age, and prior to that within anatomy laboratories. Our understanding of the types of tissues which can be found in humans is well known and the literature is vast; there has been a fair amount of exploration of the histological characteristics of other animals, including mammals, birds, and reptiles. Given our current understanding of the various kinds of tissue organization that are found, it is surprising that there are still challenges when using these characteristics to distinguish species (Shapiro and Wu, 2019). This chapter is designed to present the reader with an overview of the common tissue types found in animal bone (including human), to provide some qualitative comparisons for unmodified bone, some quantitative comparisons for unmodified bone, and then to provide a case study of burnt bone at three temperatures. This chapter may serve as a reference for individuals faced with the interpretation of burnt bone fragments. In this discussion the following questions will be addressed: 1) Can the characteristic tissue organization found in unburnt bone be found within cremated bone fragments? 2) Can comparisons of quantitative data be used to distinguish animal from human? and 3) Can other analyses be applied successfully to cremated bone histology, for example, age estimation?

Burnt Human Remains: Recovery, Analysis, and Interpretation, First Edition. Edited by Sarah Ellingham, Joe Adserias-Garriga, Sara C. Zapico and Douglas H. Ubelaker.

14.2 Bone Tissue

Macroscopically, bone is a rigid but flexible and strong material. The form of a specific bone is dependent upon its location in the body, and the various stresses applied by the actions of the associated muscles. Fossae, ridges, and vascular impressions on a smooth, dense cortical bone (except for the vertebrae) can be found on the external surfaces. The internal surface, generally, has visible bony trabeculae. The presence of this bone type diminishes towards the midshaft on the long bones and short bones and is replaced by myeloid tissue. The irregular bones, such as the innominates, vertebrae, scapulae, carpals, tarsals, and clavicles, have varying amounts of spongy bone surrounded by a thin layer of cortical bone. The cranium consists of two layers of periosteal bone between which spongy bone (diplöe) is sandwiched (Currey, 2006).

There has been a long history of describing bone tissue microscopically by describing the presence and arrangement of vessels and the orientation of collagen fibers (cf. Foote, 1916; Enlow and Brown, 1956, 1958; Smith, 1960a, 1960b; Schultz, 1997a; Locke, 2004; Cuijpers, 2006, 2009; Hillier and Bell, 2007; Greenlee and Dunnell, 2010; Mulhern and Ubelaker, 2012; Brits *et al.*, 2014; Britz *et al.*, 2014; Caccia *et al.*, 2016; Shapiro and Wu, 2019). By understanding the relationships between the vessels and collagen, there has been a broadening of our understanding of the mechanics of bone tissue. For the purposes of distinguishing nonhuman animal from human bone, it is necessary to understand the characteristics of the various bone tissue types found in vertebrates. The questionable sample will need to be viewed, described, and classified into one or more of the various tissues and from there some conclusions can be drawn as to the species origin.

There have been a number of attempts to build classification systems (c.f. Enlow and Brown, 1956; de Ricqlès, 1975; Francillon-Vieillot *et al.*, 1990; Shapiro and Wu, 2019) and to use a common terminology; however, as our understanding of the various tissues improves, it is necessary to modify those earlier systems. It is less important to know the system and more important to really understand what is being seen in the section. For example, are these lamellar structures, avascular tissues, or Haversian systems? Is it possible to interpret reticular vessel arrangement versus radial? Is the section a view of endosteal or cortical area of the bone? Knowledge of these structures will permit the development of some conclusions about the type of animal bone under assessment. So, in order to lay a common foundation in this understanding, the next section will describe the main tissue types and their characteristics. This will include familiarization with the terminology presented in the literature, while not going into extensive embryological and developmental detail.

Primary bone tissue can be described by three recognizable types. The first is known as fetal bone and is the earliest bone formed, woven bone. Primary bone can have areas of lamellar bone present, be avascular or vascular, or have primary osteons. It is common to find a combination of woven and lamellar bone together with primary osteons. This latter bone type is known as a fibrolamellar complex (woven-parallel complex bone (Shapiro and Wu, 2019)). Secondary bone tissue is divided into two types: Haversian systems (with secondary osteons) and non-Haversian lamellar bone. As will be described in the next section and seen in Table 14.1, the presence of each type of bone tissue may assist in determining the origin of a bone fragment.

14.2.1 Primary Bone Tissue

14.2.1.1 Woven Bone

Woven bone is the first form of bone to be produced, either in utero or after injury. This rapid bone synthesis is completed by the osteoblast (and possibly a specialized osteoblast known as a "mesenchymal osteoblast" (Shapiro and Wu, 2019), which distributes a 360° arc of collagen fibers in an irregular meshwork in which there are initially no lamella. Woven bone provides a "scaffold" for later bone formation into more organized lamellar tissue. Woven bone at the microscopic level appears coarse and fibrous and has a higher concentration of osteocytes than mature bone (White and Folkens, 2005). It is found during early embryological stages of bone development and is present at sites of injury as a "first response" to mending damaged skeletal tissue, such as within a bone callus. It may present in pathological bone, for example, avascular necrosis. Woven bone may be vascular or avascular and may be combined with lamellar bone. Woven bone is continually synthesized in nonhuman animals but is replaced in humans. When viewing woven bone, what is most noticeable is the lack of features. The lacuna and a rather smooth surface devoid of features (Figure 14.1) is visible. This can be complicated if there is the beginning of primary osteon development or lamellar structures. As woven bone can either be avascular or vascular, the presence of vessels is seen in the latter. If there is lamellar bone present it may be localized on the periosteal or endosteal margins of the bone and may contain primary osteons. When the fibrous woven bone and lamellar bone combine in the fibrolamellar complex, then this will be seen within the cortex of the bone (Shapiro and Wu, 2019).

14.2.1.2 Lamellar Bone

As the collagen fibers begin to be aligned and reorganized through remodeling, the bone takes on a more organized appearance. The lacunae are still visible, but instead of the smooth surface seen in woven bone, the bone begins to take on a pattern of organized lines of collagen fibers (lamella) and the associated lacuna. These fibers can be oriented parallel to each other or may take on an alternating arrangement (which leads to the birefringence of the bone). This arrangement has been described as being at right angles to each other or of twisted plywood appearance due to a variety of rotations (Greenlee and Dunnell, 2010; Shapiro and Wu,

Table 14.1 Comparison of qualitative analysis of various animals and humans.

Research Source	Species	Element studied	Qualitative Description
Deer (variety sp.)			
Foote (1916)	**Mule deer (*Odocoileus hemionus*)**	Femur	mostly composed of plexiform with few Haversian systems
	Reindeer (*Rangifer tarandus*)		
	Elk (*Cervus canadensis*)		
Singh *et al*. (1974)	**Reindeer (*Rangifer tarandus*)**	Long bones, ribs	primary vascular (non-Haversian) reticular bone neither inner nor outer circumferential lamellae
			neither inner nor outer circumferential lamellae
Owsley *et al*. (1985)	**Unidentified cervid****	Humerus	plexiform bone; primary osteons with few interstitial lamellae
Skedros *et al*. (2003)	**Rocky Mountain mule deer (*Odocoileus hemionus*)**	Forearm (metacarpal, radius, humerus)	plexiform with incompletely remodeled secondary osteons occupying 30% of mid-diaphyseal cortex
Hillier and Bell (2007)	**White-tailed deer (*Odocoileus virginianus*)**	Long bones	dense Haversian bone
			small Haversian canal diameter and low osteon density compared to other mammals of relative size
Morris (2007)	**White-tailed deer (*Odocoileus virginianus*)**	Femur, humerus, rib	plexiform present in all femora, 2/3 of humeri, and 1/6 ribs
			osteon banding found in 66.7% femora and 33.3% humeri

Table 14.1 (Continued)

Horocholyn (2013)	**White-tailed deer (*Odocoileus virginianus*)**	Femur – dry bone	mid-cortical – Haversian and some plexiform, periosteal – plexiform,
		Femur (600°C)	cortical region too black to see anything but canals, periosteal region with plexiform structure, primary vascular (laminar, plextform, and
		Femur (800°C)	mid-cortical region blackened, endosteal margin viewable, periosteal – Haversian and plexiform bone, endosteal margin –plexiform
		Femur (1000°C)	cortical and margin areas clearly visible, Carbon remnants still a problem. Laminar, plexiform, and scattered Haversian bone seen in
	Pig (*Sus scrofa*)		
Foote (1916)		Femur	predominantly plexiform structure with dense clusters of secondary
Enlow and Brown (1958)		Long bone, Rib	primary plexiform with few scattered secondary osteons in older
Mulhern and Ubelaker (2001)		Femur	4 out of 6 specimens displayed osteon banding widespread plexiform structures
Martiniaková *et al.* (2006a, 2007)		Femur	primary vascular plexiform and dense Haversian bone
Horocholyn (2013)		Femur	plexiform and Haversian, reticular found throughout, reticular most
		Femur (600°C)	N/A as carbonization
		Femur (800°C)	some visible plexiform, and reticular bone seen, a few Haversian systems were visible overall similar to control, but obscured by carbon
		Femur (1000°C)	porous with carbon present, plexiform and Haversian systems
	Cow (*Bos taurus*)		
Enlow and Brown (1958)		Long bone, Rib	primary plexiform bone with some scattered secondary osteons dense Haversian bone present in cortex of ribs

(Continued)

Table 14.1 (Continued)

Research Source	Species	Element studied	Qualitative Description
Martiniaková *et al.* (2006a)		Femur	non-vascular bone present around medullary cavity with concentric dense Haversian structures in mid-cortex primary vascular plexiform bone with primary osteons found near
Cuijpers (2006)		Femur	primary lamellar non-vascular bone
			reticular and plexiform with primary osteons
			scattered secondary osteons with little to no organization
			longitudinal and reticular Haversian canals
Martiniaková *et al.* (2006b)		Femur	primary vascular plexiform
			non-vascular bone at endosteal and periosteal borders
Martiniaková *et al.* (s2007)		Femur	primary vascular plexiform
			non-vascular bone at endosteal and periosteal borders
			middle of cortex housed irregular and/or dense Haversian structures
Cuijpers and Lauwerier (2008)		Diaphyses of femur, tibia, metatarsus, metacarpus, radius	fibrous fibro-lamellar bone complex

Table 14.1 (Continued)

Zedda *et al.* (2008)		Femur, Humerus	elliptically shaped osteons that are irregularly scattered- vascular canals irregularly arranged longitudinally or slightly obliquely
Castrogiovanni *et al.* (2011)		Femur	homogenous appearance of bone with few borders between adjacent lamellae visible
Horocholyn (2013)		Femur	endosteal region -woven, primary osteon, periosteal and midcortical –
		Femur (600°C)	primary osteon and plexiform, Haversian in midcortical visible
		Femur (800°C)	carbon in midcortical region, plexiform and Haversian, endosteal not viewable in most instances, plextform in periosteal region
		Femur (1000°C)	virtuallly all Haversian structure in samples
	Horse (Perissodactyla)		
Enlow and Brown (1958)		mandible	reticular and some plexiform
		diapyses	reticular and dense Haversian bone
Cuijpers (2006)		Diaphyses of femur, humerus, metatarsus	reticular and some plexiform some osteon banding
	Sheep (Artiodactyla)		
Cuijpers (2009)		Femur, Humerus	reticular and radial tissue, scattered and dense Haversian systems
Martiniaková *et al.* (2007)		Femur	plexiform with irregular secondary osteons located periosteal and
Mulhern and Ubelaker (2001)		subadult Femur	plexiform with possibly band of primary osteons
Mori *et al.* (2005)		Tibia	no secondary osteons under one year, but then after a year present in midcortex

(Continued)

Table 14.1 (Continued)

Research Source	Species	Element studied	Qualitative Description
Mayne Correia *et al.*		Femur (650°C)	non vascular bone on the periphery, while plexiform can be seen midcortex, but the overwhelming appearance is solid black
		Femur (750°C)	only the margins retain any discemable structure, p exiform, primary
		Femur (900°C)	larger areas of tissue are available for viewing, and nclude those
	Rabbit (Lagomorph)		
Martiniaková *et al.* (2006b)		Femur	primary vascular longitudinal bone
			irregular and dense Haversian bone
	Bear (Ursus sp.)		
Foote (1916)		Femur	plexiform, and some secondary osteons
Enlow and Brown (1958)		Rib	dense Haversian
		Mandilble	reticular bone
		Long bones	plexiform amd scattered primary osteons in outer layer
			dense Haversian in midcortex
	Dog (Canis domesticus)		
Foote (1916)		Femur	plexiform
Enlow and Brown (1958)		Rib	dense haversian
		Long bones	plexiform amd scattered primary osteons in outer layer
			dense Haversian in midcortex

Table 14.1 (Continued)

Morris (2007)		Femur	plexiform
	Fox		
Foote (1916)	*Urocyon cinereoargenteus*		plexiform periosteal, Haversian in midcortex
Singh *et al*. (1974)	***Fennecus zerda***		inner circumferential layers pronounced, lacking on the outer margin
	Cat (Felidae)		
Enlow and Brown (1958)	*Fells*	Ribs and long bones	Haversian in mid cortex, circumferential lamella in outer layer
Singh *et al*. (1974)	Siberian tiger, jaguar	Femur	primary longitudinal canals, primary osteons, and reticular bone
	Human (*Homo sapiens*)		
Mulhern and Ubelaker (2001)		Femur	limited secondary osteons in rows (bands, 5 or less)
			dense Haversian and circumferential lamella
Pfeifer (2006)		Ribs	young bone lines of primary osteons – woven bone
			fragmentary interstitial lamella
Mulhern and Van Gerven (1997)		Femur adult	Haversian osteons, interstitial lamellae, thinner cortices, more resorption spaces
Pointer (2014)		Femur adult	dense Haversian osteons
		Femur (600°C)	high amounts of carbon, Haversian canals visible, but no lamellae,
		Femur (800°C)	margins more visible, mid cortex had lots of carbon still, Haversian
		Femur (1000°C)	Haversian osteons, but cloudy appearance

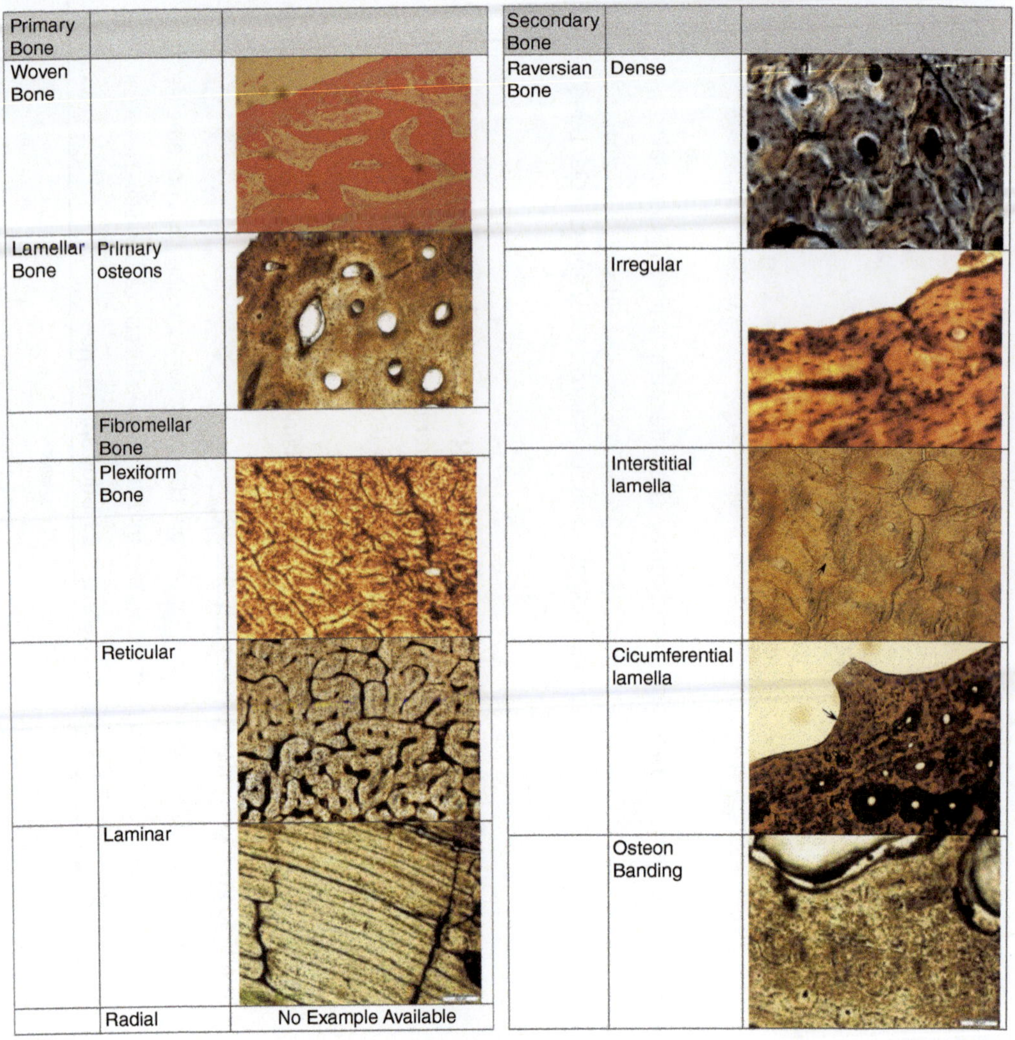

Figure 14.1 Examples of each bone tissue type.

2019). It is in this organization that the range of options across the species is seen. This primary lamellar bone may have vessel structures arranged in a radial, circular, or longitudinal orientation. This organization results in the unique appearances of this primary bone. One further aspect of this new organization is the potential for the primary osteons to be organized in a linear fashion. For some animals this means multiple rows of osteons (known as osteon banding), or it may mean just a few osteons (less than five in one row) as has been documented for humans (Mulhern and Ubelakar, 2001; Caccia *et al.*, 2016). It is important to note that there is variation in the position of these types of organizations across the bone section. Some types are more frequently seen in the perimeter of the bone (e.g. circumferential lamella in the periosteal region) while others are found predominately in the cortical regions (e.g. radially oriented lamellae).

14.2.1.3 Fibrolamellar Bone

It is interesting that there is yet one more variation on primary bone, and this is the fibrolamellar complex or woven parallel-complex. This tissue is a mixture of the fibrous woven bone and lamellar bone. Fibrolamellar bone is found in many fast-growing animals and is thought to relate to the need to grow rapidly. Woven bone is thought to be produced at a rate of 4 μm/day, while lamellar bone is thought to be produced at 1 μm/day (Mulhern and Ubelaker, 2012). Fibrolamellar bone is produced at a rate of 7–171 μm/day (de Magerie *et al.*, 2004). Fibrolamellar bone can be divided into four variations; however, the one most often referred to is plexiform bone. Laminar, reticular, and radial bone are the three other forms of fibrolamellar bone (Shapiro and Wu, 2019).

14.2.1.3.1 Plexiform Bone

According to Enlow and Brown's (1956, 1958) classification of bone structures, plexiform bone appears as the layering of rectangular primary vascular canals (also called primary osteons) in a well-organized network known as a plexus. These rectangular sections are layered in a horizontal direction (Mulhern and Ubelaker, 2001). Brits and colleagues (2014:371) describe plexiform bone as "primary bone with a dense network of vascular canals arranged longitudinally, circumferentially, and radially." While Shapiro and Wu (2019) describe plexiform bone as "laminar bone [that] has differing vascular orientations – longitudinal canals connected by radial and circular canals" (p. 141). Others have confirmed this interpretation in their studies observing various animal bone tissue (Cuijpers, 2006, 2009; Martiniaková *et al.*, 2007; Crescimanno and Stout, 2012).

Plexiform bone is typically cited as a form of bone structure that is indicative of nonhuman origin. It is not prevalent in all nonhuman groups, and can occasionally occur in rapidly growing human infants and children (Enlow and Brown, 1958; Enlow, 1963; Cuijpers, 2009), so its usage in species verification must be in conjunction with other features. A cautionary note is made here upon its reliance as a sole indicator for species.

14.2.1.3.2 Reticular Bone

Perhaps one of the clearest descriptions of reticular bone is provided by Brits and colleagues (2014), "as primary vascular bone…with unorganized display of branching vascular canals," but it is most helpful to think of a structure with vessels oriented in a variety of directions with the woven bone and lamellar bone oriented around them. Shapiro and Wu (2019) discuss the orientation of the vessels as being obliquely oriented. As well, there are numerous primary osteons associated with reticular bone. Locke (2004) provides an excellent discussion of laminar and reticular bone in mammals.

14.2.1.3.3 Laminar Bone

To visualize laminar bone, consider rings of lamellar bone alternating with rings of primary osteons. Shapiro and Wu (2019) describe laminar bone as composed of "fibrolamellar complexes of woven bone with primary osteons with a circumferential orientation of vascular canals" (p. 141). The key to identification here is the presence of the continuous lamellar organization around the bone in strata alternating with the primary osteons (Enlow and Brown, 1956; Martiniaková *et al.*, 2007).

14.2.1.3.4 Radial Bone

The final type of fibrolamellar bone to be discussed here is radial fibrolamellar bone. This bone tissue is loaded with "primary osteons with radially oriented canals" (Shapiro and Wu, 2019). The radiating canals extend across the periosteal and cortical regions of the bone. In a vast coverage of animals, Hillier and Bell (2007) only note radial bone in raccoon dogs; Cuijpers (2009) found it in sheep. It is seen in dinosaurs, though not likely a concern for anthropologists (Jentgen-Ceschino et.al., 2020).

14.2.2 Secondary Bone

Once the bone tissue begins to mature, in some species like humans, secondary bone replaces the earlier woven and lamellar bone. In other species this early bone is continually remodeled but is remodeled with woven and lamellar bone and primary osteons, not secondary osteons. The characteristic appearance of cortical bone in humans is the result of this remodeling. Several species have this secondary bone present in the cortical region (Table 14.1). Two types of secondary bone are recognized: Haversian bone, and non-Haversian lamellar bone (Ricqlès, 1975; Shapiro and Wu, 2019).

14.2.2.1 Haversian Bone

As primary osteons are replaced by new bone growth, longitudinal vessels tunnel through the bony matrix. They supply nutrients to the organic components of the bone. As old bone is resorbed and new bone is produced during remodeling, it is organized in concentric lamellae around the blood vessel situated in a longitudinal canal, now referred to as the Haversian canal. The cells producing the osteoid (bone protein) become entrapped in the inorganic matrix; and because of the need for nutrients, they must maintain a connection with the Haversian canal through channels known as canaliculi. The whole process produces the structural unit of bone: the secondary osteon. The secondary osteon consists of the Haversian canal, concentric lamellae, elongated lacunae (housing the cell), and canaliculi, as well as transverse or radial canals. These canals lack the concentric lamellae and are referred to as Volkmann's canals (Shapiro and Wu, 2019). The outer ring of the osteon has a layer of modified matrix; this zone is called the cement line. In a cross section of cortical bone, it is possible to identify new osteons and the remains of the old osteons – the interstitial lamellae (Ortner and Putschar, 1981; Currey, 2006). Primary osteons do not have a cement line.

14.2.2.1.1 Special/Dense Haversian Systems

The Haversian canal and associated concentric lamellae make up a complex which is known as a Haversian system or a secondary osteon. The concentric lamellae are made of rows of alternating collagen fibers. In a histological cross section, the Haversian system can be described as similar to tree rings circulating outwards from a central canal. In between the concentric lamellar layers are small cavities called lacunae in which osteocytes reside. These lacunae are in turn connected to each other through canaliculi, allowing direct networking between osteocytes to coordinate the bone remodeling unit's (BMU) actions in bone remodeling and maintenance (Schultz, 1997a). Dense Haversian or special lamellae (Schultz, 1997b) are recognized by the density of the osteons in the cortical tissue. In some cases, there is very little evidence of the interstitial lamellae as the Haversian osteons are packed in so tightly (Enlow and Brown, 1956; Smith, 1960a, 1960b; Hillier and Bell, 2007; Brits *et al.*, 2014).

14.2.2.1.2 Irregular Haversian Systems

Irregular Haversian systems only differ from the dense systems regarding the number of secondary osteons found in the tissue; there are less and they are irregularly distributed. Irregular Haversian systems are likely to be scattered across the cortical region in clusters or may stand alone (Hillier and Bell, 2007).

14.2.2.1.3 Basic, Surface, Endosteal, Circumferential Lamellae

On the outer edges of the cortical bone, the lamellae abandon the need to form around the blood vessels, because of the proximity to the marrow cavity or external vascularization. The result is the formation of layers of lamellar bone without the Haversian systems. These layers of bone form the inner (endosteal) and outer (periosteal) margins of the cortical bone. The cellular function of these bone types is slightly modified; endosteal bone, situated on the inner perimeter of the cortical bone, contains cells which function osteogenically and hemopoietically. The outer perimeter, the periosteum, contains osteoprogenitor cells; therefore, the periosteal lamellar bone is stimulated by injury to produce osteoblasts (bone forming cells) to initiate repair (Enlow and Brown, 1956; Smith, 1960a; Leeson *et al.*, 1981; Schultz, 1997a).

14.2.2.1.4 Interstitial Lamellae

The bony matrix between Haversian systems is occupied by interstitial lamellae. The process of remodeling (removal of primary bone and replacement by new osteons) leaves behind fragments of old osteons. These fragments of osteons are known as the interstitial lamellae (Smith, 1960a; Schultz, 1997a; Mulhern and Ubelaker, 2012).

14.2.2.1.5 Osteon Banding

When osteons (primary or secondary) present in a linear fashion, this is referred to as osteon banding. These linear clusters of osteons may number a few (~3–5), as is sometimes seen in human tissue, or in multiple lines of several osteons (~ 5–20). Bands of osteons are divided by lamellar bone (Mulhern and Ubelaka, 2001). Multiple bands of osteons are more likely to be indicative of a nonhuman bone fragment.

14.3 Vertebrate Histology

A substantial literature exists on the histological differentiation of medium-large sized mammals (Enlow and Brown, 1956, 1958; Urbanová and Novotný, 2005; Martiniáková *et al.*, 2006a, 2006b, 2007; Morris, 2007) including humans (Owsley *et al.*, 1985; Mulhern and Ubelaker, 2001, 2012; Hillier and Bell, 2007). These studies do not address all species but highlight many of the common mammals found in archaeological and modern forensic scenes. In this chapter, there is a discussion of several common species specifically and others more generally (see Table 14.1). Unidentifiable bone fragments tend to originate from long bones; this is a result of animal scavenging of the remains. These fragments often come from a variety of domestic animals, such as pig, cow, dog, and in the bush, those of coyote, deer, moose, and bear. It is recommended that some comparative samples from regional species be obtained for comparison.

Artiodactyls (cloven-hooved mammals) typically have plexiform structures forming the bulk of the compact bone, while older individuals may display scattered secondary osteons; these Haversian systems, however, are few throughout the plexiform layers. The area near the endosteum of the bone is often dense Haversian bone and is characterized by a greater concentration of Haversian systems, frequently superimposing previous generations of osteons (Hillier and Bell, 2007).

As can be expected, there are still structural differences between artiodactyls. Hillier and Bell (2007) succinctly summarize the typical pattern of deer as plexiform bone that originates near the periosteal surface, while Haversian structures extend from the endosteal edge. Immature cervids predominantly display plexiform bone, while mature individuals have a higher proportion of dense Haversian structures, indicating that Haversian bone replaces plexiform structures throughout growth and aging. Besides plexiform bone with few secondary osteons and few interstitial lamellae (Foote, 1916; Owsley *et al.*, 1985), deer also display primary vascular reticular bone (Singh *et al.*, 1974), an absence of inner and outer circumferential lamellae (Singh *et al.*, 1974), and osteon banding (Morris, 2007). The primary vascular reticular bone found in reindeer (Singh *et al.*, 1974) is bone with irregular and disorganized primary vascular canals (Enlow and Brown, 1956). Osteon banding, as found in the femur and humeri of white-tailed deer (Morris, 2007), is described as a "distinct row of five or more primary and/or secondary osteons" (Mulhern and Ubelaker, 2001:221). Unfortunately, most studies done on cervids (Table 14.1) lack consensus on which species to focus on, resulting in the possibility of potentially conflating histological features across species.

Research on the bone structures in domestic pigs (Table 14.1) confirms the artiodactyl pattern of predominantly plexiform bone with few scattered secondary osteons. This compact bone is made up of dense Haversian structures (Foote, 1916; Martiniaková *et al.*, 2006a, 2006b), and osteon banding is present in roughly half of the specimens analyzed (Mulhern and Ubelaker, 2001; Morris, 2007; Cuijpers, 2009). A feature that is unique to domestic pigs is the presence of resorption lacunae found in the spaces between Haversian systems (Martiniaková *et al.*, 2006a, 2006b). These lacunae, housing osteocytes, indicate that pigs have a higher turnover rate of bone development compared to other artiodactyls (Martiniaková *et al.*, 2006b); however, Hillier and Bell (2007) include pigs and cows in the same category as humans based on the similar appearance of dense Haversian bone. This stresses the importance of these other features, especially plexiform bone and osteon banding, in reliably differentiating pig bones from human bones.

Domestic cattle (Table 14.1) likewise display the same artiodactyl features of primary vascular plexiform bone with few scattered secondary osteons. The middle of the cortex contains dense Haversian structures (Enlow and Brown, 1958; Martiniaková *et al.*, 2006a, 2007), while the endosteal and periosteal layers house non-vascular bone (Cuijpers, 2006; Martiniaková *et al.*, 2006a, 2006b, 2007) which is unique to bovids. This histological type is characterized by concentric lamellae absent of vascular canals (Enlow and Brown, 1956).

In studies differentiating cow bone from horse (Perissodactyla), Cuijpers (2006) and Cuijpers and Lauwerier (2008) describe the fibrolamellar bone type in cows as being more fibrous than in horses, which has a more predominant lamellar component to the same structure type. The lamellar matrix creates primary osteons which densely vascularize the woven bone. This shows the variability of structure types in terms both of type of deposition and type of vascularization (Francillon-Viellot *et al.*, 1990). The horse diaphysis exhibits reticular bone and some dense Haversian bone (Enlow and Brown, 1958), but may have plexiform and possibly osteon banding (Cuijpers, 2006).

The subadult domestic sheep femora displays plexiform bone with primary osteons and possibly osteon banding in observations by Mulhern and Ubelaker (2001). Mori and colleagues (2005) identify secondary osteons in sheep tibia over one year old. In rib sections, secondary osteons along with plexiform bone are recorded by Enlow and Brown (1958).

Martiniaková and colleagues (2006b) identify primary longitudinal vascular bone present, along with areas of irregular and dense Haversian bone in the femora of the rabbit they assessed.

Bear femora have been identified with plexifom bone with some Haversian osteons (Foote, 1916) and with dense Haversian bone in the midcortex (Enlow and Brown, 1958). They observe reticular bone in the mandible and dense

Haversian bone in the rib. The dog is seen to have a similar pattern, as is the fox; however, there is no mention of reticular bone in the latter two genera. Enlow and Brown (1958) describe the ribs and long bones of a cat (Felidae) as having circumferential lamella in the outer layer, but Haversian bone in the mid cortex. Singh and colleagues (1974) describe the tissue from a Siberian tiger and Jaguar femora as dominated by primary longitudinal canals and some reticular structures, with some primary osteons.

14.4 Burnt Bone Histology

The earliest work located which attempts to describe the histological changes found in cremated bone is that of Forbes (1941). His study results from a medicolegal case in which he determines whether a burnt sample is bone. He supplies us with a description of compact and cancellous tissue exposed to the heat of a Bunsen burner. The general observations were made with decalcified thin sections under normal light microscopy. For compact bone, he describes an initial prominence of the canaliculi which disappear as the lamellae become coarse and granular. The lacunae are described as changing from flat and distorted to mere hazy outlines. The lamellae gradually disappear, leaving a uniformly granular matrix with Haversian canals throughout. The Haversian systems decreased in size, but the Haversian canals increase in diameter and fill with debris. He notes the presence of cracks which are irregular in width; they tend to travel along the periphery of the Haversian system to join with other cracks. The cancellous bone undergoes similar changes, except for those noted for the Haversian systems.

This early experiment demonstrates that an important issue that arises in burnt bone is the alteration in the dimensions of bone which could potentially impact histological analysis. In a study using spongy bone, Grupe and Herrmann (1983) record a 12% reduction in various measurements. In compact bone, Bradtmiller and Buikstra (1984) observed a statistically significant *increase* in osteon size of bone burned at 600°C; and Buikstra and Swegle (1989) suggest a correction factor of 0–10%. They demonstrated a narrow range of shrinkage from -0.7% to -5.6%, with a maximum temperature that reached 1060°C. They noted that most altered bones shrank less than 3% at 700–800°C. In temperatures up to 1000°C, Hummel and Schutkowski (1986) record a 5% shrinkage in the proximo-distal length of the compact bone, but a 27% reduction in the cross-sectional diameter. The identification technique which uses wall thickness for sex determination may, therefore, be adversely affected. The study by Holland (1989) claims that the cranial base is expected to shrink by 1–2.25%, but he notes that above 800°C this figure may be an underestimate, as measurements were more difficult to make on the severely calcined bone. These amounts are inconsistent with those found by Gilchrist and Mythum (1986); they suggested different elements of the same species will vary drastically, for example the cow femur shrunk 5.8%, while the rib shrunk as much as 29%, and the sheep rib up to 32%. Nelson observed in his study that mean osteon diameter decreased by 16.7% while mean canal diameter *increased* by 10.5% (1992). Thompson (2005) tested the extent of distortion at a similar range of temperatures (500°C, 700°C, and 900°C). He found that the percentage of shrinkage of bone was linked to the temperature as well as duration of exposure. Thompson (2005) showed that less than 9% of the bone samples studied demonstrated changes in dimension; however, in the same experiment, burning bone at 900°C could account for a shrinkage of 15–40%, suggesting a lowered threshold of 700–1000°C for potential alteration in bone dimensions. Sawada and colleagues (2014) found that by using the 17% suggested shrinkage (from Nelson, 1992) they were successful in distinguishing a variety of animal species based on the histomorphometry. While Absolonova and associates (2013) were assessing the usefulness of estimating age on burnt bone, they noted that heat changes mimic age changes to osteons, yielding a decrease in dimension and an increase in the osteon number per mm^2.

Herrmann (1972a, 1972b, 1977) used histological techniques to examine the microstructural responses of archaeological bone to extreme heat exposure. In these studies, Herrmann determined the temperatures at which the organic components of bone were completely burned, resulting in the fusion of bone mineral crystals. This "critical level" was set at 700–800°C (Herrmann, 1972a), at which point the fusion of the inorganic components of bone impacts the macroscopic appearance due to shrinkage. Below this critical level is "incomplete cremation" which is characterized by darker coloration of the bone in shades of black, brown, and blue-gray (Herrmann, 1972b) due to the carbonization of the organic material remaining in the bone material. Despite the remarkable changes occurring around the critical level, the histological makeup of completely cremated bone is still identifiable using scanning electron microscopic (SEM) analysis. Herrmann (1977) referred to the shrunken dimensions of osteons at higher temperatures (past the critical level) which was determined to be a result of the inorganic crystal fusion.

Castillo and his fellow researchers (2013) investigated the histological appearance of human iliac bone from 100°C to 1100°C. In the first range of temperatures (100–300°C), the deformation of collagen fibers was observed. The second range (400–600°C) produced the degradation of collagen and beginnings of crystallization. Heterogenous crystalline structures were present within the third range (700–800°C), and the last stage (900–1100°C) showed a compact bone surface made up of irregular microcrystals. These results are comparable to other studies focused on crystalline appearance (Shipman *et al.*, 1984; Holden *et al.*, 1995; Hiller *et al.*, 2003; Piga *et al.*, 2008), yet do not address any of the factors in using light microscopy for identification purposes similar to those in Beckett *et al.* (2011). This demonstrates the necessity of testing whether light microscopy is a valid technique in differentiating human and faunal material after cremation.

Responding to the recognition that burning could affect methods used to discriminate between animals, Cattaneo and colleagues (1999) compared the accuracy of DNA, immunological, and histological approaches and they created a new discriminant function for several domestic species and humans. They claimed a 79.4% (human) and 79.2% (for nonhuman) success for human and animal discrimination by using their function. They claimed that metric analysis is the most accurate of the methods compared. No DNA was detectable in the samples and albumin was largely undetectable. They later tested this conclusion in 2009 in a study that focused on the analysis of flat and subadult bones compared to values derived from long and adult bones. The nonhuman collection was composed of dog, cat, cow, rabbit, sheep, pig, quail, chicken, and turkey samples. Discriminant function analysis was performed using Haversian canal area and minimum-maximum diameters of Haversian canals. An algorithm generated from the previous study was used to verify the accuracy of differentiating between human and nonhuman samples; a negative value denoted nonhuman origin while a positive value implied human origin. The type of element or age played no factor in correctly identifying nonhuman origin, but these two variables were necessary for proper diagnosis of human samples. Metric analysis performed on adult human long bones had 70% accuracy, while adult flat bones had 28.2% accuracy. Incorrect identification was especially high in neonate remains (93.3% on long bone and 68% on flat bone). Subadult analysis had a high failure, with 56.1% of long bones incorrectly identified and 60% of flat bones incorrectly assigned.

A further concern when analyzing animal and human burnt bone are the taphonomic changes which may impact our ability to interpret the histology. Hanson and Cain (2007) created a scale to describe the observed taphonomic changes seen in burnt archaeological bone. Diagenetic changes are an issue to be expected when dealing with non-experimental bone, as with archaeological or forensic case bone (cf. Garland, 1987). An important point made by these authors is that "several types (non-burning diagenetic destruction) were observed, were easily distinguished from burning damage" (Hanson and Cain, 2007:1911). As early as 1993, Nicholson indicated that diagenesis would complicate how we viewed burnt bone macroscopically. Hanson and Buikstra (1987) recognized fungal damage in the unburnt bones that precluded the analysis of the histological morphology. Pitre and colleagues (2012) identified biofilms in archaeological bone and Bell (2012) and Schultz (1997b) remind us as well that bone damage resulting from fungal, bacterial, and algae damage is important to consider when viewing the histomorphology. Others noted the presence of soil debris infiltrate in the bone samples affecting the ability to successfully observe the histology (Sawada *et al.*, 2014).

Partially in response to the issues noted around the understanding of the change in bone structure due to shrinkage, bone mineral crystallization, and taphonomic changes, the contributions of further investigations may help to identify any issues in applying standard histological methods to burnt remains. Initial work by Horocholyn (2013) on burnt animal bones was supplemented by Pointer's (2014) similar experiment on human bone. A case study based upon these studies is presented here, along with a small test of sheep bone histology taken from the experimental sheep bones (Mayne, 1990).

14.5 Case Study for Comparison of Histology of Cremated Bone

The case study presented here is drawn from several projects originating in the Department of Anthropology at the University of Alberta. As part of continuing interest in the histology of bone, the first author sampled some cremated sheep femora with known burn temperatures and times in order to see the histological characteristics; the second author has provided the data for the cow, pig, and deer femora (Horocholyn, 2013); and finally, the third author has contributed data from the burning of five human femora (Pointer, 2014). These samples provide the basis for conclusions about the utility of histological analysis after remains have been cremated.

The samples used in this case study consist of young sheep, cow, pig, and deer, and mature adult human femora. All samples were heated in electric furnaces (Fisher IsoTemp Muffle Furnace, Barnstead-Thermolyne Type F62700 Furnace, ventilated fire-Asane furnace) for a period of 15 minutes, except the sheep, which were burned for one hour. The temperatures used in the studies were 600–1000°C. The sheep was fresh with fleece; the pig, cow, and human were all fresh bone; and the deer was dry bone (Mayne, 1990; Horocholyn, 2013; Pointer, 2014). Thin sections of the cremated samples were completed after embedding the samples in resin, and then producing 100 µm thin sections. The sheep samples were not embedded in resin before sectioning. These sections were viewed using a digital light microscope (Leitz Laborlux 12 POL S) at 100× magnification. Images for this chapter were captured using an Olympus BX53 light microscope with digital camera. *Celllsens* or *Image J* software was used to measure the minimum/maximum diameters and areas of Haversian canals and Haversian systems. A minimum of 30 osteons and Haversian canals for each species per temperature were measured to meet the requirements for adequate sample sizes.

14.5.1 Qualitative and Quantitative Analysis for Case Study

For each of these species, both qualitative and quantitative observations were made to determine what characteristics could still be observed after cremation and how the mean Haversian osteon area and mean Haversian canal area compared to other publications (c.f. Tables 14.1 and Table 14.2) on unburnt and burnt remains.

Table 14.2 Comparison of quantitative analysis of various animals and humans.

Research Source	Species	Element Studied	Mean Osteon Area (mm2)	Mean Haversian Canal Area (mm2)
	Deer (*Cervidae*)			
Urbanova and Novotny (2005)	**Red deer**		0.007410	0.000409
	Roe deer		0.009900	0.000328
Moms (2007)		Femur	0.013900	0.000387
		Humerus	0.014700	0.000401
Horocholyn (2013)	**White-tailed deer (*Odocoileus virginianus*)**	Femur	0.015310	0.000313
		Femur 600°C	0.011977	0.000228
		Femur 800°C	0.016259	0.000286
		Femur 1000°C	0.013668	0.000254
	Pig domestic (*Sus scrofa*)			
Urbanova and Novotny (2005)			0.033118	0.000826
Martiniaková *et al*. (2006a)			0.029194	0.001009
Martiniaková *et al*. (2006b)			0.028310	0.001015
Mortis (2007)			0.019700	0.000645
Horocholyn (2013)		Femur	0.020622	0.000465
		Femur 600°C	N/A	N/A
		Femur 800°C	0.015382	0.000429
		Femur 1000°C	0.018110	0.000443
	Cow domestic (*Bos taurus*)			
Urbanova and Novotny (2005)			0.036067	0.001176
Martiniaková *et al*. (2006a)			0.031725	0.001197
Martiniaková *et al*. (2006b)			0.032664	0.001225
Zedda *et al*. (2008)			0.023576	0.000717
Horocholyn (2013)		Femur	0.031727	0.000717
		Femur 600°C	0.032948	0.000790
		Femur 800°C	0.026178	0.000658
		Femur 1000°C	0.026226	0.000634

Table 14.2 (Continued)

	Sheep domestic (Ovis aries)			
Horni (2012)		Femur (but goat)	0.028220	N/A
Castrogiovanni *et al*. (2011)		Femur	~0.031416	N/A
Mayne (1990)		Femur 650°C	N/A	N/A
		Femur 750°C	N/A	N/A
		Femur 900°C	0.001904	0.000085
	Human (*Homo sapiens*)			
Thompson (1980)		Femur female	N/A	0.006300
		Femur male	N/A	0.004100
Burr *et al*. (1990)		Femur female	0.041000	0.002400
		Femur male	0.034000	0.002300
Mulhem and Van Gerven (1998)		Femur	0.037620	0.000214
		Femur female	0.040000	0.002000
		Femur male	0.036000	0.002100
Pfeifer *et al*. (2006)		Rib	0.034080	
Blitz *et al*. (2009)		Femur	0.060750	
Dominguez and Crowder (2012)		Rib	0.036000	
Dominguez and Agnew (2016)		Rib	0.036000	
Absolonova *et al*. (2013)		Rib	0.028090	0.002172
		Rib 700°C	0.021505	0.001659
		Rib 800°C	0.014926	0.001211
Nelson (1992)		Femur	0.036087	0.003499
		Femur 537–815°C	0.025539	0.004072
Pointer (2014)		Femur	0.053462	0.005093
		Femur 600°C	0.042796	0.005058
		Femur 800°C	0.038603	0.004530
		Femur 1000°C	0.061299	0.005316

14.5.1.1 Qualitative Results

The literature predicts that histological structures will be visible at all temperatures, allowing for qualitative analysis in the burnt samples. As well, the literature indicates that given the structures will be visible, they should be measurable (Bradtmiller and Buikstra, 1984; Nelson, 1992; Cattaneo *et al.*, 1999; Absolonova *et al.*, 2013). The case study discussed here had variable success in completing these observations, which are summarized alongside other studies in Table 14.1.

In the sheep sections, several disheartening observations can be made. These samples were not embedded in resin, and thus did not survive the grinding process well. The remaining samples were viewed using light microscopy and 100× magnification. The overall impression of each of the samples was an intense concentration of carbon present within the structures, especially in the mid-cortex. Some structures are visible on the endosteal and periosteal margins. When the bone tissue is visible to see and not saturated with carbon, then the expected tissue is seen. Plexiform, irregular primary vascular, and sections of nonvascular tissue were all observed; the most difficult specimens were those burned at 650°C and 750°C, while the clearest section had been heated to 900°C.

In the deer, pig, and cow sections, a similar set of observations were made (Horocholyn, 2013). Carbonization was prevalent at all three temperatures but was most extensive at 600°C due to residual organic content (Figure 14.2). A

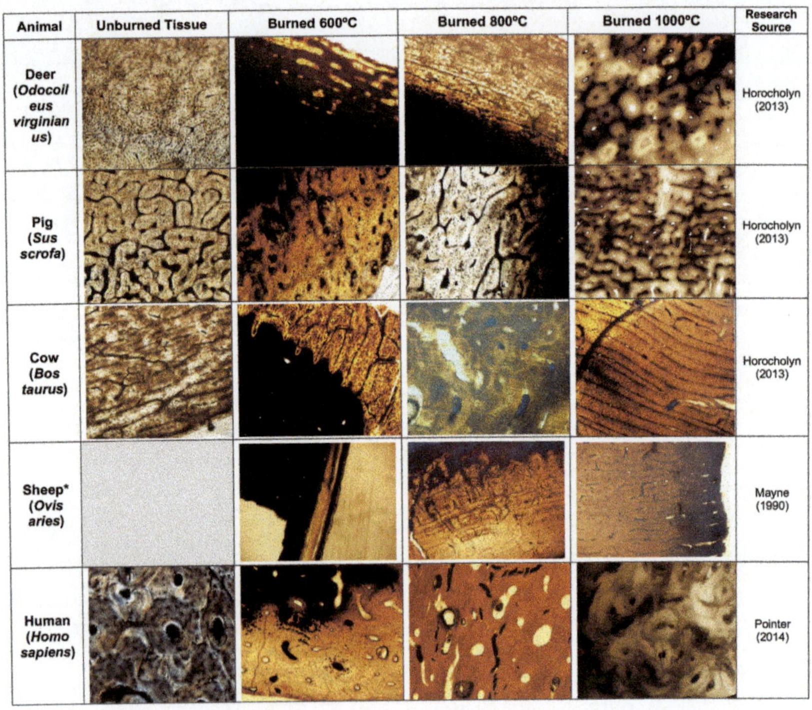

Figure 14.2 Images of species at various temperatures (*Sheep burned at 650°C, 750°C, and 900°C).

gray-white cloudiness was visible in samples burned at 800°C and 1000°C. In the deer specimens this cloudiness obscured the view enough that plexiform structures took on the appearance of laminar structures. Alternatively, this would be the first evidence of laminar bone in deer. An interesting find in the pig samples, is the presence of reticular tissue, previously only mentioned by Enlow and Brown (1958). The reticular tissue was clearly identifiable at both the 600°C and 800°C samples; although at 1000°C, no reticular bone was identified in this section. Plexiform and Haversian systems were identified at all temperatures. In the cow bone, the control exhibited non-vascular structures; however, these tissues were not identified in any other temperatures. It is argued by Horocholyn (2013) that the non-vascular bone is either concealed by carbon or has undergone some change in the heating process. The mid-cortex area is obscured by carbon, while the margins are less affected by carbon. Non-vascular bone is most likely to be in the endosteal and periosteal margins, the clearest area on these sections.

The human samples resulted in sections which had about a 50% visibility. As with the other examples, the samples burned at 600°C and 800°C were the most obscured by carbon (Figure 14.2). The mid-cortex was very difficult to see in these specimens. At 1000°C there was more visibility and this was enhanced by modifying the microscope settings. Pointer (2014) indicates that Haversian canals were visible; however, the circumferential lamellae were less distinct, and the cement lines are clearly demarcated at 600°C. In the endosteal and periosteal regions at 800°C, these structures were shaded by a chalky, translucent film. At 1000°C, the lighter gray-white, chalky appearance was found in the margins, but the mid-cortical area remained blackened. Dense Haversian systems were identifiable in all regions of the bone.

14.5.1.2 Quantitative Observations

Overall, the cremation process tends to result in lower osteon areas and Haversian canal areas in this case study. The most notable exception is with the human sample that shows an *increase* in mean size of osteons for one individual. Mean osteon areas and mean Haversian canal areas are presented in Table 14.2, along with published reference samples.

For the human Haversian osteon areas, generally, there was a pattern of overall decrease in the area from as much as 44.5% (600°C) to as low 3.4% (1000°C), but the amounts were variable, and did not meet statistical significance tests. In one individual, there was an increase by 21% in the osteon area (800°C). For the Haversian canal size there were no identified patterns, as increases of up to 20.6% were seen, but also reductions in size were recorded. This inconsistency was seen at all temperatures. One important observation identified when completing these measurements relates to the visibility of the osteons and canals using the light microscopy. Carbon deposits within the tissue obscures the histological structures. It may be necessary to experiment with the lighting and the filters to view structures through the carbon.

The amount of carbonization affected the availability of structures to be measured. Sampling was biased, as visible osteons were predominately located on the margins of the samples. For the lower temperatures the carbon was the most problematic. Margins and fractured areas provided viewable osteons, but due to the carbon it was difficult to determine what percentage of the osteons were visible. In some cases, the osteon was visible, but the cement line was obscured by the cloudy or foggy surface. So, it might be possible to recognize an osteon but not measure it. For deer samples, the osteons both decreased in size (~4%) and increased (as much as 16% at 800°C), in size canals decreased in size from the control (up to 11.5% at 800°C). The pig samples, limited as they were, demonstrated a decrease in size both in the osteons and canals. For the cow samples, osteons and canals increased in size at 600°C, but there were decreases at higher temperatures (1–5%). Only the osteons were observed for the sheep as the carbonization was too excessive. The measurements that were possible indicated that the osteons did decrease in size when compared with the meagre published data for osteon size in unburnt sheep.

14.6 Discussion

Observations on the case study's cremated bone samples provide mixed conclusions regarding the possibility of using methods for discriminating animal from human remains and of histomorphometric analysis. In forensic situations, it may be necessary to try any methods available to provide evidence to draw conclusions regarding the origin of a bone fragment. While conclusions are not overwhelmingly positive, there is a potential to still distinguish animal from human bone using qualitative observations. Less promising are the observations from quantitative data. Depending on the heat of the fire exposure, the carbon may have been burned away sufficiently to provide a clearer view of the bone structure. One thought, though it may seem outrageous, may be to purposefully extend the heat damage to the point of fusion as the higher temperature may result in clearer histological features.

While it is generally common practice to embed burnt bone samples, this process makes them useless for further DNA analysis, so sampling without embedding was explored here to look at the viability of such an approach. Results confirmed that samples disintegrate too rapidly to be ground unembedded; therefore, if there is an intent to complete DNA extraction for the burnt samples, that component should be preserved separately. The experience of this investigator has been such, that the samples from forensic cases that require histological analysis are already too small to be split for this purpose. This is relevant for those samples only exposed to very low heat temperatures but must be kept in mind when thinking about this destructive approach (c.f. Chapter 12 in this text). Resources available for analyses are often limited and histological analysis is less expensive than DNA analysis, so when many bone samples need to be assessed to determine the presence of human remains this becomes a consideration.

As seen in the case study, cremation limits the area of bone that is observable for qualitative analysis. Endosteal and periosteal margins are frequently all that is left to observe, as the cortical area is obscured by carbon. This situation and heat fracturing of the bone impact the ability to identify the cement lines around the Haversian systems and carbon may line the Haversian canals, thus impacting the measurement of those features. As the common mantra in histological analysis of human and animal remains is to "use both qualitative and quantitative" methods (Cuijpers, 2006; Brits *et al.*, 2014; Sawada *et al.*, 2014:271), it is important to understand the limitations on the observations we make due to sampling bias. If the cortical area is unavailable to view, then certain tissue types typically located there will not be accounted for in the sample. Researchers have noted that the presence of a particular tissue type is related to the bone or portion of bone (Caccia *et al.*, 2016). In cases with fragmentary bone, those too small to identify as human are also often difficult to specify to particular bone. A radial, humeral, or femoral shaft fragment may not be distinguished whether burned or not, and it must be recognized that most studies indicating bone tissues for various animals are based on mid-femoral shaft analysis. An even greater issue occurs when trying to compare to rib bone, as the cremation process affects the thin cortical surface of ribs, ilia, mandibular, tarsal, and carpal bone by causing this surface to delaminate. At this time, there is no clear picture of the variation in humans, let alone all relevant nonhuman animals. There is little to no idea of the common bone tissue structures found in irregular and flat bones (e.g. diploe, scapula, vertebrae). These facts complicate any analysis on burnt remains and, therefore, caution must be taken with the conclusions drawn from histological analysis.

For quantitative analysis there are even more issues. Most important is the ability to assess enough Haversian osteons successfully for discrimination between animals. Dense Haversian bone is often located in the mid-cortical regions, and; therefore, often not visible in cremated bone. Irregular Haversian osteons may be more helpful as they are found in the margins. Haversian canals are visible, but the margins are ill-defined and cannot be reliably measured for fear of debris buildup within the canal. This fact is impacted by issues recognized in unburnt bone differentiation.

Although this chapter does not directly address age assessment methods using histology (cf. Chapter 5 in this text), it is important to consider the implications of burning bone on age assessment. Crowder and Pfeifer (2012) and Crowder *et al.* (2018) state that there may be issues in reliability of age estimation depending on the human bone section. Pfeiffer (1998, Pfeifer *et al.*, 2006) draws our attention to the issues of aging and sex when completing age estimation on human remains via histomorphometry. Age has been demonstrated to have a direct relationship with the prevalence of plexiform and Haversian bone in nonhuman animals. Hillier and Bell (2007) indicate that there are differences between mature and immature cervids in the relative proportion of plexiform bone. In mature cervids, dense Haversian structures replace plexiform bone, especially near the endosteal area of the cortex (Hillier and Bell, 2007). Morris (2007) notes that in her study, the limited availability of pig Haversian structures for analysis was most likely related to the young age of her pig specimens. These two studies, along with Enlow and Brown (1956) suggest that plexiform bone is more abundant in immature artiodactyls, while proportions of Haversian structures increase in mature individuals. So, if applying histological age assessment is considered problematic in unburnt bone, then greater care must be taken when assessing cremated bone for these characteristics when completing animal versus human bone analysis.

A second issue that impacts quantitative analysis is our lack of consistent results in the amount of shrinkage or expansion of the Haversian osteon and Haversian canals (Table 14.2). There appears to be shrinkage of the two features generally, but there is a huge amount of variation between species (Horocholyn, 2013) and between individuals within a species (Pointer, 2014) in the amount to be expected and, therefore, accounted for in any calculation or comparison with unburnt samples. Rates of shrinkage from over 45% to as little as 3% have been recorded in the literature. Given this situation, it must be strongly recommended to avoid quantitative interpretation of histological features in burnt bone. At this time, we do not have enough research to predict if there will be expansion (as seen in the case study samples: osteons and canals of humans at 1000°C, cow at 600°C, and osteons of deer at 800°C), or shrinkage of the features (Thompson, 2005).

One final issue that must be addressed when undertaking histological analysis of burnt bone (and unburnt bone) is the effect of diagenesis on the sample. Taphonomic processes beyond burning will impact on samples exposed to the environment after cremation. Biofilms, and fungal and bacterial destruction may be present, as well as infiltrations from carbon and soil particles (Garland, 1987; Schultz, 1997b; Bell, 2012; Pitre *et al.*, 2012). It is important to know how these changes will affect the normal appearance.

14.7 Conclusion

There is still a lot to learn about the application of histology to cremated bone. These early studies (Hermann, 1977; Bradtmiller and Buikstra, 1984; Nelson, 1992; Cattaneo *et al.*, 1999; Thompson, 2005; Horocholyn, 2013; Pointer, 2014) have clearly shown that there are issues in applying methodology developed on unburnt remains to those cremated at various temperatures. There is not enough known about the variation in type and location of tissue types in all relevant species. It can be argued that there is no good temperature when it is possible to use these interpretive methods. It has been shown that there are discrepancies under the "critical" temperature at 750°C as well as for all higher temperatures. There are several questions arising from the various experimental projects. How does the experimental design impact the results? Does the burning of sections versus whole bones affect how the bone matrix reacts to the heat? How does the length of the burn affect the understanding, for example is it enough to say that something was burned at 1000°C given the understanding of the impact of time on this process?

At this point, the use of histomorphology and histomorphometrics can be used with extreme caution and with the discretion of the scientist assessing the condition of the samples and their ability to confidently recognize the necessary features for both metric and non-metric analyses.

References

Absolonova, K., Veleminsky, P., Dobisikova, M., Beran, M., and Zocova, J. (2013) Histological estimation of age at death from the compact bone of burned and unburned human ribs. *Journal of Forensic Sciences*, **58**(S1), S135–S145.

Beckett, S., Rogers, K.H., and Clement, J.G. (2011) Inter-species variation in bone mineral behavior upon heating. *Journal of Forensic Sciences*, **56**(3), 571–579.

Bell, L. (2012) Histotaphonomy. In: *Bone Histology: An Anthropological Perspective* (eds. C. Crowder and S. Stout). CRC Press, Boca Raton, FL, pp. 241–251.

Bradtmiller, B. and Buikstra, J.E. (1984) Effects of burning on human bone microstructure: A preliminary study. *Journal of Forensic Sciences*, **29**(2), 535–540.

Brits, D., Steyn, M., and L'Abbé, E.N. (2014) A histomorphological analysis of human and non-human femora. *International Journal of Legal Medicine*, **128**, 369–377.

Britz, H.M., Thomas, C.D., Clement, J.G., and Cooper, D.M. (2009) The relation of femoral osteon geometry to age, sex, height and weight. *Bone*, **45**(1), 77–83.

Buikstra, J.F. and Swegle, M. (1989) Bone modification due to burning: Experimental evidence. In: *Bone Modification* (ed. R. Bonnischen). Peopling of the Americas Publication, Centre for the Study of the First Americans, Institute Quaternary Studies, University of Maine, ME, pp. 247–258.

Caccia, G., Magli, F., Tagi, V.M., Porta, D.G., Cummaudo, M., Márquez-Grant, N., *et al.* (2016) Histological determination of the human origin from dry bone: A cautionary note for subadults. *International Journal of Legal Medicine*, **130**, 299–307.

Castillo, R.F., Ubelaker, D., Acosta, J., and Canãdas de la Fuente, G.A. (2013) Effects of temperature on bone tissue. Histological study of the changes in the bone matrix. *Forensic Science International*, **226**, 33–37.

Castrogiovanni, P., Imbesi, R., Fisichella, M., and Mazzone, V. (2011) Osteonic organization of limb bones in mammals, including humans, and birds: A preliminary study. *Italian Journal of Anatomy and Embryology*, **116**(1), 30–37.

Cattaneo, C., DiMartino, S., Scali, S., Craig, O.E., Grandi, M., and Sokol, R.J. (1999) Determining the human origin of fragments of burnt bone: A comparative study of histological, immunological and DNA techniques. *Forensic Science International*, **102**, 181–191.

Crescimanno, A. and Stout, S.D. (2012) Differentiating fragmented human and non-human long bone using osteon circularity. *Journal of Forensic Sciences*, **57**(2), 287–294.

Crowder, C. and Pfeiffer, S. (2012) The application of cortical bone histomorphometry to estimate age at death. In: *Bone Histology: An Anthropological Perspective* (eds. C. Crowder and S. Stout). CRC Press, New York, pp. 193–215.

Crowder, C., Pinto, D.C., Andronowski, J.M., and Dominguez, V.M. (2018) Theory and histological methods. In: *Forensic Anthropology: Theoretical Framework and Scientific Basis*, 1st edn. (eds. C.C. Boyd and D.C. Boyd). Wiley and Sons Ltd, NJ, pp. 113–126.

Cuijpers, A.G. (2006) Histological identification of bone fragments in archaeology: Telling humans apart from horses and cattle. *International Journal of Osteoarchaeology*, **16**, 465–480.

Cuijpers, S. (2009) Distinguishing between the bone fragments of medium-sized mammals and children. A histological identification for archaeology. *Anthropologischer Anzeiger*, **67**(2), 181–203.

Cuijpers, S. and Lauwerier, R. (2008) Differentiating between bone fragments from horses and cattle: A histological identification method for archaeology. *Environmental Archaeology*, **13**(2), 165–179.

Currey, J.D. (2006) *Bones: Structures and Mechanics*. Princeton University Press, NJ.

de Margerie, E., Robin, J.-P., Verrier, D., Cubo, J., Groscolas, R., and Castanet, J. (2004) Assessing a relationship between bone microstructure and growth rate: A fluorescent labelling study in the king penguin chick (*Aptenodytes patagonicus*). *Journal of Experimental Biology*, **207**, 869–879.

de Ricqlès, A. (1975) Recherches paléohistologiques sur les os longs des tétrapodes. VII.- Sur la classification, la signification fonctionelle et l'histoire des tissus osseux des tétrapodes. Première partie. *Annales de Paléontologie (Vertébrés)*, **61**, 51–129.

Dominguez, V.M. and Crowder, C.M. (2012) The utility of osteon shape and circularity for differentiating human and nonhuman Haversian bone. *American Journal of Physical Anthropology*, **149**, 84–91.

Dominguez, V.M. and Agnew, A.M. (2016) Examination of factors potentially influencing osteon size in the human rib. *The Anatomical Record*, **299**, 313–324.

Enlow, D. (1963) *Principles of Bone Remodeling*. C.C. Thomas Publishing, Springfield, IL.

Enlow, D.H. and Brown, S.O. (1956) A comparative histological study of fossil and recent bone tissues, part I. *The Texas Journal of Science*, **7**(4), 405–443.

Enlow, D.H. and Brown, S.O. (1958) A comparative histological study of fossil and recent bone tissues, part III. *The Texas Journal of Science*, **10**(2), 187–230.

Foote, J.S. (1916) A contribution to the comparative histology of the femur. *Smithsonian Contributions to Knowledge*, **35**(3).

Forbes, G. (1941) The effects of heat on the histological structure of bone. *Police Journal*, **14**, 50–60.

Francillon-Vieillot, H., de Buffrénil, V., Castanet, J., Géraudie, J., Meunier, F.J., Sire, J., *et al.* (1990) Microstructure and mineralization of vertebrate skeletal tissues. In: *Skeletal Biomineralization: Patterns, Processes and Evolutionary Trends* (ed. J.G. Carter). Van Nostrand Reinhold, New York, pp. 471–530.

Garland, A.N. (1987) A histological study of archaeological bone decomposition. In: *Death, Decay and Reconstruction: Approaches to Archeology and Forensic Sciences* (eds. A. Boddington, A.N. Garland, and R.C. Janaway). Manchester University Press, Manchester, pp. 109–126.

Gilchrist, R. and Mytum, H.C. (1986) Experimental archaeology and burnt animal bone from archaeological sites. *Circaea*, **4**(1), 29–38.

Greenlee, D.M. and Dunnell, R.C. (2010) Identification of fragmentary bone from the Pacific. *Journal of Archaeological Science*, **37**, 957–970.

Grupe, G. and Herrmann, B. (1983) Über das Schrumpfungsverhalten experimentell verbrannter spongiöser Knochen am Beispiel des Caput femoris. *Zeitschrift für Morphologie und Anthropologie*, **74**(2), 121–127.

Hanson, D.B. and Buikstra, J.E. (1987) Histomorphological alteration in buried human bone from the lower Illinois Valley: implications for palaeodietary research. *Journal of Archaeological Science*, **14**(5), 549–563.

Hanson, M. and Cain, C.R. (2007) Examining histology to identify burned bone. *Journal of Archaeological Science*, **34**, 1902–1913.

Herrmann, B. (1972a) Das Combe Capell-Skelet. Eine Untersuchung der Brandreste unter Berucksichtigung thermoinduzierter veranderungen am Knochen. *Ausgrabungen in Berlin*, **3**, 769.

Herrmann, B. (1972b) Zur Beurteilung von Kohlenstoffverfäbungen bei Leichenbränden. *Ausgrabungen und Funde*, **17**(6), 275–277.

Herrmann, B. (1977) On histological Investigations of cremated human remains. *Journal of Human Evolution*, **6**, 101–103.

Hiller, J.C., Thompson, T.J., Evison, M.P., Chamberlain, A.T., and Wess, T.J. (2003) Bone mineral change during experimental heating: an X-ray scattering investigation. *Biomaterials*, **24**(28), 5091–5097.

Hillier, M.L. and Bell, L. (2007) Differentiating human bone from animal bone: A review of histological methods. *Journal of Forensic Sciences*, **52**(2), 249–263.

Holland, T.D. (1989) Use of the cranial base in the identification of fire victims. *Journal of Forensic Sciences*, **34**(2), 458–460.

Holden, J.L., Phakey, P.P., and Clement, J.G. (1995) Scanning electron microscope observations of heat-treated human bone. *Forensic Science International*, **74**(1–2), 29–45.

Horocholyn, K. (2013) *Comparative Histology of Burned Mammals using Light Microscopy*. Master of Arts Thesis, University of Alberta, Alberta.

Hummel, S. and Schutkowski, H. (1986) Das Verhalten von Knochengewebe unter dem Einfluss höherer Temperaturen, Bedeutungen für die Leichenbranddiagnose. *Zeitschrift für Morphologie und Anthropologie*, **77**(1), 1–9.

Jentgen-Ceshino, B., Stein, K., and Fischer, V. (2020) Case study of radial fibrolamellar bone tissues in the outer cortex of basal sauropods. *Philosophical Transactions of the Royal Society of B*, **375**, 20190143.

Leeson, C.R., Leeson, T.S., and Paparo, A.A. (1981) *Textbook of Histology*. WB Saunders Company, Philadelphia, PA.

Locke, M. (2004) Structure of long bones in mammals. *Journal of Morphology*, **262**, 546–565.

Martiniaková, M., Grosskopf, B., Omelka, R., Dammers, K., Vondráková, M., and Bauerova, M. (2006a) Differences among species in compact bone tissue microstructure of mammalian skeleton: Use of a discriminant function analysis for species identification. *Journal of Forensic Sciences*, **51**(6), 1235–1239.

Martiniaková, M., Grosskopf, B., Vondráková, M., Omelka, R., and Fabis, M. (2006b) Differences in femoral compact bone tissue microscopic structure between adult cows (*Bos taurus*) and pigs (*Sus scrofa domestica*). *Anatomia, Histologia, Embryologia*, **35**, 167–170.

Martiniaková, M., Grosskopf, B., Omelka, R., Dammers, K., Vondráková, M., and Bauerova, B. (2007) Histological study of compact bone tissue in some mammals: A method for species determination. *International Journal of Osteoarchaeology*, **17**, 82–90.

Mayne, P.M. (1990) *The Identification of Precremation Trauma in Cremated Bone*, Master of Arts Thesis, University of Alberta, Alberta.

Mori, R., Tetsuo, K., Soeta, S., Sato, J., Kakino, J., Hamato, S., *et al.* (2005) Preliminary study of histological comparison on the growth patterns of long-bone cortex in young calf, pig, and sheep. *Journal Veterinary Medicine Science*, **67**(12), 1223–1229.

Morris, Z.H. (2007) *Quantitative and Spatial Analysis of the Microscopic Bone Structures of deer (Odocoileus virginianus), dog (Canis familiaris), and pig (Sus scrofa domesticus)*, Master of Arts Thesis, Department of Geography and Anthropology, University of Toronto, Toronto.

Mulhern, D.M. and Ubelaker, D.H. (2001) Differences in osteon banding between human and nonhuman bone. *Journal of Forensic Sciences*, **46**(2), 220–222.

Mulhern, D.M. and Van Gerven, D. (1997) Patterns of femoral bone remodeling dynamics in a medieval Nubian population. *American Journal of Physical Anthropology*, **104**, 133–146.

Mulhern, D.M. and Ubelaker, D.H. (2012) Differentiating human and nonhuman bone microstructure. In: *Bone Histology: An Anthropological Perspective* (eds. C. Crowder and S. Stout). CRC Press, New York, pp. 109–134.

Nelson, R.A. (1992) Microscopic comparison of fresh and burned bone. *Journal of Forensic Sciences*, **37**(4), 1055–1060.

Ortner, D.J. and Putschar, W.G.J. (1981) *Identification of Pathological Conditions in Human Skeletal Remains*. Smithsonian Institute Press, Washington, DC.

Owsley, D.S., Mires, A.M., and Keith, M.S. (1985) Case involving differentiation of deer and human bone fragments. *Journal of Forensic Sciences*, **30**(2), 572–578.

Pfeiffer, S. (1998) Variability in osteon size in recent human populations. *American Journal of Physical Anthropology*, **106**, 219–227.

Pfeifer, S., Crowder, C., Harrington, L., and Brown, M. (2006) Secondary osteons and Haversian canal dimensions as behavioral indicators. *American Journal of Physical Anthropology*, **131**, 460–468.

Piga, G., Malgosa, A., Thompson, T.J.U., and Enzo, S. (2008) A new calibration of the XRD technique for the study of archaeological burned human remains. *Journal of Archaeological Science*, **35**, 2171–2178.

Pitre, M.C., Mayne Correia, P.M., Mankowski, P.J., Klassen, J., Day, M.J., Lovell, N.C., *et al.* (2012) Examining biofilm formation in human skeletal remains from ancient Mesopotamia. *Journal of Archaeological Science*, **40**(1), 24–29.

Pointer, K. (2014) *Histological Analysis of Cremated Human Bone*. Honors Thesis, Department of Anthropology, University of Alberta, Alberta.

Sawada, J., Nara, T., Fukui, J., Dodo, Y., and Hirata, K. (2014) Histomorphological species identification of tiny bone fragments from a Paleolithic site in the Northern Japanese Archipelago. *Journal of Archaeological Science*, **46**, 270–280.

Schultz, M. (1997a) Microscopic structures of bone. In: *Forensic Taphonomy: The Postmortem Fate of Human Remains* (eds. W. Haglund and M.H. Sorg). CRC Press, New York, pp. 187–199.

Schultz, M. (1997b) Microscopic investigation of excavated skeletal remains: A contribution to paleopathology and forensic medicine. In: *Forensic Taphonomy: The Postmortem Fate of Human Remains* (eds. W. Haglund and M.H. Sorg). CRC Press, New York, pp. 201–222.

Shapiro, F. and Wu, J.Y. (2019) Woven bone overview: Structural classification based on its integral role in developmental, repair and pathological bone formation throughout vertebrate groups. *European Cells and Materials*, **38**, 137–167. https://doi.org/10.22203/eCM.v038a11

Shipman, P., Foster, G., and Schoenlinger, M. (1984) Burnt bones and teeth: An experimental study of color, morphology, crystal structure and shrinkage. *Journal of Archaeological Science*, **11**, 307–325.

Singh, I.J., Tonna, E.A., and Gandel, C.P. (1974) A comparative histological study of mammalian bone. *Journal of Morphology*, **144**, 421–438.

Skedros, J.G., Sybrowksky, C.L., Parry, T.R., and Bloebaum, R.D. (2003) Regional differences in cortical bone of organization and microdamage prevalence in Rocky Mountain Mule Deer. *The Anatomical Record*, Part A, **274A**, 837–850.

Smith, J.W. (1960a) Collagen fibre patterns in mammalian bone. *Journal of Anatomy*, **94**, 329–344.

Smith, J.W. (1960b) The arrangement of collagen fibers in human secondary osteons. *Journal of Bone and Joint Surgery*, **42**, 588–605.

Thompson, D.D. (1980) Age changes in bone mineralization, cortical thickness and Haversian canal area. *Calcified Tissue International*, **31**, 5–11.

Thompson, T.J.U. (2005) Heat-induced dimensional changes in bone and their consequences for forensic anthropology. *Journal of Forensic Science*, **50**(5), 1–8. Paper ID JFS2004297.

Urbanová, P. and Novotný, V. (2005) Distinguishing between human and non-human bones: Histometric method for forensic anthropology. *Anthropologie*, **43**(1), 77–85.

White, T.D. and Folkens, P.A. (2005) *The Human Bone Manual*. Elsevier Academic Press, San Diego, CA.

Zedda, M., Lepore, G., Manca, P., Chisu, V., and Farina, V. (2008) Comparative bone histology of adult horses (*Equus callabus*) and cows (*Bos taurus*). *Anatomia Histologia Embryologia*, **37**, 442–445.

CHAPTER 15

Isotope Analysis from Cremated Remains

Christophe Snoeck, PhD

Research Professor, Research Unit: Analytical, Environmental and Geo-Chemistry, Department of Chemistry, Vrije Universiteit Brussel, AMGC-WE-VUB, Belgium

Maritime Cultures Research Institute, Department of Art Sciences & Archaeology, Vrije Universiteit Brussel, MARI-LW-VUB

15.1 Introduction

The year 1998 represents a turning point in the analytical study of burnt bone. Indeed, the pioneering work of Lanting and Brindley (1998) demonstrated the reliability of calcined bone from archaeological contexts for radiocarbon dating, further confirmed by an international inter-laboratory comparison (Naysmith *et al.*, 2007). Still, doubts remained regarding the validity of some dates obtained from calcined bone (e.g. Olsen *et al.*, 2013; Zazzo *et al.*, 2013; Snoeck *et al.*, 2014a; Annaert *et al.*, 2020). Nevertheless, thanks to this development many archaeological sites, where cremation was practiced, can now be dated and placed in a chronological time frame (e.g. De Reu *et al.*, 2012; De Mulder *et al.*, 2013). This new opportunity finally allowed the radiocarbon dating of the cremated bone excavated at Stonehenge, showing that the site was used for over 400 years as a burial ground (Willis *et al.*, 2016), making it one of the largest Late Neolithic burial sites known in Britain.

Identifying and assessing heat transformations of bone has also received increasing attention, as evidenced by two important edited volumes summarizing macro- and microscopic studies of burnt bones from a wide range of archaeological and forensic contexts (Schmidt and Symes, 2008; Thompson, 2015). Combined, these studies and subsequent ones have improved our understanding of funerary practices (e.g. Carroll and Squires, 2020; Paba *et al.*, 2021) and helped in better assessing the age and sex of cremated individuals, which is particularly challenging due to the high fragmentary state and shrinkage of burnt human remains (e.g. Cavazzuti *et al.*, 2019a; Veselka *et al.*, 2021b). Statistical analyses are also more often used to improve sex and age classification rates (e.g. Gonçalves *et al.*, 2020; Hlad *et al.*, 2021). The increasing number of sex and age identifications allows a better

Burnt Human Remains: Recovery, Analysis, and Interpretation, First Edition. Edited by Sarah Ellingham, Joe Adserias-Garriga, Sara C. Zapico and Douglas H. Ubelaker.

understanding of demography and age / sex related differences in populations practicing cremations and, also, helps in the identification of fire victims.

In 2015, another important step occurred that boosted the importance of calcined bone in archaeological studies when it was demonstrated that any type of calcined bone (not only the petrous parts of the temporal bone – Harvig *et al.*, 2014) could provide a reliable substrate for strontium isotope analyses (Snoeck *et al.*, 2015). This development at last enabled palaeomobility studies in times and places where cremation was practiced (e.g. Snoeck *et al.*, 2016a, 2018; Grupe *et al.*, 2018; Price *et al.*, 2018; Sebald *et al.*, 2018; Cavazzuti *et al.*, 2019b; Graham and Bethard, 2019; Sabaux *et al.*, 2021; Veselka *et al.*, 2021a). The potential to use calcined dentine, which is more often recovered after cremation than enamel, for strontium isotope analyses was also shown (Sebald *et al.*, 2018). The combined use of strontium and lead isotopes in calcined bone has also been recently carried out (Grupe *et al.*, 2018), though more experimental work is needed to comprehensively demonstrate the resistance of calcined bone to the incorporation of exogenous lead from the burial environment.

Here, an overview of the current state-of-the art for the isotopic, elemental, and structural studies of burnt bone is presented, with a focus on infrared analyses, radiocarbon dating, carbon, oxygen, and strontium isotope ratios. Together, they provide new insight into past funerary practices (i.e. burning condition) and palaeomobility of populations that practiced cremation, helping forensic investigations dealing with burnt human remains.

15.2 Infrared Analyses

Bones and teeth are composed of an organic and inorganic fraction as well as water. During heating, the water is lost and most of the organic matter is destroyed (Van Strydonck *et al.*, 2010; Snoeck *et al.*, 2014a). As such, the focus when dealing with burnt human remains lies on the inorganic fraction, a carbonate-substituted apatite often called bioapatite (Skinner, 2005).

Infrared analyses of bioapatite have been carried out for a long time to assess diagenetic alterations (Sponheimer and Lee-Thorp, 1999) and a wide range of infrared indices have been developed to characterize these diagenetic changes (Lebon *et al.*, 2010; Roche *et al.*, 2010; Salesse *et al.*, 2014). These indices have also been shown to help in identifying heat-induced alterations in bioapatite as some of these indices are temperature dependent (Figure 15.1, 15.2) (Thompson *et al.*, 2009; Snoeck *et al.*, 2014b; Ellingham *et al.*, 2015b). Furthermore, a peak in the infrared spectrum related to the presence of cyanamide ($-CN_2H$) seems exclusively present in burnt bone and has been suggested to be the consequence of bones burned in the presence of ammonia and / or under reducing conditions (i.e. lower availability of O_2) (Habelitz *et al.*, 2001; Zazzo *et al.*, 2013; Snoeck *et al.*, 2014b; Marques *et al.*, 2021). However, more research is needed to better understand the reasons for the presence of cyanamide in burnt bone.

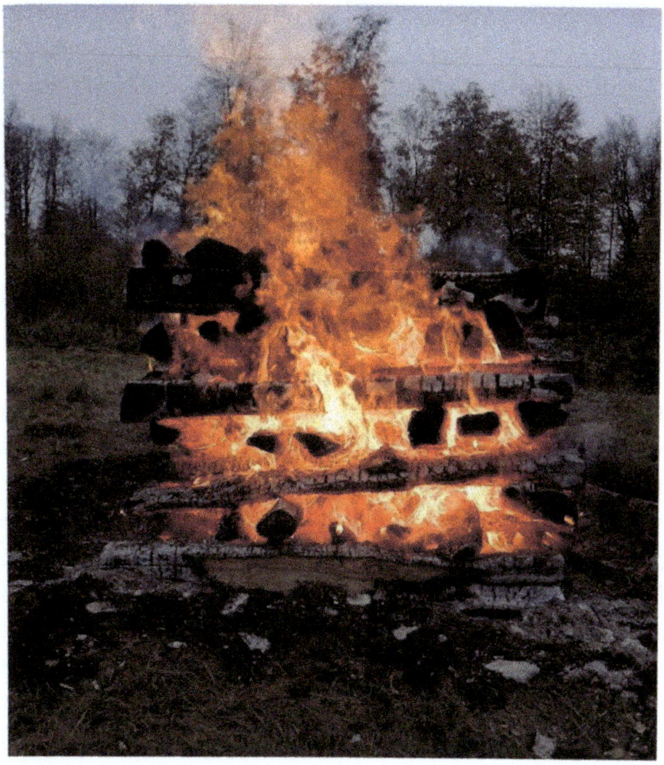

Figure 15.1 Experimental pyre from the CRUMBEL Project (Cremation, Urns and Mobility, population dynamics in Belgium).

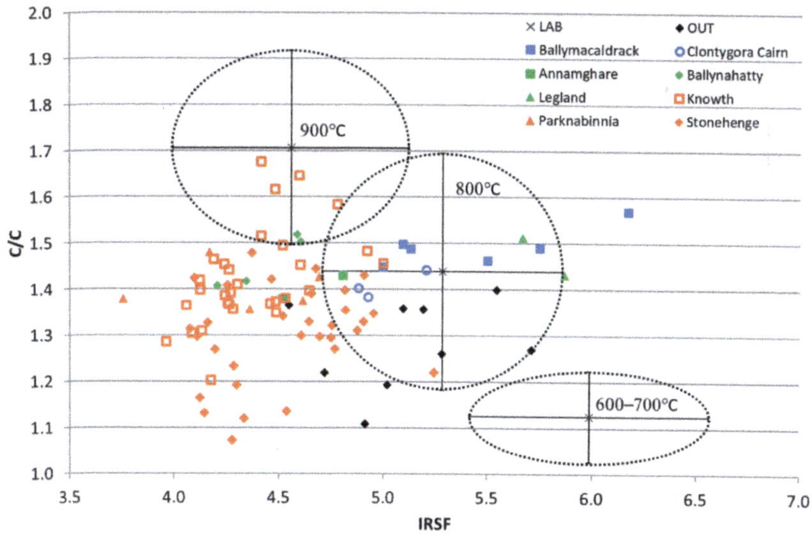

Figure 15.2 C/C vs. IRSF for modern cow tibia fragments heated in a laboratory muffle furnace (LAB) at different temperature together with lamb, chicken, pig, and cow bones (OUT) burned on outdoor experimental pyres and archaeological human calcined bone fragments from Neolithic and Bronze Age Ireland and UK (based on Snoeck *et al.*, 2014b and Snoeck, 2015).

Laboratory burnings and experimental cremations are also hugely informative for the better understanding of changes occurring in bones burned at different temperature and in different conditions (Figure 15.1, 15.2). Cow bone fragments heated at different temperatures clearly showed that the crystallinity of the bone (evaluated via the infrared splitting factor: IRSF) first increases to temperatures up to 600–700°C before decreasing again at higher temperatures (Figure 15.1, 15.2). This helps in assessing at which temperature bones were burned and potentially infers the conditions under which the individuals were burned. Still, some questions remain as some modern animal bones burned on outdoor pyres have different values compared to the samples heated in a muffle furnace, while a large number of archaeological human calcined bone fragments returned values that are inconsistent with the experimental results (Figure 15.1, 15.2). This could potentially be explained by differences between species (different animals; animal vs. human bone) or by the impact of post-burial alterations (or diagenesis) on the archaeological samples. More experimental work is currently under way to better assess these differences. Furthermore, sieving to avoid the "particle size effect" (see Kontopoulos *et al.*, 2018 for more details) and analyzing the samples under vacuum might help further improve the quality of the infrared spectra and detect more subtle variations in the chemical composition and structure of burnt animal and human bones.

Infrared analyses applied on the human remains found in stone chambers close to the beach of Herculaneum, Italy, showed that, because they sought refuge in a stone chamber, they were exposed to lower temperature and did not undergo instantaneous soft tissue vaporization as was the case for others found in the street or on the beach of Herculaneum (Martyn *et al.*, 2020). These results highlight the importance of carrying out infrared analyses of bones that underwent heat transformation, as macroscopic data is often biased by the context in which the bones were found. Infrared analyses, however, on their own offer only a limited view of the changes occurring in bone during heating. Nevertheless, they become increasingly more powerful when combined with information obtained from other types of analyses, such as thermogravimetric analysis (TGA) (Ellingham *et al.*, 2015a), carbon and oxygen isotope analyses (Snoeck *et al.*, 2016b), or micro-CT scans (Ellingham and Sandholzer, 2020).

15.3 Radiocarbon Dating

An increasing number of archaeological sites are now dated using the carbon left in bone apatite carbonates of cremated human remains following the initial work of Lanting and colleagues (Lanting and Brindley, 1998; Lanting *et al.*, 2001) and an intercomparison study between six radiocarbon laboratories (Naysmith *et al.*, 2007). Several experimental studies have, however, shown that the carbon present in bio-apatite carbonates after cremation is mostly composed of fuel carbon rather than endogenous bone carbon, although the amount of fuel carbon is heavily variable, between 39 and 95% (Hüls *et al.*, 2010; Zazzo *et al.*, 2012; Snoeck *et al.*, 2014a). This means that, when dating cremated human remains, it is a mixture of fuel and bone carbon that is being dated. Therefore, it is crucial to keep in mind that the dates obtained on calcined bone provide a reliable date only if it can be assumed that the fuel used for cremation and the body have a similar age. If, however, the anthracological analysis of the pyre remains suggests that older wood could have been used, it is likely that the date obtained will be too old (Rose *et al.*, 2020).

An extensive radiocarbon study at the Early Medieval site of Broechem, Belgium, raised new questions in relation to the validity of radiocarbon dating of calcined human remains (Annaert *et al.*, 2020). Calcined human and pig bones were dated from the same graves and, overall, there was an average different of ca. 100 radiocarbon years between the human and pig bones, where the pig bones were systematically younger. It is unclear why this is the case and while aquatic reservoir and old wood effects are mentioned as possible explanations, more experimental work is needed to reach a conclusive interpretation. Still, in most cases, it can be assumed that short-lived wood species had been used for cremation.

Radiocarbon dating of cremation cemeteries has enabled a decrease in the bias linked to the over-representation of inhumations in radiocarbon databases (Capuzzo *et al.* 2020). In Belgium, for example, when compiling the existing radiocarbon dates of inhumation and cremation contexts from the Roman Period and the Early-High Middle Ages (Figure 15.3) it becomes clear that, even though there is a lack of radiocarbon dated cremation contexts for the south of Belgium (Figure 15.3b), cremation seems to disappear almost entirely around AD 700 (Figure 15.3d) and a significant increase in inhumation is observed (Figure 15.3c). In Ireland, radiocarbon dating of cremated bone also confirmed the re-use of the Neolithic Court tomb of Parknabinnia, Co. Clare, during the Bronze Age, more than a thousand years after the construction of the monument and its use as inhumation burial site (Figure 15.4; Snoeck *et al.*, 2020).

15.4 Isotope Analyses

15.4.1 Carbon and Oxygen Isotope Ratios

Carbon exchanges observed during radiocarbon dating studies sparked an interest not only in understanding the impact of carbon exchange on radiocarbon dating but also on the potential of carbon (and by extension oxygen) isotope ratios to gain insights into the burning conditions of corpses. A better understanding of the carbon exchanges occurring during the burning of bone could provide key information about the size of the pyre, the type of wood used, the position of the pyre within the landscape (i.e. open or enclosed area), etc. Still, this is a very complex process as it requires the characterization of different losses, exchanges, and potential fractionation mechanisms taking place during cremation (Figure 15.5). Indeed, carbon is

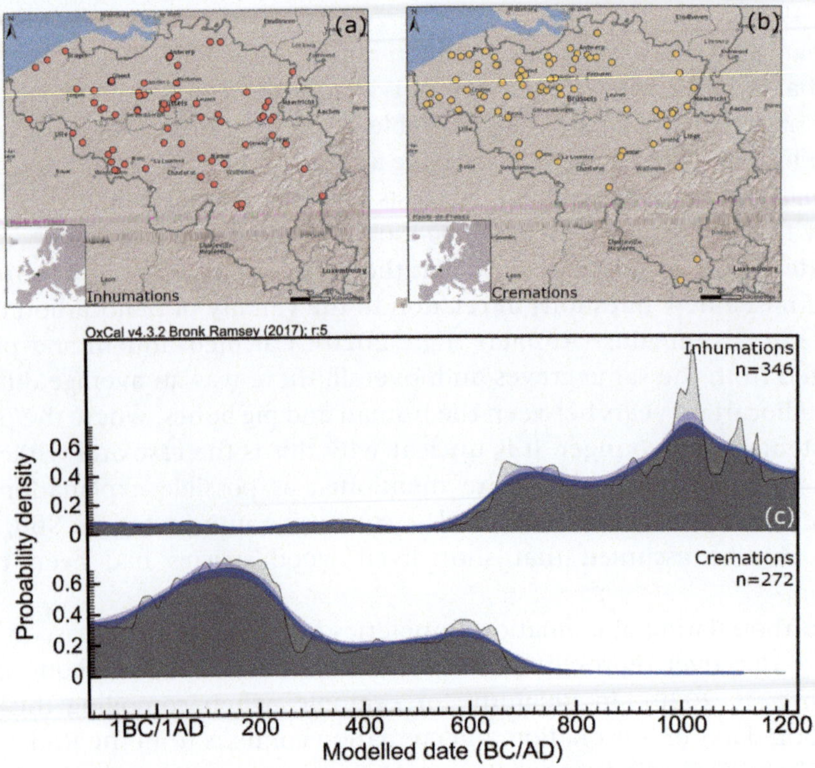

Figure 15.3 Maps with the spatial distribution of Roman and medieval 14th-century dated funerary contexts and KDE (Kernel Density Estimation) plots showing the temporal distribution of the data for (a, c) inhumations and (b, d) cremations (based on Capuzzo *et al.* 2020, updated with CRUMBEL dates).

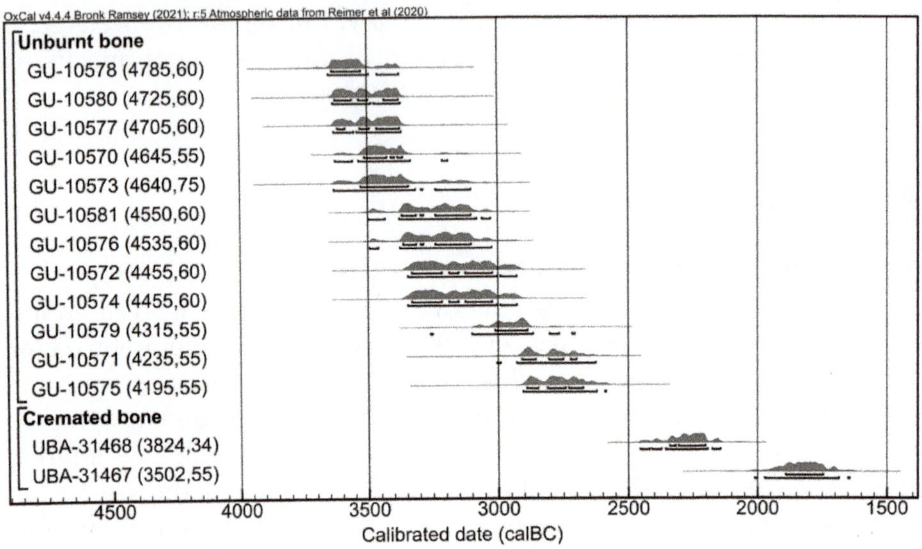

Figure 15.4 Radiocarbon dates obtained on uncremated (Schulting *et al.*, 2012) and cremated bone from the Neolithic Court tomb of Parknabinnia, Co. Clare, Ireland (Snoeck *et al.*, 2020) recalibrated using IntCal20 (Reimer *et al.*, 2020).

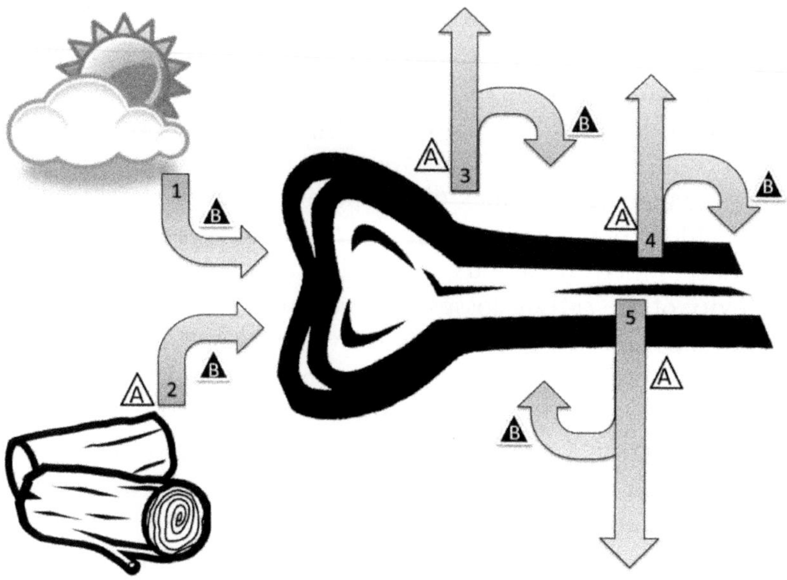

Figure 15.5 Potential carbon exchanges, losses, and fractionations that have to be taken into account when studying the carbon isotope composition of bone apatite during heating: (1) atmospheric carbon dioxide; (2) carbon dioxide released during the combustion of fuels; (3) carbon dioxide released by the combustion of flesh, fat, skin, and marrow; (4) carbon dioxide released by the heating of bone apatite carbonates; (5) carbon dioxide released by the combustion of collagen; (A) potential fractionation between the carbon present in fuels, organic matter or bone apatite carbonates, and the carbon dioxide released into the combustion atmosphere; (B)potential fractionation between the carbon dioxide from the combustion atmosphere around bone apatite and bone apatite carbonates; the arrows indicate the different carbonate / carbon dioxide flows (based on Snoeck, 2015).

present in both the organic and inorganic fraction of bone, as well as in skin, muscles, organs, etc. Furthermore, there is a very large amount of carbon present in the wood that is released as carbon dioxide (CO_2) during the burning process. To a lesser extent, there is also carbon present in the atmosphere under the form of CO_2 that could participate in these exchanges, although it can be assumed that, compared to the large amounts of CO_2 produced by the body and the fuel (i.e. wood) during the burning process, the atmospheric CO_2 contribution will be negligeable.

As such, the main pools of carbon present during burning are CO_2 from the fuel, and that released by the burning of flesh, skin, and bone organic matter (i.e. collagen), and the carbon present in the form of carbonates in bone apatite, all of which have different carbon isotope values. When comparing the carbon isotope ratios ($\delta^{13}C$) of samples heated in a muffle furnace (without any fuel) with those of samples burned on experimental pyres (Figure 15.5), the latter have much lower $\delta^{13}C$ values. This shows the impact of the presence of fuel carbon in the burning environment. Indeed, wood (which is a C3-plant) has lower $\delta^{13}C$ values compared to the organic carbon pool of a human or animal individual. The impact of fuel carbon on the $\delta^{13}C$ values of burnt bone apatite is further evidenced by the much higher $\delta^{13}C$ values of bones heated in the presence of millet seeds which is a C4 plant that has much higher $\delta^{13}C$ values compared to C3-plants (Vogel and Van Der Merwe, 1977). The experimental burning of a corn-fed chicken (corn being a C4-plant) also revealed interesting information about the impact of the carbon present in the animal before burning on the final $\delta^{13}C$ values of burnt bone. Indeed, the corn-fed chicken has the highest $\delta^{13}C$ values of all the animal bone fragments burned on experimental outdoor pyres (Figure 15.5), confirming that the final $\delta^{13}C$ values of burnt bone reflect of mixture of body and fuel carbon (Snoeck *et al.*, 2016b).

The complexity of the carbon losses and exchanges described above shows the need for more experimental work. This is even more true when attempting to understand the oxygen isotope ratios ($\delta^{18}O$) of burnt bones. While all the sources mentioned for carbon exchanges need to be considered, in the case of oxygen there are several additional reservoirs of oxygen present around the body during burning, one of which is atmospheric dioxygen (O_2), which, in contrast to atmospheric CO_2, cannot be ignored as it represents about 21% of the atmospheric gases. An interesting aspect that can be investigated using oxygen isotope ratios of burnt bones is the ventilation (i.e. amount of oxygen) of the burning process and / or the position of a bone / body on a pyre. A large variation in $\delta^{18}O$ values can indeed be seen in bone fragments burned the same day on the same pyre but not placed exactly at the same place on the pyre (Figure 15.6). It is, however, unclear at the moment which parameters of the burning process (type of wood, size of the pyre, position of the body, position of the pyre in the environment, etc.) are responsible for these variations (Snoeck *et al.*, 2016b) and more experimental

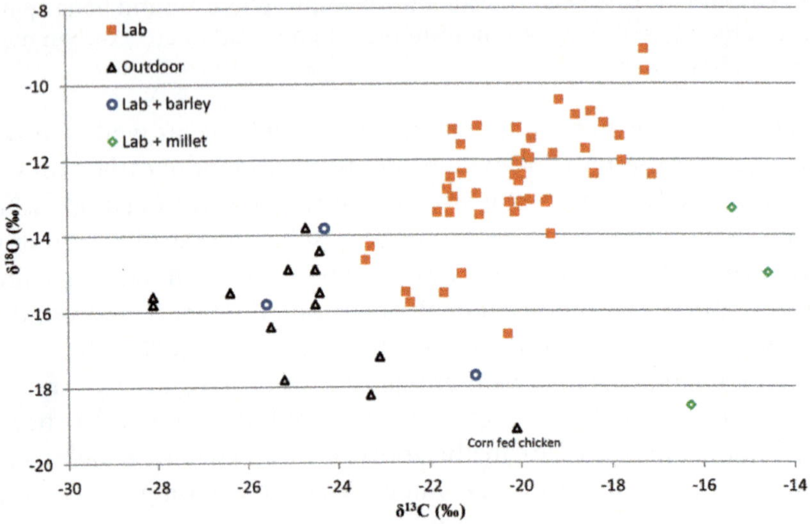

Figure 15.6 Carbon and oxygen isotope ratios of modern animal bones heated in a muffle furnace without fuel (Lab), with additional barley (Lab + barley) or millet seeds (Lab + millet), and animal bone fragments burned on experimental pyres (outdoor) (based on Snoeck, 2015 and Snoeck *et al.*, 2016b).

studies are required to gain more insights into these questions and to achieve a better understanding of cremation settings and, by extension, funerary practices.

15.4.2 Strontium Isotope Ratios and Concentrations

Strontium isotope ratios measured in human and animal bone and teeth record mostly the origin of the foods consumed by those humans and animals. Due to its porosity and low crystallinity, and hence, possible strontium exchanges with the environment after burial (e.g. Tuross *et al.*, 1989), unburnt bone from archaeological contexts has been excluded from such studies. More crystalline tooth enamel, however, has been successfully analyzed to highlight, for example, the important degree of mobility between childhood and death of the Beaker people of Britain (Parker Pearson *et al.*, 2016). As unburnt bone, cremated bone was discarded from such isotopic studies, until recently, when it was demonstrated that, due to its much higher crystallinity compared to unburnt bone, fully calcined bone (white bone burned at temperatures above 650°C) is immune from post-burial strontium exchanges (Snoeck *et al.*, 2015). The possibility of measuring strontium isotope ratios from fully calcined bone opened the door to the analyses, using isotopic systems as tracers of mobility, migration, and landscape use, of the vast existing collection of cremated bones, which have often lain dormant in both museums and university collections. Recently, new understandings of landscape use and population mobility in Neolithic and Bronze Age Ireland have been gained. For example, at Ballynahatty, Co. Down (Northern Ireland), both cremated bone and unburnt skulls were found in the same circular chamber. The strontium isotope ratios showed that those inhumed at the site used parts of the landscape situated to the north of the site, while those cremated were consuming food growing south and / or west of the site (Snoeck *et al.*, 2016a).

The combination of strontium isotope ratios and strontium concentration measurements can be particularly useful to identify different food sources (Montgomery, 2010), especially when marine resources are being consumed. Modern day seawater and marine resources have a specific strontium isotope ratio of 0.7092 (Hess *et al.*, 1986) and generally higher strontium concentrations compared to terrestrial resources. For example, two Mesolithic cremated bone fragments from Langford (Essex, England) had strontium isotope ratios of 0.7094 and 0.7095 (Schulting *et al.*, 2016), very close to the value of seawater, and had strontium concentrations higher than 300 ppm. This is much higher than observed in Neolithic calcined bone from Stonehenge, where strontium concentrations of 25 calcined bone fragments varied between 40 and 110 ppm (Snoeck *et al.*, 2018). These results highlight the potential of using strontium concentrations to look at the diet of past populations that practiced cremation (as all organic matter usually used for such studies is destroyed), though more work is required to better understand how strontium concentrations vary within an individual and across the landscape.

The possibility of extracting reliable strontium isotope ratios from calcined bone fragments not only gives the opportunity to study mobility in populations that practice cremations, but also to assess changes throughout the lives of individuals.

Indeed, by measuring strontium isotope ratios in different skeletal elements with different turnover rates, it becomes possible to compare childhood and adulthood signals (Veselka *et al.*, 2021a, 2021c). The inner cortex of the otic capsule (IC), tooth dentine, and enamel represent different stages of childhood as, once formed, they do not remodel (see Veselka *et al.*, 2021c for more details). Bone, on the other hand (with the exception of the inner cortex of the otic capsule), remodels (Hedges *et al.*, 2007; Jørkov *et al.* 2009). The strontium isotope ratios measured on bone represent an average of the food consumed over the last 5–20 years of life, depending on which bone is being analyzed (rib, femurs, cranial fragments). It is, however, still unclear how much difference in turnover rates exists between the different adult bones and even between different parts of the same bone (e.g. spongious vs. cortical). A recent study further demonstrated the importance of carefully sampling the inner cortex of calcined otic capsules as only the IC (IC, purple in Figure 15.7) does not remodel. The outer layer (EC, blue in Figure 15.6) does remodel and should be avoided when aiming to obtain a strontium isotope ratio reflecting early childhood (Veselka *et al.*, 2021c). While opening a plethora of new opportunities for the study of past population that practiced cremation, these new developments also raised several questions that need to be answered before a comprehensive understanding of individual life histories can be obtained.

15.5 Archaeological Case Studies

15.5.1 Stonehenge

Between 1919 and 1926, more than 50 cremated individuals were found in the "Aubrey Holes" of Stonehenge, making it one of the largest burial sites from Late Neolithic Britain (Parker Pearson *et al.* 2009). After the excavation, all the cremated bone fragments were re-interred in a single Aubrey Hole (AH7) mixing the remains

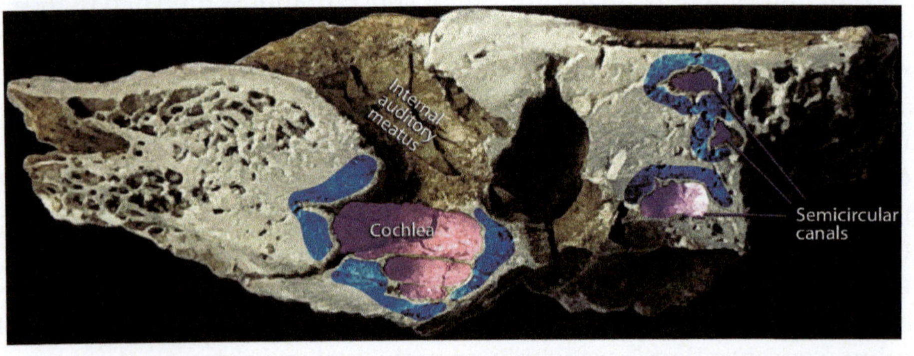

Figure 15.7 A midmodiolar section of a right burnt human pars petrosa, exposing the cochlea and semicircular canals which are part of the otic capsule. Purple colored areas experience virtually no remodeling rate, while the blue colored areas, still part of the otic capsule, do remodel (image by B. Veselka and L. van Maren, 2021).

of the different individuals. The re-excavation of AH7 in 2008 allowed a study of these cremated human remains and, through careful osteoarchaeological work, it was possible to identify 25 distinct individuals based on central occipital bone fragments (Willis *et al.*, 2016). These 25 central occipital bone fragments were analyzed for strontium isotope ratios (Snoeck *et al.*, 2018) and the results were compared to the biologically available strontium baseline of Britain (Evans *et al.*, 2010). This comparison highlighted that from 25 individuals buried at Stonehenge, at least 40% (10 out of 25) came from much further afield, perhaps as far as West Wales, where the blue stones used to build part of the monument came from (Figure 15.7; Snoeck *et al.*, 2018). Other origins are, of course, possible as similar strontium isotope ratios are found in different part of Britain (Figure 15.8). Furthermore, it is also important to highlight that cranial bone fragments represent the last decade or so of an individual's life and, therefore, their strontium isotope ratios represent a mixture of all the foods consumed over that period. Still, the combination of archaeological and isotopic evidence suggests that some of the cremated individuals buried at Stonehenge could indeed have lived parts of their lives in West Wales.

15.5.2 Meuse Basin, Belgium and the Netherlands

Large-scale application of strontium isotope analyses on two cremation cemeteries situated close to the River Meuse in Belgium and the Netherlands

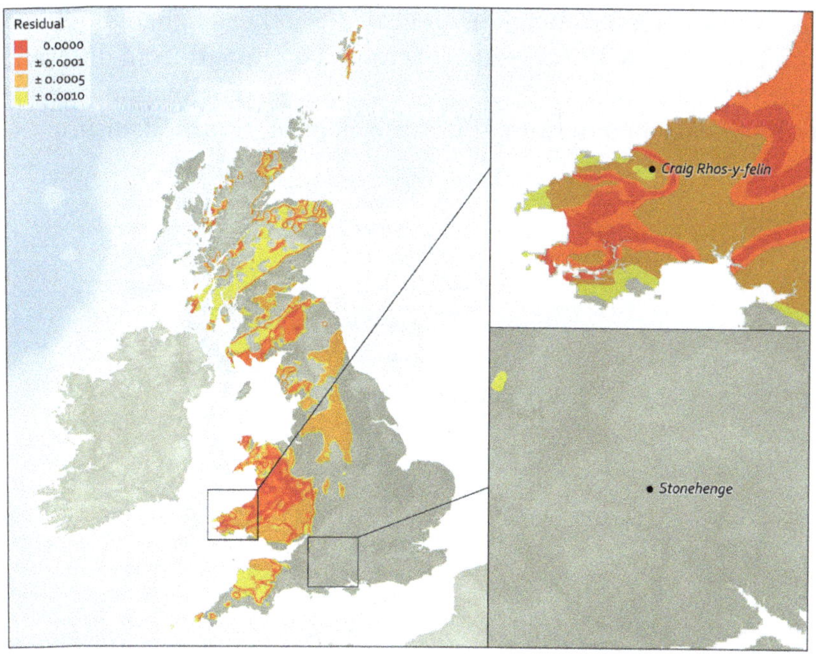

Figure 15.8 Geographic assignments of individual 596 from Stonehenge based on the residuals between the measured $^{87}Sr/^{86}Sr$ isotope ratio and the focal mean of the biologically available strontium baseline (5 km search radius) (based on Snoeck *et al.*, 2018; image by J. Pouncett).

highlighted the complexity of studying cremation deposits using strontium isotope ratios of multiple skeletal elements and radiocarbon dating (Sabaux *et al.*, 2021; Veselka *et al.*, 2021a). At the Late Bronze Age cremation cemetery of Herstal, Belgium, a total of 98 calcined bone fragments from 21 different graves have been analyzed using strontium isotope ratios, of which 16 have also been radiocarbon dated (Sabaux *et al.*, 2021). The strontium isotope ratios show a very large spread in values, going from 0.7109 to 0.7138 (Figure 15.8). This huge spread in values is actually similar to the variation in biologically available strontium within 15 km of the site (Veselka *et al.*, 2021a). In this case, it is particularly complex to identify mobility as all the individuals have values consistent with the "local" area. Still, the large spread in data clearly shows that they were not consuming the same food and that the food was not all grown in the same location. A similar pattern is seen at the Early Medieval cremation cemetery of Echt, the Netherlands, where the spread in values obtained from more than 100 calcined bone fragments taken from 73 cremation deposits is even larger (0.7096–0.7139), but still within the variations seen in the "local area" (Veselka *et al.*, 2021a). This range is similar to that seen in Neolithic Stonehenge (0.7079–07118), but in Stonehenge it was clear that some individuals were "non-locals" (Figure 15.9). These results show the importance of creating an adequate biologically available strontium baseline to correctly interpret the results obtained on human remains (cremated or not).

The combination of strontium isotope ratios and radiocarbon dating on the cremation deposits of Herstal, Belgium, revealed another challenge when working with cremation deposits: the presence of cremated remains from different individuals within the same deposit (Sabaux *et al.*, 2021). For example, two calcined diaphysis fragments taken from the same deposit returned distinct strontium

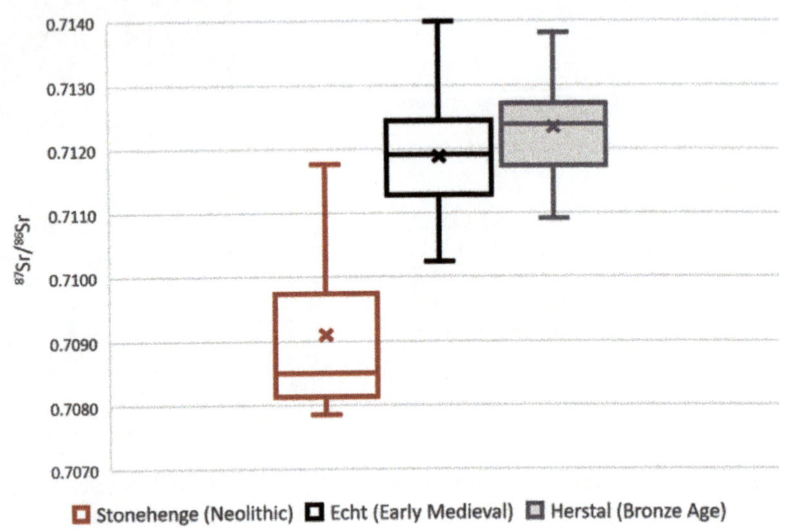

Figure 15.9 Strontium isotope ratios in calcined bone remains from Neolithic Stonehenge (Snoeck *et al.*, 2018), Early Medieval Echt (Veselka *et al.*, 2021a), and Bronze Age Herstal (Sabaux *et al.*, 2021).

isotope ratios (0.7121 and 0.7134) and radiocarbon dates (1201–1008 cal. BC and 1043–899 cal. BC – 2σ / 95.4%) clearly showing that the remains of two different individuals were present in the same deposit, which was not observed through classical osteological analyses (Sabaux *et al.*, 2021). It remains, however, unknown if the presence of the remains of two individuals was intentional or not. Exploring all the isotopic data stored in open access databases such as IsoArcH (www.isoarch.eu; Salesse *et al.*, 2018) will allow big data approaches and strengthen our interpretation and help to draw large-scale trends in such data.

15.6 Conclusions

The interdisciplinary study of cremated human remains from archaeological and forensic contexts has enabled an increase in our understanding of changes (or lack thereof in the case of strontium isotope ratios) occurring in bone during burning. These have been successfully used to reconstruct the way in which bodies were burned in past and modern populations and has enabled new insights into mobility patterns and landscape use of past populations that practiced cremations as a funerary ritual. It goes without saying that more research is needed to refine our understanding of different aspects of the impact of heat and time on bone (and teeth) and future research should keep these goals in mind. Statistical analyses and big data are also becoming increasingly important to interpret the larger and larger amounts of osteological, infrared, and isotope data.

Acknowledgments

The research presented here was supported by the Philippe Wiener-Maurice Anspach foundation (FWA), the Fonds Wetenschappelijk Onderzoek-Vlaanderen (FWO), and the Fonds de la Recherche Scientifique (F.R.S.-FNRS). The author would also like to thank Barbara Veselka, Giacomo Capuzzo, and Kevin Salesse for their useful comments. We thank John Pouncett, Barbara Veselka, Laurens van Maren (maren74 DTP & vormgeving), and Giacomo Capuzzo for their help with creating the figures.

References

Annaert, R., Boudin, M., Deforce, K., Ervynck, A., Haneca, K., Lentacker, A., *et al.* (2020) Anomalous radiocarbon dates from the Early Medieval cremation graves from Broechem (Flanders, Belgium): Reservoir or old wood effect? *Radiocarbon*, **62**(2), 269–288.

Capuzzo, G., Snoeck, C., Boudin, M., Annaert, R., Dalle, S., Hlad, M., *et al.* (2020) Cremation vs inhumation, modelling cultural changes in funerary practices from the Mesolithic to the Middle Ages in Belgium using Kernel Density Analysis. *Radiocarbon*, **62**(6), 1809–1832.

Carroll, E.L. and Squires, K.E. (2020) The application of quantitative petrography and macroscopic colour change in a comparative analysis of Roman and Anglo-Saxon cremation practices. *International Journal of Osteoarchaeology*, **30**(6), 882–890.

Cavazzuti, C., Bresadola, B., d'Innocenzo, C., Interlando, S., and Sperduti, A. (2019a) Towards a new osteometric method for sexing ancient cremated human remains. Analysis of Late Bronze Age and Iron Age samples from Italy with gendered grave goods. *PloS One*, **14**(1), e0209423.

Cavazzuti, C., Cardarelli, A., Quondam, F., Salzani, L., Ferrante, M., Nisi, S., *et al.* (2019b) Mobile elites at Frattesina: Flows of people in a Late Bronze Age 'port of trade' in northern Italy. *Antiquity*, **93**(369), 624–644.

De Mulder, G., Van Strydonck, M., and De Clercq, W. (2013) 14C dating of "Brandgrubengräber" from the Bronze Age to the Roman period in western Flanders (Belgium). *Radiocarbon*, **55**(2–3), 1233–1245.

De Reu, J., De Mulder, G., Van Strydonck, M., Boudin, M., and Bourgeois, J. (2012) 14C dates and spatial statistics: Modeling intrasite spatial dynamics of urnfield cemeteries in Belgium using case study of Destelbergen cemetery. *Radiocarbon*, **54**(3–4), 635–648.

Ellingham, S.T.D. and Sandholzer, M.A. (2020) Determining volumetric shrinkage trends of burnt bone using micro-CT. *Journal of Forensic Sciences*, **65**(1), 196–199.

Ellingham, S.T.D., Thompson, T.J.U., and Islam, M. (2015a) Thermogravimetric analysis of property changes and weight loss in incinerated bone. *Palaeogeography, Palaeoclimatology, Palaeoecology*, **438**, 239–244.

Ellingham, S.T.D., Thompson, T.J.U., Islam, M., and Taylor, G. (2015b) Estimating temperature exposure of burnt bone – A methodological review. *Science & Justice*, **55**(3), 181–188.

Evans, J.A., Montgomery, J., Wildman, G., and Boulton, N. (2010) Spatial variations in biosphere 87Sr/86Sr in Britain. *Journal of the Geological Society*, **167**(1), 1–4.

Gonçalves, D., Vassalo, A.R., Makhoul, C., Piga, G., Mamede, A.P., Parker, S.F., *et al.* (2020) Chemosteometric regression models of heat exposed human bones to determine their pre-burnt metric dimensions. *American Journal of Physical Anthropology*, **173**(4), 734–747.

Graham, D.D. and Bethard, J.D. (2019) Reconstructing the origins of the Perrins Ledge cremains using strontium isotope analysis. *Journal of Archaeological Science: Reports*, **24**, 350–362.

Grupe, G., Klaut, D., Mauder, M., Kröger, P., Lang, A., Mayr, C., *et al.* (2018) Multi-isotope provenancing of archaeological skeletons including cremations in a reference area of the European Alps. *Rapid Communications in Mass Spectrometry*, **32**(19), 1711–1727.

Habelitz, S., Pascual, L., and Durán, A. (2001) Transformation of tricalcium phosphate into apatite by ammonia treatment. *Journal of Materials Science*, **36**(17), 4131–4135.

Harvig, L., Frei, K.M., Price, T.D., and Lynnerup, N. (2014) Strontium isotope signals in cremated petrous portions as indicator for childhood origin. *PloS One*, **9**(7), e101603.

Hedges, R.E., Clement, J.G., Thomas, C.D.L., and O'Connell, T.C. (2007) Collagen turnover in the adult femoral mid-shaft: Modeled from anthropogenic radiocarbon tracer measurements. *American Journal of Physical Anthropology*, **133**(2), 808–816.

Hess, J., Bender, M.L., and Schilling, J.G. (1986) Evolution of the ratio of strontium-87 to strontium-86 in seawater from Cretaceous to present. *Science*, **231**(4741), 979–984.

Hlad, M., Veselka, B., Steadman, D.W., Herregods, B., Elskens, M., Annaert, R., *et al.* (2021) Revisiting metric sex estimation of cremated human remains via supervised learning using a reference collection of modern identified individuals (Knoxville, USA). *American Journal of Physical Anthropology*, **175**(4), 777–793.

Hüls, C.M., Erlenkeuser, H., Nadeau, M.J., Grootes, P.M., and Andersen, N. (2010) Experimental study on the origin of cremated bone apatite carbon. *Radiocarbon*, **52**(2), 587–599.

Jørkov, M.L.S., Heinemeier, J., and Lynnerup, N. (2009) The petrous bone – A new sampling site for identifying early dietary patterns in stable isotopic studies. *American Journal of Physical Anthropology,* **138**(2), 199–209.

Kontopoulos, I., Presslee, S., Penkman, K., and Collins, M.J. (2018) Preparation of bone powder for FTIR-ATR analysis: The particle size effect. *Vibrational Spectroscopy,* **99**, 167–177.

Lanting, J.N., Aerts-Bijma, A.T., and van der Plicht, J. (2001) Dating of cremated bones. *Radiocarbon,* **43**(2A), 249–254.

Lanting, J.N. and Brindley, A.L. (1998) Dating cremated bone: The dawn of a new era. *The Journal of Irish Archaeology,* **9**(9), 1–7.

Lebon, M., Reiche, I., Bahain, J.J., Chadefaux, C., Moigne, A.M., Fröhlich, F., *et al.* (2010) New parameters for the characterization of diagenetic alterations and heat-induced changes of fossil bone mineral using Fourier transform infrared spectrometry. *Journal of Archaeological Science,* **37**(9), 2265–2276.

Marques, M.P.M., Gonçalves, D., Mamede, A.P., Coutinho, T., Cunha, E., Kockelmann, W., *et al.* (2021) Profiling of human burned bones: Oxidising versus reducing conditions. *Scientific Reports,* **11**(1), 1361.

Martyn, R., Craig, O.E., Ellingham, S.T., Islam, M., Fattore, L., Sperduti, A., *et al.* (2020) A re-evaluation of manner of death at Roman Herculaneum following the AD 79 eruption of Vesuvius. *Antiquity,* **94**(373), 76–91.

Montgomery, J. (2010) Passports from the past: Investigating human dispersals using strontium isotope analysis of tooth enamel. *Annals of Human Biology,* **37**(3), 325–346.

Naysmith, P., Scott, E.M., Cook, G.T., Heinemeier, J., van der Plicht, J., Van Strydonck, M., *et al.* (2007) A cremated bone intercomparison study. *Radiocarbon,* **49**(2), 403–408.

Olsen, J., Heinemeier, J., Hornstrup, K.M., Bennike, P., and Thrane, H. (2013) 'Old wood' effect in radiocarbon dating of prehistoric cremated bones? *Journal of Archaeological Science,* **40**(1), 30–34.

Paba, R., Thompson, T.J.U., Fanti, L., and Lugliè, C. (2021) Rising from the ashes: A multi-technique analytical approach to determine cremation. A case study from a Middle Neolithic burial in Sardinia (Italy). *Journal of Archaeological Science: Reports,* **36**, 102855.

Parker Pearson, M., Chamberlain, A., Jay, M., Marshall, P., Pollard, J., Richards, C., *et al.* (2009) Who was buried at Stonehenge? *Antiquity,* **83**(319), 23–39.

Parker Pearson, M., Chamberlain, A., Jay, M., Richards, M., Sheridan, A., Curtis, N., *et al.* (2016) Beaker people in Britain: Migration, mobility and diet. *Antiquity,* **90**(351), 620–637.

Price, T.D., Arcini, C., Gustin, I., Drenzel, L., and Kalmring, S. (2018) Isotopes and human burials at Viking Age Birka and the Mälaren region, east central Sweden. *Journal of Anthropological Archaeology,* **49**, 19–38.

Reimer, P.J., Austin, W.E., Bard, E., Bayliss, A., Blackwell, P.G., Ramsey, C.B., *et al.* (2020) The IntCal20 Northern Hemisphere radiocarbon age calibration curve (0–55 cal kBP). *Radiocarbon,* **62**(4), 725–757.

Roche, D., Ségalen, L., Balan, E., and Delattre, S. (2010) Preservation assessment of Miocene–Pliocene tooth enamel from Tugen Hills (Kenyan Rift Valley) through FTIR, chemical and stable-isotope analyses. *Journal of Archaeological Science,* **37**(7), 1690–1699.

Rose, H.A., Meadows, J., and Henriksen, M.B. (2020) Bayesian modeling of wood-age offsets in cremated bone. *Radiocarbon,* **62**(2), 379–401.

Sabaux, C., Veselka, B., Capuzzo, G., Snoeck, C., Sengeløv, A., Hlad, M., *et al.* (2021) Multi-proxy analyses reveal regional cremation practices and social status at the Late Bronze Age site of Herstal, Belgium. *Journal of Archaeological Science,* **132**, 105437.

Salesse, K., Dufour, E., Lebon, M., Wurster, C., Castex, D., Brůžek, J., *et al.* (2014) Variability of bone preservation in a confined environment: The case of the catacomb of Sts Peter and Marcellinus (Rome, Italy). *Palaeogeography, Palaeoclimatology, Palaeoecology*, **416**, 43–54.

Salesse, K., Fernandes, R., de Rochefort, X., Brůžek, J., Castex, D., and Dufour, É. (2018) IsoArcH.eu: An open-access and collaborative isotope database for bioarchaeological samples from the Graeco-Roman world and its margins. *Journal of Archaeological Science: Reports*, **19**, 1050–1055.

Schmidt, C.W. and Symes, S.A. (eds.) (2008) *The Analysis of Burnt Human Remains*. Academic Press, London.

Schulting, R., Snoeck, C., Loe, L., and Gilmour, N. (2016) Strontium isotope analysis of the Mesolithic cremation from Langford, Essex, England. *Mesolithic Miscellany*, **24**(1), 19–21.

Schulting, R.J., Murphy, E., Jones, C., and Warren, G. (2012) New dates from the north and a proposed chronology for Irish court tombs. *Proceedings of the Royal Irish Academy. Section C: Archaeology, Celtic Studies, History, Linguistics, Literature*, 1–60.

Sebald, S.V., Zeiler, M., and Grupe, G. (2018) Provenance analysis of human cremations by 87Sr/86Sr isotopic ratios: Migration into an Iron Age mining region in North-Rhine Westphalia. *Open Journal of Archaeometry*, **4**(1).

Skinner, H.C.W. (2005) Biominerals. *Mineralogical Magazine*, **69**(5), 621–641.

Snoeck, C. (2015) A burning question: Structural and isotopic analysis of cremated bone in archaeological contexts (Doctoral dissertation, University of Oxford).

Snoeck, C., Brock, F., and Schulting, R.J. (2014a) Carbon exchanges between bone apatite and fuels during cremation: Impact on radiocarbon dates. *Radiocarbon*, **56**(2), 591–602.

Snoeck, C., Lee-Thorp, J.A., and Schulting, R.J. (2014b) From bone to ash: Compositional and structural studies of burned bone. *Palaeogeography, Palaeoclimatology, Palaeoecology*, **416**, 55–68.

Snoeck, C., Jones, C., Pouncett, J., Goderis, S., Claeys, Ph., Mattielli, N., *et al.* (2020) Isotopic evidence for shifting mobility and landscape use between the Neolithic and Early Bronze Age in western Ireland. *Journal of Archaeological Science: Reports*, **30**, 102214.

Snoeck, C., Pouncett, J., Claeys, Ph., Goderis, S., Mattielli, N., Parker Pearson, M., *et al.* (2018) Strontium isotope analysis on cremated human remains from Stonehenge support links with west Wales. *Scientific Reports*, **8**, 10790.

Snoeck, C., Pouncett, J., Ramsey, G., Meighan, I., Mattielli, N., Goderis, S., *et al.* (2016a) Mobility during the Neolithic and Bronze Age in Northern Ireland explored using strontium isotope analysis of cremated human bone. *American Journal of Physical Anthropology*, **160**(3), 397–413.

Snoeck, C., Schulting, R.J., Lee-Thorp, J.A., de Jong, J., Debouge, W., and Mattielli, N. (2015) Calcined bone provides a reliable substrate for strontium isotope ratios as shown by an enrichment experiment. *Rapid Communications in Mass Spectrometry*, **29**, 107–114.

Snoeck, C., Schulting, R.J., Lee-Thorp, J.A., Lebon, M., and Zazzo, A. (2016b) Impact of heating conditions on the carbon and oxygen isotope composition of calcined bone. *Journal of Archaeological Science*, **65**, 32–43.

Sponheimer, M. and Lee-Thorp, J.A. (1999) Alteration of enamel carbonate environments during fossilization. *Journal of Archaeological Science*, **26**, 143–150.

Thompson, T. (2015) *The Archaeology of Cremation: Burned Human Remains in Funerary Studies*, Vol. **8**. Oxbow Books, Oxford.

Thompson, T.J.U., Gauthier, M., and Islam, M. (2009) The application of a new method of Fourier Transform Infrared Spectroscopy to the analysis of burned bone. *Journal of Archaeological Science*, **36**(3), 910–914.

Tuross, N., Behrensmeyer, A.K., and Eanes, E.D. (1989) Strontium increases and crystallinity changes in taphonomic and archaeological bone. *Journal of Archaeological Science*, **16**(6), 661–672.

Van Strydonck, M., Boudin, M., and De Mulder, G. (2010) The carbon origin of structural carbonate in bone apatite of cremated bones. *Radiocarbon*, **52**(2), 578–586.

Veselka, B., Capuzzo, G., Annaert, R., Mattielli, N., Boudin, M., Dalle, S., *et al.* (2021a) Divergence, diet, and disease: The identification of group identity, landscape use, health, and mobility in the 5th to 6th-century burial community of Echt, the Netherlands. *Archaeological and Anthropological Sciences*, **13**(6), 1–14.

Veselka, B., Hlad, M., Steadman, D.W., Annaert, R., Boudin, M., Capuzzo, G., *et al.* (2021b) Estimating age-at-death in burnt adult human remains using degenerative phases of the sternal clavicle end. *American Journal of Physical Anthropology*, **175**(1), 128–136.

Veselka, B., Locher, H., de Groot, J.C.M.J., Davies, G.R., Snoeck, C., and Kootker, L.M. (2021c) Strontium isotope ratios related to childhood mobility: Revisiting sampling strategies of the calcined human pars petrosa ossis temporalis. *Rapid Communication in Mass Spectrometry*, **35**(7), e9038.

Vogel, J.C. and Van Der Merwe, N.J. (1977) Isotopic evidence for early maize cultivation in New York State. In: *American Antiquity*, **42**, 238–242.

Willis, C., Marshall, P., McKinley, J., Pitts, M., Pollard, J., Richards, C., *et al.* (2016) The dead of Stonehenge. *Antiquity*, **90**(350), 337–356.

Zazzo, A., Lebon, M., Chiotti, L., Comby, C., Delqué-Količ, E., Nespoulet, R., *et al.* (2013) Can we use calcined bones for radiocarbon dating the Paleolithic? *Radiocarbon*, **55**(2–3), 1409–1421.

Zazzo, A., Saliege, J.-F., Lebon, M., Lepetz, S., and Moreau, C. (2012) Radiocarbon dating of calcined bones: Insights from combustion experiments under natural conditions. *Radiocarbon*, **54**(3–4), 1–12.

CHAPTER 16
The Application of Imaging to Heat-Induced Bone

Rachael M. Carew[1], PhD and David Errickson[2], PhD
[1] *Lecturer in Forensic Science, School of Life Sciences, Coventry University, Coventry, UK*
[2] *Senior Lecturer in Forensic Archaeology, Cranfield Forensic Institute, Cranfield University, Bedford, UK*

16.1 Introduction

The human body is studied and assessed in a wide range of disciplines for various purposes. The body takes on the role of a database containing the information of the once living individual; this can be distinctive yet also complex. In recent decades a multitude of techniques have been developed to understand and interpret the life course of a body, including events that occurred before, during, and after death. Extrinsic changes such as taphonomic factors can severely impact our ability to examine a body post-mortem; one of these biggest factors is heat-induced change or burning.

As technology progresses there is a growing interest in new methodologies for visualizing and analyzing the part of the human body that is more often left behind, the osteological remains (Thompson, 2017). Three-dimensional (3D) visualization techniques provide an enhanced approach to digitizing, exposing, comparing, reconstructing, materializing, and sharing data from remains (Weber, 2015). As a result of these various applications, 3D technology has been successfully applied to the body across fields that are osteologically related, such as medicine, forensic anthropology, osteoarchaeology, paleoanthropology, and zooarchaeology.

Although there is a substantial amount of literature pertaining to imaging the human body and osteological remains post-mortem, the application of these technologies to heat-induced and burnt bone is limited. Nevertheless, imaging techniques can provide opportunities to expose hidden details, perform ethical analyses, and create permanent digital records. Imaging can provide and preserve valuable information for species determination, histological analysis, and aid in the interpretation of traumatic and taphonomic changes, as well as facilitate 3D visualization of the body at the macro, micro, and nano level. In each of these

Burnt Human Remains: Recovery, Analysis, and Interpretation, First Edition. Edited by Sarah Ellingham, Joe Adserias-Garriga, Sara C. Zapico and Douglas H. Ubelaker.

instances, the data can be utilized to create visually appealing digital and physical replicas for documentation, display, and archiving purposes.

This chapter discusses the technological progression of imaging with specific application to burnt human remains, with a discussion on two-dimensional (2D) imaging methodologies, but with a focus on those using 3D formats. Furthermore, this chapter demonstrates how different imaging techniques can be applied to burnt human remains, as well as the advantages and disadvantages that the user is likely to encounter. It is hoped that this work will be used as a guide for researchers and practitioners who may want to apply imaging in their practice.

16.2 Technological Progression

The application of imaging in forensic science has evolved since the development of an early mugshot database. At the turn of the twentieth century, photography was used to methodically document crime scenes and to demonstrate the spatial relationships between objects and people (Blitzer and Jacobia, 2002; Platt, 2005). Nowadays, it is hard to imagine any forensic case or evidence that does not include capture in the form of images. For example, the documentation of human remains provides a lasting asset to a court of law, offering an accurate snapshot of a body prior to any changes that may occur during or after recovery (e.g. due to decomposition or intervention during autopsy). Furthermore, long after a body has been interred, the images serve as a near-everlasting reminder of how the body looked upon its discovery.

Traditionally, imaging has been applied to forensic science with the use of microscopy, radiographs, and photographic documentation. However, each of these techniques have developed exponentially into several specialized areas under the umbrella of imaging, and in some cases even created new disciplines (Weber, 2015). For example, the late 1990s and early 2000s saw radiographic imaging increase in popularity through its application to imaging mummified remains and museum specimens as a non-destructive technique that permitted visualization of internal anatomical structures. Interestingly, because of the advancement in technology there has also been an increase in the different types of materials that can be assessed. For example, this includes peri- and post-mortem alterations created by extrinsic taphonomic factors such as weathering, animal scavenging, and heat-induced changes. The use of 3D imaging in the criminal justice system has even been established as a new field termed "3D forensic science" (Carew *et al.*, 2021b). However, the literature currently available surrounding 3D imaging of bodies that have been modified by fire or explosions is scattered.

Presently, imaging is being used in forensic investigations more and more frequently, particularly following mass disaster events where intense heat can often be associated with the incident. For example, following the September 11, 2001, terrorist attacks on the World Trade Center in New York, radiography was used to help identify the remains of victims (Mackinnon and Mundorff, 2006). Likewise, following the 2009 Victorian bushfires in Australia, post-mortem computed tomography was used to examine and identify fragmented human remains, including calcined bone (O'Donnell *et al.*, 2011). Furthermore, mobile computed tomography in conjunction with radiography aided the identification of the fatalities from the Grenfell Tower fire in London, UK, in 2017 (Rutty *et al.*, 2019).

The material properties of the target that is to be imaged will influence the recording technique used, as will the aim of the imaging. It can be difficult to navigate the numerous techniques available, and individuals tend to be biased and can either stick to what they know or what is readily available to them. This is further complicated by the current rate at which new imaging techniques and instruments are becoming available. This technological succession is a double-edged sword, as while imaging techniques have steadily improved, so has its technical ability (such as in the degree of magnification available, or the use of filters to enhance CT scans), as well as its affordability and accessibility. However, it therefore becomes difficult to keep up to date with the technology available; training and knowledge can quickly become outdated and knowing how to apply these different techniques in different scenarios can be challenging.

In many UK day-to-day forensic cases the use of imaging technology is often down to what is available and / or convenient, that is, limited to those techniques that are available in-house or at known clinical or academic institutes. Further, most cases of forensic imaging of a victim will be conducted within a hospital or clinical setting, where pre-surgery assessment or medical intervention is undertaken, or during post-mortem analysis. Medical imaging equipment can also be made available through associated universities, particularly if affiliated with a teaching hospital. On the other hand, it is not unusual to utilize private companies, although this is likely to be higher cost than universities. Likewise, large museums often have the capability to apply methods such as radiography, micro-CT, and surface capture; however, regarding forensic analysis, the availability of the techniques will depend on the circumstances of a case.

The main considerations for the selection of imaging techniques to record human remains, include the size of the remains (whether they will fit inside an imaging chamber, on a stage, or through gantry); the accessibility (whether the remains are transportable and can be taken to another location); the visibility (whether the remains are visible or contained within a substrate); and contamination (including whether the remains form a chemical, biological, radiological, or nuclear hazard). Depending upon these factors, techniques such as laser scanning, micro-CT, or scanning electron microscopy can be selected further, depending on the desired output from the imaging. Outputs can include visualization of surfaces (e.g. to interpret burn or trauma patterns) or internal features (e.g. bones inside a body, or internal bone morphology); magnification for viewing cell structures (e.g. for species identification), or further analysis (e.g. for elemental profiling).

16.3 The Current Technology

This section briefly discusses the imaging techniques available for assessing human remains. This is supported by Figure 16.1, which illustrates some of the decisions considered when selecting an imaging modality and provides a useful decision tree for selecting techniques. For further detail, a helpful table outlining the advantages and limitations of 3D recording techniques is provided in Carew and Errickson (2019), which includes the destructive and invasive nature of the methods.

16.3.1 Two-Dimensional Imaging

For this chapter, 2D imaging methods are generally associated with non-contact techniques that are concerned with visualization alone. It should also be noted that thin sections for use with light microscopes will involve destructive sampling processes. Generally, these 2D methods involve viewing the surface or a slice through a body, and these often require basic equipment. Thus, 2D methods can be more affordable, transportable, and straightforward to use. The techniques discussed in this section are photography, microscopy, and radiography.

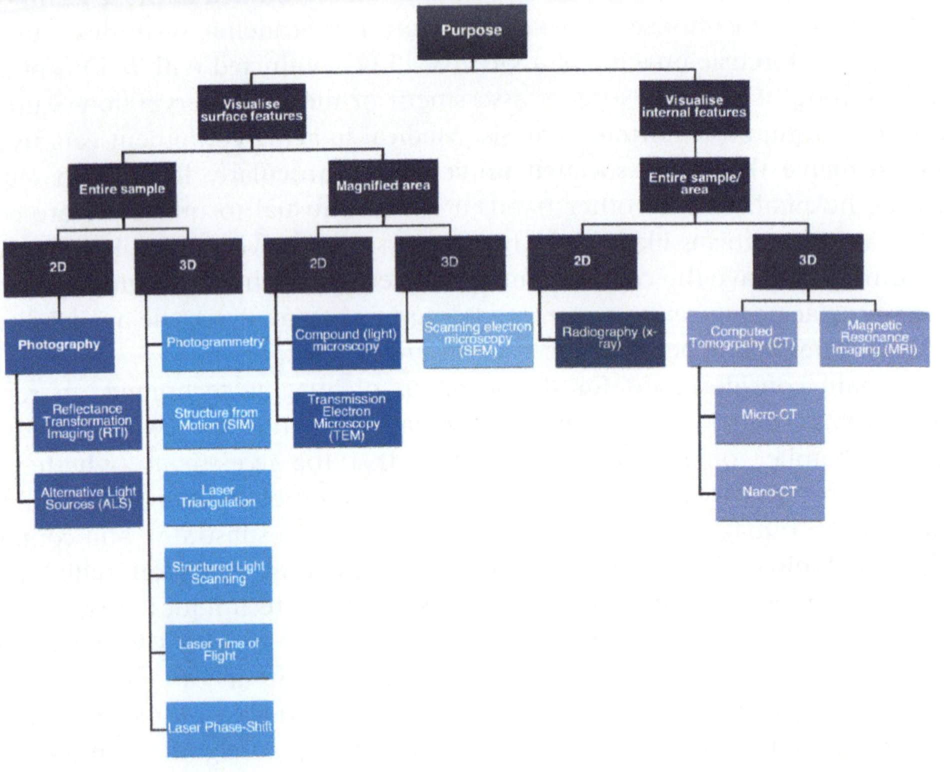

Figure 16.1 Flowchart illustrating choices made when selecting different imaging techniques.

A digital camera is the most readily available tool and digital photography is a rapid and effective way for recording materials at a scene or in a controlled environment. Deceased bodies and body parts will degrade and change over time, and photography allows the documentation of the object at the time of discovery and prior to any further change. Similarly, photography can be effectively utilized to demonstrate how objects and materials change. This form of immediate documentation is valuable and photographic documentation should precede all other imaging techniques to establish a focal point and timeline (Redsicker, 2000).

For microscopic analysis, conventional microscopy is commonly used as a readily available, cost-effective technique. However, methods have developed considerably from the use of "light microscopes" that magnify from centimeters to micrometers, to scanning electron and transmission electron microscopes (SEM and TEM, respectively) providing magnified images in the nanometer scale. These techniques are widely used and accepted in both forensic and archaeological contexts; however, the type of sample may be limited due to the stand-off height of each technique and in some instances samples may need to be coated prior to analysis. Nevertheless, higher magnification methods also have the capability to provide elemental identification of materials within or upon samples, as well as information on material and chemical composition.

Traditional X-radiography provides 2D images, known as radiographs. Radiographs can be in the form of the traditional plain film radiographs (the type often found in academic archaeology departments) as well as digital images; either format of radiograph is straightforward to interpret and does not require specialist reconstruction software. X- radiography facilitates the documentation of internal structures of a body without invasive intervention and can be used to aid identification of foreign objects within a body, which is particularly beneficial when looking for metallic fragments or surgical implants. Although the use of radiation itself can be a hazard and potential limitation, this is of less concern when imaging non-living subjects. A wider concern with traditional X-radiography is the superimposition of structures. As a radiograph is taken in only one plane, anatomical structures become stacked on top of one another. For this reason, it is always recommended to take radiographs from at least two viewpoints. However, this should not generally pose an issue given the low cost associated with the technique.

16.3.2 Three-Dimensional Imaging

The 3D imaging techniques involve taking multiple scans or images where either the sample or the instrument rotates about the other. Thus, a picture of an entire sample can be built up and reconstructed as one 3D model for 360-degree visualization. Techniques can involve the instrument rotating about the sample, or conversely the sample can be rotated to reveal all surfaces while the imaging equipment remains stationary. Techniques such as photogrammetry and laser scanning can be performed in either manner, depending on the set-up of the equipment. For example, photogrammetry can be performed with the sample on a turntable and the use of a single camera to capture the images, or a photogrammetry suite can be set up to provide image capture from multiple angles with the sample staying stationary in the centre (Carew and Errickson, 2019). If multiple viewpoints have been acquired, a model can be built up from multiple angles and thus a 3D model can be generated. Although, such techniques often do not capture the entire model, such as the base (or the face touching the platform / surface), which can be missed during the imaging process. The progression of radiography for imaging has developed around this aspect of moving elements, with traditional radiographs being taken from fixed positions with the subject moved to obtain multiple viewpoints, through to the use of multi detector CT (MDCT) being developed so that a subject is moved through the imaging equipment whilst the imaging equipment itself also rotates around the subject, to generate a full set of images around 360 degrees.

It is also important to note that while the term 3D is used to describe a 3D digital model, a 3D model viewed on a screen is only stereoscopic and presents with an illusion of depth using features such as shadows and light (Carew *et al.*, 2019). A physical 3D model such as a 3D printed replica, holds true 3D properties and thus has genuine depth as well as greater cognitive feedback from haptic and spatial awareness. An important distinction between 3D imaging techniques are methods that capture surfaces (external techniques) and those that are volumetric (internal techniques); these are discussed in the next section.

16.3.2.1 3D Volumetric Scanning

Micro-CT is a radiographic technique with a high resolution, greater than seen with traditional MDCT. During a micro-CT scan, the sample is fixed to a mount that rotates 360 degrees. The X-radiation source is fixed and has a limited field of view towards the sample mount. The resolution of a micro-CT scan is influenced by X-ray tube potential (kV), X-ray tube current (μ), number of projections, and number of images per projection (number of frames). Thus, an image can be gained in quick time (within minutes) if certain parameters are sacrificed or not needed, or a longer scan time (hours) can enable higher resolution or larger data capture (e.g. with a wide or thick sample). As with CT, micro-CT scan data can be visualized as 2D planes or reconstructed as 3D volume renders. A limitation of micro-CT is the size of the sample and the scan chamber, the latter varies with models (e.g. some instruments will fit a human skull, while others will not) (Figure 16.2). Micro-CT sample chambers are smaller than clinical CT scanner beds and the decision can sometimes be made to destructively downsize a sample to gain higher resolution in a micro-CT scanner. Data storage of micro-CT images will require consideration due to the large scan files obtained. Likewise, a nano-CT uses the same principles. However, the imaging quality is increased when using a nano-CT for samples that are smaller than 10 mm. Nano-CT is useful for providing a clear view of bone microstructure and allowing accurate measurements to be obtained (du Plessis *et al.*, 2017).

Magnetic resonance imaging (MRI) is seldom used for imaging bony material; however, there are useful examples of MRI applications. MRI is an imaging technique that

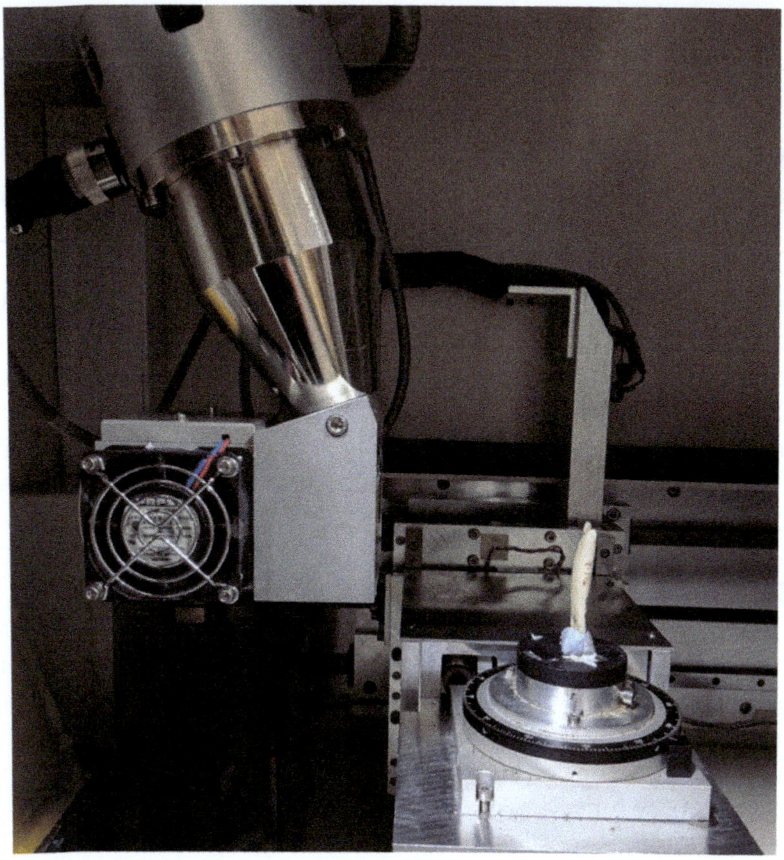

Figure 16.2 Photograph illustrating the size of an imaging mount and chamber of a micro-CT scanner (bone is around 70 mm in length).

exploits the interaction of radio waves with hydrogen atoms. Through observing the excitation of hydrogen atoms with a strong magnetic field, it is possible to create an image of a subject. Due to this interaction with hydrogen atoms, MRI works well to image soft tissues (that contain greater quantities of hydrogen, i.e. water), and is less effective for visualizing hard tissues such as bones. Nevertheless, MRI may be used to capture osteological material and studies have shown that this can help visualize heat-induced structural change in bone (Thompson and Chudek, 2007).

16.3.2.2 3D Surface Scanning

16.3.2.2.1 Scanning Electron Microscopy

SEM is a surface imaging method that facilitates visualizations in three-dimensions. SEM uses electron beams to scan across the surface of a sample; these electrons interact with the sample, generating backscattered and secondary electrons that subsequently provide an image of the sample. However, SEM usually only captures images from the view that was imaged and does not usually provide a 360-degree view. It can be possible to use additional techniques such as photogrammetry to take further images of a sample at differing angles (e.g. through using a tilt stage), to obtain 3D "moving" models.

16.3.2.2.2 Photogrammetry

Photogrammetry has become increasingly accessible in comparison to other surface scanning techniques. This is due to the availability of open source software applications that are capable of processing high-resolution data (Urbanova *et al.*, 2015). Photogrammetry uses standard digital photographic images (even taken using mobile phones) that have captured all surfaces of an object. Similar coordinates on each image are identified and from this, a computer can semi-automatically build up a 3D model. Regarding human remains, photogrammetry has been used in skin and mark documentation (Thali *et al.*, 2000, 2002; Schweitzer *et al.*, 2013), as well as with osteological remains (Wilson *et al.*, 2017; Edwards and Rogers, 2018; Villa *et al.*, 2018; Morgan *et al.*, 2019).

16.3.2.2.3 Structure from Motion

Structure from motion (SfM) is a photogrammetric range imaging technique that uses the principles of photogrammetry but documents an object such as a body using video rather than still photographic images. Essentially, the method uses the frames from a video as an alternative to the photos, where similar coordinates on these stills are identified to build up a 3D model. SfM is capable of documenting large areas but has also been applied to human skeletal material for documentation and visualization purposes (Morgan *et al.*, 2019).

16.3.2.2.4 Laser Scanning

Laser scanning is another popular method; this involves a laser beam that is passed over an object to create a set of vertices known as a point cloud. Triangulation is the laser scanning method used to obtain 3D coordinates; due to its simple and robust approach, laser scanning tends to give results with high accuracy (Zeng *et al.*, 1999). Once an entire object has been documented in this way, a computer will merge the points in the point cloud to create a high-resolution surface. There are many laser scanners available, each with various advantages and disadvantages (see Carew and Errickson, 2019). However, it is useful as a technique that requires minimal training. Laser scanning has extensive applications and has been used to document and reconstruct injuries on the deceased (Cattaneo, 2007; Komar *et al.*, 2012), conserve skeletal remains (Kuzminsky and Gardiner, 2012), for biological assessment (Dennis *et al.*, 2004; Shearer *et al.*, 2012), and for teaching and research purposes (Mallison, 2011; Attard and Rogers, 2015).

16.3.2.2.5 Laser Time of Flight

On the other end of the scale, laser time of flight or phase-shift measurement are methods used to image larger objects, scenes, or landscapes. For time of flight, a transmitter sends out a laser beam and a receiver documents how long it takes for the laser to reflect off an object and back to the device. This is different to phase-shift, where a signal is transmitted and returned to a receiver. In the context of imaging human remains, these techniques are primarily used to document mass disaster sites such as mass graves, airplane crashes, and fire investigation scenes (Buck *et al.*, 2013), rather than individual bodies or elements.

16.3.2.2.6 Structured Light Scanning

Rather than a laser stripe, structured light scanners project a plain of patterned light. This patterned light is distorted by the object it is recording, and a camera picks up these changes and creates a digital 3D surface of the object. Structured light scanning is often preferred over laser scanning due to its ability to record color and texture during capture. The main use of the method has been in recording and archiving human remains (Errickson *et al.*, 2017) and for documenting surface injuries (Shamata and Thompson, 2018, 2020).

16.4 The Application of Imaging to Heat-Induced and Burnt Bodies

The application of imaging to human remains is well demonstrated; however, the literature regarding its application to heat-induced bone and burnt bodies is limited and often lost in the wider literature. Therefore, the following section details how imaging can be applied to human remains that have been exposed to fire or impacted by blast trauma.

16.4.1 Locating and Identifying Burnt Bone

Locating bone within mixed samples, such as debris or cremations, can be challenging using the naked eye alone. Several imaging techniques can aid this through exploiting the properties of (human) bone. Radiography can aid determination of bone in mixed samples due to osseous and dental tissues having high radiopacity due to their mineral content (Christensen *et al.*, 2014). As such, this high radiopacity means that bone and dental tissues will appear bright white on radiographs, providing a stark contrast to surrounding materials. Radiography provides an accessible 2D technique that is more affordable than advanced imaging methods; it can also be portable and recorded digitally for on-site or remote analysis.

Routine digital photography is typically not examined in this chapter; however, it is worth noting the benefits of using reflectance transformation imaging (RTI), as well as alternative light sources (ALS) for locating human remains as well as distinguishing burning temperatures. RTI is a photographic method that can enhance surface details, including shape and color, and this has been shown to enhance visibility of burnt bone surfaces (Newman, 2015). Similarly, the use of ALS with photography can aid recovery and identification of thermally altered human remains using the fluorescent or luminescent properties of burnt bone when viewed under different wavelengths of light (Green *et al.*, 2019). ALS has shown to be valuable for distinguishing between human and non-human material, as well as between different burning temperatures (Green *et al.*, 2019).

Transmissive CT techniques can be useful for locating skeletal elements within a burnt body or body parts. During CT imaging a sample does not need to be unpackaged or manually handled, a valuable consideration when working with hazardous or forensically relevant materials. Micro-CT has previously been used to "virtually dissect" burnt human remains from surrounding charred tissues for reconstruction and toolmark analysis (Baier *et al.*, 2017). Additionally, following a mass fatality incident in the UK, forensic pathologists utilized post-mortem CT imaging and 3D printing as a method to visualize the dentition from a severely charred body (Biggs and Marsden, 2019). This use of imaging and 3D printing avoided dissection and disfiguring facial incisions and instead offered a more ethical visualization method that ultimately helped to positively identify the individual (Biggs and Marsden, 2019).

Most techniques useful for locating and identifying bone need to be applied in specific manners to undertake full documentation. For instance, CT scanning could not be undertaken directly at a crime scene to document a body in situ. To utilize CT scanning, a body would need to be initially documented at the scene (e.g. using digital photography), following which there would have to be some movement of the evidence before scanning. On the other hand, a body concealed within a container (such as a suitcase) could be captured prior to opening if the object were to fit within a scanner. This could be advantageous in informing the investigators of any hazards contained within, or for informing on the best approach for removal. With these considerations in mind, generic in situ visual scene capture and documentation can still be achieved by surface scanning techniques.

16.4.2 Visual Capture and Documentation for Recording and Archiving

Due to the fragile nature of burnt samples, in situ modelling and documentation is recommended so that surfaces can be accurately captured prior to handling (Collings and Brown, 2020).

Photogrammetric documentation is useful to create a 3D model, especially when debris is present and remains have been subjected to varying conditions (such as a building explosion or fatal fire) (de Boer *et al.*, 2020). Photogrammetry and structure from motion can be used to document a whole area, including the remains within the scene (Baier and Rando, 2016), or to focus only on the remains. However, photogrammetry does not record dimensions in microns, and in a legal context this may present an issue. For example, during post-processing of photogrammetry data, a scale may need to be manually added to the model, which may add a degree of uncertainty around the accuracy of a model. Nevertheless, this error can be reduced by including measurement scales within the initial data capture – as is performed with traditional photography.

The application of hand-held surface scanning techniques in the field can be problematic. This will vary from scene to scene; however, the most important factors often include the lighting available and the location of the target material within the capture area. Structured light scanners are particularly affected by light, meaning that bright and ambient light environments can be problematic to capture (Kuzminsky and Gardiner, 2012). Similarly, the color of the target surface can affect the ability to accurately capture that surface, for example skin or burnt bone may present as dark-colored surfaces that absorb light or light-colored surfaces that reflect light. Using either laser or structured light scanning to document carbonized and calcined remains in situ would be extremely difficult to do, because of the potential errors created within the data sets gathered in uncontrolled environments (Errickson *et al.*, 2017). However, these techniques would still be useful for generic documentation in a laboratory or clinical environment under controlled conditions.

Computed tomography (CT) is an extremely useful tool for documenting burnt human remains. CT imaging can be performed to visualize whole bodies to capture surface details or to view skeletal elements within a burnt body. This technique could also be used to document and obtain data from foreign objects within a body, such as explosive material from a terrorism incident, ballistics from a gunshot wound, or even serial numbers on a medical prothesis. Further advantages to the approach of documentation include that CT scanning can also be combined with surface scanning techniques such as photogrammetry to accurately capture both internal and external features (Villa *et al.*, 2018). The resulting 3D models from each technique can be combined to create one composite model that provides a complete view of an object. On the other hand, the limitations to CT scanning include unwanted noise in a data set from metallic artifacts, and difficulty in positioning burnt bodies if, for example, in the pugilistic pose (O'Donnell *et al.*, 2011). Similarly, sometimes the accessibility of CT scanning may be difficult to obtain or provide outside "normal working hours"; a radiographer is needed for undertaking the data capture and a professional trained in 3D methods and anatomical modelling should be utilized for processing and interpretation of the CT data.

16.4.3 Quantifying and Analyzing Burnt Remains

Digital imaging techniques themselves can be used for analytical purposes, particularly for viewing and interpreting trauma or burning patterns, as well as for histology and histomorphometry. Moreover, digital imaging can also be combined with analytical techniques for complementary data capture.

SEM provides high magnification images of a sample and is useful for viewing the topology of burnt bones, as well as any fractures and even mineral deposits upon a surface. SEM is thus also useful for interpreting burning patterns on a sample (Ellingham *et al.*, 2018; Fernández-Jalvo *et al.*, 2018). SEM can also be used in conjunction with analytical techniques such as combined with energy dispersive X-ray analysis (EDX) (or energy dispersive X-ray spectroscopy (EDS)).

SEM-EDX can provide analytical information from burnt bones, such as elemental analysis or chemical characterization (Ellingham *et al.*, 2018).

Due to the high resolution of micro-CT, this imaging technique is often used for histological analysis, and can be used for histomorphology and species identification (Boschin *et al.*, 2015; Franklin *et al.*, 2016; Cummaudo *et al.*, 2020). Micro-CT has also been used to observe internal bone porosity to examine the effects of different burning temperatures (McKinnon *et al.*, 2021) as well as to visualize macroscopic heat-induced changes such as cracks in teeth (Sandholzer *et al.*, 2014). Comparisons between micro-CT and more traditional cost-effective imaging methods are common and can provide useful notes on the advantages and limitations of each. For example, microbial bioerosion features in burnt bones were assessed using transmitted light microscopy and backscattered scanning electron microscopy (Végh *et al.*, 2021). The effects of heat on cut mark characteristics on burnt bones has been explored, with research indicating that both digital microscopy and micro-CT are suitable tools (Baier *et al.*, 2017; Waltenberger and Schutkowski, 2017) that should even be used in conjunction (Waltenberger and Schutkowski, 2017).

While of a lower resolution than micro-CT, MDCT has been used to calculate and describe archaeologically recovered cremated bone volume as a method for estimating the original prehistoric post-cremation weight (Harvig and Lynnerup, 2013). The authors CT scanned remains in situ and remains that were ex situ (in urns) and were able to segment the remains as well as distinguish between trabecular and compact bone (Harvig and Lynnerup, 2013).

16.4.4 Reconstruction

The term *reconstruction* can have several meanings or purposes in virtual anthropology. Digital scan data is *reconstructed* from raw data into volumetric or cloud point data, and then into surface renderings or 3D models. However, digital models can also be used to virtually *reconstruct* fragmented remains into a whole object. This latter type of reconstruction can be useful for demonstrating how objects may have looked prior to fragmentation or burning (Figure 16.3). Software packages, such as MeshLab or CloudCompare, can be utilized to "manually" reconstruct fragments into a single whole or complete object. This software can further be used to perform mesh to mesh comparisons, whereby data can be obtained detailing how closely aligned fragments or objects are to each other. Similarly, scans of the same object can be aligned and compared to obtain mesh distance values, that can provide information on how accurate the scans or models are to each other (Figure 16.4). This is particularly useful for comparing scan techniques, scan instruments, or for observing changes over time. Mesh comparison methods can also be used to perform pair matching of skeletal elements or to obtain geometric data from elements for modern, metric, biological, profiling methods (Griffith and Thompson, 2017).

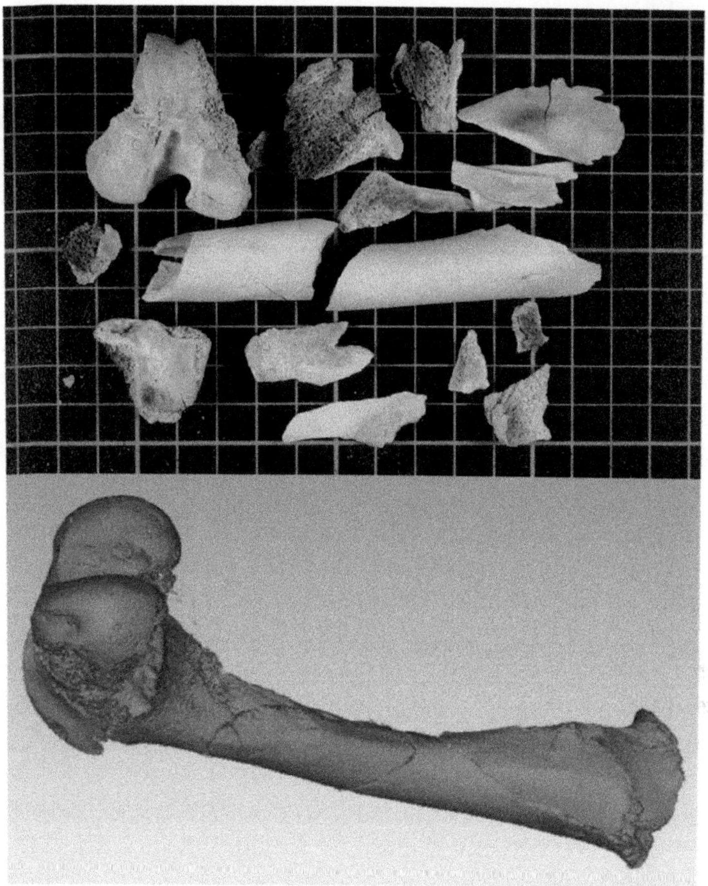

Figure 16.3 Depiction of a sheep femur that was burned at 700°C, resulting in fragmentation (upper burnt bone fragments; lower reconstructed 3D model). Six individual fragments were laser scanned and virtually reconstructed to demonstrate how the bone may have looked prior to burning (Errickson, 2016).

Three-dimensional printing (or additive manufacturing) is a complementary technique to digital imaging that extends the utility of digital 3D models by bringing models back into true 3D space. Within 3D printing, *reconstruction* can also mean the creation of a physical replica using 3D printing methods (for types of 3D printing see Carew and Errickson (2020)). Digital models can be 3D printed to scale to enable visualization of small features, or to enable larger objects to fit within a printer or become handheld. Replicas can also be printed to a true 1:1 size, providing accurate scan and printing techniques are chosen. Reconstructed replicas can also be 3D printed at this stage. Mirroring is a useful technique within digital imaging that can be used to replicate mirror images of missing objects, and this mirrored object can be 3D printed in situ to, for example, fill in missing gaps of data. It is worth noting that this aspect should be carefully documented, and it is recommended that mirrored aspects are replicated in different colors to provide

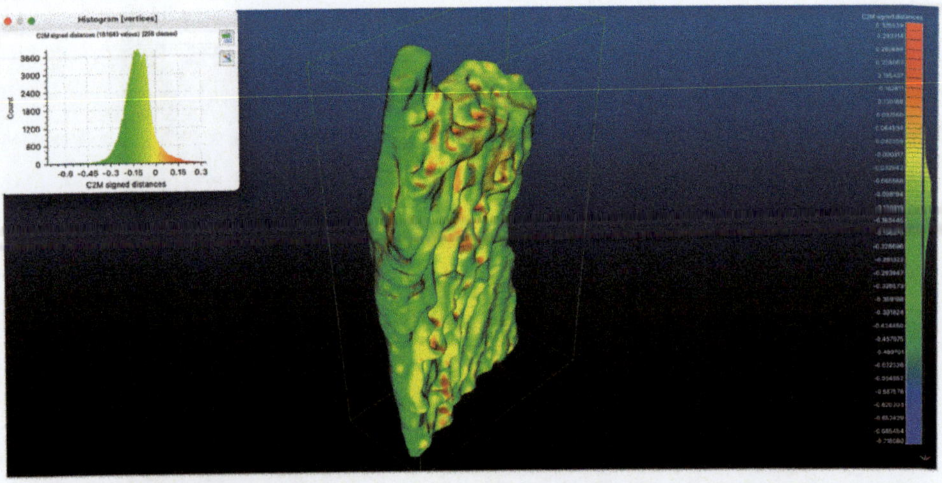

Figure 16.4 A mesh comparison performed in CloudCompare between a 3D model from micro-CT scanned burnt bone fragment with a scan of the 3D printed replica (Carew *et al.*, 2022). Distance values (mm) between the two models are illustrated in color scale and as a histogram.

transparency to this process. The 3D prints may be created in different colors and even in photo-realistic full color, depending on the scanning and printing techniques selected.

Three-dimensional printing also offers the opportunity to create a physical replica of a fragile object that is threatened by fragmentation. The 3D prints can be continually handled without any fear of degradation or cross-contamination; they can also be re-printed as needed, or digitally shared for remote 3D printing.

The use of surface scanning methods (specifically laser scanning) has been advocated as a reliable technique to reconstruct fragmented teeth that can subsequently be 3D printed whole (Jani *et al.*, 2020). Burnt human bone fragments have also been successfully replicated using 3D printing to provide a medium to conduct physical fit analysis by Collings and Brown (2020). The authors provided a comparison between structured light scanning and micro-CT for recording burnt bone fragments and found that micro-CT provided higher resolution data, but also that there were limitations associated with the requirement to use a mattifying spray on the bone fragments for the structured light scanning (Collings and Brown, 2020). The use of a mattifying spray is common with shiny or reflective objects and helps to enhance the visibility of a surface to improve data capture with a structured light scanner. However, the application of a spray requires consideration around potential interference and trace material recovery, as well as any subsequent analysis of the bone (such as DNA recovery).

Of course, there are further limitations with reconstruction. For instance, when subjected to burning bones and bodies undergo physical changes. The documentation process using imaging techniques cannot surmise the change prior warping and modification and can only serve as a record of the object at the time of analysis. Therefore, any virtual reconstruction undertaken (when piecing together samples) will have a degree of uncertainty and error, including systematic and observer error. It is vital to provide transparency and full reporting of errors within the medicolegal system.

Digital imaging can additionally provide opportunities for enhanced public engagement, from the display of CT scans of mummified remains to virtual and augmented reality of remains in museum and outreach settings. Through increasing use of technology and different approaches, objects move from the physical world to the digital world, before emerging back into the physical world (Figure 16.5). Thus, the perceptual presence and level of interaction with a model alters with each technique. Further, the use of 3D printed replicas allows for increased accessibility due to their increased perceptual presence (as a physical object), where 3D printed replicas of objects such as remains, urns, or artifacts can be produced for tactile interaction for individuals with visual impairments, for children, or simply used for sanitized display purposes.

16.4.5 Ethical and Legal Considerations within the Forensic Context

In an archaeological and historical context, imaging should be considered for the aspects of documentation (digitization and exposing remains), comparison (quantitative evaluation), reconstruction, 3D printing, and dissemination of data (Weber, 2015). Likewise, there are several benefits that are also advantageous for

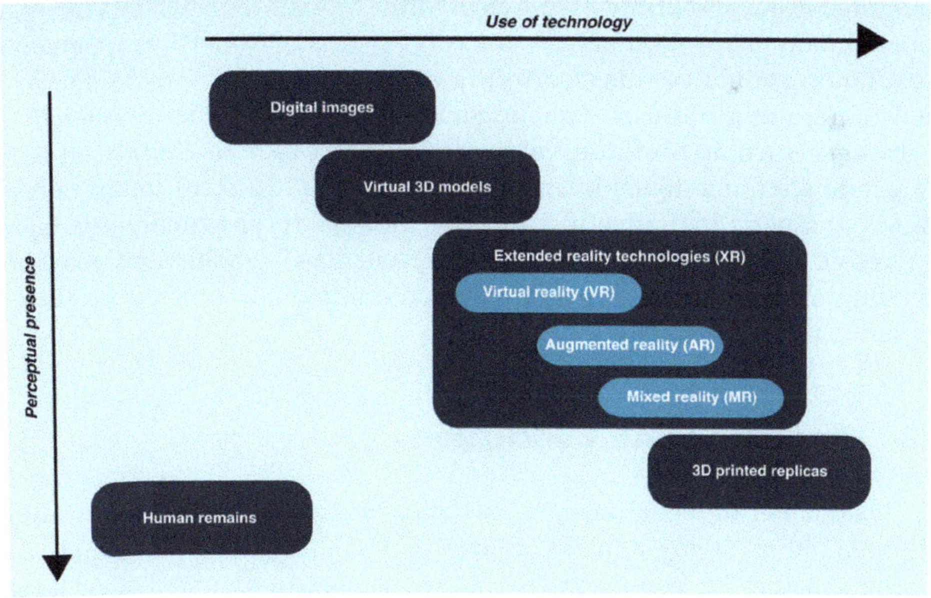

Figure 16.5 Representation of increasing perceptual presence with increasing use of technology.

the forensic context. However, it should be noted that this chapter does not suggest that the use of imaging techniques replaces standard photographic documentation, but rather they should be used in conjunction with them.

Traditionally in courts of law, photographs are used to display burnt remains, human bone, and other types of graphic evidence as a more sanitized method (Errickson *et al.*, 2014). However, understanding of evidence is important for decision making (Burgoon *et al.*, 2000), and information within a court of law should be visualized and presented in an accurate and meaningful way (March *et al.*, 2004). Interestingly, in the UK there are no guidelines for the use of 3D models in courtrooms. Yet, 3D visualizations of human remains are being used in UK courts of law as demonstrative evidence (Baier *et al.*, 2018). There is evidence that 3D visual methods offer a better medium for lay people to understand technical language, as a method that is more engaging than traditional 2D imaging techniques (Errickson *et al.*, 2019). For burnt remains, a 3D visualization that can be moved around on a screen in front of a jury may offer an enhanced spatial awareness of a finding, body, or of a scene containing remains. Similarly, a 3D visualization may help jurors understand a possible burning process or scenario. However, caution should again be applied to the use of 3D printed materials in courtrooms, as the effect that 3D prints may have on a judge or jury is currently not fully understood and further research is needed (Belau; Errickson *et al.*, 2019; Carew *et al.*, 2021a). It is recommended that further psychological studies are undertaken to understand whether these types of examples negatively impact or unfairly bias members within a court of law.

There are also ethical considerations that should be considered with regards to creating virtual and printed replicas of burnt human remains. Of course, any documentation of burnt human remains are replicas of a once living person and consideration should be afforded to the capture, analysis, and storage of any digital or resulting physical data (including long-term). The associated legal implications (such as continuity of evidence) must also be considered before, during, and after any digital imaging; see Carew *et al.* (2021b) for an overview of different aspects that affect the integrity of a 3D reconstruction throughout the forensic science process. Further, different legal jurisdictions may apply depending on where data is being gathered and stored, which pose issues in international casework.

16.5 Discussion and Conclusion

The development of digital imaging has opened many possibilities for locating, capturing, and recording remains, as well as visualizing, analyzing, and reconstructing remains. The non-destructive and non-invasive nature of many imaging techniques affords benefits with fragile heat-induced remains.

An example is presented that depicts many of the advantages of digital imaging (for full details, see Carew *et al.* 2022). In this example presented in Figure 16.6, two fragments of burnt non-human archaeological bone were imaged using micro-CT. Sample A was a calcined fragment and both samples exhibited very intricate surface details, including hoop fractures and microporosity from burning, as well as exposed trabecular bone. These surface details were successfully captured using micro-CT and the resulting digital models displayed a comparable level of detail. The digital models were also replicated using 3D printing (using selective laser sintering), where some loss of detail was observed on the 3D prints, in particular a degree of microporosity was lost from the external surface of sample A (see Figure 16.6).

Digital imaging has many applications with heat-induced remains, the extent of which will only increase with further research and the development of new imaging techniques. The ethical and legal considerations surrounding the use of imaging techniques in the criminal justice system needs greater input and collaboration from multiple disciplines, including archaeology, forensic anthropology, radiography, and medicine. Exciting new possibilities for automated analysis, reconstruction of fragmented remains, and biological profiling using machine learning and artificial intelligence methods are in the pipeline and may be suitable for use soon. The possibilities created when integrating osseous materials into the digital world present valuable approaches and an exciting future for the application of imaging to heat-induced bone.

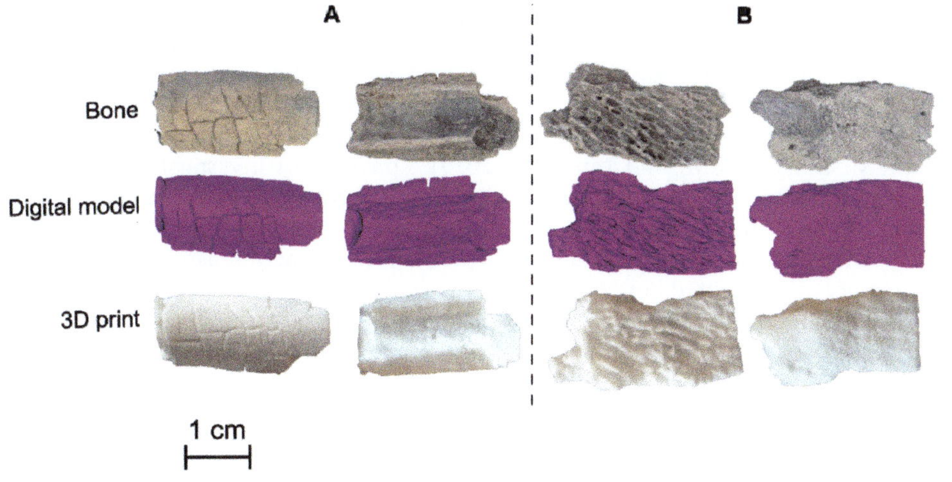

Figure 16.6 Representation of surface detail obtained from external and internal surfaces of two burnt bone fragments (A and B). Upper: photographs depicting the dry bone surface; Centre: screenshot of digital STL model taken in 3D Slicer; Lower: photographs of 3D printed bone produced using selective laser sintering. For further details see Carew *et al.* (2022).

References

Attard, S.M. and Rogers, K.A. (2015) Design and implementation of an online systemic human anatomy course with laboratory. *Anatomical Sciences Education*, **8**(1), 53–62. https://doi.org/10.1002/ase.1465.

Baier, W. and Rando, C. (2016) Developing the use of Structure-from-Motion in mass grave documentation. *Forensic Science International*, **261**, 19–25. https://doi.org/10.1016/j.forsciint.2015.12.008.

Baier, W., Norman, D.G., Warnett, J.M., Payne, M., Harrison, N.P., Hunt, N.C., *et al.* (2017) Novel application of three-dimensional technologies in a case of dismemberment. *Forensic Science International*, **270**, 139–145. https://doi.org/10.1016/j.forsciint.2016.11.040.

Baier, W., Warnett, J.M., Payne, M., and Williams, M.A. (2018) Introducing 3D printed models as demonstrative evidence at criminal trials. *Journal of Forensic Sciences*, **63**(4), 1298–1302. https://doi.org/10.1111/1556-4029.13700.

Biggs, M. and Marsden, P. (2019) Dental identification using 3D printed teeth following a mass fatality incident. *Journal of Forensic Radiology and Imaging*, **18**, 1–3. https://doi.org/10.1016/j.jofri.2019.07.001.

Blitzer, H. and Jacobia, J. (2002) *Forensic Digital Imaging and Photography*. Academic Press, San Diego, CA.

Boschin, F., Zanolli, C., Bernardini, F., Princivalle, F., and Tuniz, C. (2015) A look from the inside: MicroCT analysis of burned bones. *Ethnobiology Letters*, **6**(2), 258–266. https://doi.org/10.14237/ebl.6.2.2015.365.

Buck, U., Naether, S., Räss, B., Jackowski, C., and Thali, M.J. (2013) Accident or homicide – virtual crime scene reconstruction using 3D methods. *Forensic Science International*, **225**(1–3), 75–84. https://doi.org/10.1016/j.forsciint.2012.05.015.

Burgoon, J.K., Bonito, J.A., Bengtsson, B., Cederberg, C., Lundeberg, M., and Allspach, L. (2000) Interactivity in human–computer interaction: A study of credibility, understanding, and influence. *Computers in Human Behavior*, **16**(6), 553–574.

Carew, R.M. and Errickson, D. (2019) Imaging in forensic science: Five years on. *Journal of Forensic Radiology and Imaging*, **16**, 24–33. https://doi.org/10.1016/j.jofri.2019.01.002.

Carew, R.M. and Errickson, D. (2020) An overview of 3D printing in forensic science: The tangible third-dimension. *Journal of Forensic Sciences*, **65**(5), 1752–1760. https://doi.org/10.1111/1556-4029.14442.

Carew, R.M., Morgan, R.M., and Rando, C. (2019) A preliminary investigation into the accuracy of 3D modeling and 3D printing in forensic anthropology evidence reconstruction. *Journal of Forensic Sciences*, **64**(2), 342–352. https://doi.org/10.1111/1556-4029.13917.

Carew, R.M., Morgan, R.M., and Rando, C. (2021a) Experimental assessment of the surface quality of 3D printed bones. *The Australian Journal of Forensic Sciences*. https://doi.org/10.1080/00450618.2020.1759684.

Carew, R.M., Morgan, R.M., and Rando, C. (2021b) 3D forensic science: A new field integrating 3D imaging and 3D printing in crime reconstruction. *Forensic Science International: Synergy*, **3**. https://doi.org/10.1016/j.fsisyn.2021.100205.

Carew, R.M., Iacoviello, F., Rando, C., Moss, R.M., Speller, R., French, J., *et al.* (2022) A multi-method assessment of 3D printed micromorphological osteological features. *International Journal of Legal Medicine*, 1–16.

Carew, R.M. and Errickson, D. (2020) An overview of 3D printing in forensic science: The tangible third-dimension. *Journal of Forensic Sciences*, **65**(5), 1752–1760. https://doi.org/10.1111/1556-4029.14442.

Cattaneo, C. (2007) Forensic anthropology: Developments of a classical discipline in the new millennium. *Forensic Science International*, **165**(2–3), 185–193. https://doi.org/10.1016/j.forsciint.2006.05.018.

Christensen, A.M., Passalacqua, N.V., and Bartelink, E.J. (2014) Medicolegal significance. In: *Forensic Anthropology: Current Methods and Practice* (eds. A.M. Christensen, N.V. Passalacqua, and E.J. Bartelink). Academic Press, Oxford, UK, pp. 91–117.

Collings, A.J. and Brown, K. (2020) Reconstruction and physical fit analysis of fragmented skeletal remains using 3D imaging and printing. *Forensic Science International: Reports*. https://doi.org/10.1016/j.fsir.2020.100114.

Cummaudo, M., Raffone, C., Cappella, A., Márquez-Grant, N., and Cattaneo, C. (2020) Histomorphometric analysis of the variability of the human skeleton: Forensic implications. *Legal Medicine (Tokyo)*, **45**, 101711. https://doi.org/10.1016/j.legalmed.2020.101711.

de Boer, H.H., Roberts, J., Delabarde, T., Mundorff, A.Z., and Blau, S. (2020) Disaster victim identification operations with fragmented, burnt, or commingled remains: Experience-based recommendations. *Forensic Science Research*, **5**(3), 191–201. https://doi.org/10.1080/20961790.2020.1751385.

Dennis, J.C., Ungar, P.S., Teaford, M.F., and Glander, K.E. (2004) Dental topography and molar wear in Alouatta Palliata from Costa Rica. *American Journal of Physical Anthropology*, **125**, 152–161. https://onlinelibrary.wiley.com/doi/10.1002/ajpa.10379.

du Plessis, A., Broeckhoven, C., Guelpa, A., and Le Roux, S.G. (2017) Laboratory X-ray micro-computer tomography: A user guideline for biological samples. *Gigascience*, **6**(6), 1–11. https://www.ncbi.nlm.nih.gov/pmc/articles/PMC5449646/pdf/gix027.pdf.

Edwards, J. and Rogers, T. (2018) The accuracy and applicability of 3D modeling and printing blunt force cranial injuries. *Journal of Forensic Sciences*, **63**(3), 683–691. https://doi.org/10.1111/1556-4029.13627.

Ellingham, S.T., Thompson, T.J., and Islam, M. (2018) Scanning Electron Microscopy-Energy-Dispersive X-Ray (SEM/EDX): A rapid diagnostic tool to aid the identification of burnt bone and contested cremains. *Journal of Forensic Sciences*, **63**(2), 504–510. https://doi.org/10.1111/1556-4029.13541.

Errickson, D. (2016) *From Crime Scene to Court: The Application of 3D Surface Digitisation in the Forensic Anthropological Context*. Thesis.

Errickson, D., Thompson, T.J., and Rankin, B.W. (2014) The application of 3D visualization of osteological trauma for the courtroom: A critical review. *Journal of Forensic Radiology and Imaging*, **2**(3), 132–137. https://doi.org/10.1016/j.jofri.2014.04.002.

Errickson, D., Grueso, I., Griffith, S.J., Setchell, J.M., Thompson, T.J.U., Thompson, C.E.L., *et al.* (2017) Towards a best practice for the use of active non-contact surface scanning to record human skeletal remains from archaeological contexts. *International Journal of Osteoarchaeology*, **27**(4), 650–661. https://doi.org/10.1002/oa.2587.

Errickson, D., Fawcett, H., Thompson, T.J.U., and Campbell, A. (2019) The effect of different imaging techniques for the visualisation of evidence in court on jury comprehension. *International Journal of Legal Medicine*, **134**, 1–5. https://doi.org/10.1007/s00414-019-02221-y.

Fernández-Jalvo, Y., Tormo, L., Andrews, P., and Marin-Monfort, M.D. (2018) Taphonomy of burnt bones from Wonderwerk Cave (South Africa). *Quaternary International*, **495**, 19–29. https://doi.org/10.1016/j.quaint.2018.05.028.

Franklin, D., Swift, L., and Flavel, A. (2016) "Virtual anthropology" and radiographic imaging in the Forensic Medical Sciences. *Egyptian Journal of Forensic Sciences*, **6**(2), 31–43. https://doi.org/10.1016/j.ejfs.2016.05.011.

Green, H., Jabez, J., and Nelson, J. (2019) Optimizing parameters for the use of alternate light sources in detecting fragmentary bones: A pilot study. *Australian Journal of Forensic Sciences*, **51**(supl), S201–S204. https://doi.org/10.1080/00450618.2019.1571104.

Griffith, S.J. and Thompson, C.E.L. (2017). The use of laser scanning for visualization and quantification of abrasion on water-submerged bone. In: *Human Remains: Another Dimension* (eds. T. Thompson and D. Errickson). Elsevier, London, UK, pp. 103–122.

Harvig, L. and Lynnerup, N. (2013) On the volume of cremated remains – A comparative study of archaeologically recovered cremated bone volume as measured manually and assessed by Computed Tomography and by Stereology. *Journal of Archaeological Science*, **40**(6), 2713–2722. https://doi.org/10.1016/j.jas.2013.01.024.

Jani, G., Johnson, A., Parekh, U., Thompson, T., and Pandey, A. (2020) Effective approaches to three-dimensional digital reconstruction of fragmented human skeletal remains using laser surface scanning. *Forensic Science International*, **2**, 215–223. https://doi.org/10.1016/j.fsisyn.2020.07.002.

Komar, D.A., Davy-Jow, S., and Decker, S.J. (2012) The use of a 3-D laser scanner to document ephemeral evidence at crime scenes and postmortem examinations. *Journal of Forensic Sciences*, **57**(1), 188–191. https://doi.org/10.1111/j.1556-4029.2011.01915.x.

Kuzminsky, S.C. and Gardiner, M.S. (2012) Three-dimensional laser scanning: Potential uses for museum conservation and scientific research. *Journal of Archaeological Science*, **39**(8), 2744–2751. https://doi.org/10.1016/j.jas.2012.04.020.

Mackinnon, G. and Mundorff, A. (2006) The World Trade Center, September 11, 2001. In: *Forensic Human Identification*, 1st edn. (eds. T. Thompson and S. Black). CRC Press, Boca Raton, FL, pp. 485–499.

Mallison, H. (2011). Digitizing methods for paleontology: Applications, benefits and limitations. In: *Computational Paleontology* (ed. A.M.T. Elewa). Springer, Berlin, Germany, pp. 7–43.

March, J., Schofield, D., Evison, M., and Woodford, N. (2004) Three-dimensional computer visualization of forensic pathology data. *American Journal of Forensic Medicine*, **25**(1), 60–70. https://doi.org/10.1097/01.paf.0000113863.69360.42.

McKinnon, M., Henneberg, M., Simpson, E., and Higgins, D. (2021) Effects of thermal insult on bone tissue as observed by micro computed tomography. *Forensic Imaging*, **24**. https://doi.org/10.1016/j.fri.2021.200437.

Morgan, B., Ford, A.L., and Smith, M.J. (2019) Standard methods for creating digital skeletal models using structure-from-motion photogrammetry. *American Journal of Physical Anthropology*, **169**(1), 152–160. https://doi.org/10.1002/ajpa.23803.

Newman, S.E. (2015) Applications of reflectance transformation imaging (RTI) to the study of bone surface modifications. *Journal of Archaeological Science*, **53**, 536–549.

O'Donnell, C., Iino, M., Mansharan, K., Leditscke, J. and Woodford, N. (2011) Contribution of postmortem multidetector CT scanning to identification of the deceased in a mass disaster: Experience gained from the 2009 Victorian bushfires. *Forensic Science International*, **205**(1–3), 15–28. https://doi.org/10.1016/j.forsciint.2010.05.026.

Platt, R. (2005) *Forensics*. Kingfisher publications, Boston, MA.

Redsicker, D. (2000) *The Practical Methodology of Forensic Photography*. CRC Press, Endicott, NY.

Rutty, G.N., Biggs, M.J., Brough, A., Morgan, B., Webster, P., Heathcote, A., *et al.* (2019) Remote post-mortem radiology reporting in disaster victim identification: Experience gained in the 2017 Grenfell Tower disaster. *International Journal of Legal Medicine*. https://doi.org/10.1007/s00414-019-02109-x.

Sandholzer, M.A., Baron, K., Heimel, P., and Metscher, B.D. (2014) Volume analysis of heat-induced cracks in human molars: A preliminary study. *Journal of Forensic Dental Sciences*, **6**(2), 139–144. https://doi.org/10.4103/0975-1475.132545.

Schweitzer, W., Röhrich, E., Schaepman, M., Thali, M.J., and Ebert, L. (2013) Aspects of 3D surface scanner performance for post-mortem skin documentation in forensic medicine using rigid benchmark objects. *Journal of Forensic Radiology and Imaging*, **1**(4), 167–175. https://doi.org/10.1016/j.jofri.2013.06.001.

Shamata, A. and Thompson, T. (2018) Documentation and analysis of traumatic injuries in clinical forensic medicine involving structured light three-dimensional surface scanning versus photography. *Journal of Forensic and Legal Medicine*, **58**, 93–100. https://doi.org/10.1016/j.jflm.2018.05.004.

Shamata, A. and Thompson, T. (2020) Determining the effectiveness of noncontact three-dimensional surface scanning for the assessment of open injuries. *Journal of Forensic Sciences*, **65**(2), 627–635. https://doi.org/10.1111/1556-4029.14205.

Shearer, B.M., Sholts, S.B., Garvin, H.M., and Wärmländer, S.K. (2012) Sexual dimorphism in human browridge volume measured from 3D models of dry crania: A new digital morphometrics approach. *Forensic Science International*, **222**(1–3), 400.e1–400.e5. https://doi.org/10.1016/j.forsciint.2012.06.013.

Thali, M.J., Braun, M., Brüschweiler, W., and Dirnhofer, R. (2000) Matching tire tracks on the head using forensic photogrammetry. *Forensic Science International*, **113**, 281–287. https://doi.org/10.1016/s0379-0738(00)00234-6.

Thali, M.J., Yen, K., Plattner, T., Schweitzer, W., Vock, P., Ozdoba, C., *et al.* (2002) Charred body: Virtual autopsy with multi-slice computed tomography and magnetic resonance imaging. *Journal of Forensic Sciences*, **47**(6), 1326–1331. https://doi.org/10.1520/JFS15569J.

Thompson, T. (2017). Context. In: *Human Remains: Another Dimension* (eds. T. Thompson and D. Errickson). Elsevier, London, UK, pp. 1–6.

Thompson, T.J. and Chudek, J.A. (2007) A novel approach to the visualisation of heat-induced structural change in bone. *Science & Justice : Journal of the Forensic Science Society*, **47**(2), 99–104. https://doi.org/10.1016/j.scijus.2006.05.002.

Urbanová, P., Hejna, P., and Jurda, M. (2015) Testing photogrammetry-based techniques for three-dimensional surface documentation in forensic pathology. *Forensic Science International*, **250**, 77–86.

Végh, E.I., Czermak, A., Márquez-Grant, N., and Schulting, R.J. (2021) Assessing the reliability of microbial bioerosion features in burnt bones: A novel approach using feature-labelling in histotaphonomical analysis. *Journal of Archaeological Science: Reports*, 37. https://doi.org/10.1016/j.jasrep.2021.102906.

Villa, C., Flies, M.J., and Jacobsen, C. (2018) Forensic 3D documentation of bodies: Simple and fast procedure for combining CT scanning with external photogrammetry data. *Journal of Forensic Radiology and Imaging*, **12**, e2–e7. https://doi.org/10.1016/j.jofri.2017.08.003.

Waltenberger, L. and Schutkowski, H. (2017) Effects of heat on cut mark characteristics. *Forensic Science International*, **271**, 49–58. https://doi.org/10.1016/j.forsciint.2016.12.018.

Weber, G.W. (2015) Virtual anthropology. *American Journal of Physical Anthropology*, **156**(Suppl 59), 22–42. https://doi.org/10.1002/ajpa.22658.

Wilson, A.S., Holland, A.D., and Sparrow, T. (2017) Laser scanning of skeletal pathological conditions. In: *Human Remains: Another Dimension* (eds. T. Thompson and D. Errickson). Elsevier, London, UK, pp. 123–134.

Zeng, L., Yuan, F., Song, D., and Zhang, R. (1999) A two-beam laser triangulation for measuring the position of a moving object. *Optics and Lasers in Engineering*, **31**(6), 445–453. https://doi.org/10.1016/S0143-8166(99)00043-3.

CHAPTER 17

The First Reference Collection for the Research of Burnt Human Skeletal Remains Stemming from the 21st Century Identified Skeletal Collection (Portugal)

David Gonçalves[1,2,3], PhD; Calil Makhoul[2,4], MSc; Maria Teresa Ferreira[2,3], PhD and Eugénia Cunha[2,5], PhD, C-FASE

[1] *Archaeosciences Laboratory, Directorate General for Cultural Heritage (LARC/CIBIO/InBIO), Calçada do Mirante à Ajuda n.º 10A 1300-418 Lisbon, Portugal*

[2] *University of Coimbra, Centre for Functional Ecology, Laboratory of Forensic Anthropology, Department of Life Sciences, Calçada Martim de Freitas, 3000-456 Coimbra, Portugal*

[3] *Research Centre for Anthropology and Health (CIAS), University of Coimbra, Portugal*

[4] *Molecular Physical Chemistry R&D Unit, Department of Chemistry, University of Coimbra, Portugal*

[5] *National Institute of Legal Medicine and Forensic Sciences, Lisbon, Portugal*

17.1 Introduction

17.1.1 The Challenge Posed by Burnt Skeletal Remains

What should be done with a problem? Usually, one of two different things. It can either be ignored to proceed with business as usual or it can be studied critically to try to solve it. Scientists usually take the second option. However, even though it sounds like the right thing to do, some problems remain unsolved despite all attempts to resolve them. That seems to be the case with burnt human skeletal remains from an anthropological point of view. Heat exposure causes a myriad of bone and teeth changes, with a large spectrum of possibilities that end up taking researchers down weak, dead-end interpretations.

Scientists have addressed the problem encompassing the analysis of these kinds of remains for more than a century (e.g. Bemis, 1850; Lepkowski and Wachholtz, 1903; Welinder, 1908), so it would be somewhat expected that by now more would be known and understood about how heat exposure affects skeletal

Burnt Human Remains: Recovery, Analysis, and Interpretation, First Edition. Edited by Sarah Ellingham, Joe Adserias-Garriga, Sara C. Zapico and Douglas H. Ubelaker.

remains. That is not the case, however, and the most compelling demonstration of that is that anthropologists are quite unable to predict exactly what changes will occur to bones and teeth when subjected to heat. Of course, some trends can be pointed out. Bones will become whitish if aerobically burnt at very high temperatures (Bonucci and Graziani, 1975; Shipman *et al.*, 1984; Etxeberria, 1994; Walker *et al.*, 2008; Krap *et al.*, 2019). Tooth cementum annulations will overlap each other when exposed to heat (Oliveira-Santos *et al.*, 2017). Metric changes will affect both bones and teeth (Thompson, 2005; Gouveia *et al.*, 2017; Ellingham and Sandholzer, 2020). However, it has been shown time and again that bones and teeth do not always react to heat exposure as expected. And when they do, it is only because the prediction is broad enough to allow for some accuracy.

The truth is that anthropologists are mostly unable to predict exactly what precise shades will be displayed by burnt bones. Failure will most probably result from any forecast about how many tooth cementum annulations will become overlapped (Oliveira-Santos *et al.*, 2017) and experts will not be able to anticipate the precise metric shrinkage or expansion experienced by bones and teeth (Gonçalves *et al.*, 2020). All this seems to be impossible even when the exact burn conditions are known. So, the only accurate prediction that can be expected from skeletal remains exposed to heat is that they will puzzle any forensic anthropologist confronted with them.

Examples of the huge spectrum of heat-induced variability are numerous. Macroscopic features are the most noticeable and include metric change, which can range from slight expansions in bone (Bradtmiller and Buikstra, 1984; Thompson, 2005) and apparent expansion in enamel (Godinho *et al.*, 2019), to extreme shrinkages in bones (Figures 17.1 and 17.2) and dental cementum and dentin, which can be up to 40% (Huxley and Kósa, 1999; Thompson, 2005; Gonçalves *et al.*, 2020). Bone warping can also manifest itself in an extremely variable fashion. It may be almost unnoticeable or quite drastic (Figures 17.1 and 17.2) and usually manifests itself differentially within the skeleton. Heat-induced fractures are other usual features present at both the macro- and microscopic scales (Holden *et al.*, 1995; Herrmann and Bennett, 1999; Symes *et al.*, 2012; Godinho *et al.*, 2019). All these heat-induced features add a confounding effect to anthropological analyses (Dokladal, 1962; van Vark, 1974; Buikstra and Swegle, 1989; Bohnert *et al.*, 1997; Campbell and Fairgrieve, 2011; Gonçalves, 2011; Gonçalves *et al.*, 2015; Oliveira-Santos *et al.*, 2017; Rodrigues *et al.*, 2020), thus undermining any inference about the biological profile or the circumstances of death. Many other bone and teeth changes that are a consequence of heat exposure could be listed here: mass loss; color changes; porosity changes; microstructural changes, namely crystallinity changes; and composition changes. Randomness appears to be a characteristic of all of them. Several papers have been written about this and can be consulted to understand this topic in greater detail (e.g. Warren and Maples, 1997; Bass and Jantz, 2004; Thompson, 2004; Munro *et al.*, 2007; Piga *et al.*, 2008; Thompson *et al.*, 2009; Lebon *et al.*, 2010;

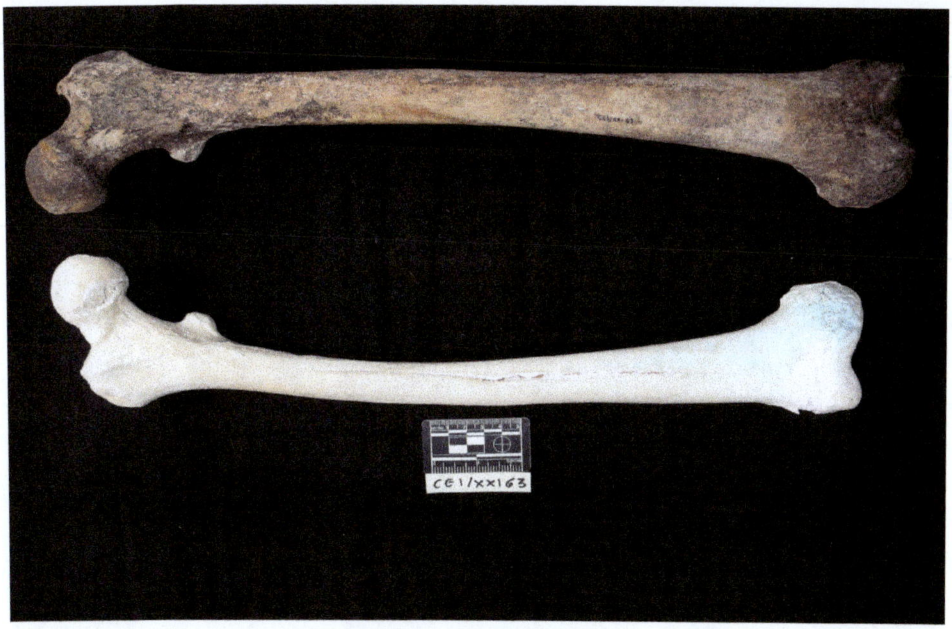

Figure 17.1 Unburnt left femur and right antimere experimentally burnt at 900°C (after a four-hour burn) of individual CEI/XXI_63, a male, 64 years old at the time of death. Heat-induced shrinkage, warping, fractures, and changes in color are clearly observed.

Snoeck *et al.*, 2014; Ellingham *et al.*, 2015; Marques *et al.*, 2016). However, despite all efforts, the latest techniques need further refinement and forensic anthropologists have little guarantee that solid conclusions can be obtained from the analysis of burnt human skeletal remains.

17.1.2 Changing the Paradigm

The bewilderment faced by anthropologists examining burnt skeletal remains appears to be mainly restricted to this kind of material. The analysis of unburnt bones and teeth, although potentially presenting other challenging taphonomic-related changes, is generally far from being affected by the systematic obstacles linked to the examination of burnt skeletal remains. The anthropological practice became increasingly standardized over the years and is mainly characterized by very solid, consistent, and reliable methods and techniques. Therefore, the gap in terms of reliability between the methodological standards used for the two kinds of remains is quite large and has not narrowed as much as needed to make the examination of burnt skeletal remains more reliable. In reality, no anthropological standards for the latter have widespread use (Gonçalves and Pires, 2017), although some efforts have been made toward that end (Gómez Bellard, 1996; Duday *et al.*, 2000; McKinley, 2004; Fairgrieve, 2008).

The contrasting abilities involved in the analysis of unburnt and burnt human skeletal remains makes sense given the usual different challenges posed by each.

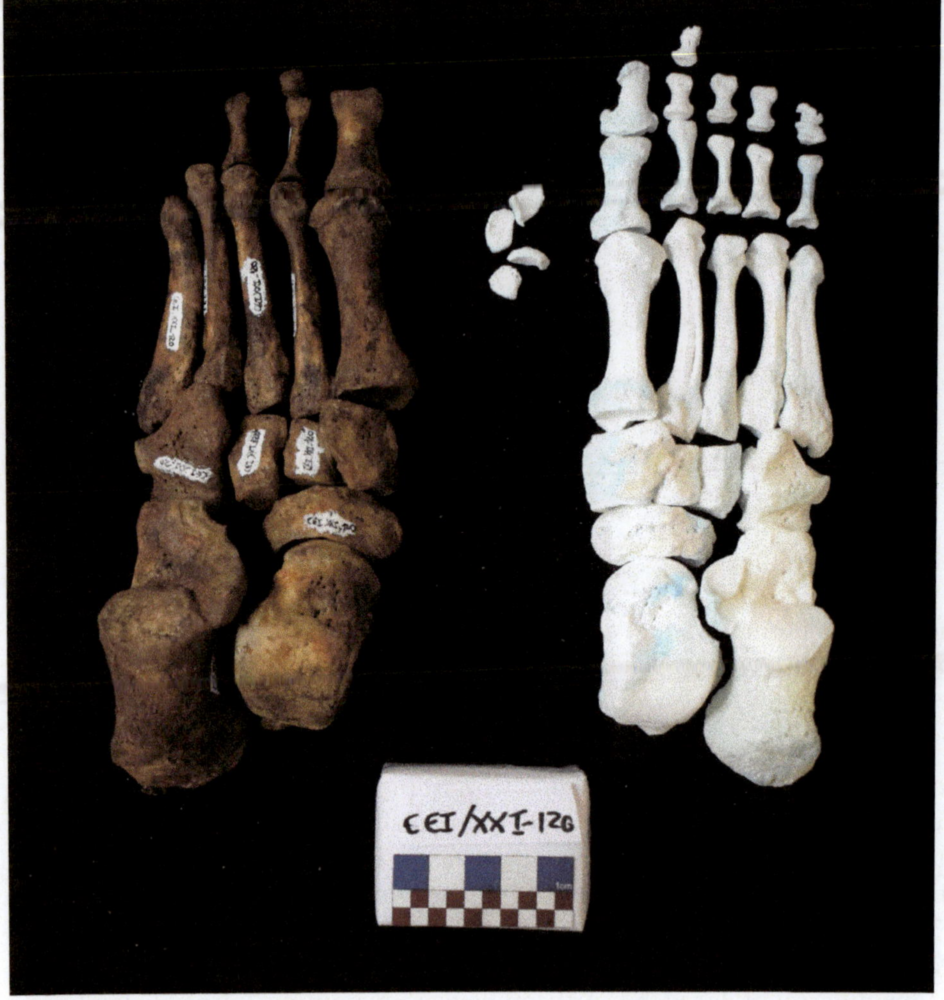

Figure 17.2 Unburnt left foot and right antimeres experimentally burnt at 800°C (after a three-hour burn) of individual CEI/XXI_120, a male, 81 years old at the time of death. Heat-induced shrinkage, fractures, and changes in color are clearly observed. Heat-induced warping is unnoticeable in most bones.

However, it is nonetheless surprising to some extent that, after more than 170 years since the first reported forensic case involving burnt skeletal remains, the Parkman-Webster murder case (Bemis, 1850; Snow, 1982), the big difference between the inference potential of the two kinds of approaches still remains. One may wonder why that is still the case.

Looking back at what has been the route to consistency regarding the analysis of both unburnt and burnt skeletal remains, one item seems to be missing from the latter: reference collections. For more than two centuries now, researchers worldwide have made a substantial effort to document the skeletal variability of the modern human species (Blumenbach, 1776; Erickson, 1997). The amassment of reference collections of human skeletons from known individuals (i.e. for which some personal details are known) led to the documentation of huge amounts of data about skeletal development, metamorphosis, degeneration, and taphonomy, providing critical insight about age at death, sex, stature, ancestry, pathology, trauma, and post-depositional impact, among other things. Numerous variables have been extensively studied and linked to skeletal features, giving researchers the opportunity to make solid predictions about unknown individuals just by examining their bones and teeth. Thanks to this approach, great trust is placed today on inferences obtained from human skeletal remains and forensic investigations rely on the expertise of forensic anthropologists to aid in positive identification and the reconstruction of circumstances of death (White *et al.*, 2015).

For obvious reasons, the "reference collection" route has not been, to a general extent, taken to boost the anthropologists' ability to draw information from burnt skeletal remains. The level of destruction to the body caused by commercial cremation has, to some degree, prevented researchers from "recruiting" cremated skeletons of known individuals to better understand them. To the authors' knowledge, the only exception has been the William M. Bass Donated Skeletal Collection, which comprises several non-pulverized cremated remains. This is a rare and priceless resource, putting scientists on the right track to improve methodological approaches concerning burnt skeletal remains. More is needed though. The cremation environment is very dynamic and eventful. Remains are sometimes handled by the operator to accelerate the removal of soft tissues (McKinley, 1994a). This leads to additional destruction of the remains.

Even when manual handling is not taking place, skeletal remains move around quite a bit during the cremation process due to the normal motions of the burning body. For instance, the pugilistic posture will elevate the hands and arms from the axial skeleton (Symes *et al.*, 2008, 2012). When heat-induced disarticulation finally occurs, frail burnt bones usually fall from pronounced heights potentially causing additional damage to them and to those below. This damage is further extended by some cremation chambers which comprise platforms at different heights, thus causing the remains to fall from one platform to the one below. Besides this, material that is not human is often present during the cremation, either due to the presence of wood and synthetic materials from the coffin, or to other objects accompanying the body, such as metal prosthetics, gold teeth, copper intrauterine devices, or pacemakers. Besides these materials becoming at times aggregated to the bones, they also promote chemical exchanges that are different from those that would occur if only skeletal materials were involved.

Deeper knowledge of burnt bones and teeth can be further obtained from experimental burns involving isolated and well-controlled variables. The burn setting must be prepared to ensure that a minimum number of factors (e.g. heat, oxygen, force of gravity) alter and cause damage to the bones and teeth, thus maximizing their preservation. Also, the exact burn dynamics need to be controlled and monitored so that variables such as temperature, burn duration, and heat increment can be tested and eventually linked to heat-induced changes. Although there is much to offer in terms of research by remains resulting from commercial cremations, for example regarding bone and teeth heat-induced changes in the presence of soft tissues, the described requirements cannot, unfortunately, be entirely guaranteed under those circumstances. Therefore, experimental research involving the burning of human skeletal remains appears to be an optimal way to amass a reference collection of this nature. For this reason, skeletons from the 21st Century Identified Skeletal Collection (CEI/XXI) housed at the Laboratory of Forensic Anthropology of the University of Coimbra (Ferreira *et al.*, 2014, 2020) are being experimentally burnt under controlled conditions. These constitute the first reference collection of this kind to enhance research in burnt human skeletal remains.

A collection of experimentally burnt skeletons raises ethical questions as, to be fair, do all human reference collections. Indeed, this issue is so sensitive that most researchers are bound to develop their research on less restrictive non-human animal skeletal remains, although their focus is on human skeletal remains. However, it is becoming increasingly clear that faunal skeletal remains constitute a limited proxy for humans. Humans have anatomies, genetic material, bone type distributions, bone architectures, bone and teeth compositions, and (possibly) bone microstructures that are different from the usual animals used as proxies (e.g. cattle, pigs, sheep, goat, deer, horse). As a result, it is no wonder that there are often doubts regarding the extrapolation of results obtained on them compared to their human counterparts (Martiniaková *et al.*, 2006; Mulhern and Ubelaker, 2012; Pfeiffer and Pinto, 2012; Gonçalves *et al.*, 2018b). General trends about the impact of heat exposure on the skeleton may indeed be obtained in this fashion, but the level of resolution must be higher to allow for the development of refined methodological approaches able to confer consistency and reliability to the examination of burnt human skeletal remains. Decades of research based on faunal proxies has failed to do so and no major breakthroughs are foreseeable now based on this approach being adopted, because extrapolability will always be debatable. Research carried out directly on human skeletal remains is the next step to guarantee more reliable inferences directly obtained by anthropologists.

The first assemblage of experimentally burnt identified human skeletons is being amassed at the University of Coimbra (more details are given in Section 17.1.3). It is composed of dry skeletons, thus reflecting only one slice of the entire spectrum involving the burning of human remains. Soft tissues are here left out of the picture since the skeletons are already free from them when they are brought to the Laboratory of Forensic Anthropology. However, their research value is not diminished by this fact since, as we stated above, controlled experiments to better understand the effect of heat on bones and teeth must be undertaken under minimal potential variables. Bones are composite materials whose properties must first be tested and documented before adding another variable such as soft tissues. This is common practice regarding all kinds of materials. To make an analogy with the study of a chemical element, the physical properties of iron (e.g. melting point or boiling point) are documented by testing iron alone. No other materials are added to the equation since they would constitute a confounding effect. The same must be done with bones and teeth. A baseline must be obtained for these composite materials before, step by step, studying other potential variables to the experiments, such as soft tissues.

In addition, not all research topics require the presence of soft tissues. For example, creating a baseline for heat-induced color changes according to heat increment must necessarily be done on dry bones and that has been the case for multiple previous researches (Shipman *et al.*, 1984; Etxeberria, 1994; Walker *et al.*, 2008; Wahl, 2008; Krap *et al.*, 2019). The presence of soft tissues would prevent anthropologists from carrying out a correct assessment because of their protective effect towards bone. The temperature affecting the bone would clearly be lower than the one registered by the thermocouple. It goes without saying that rare and precious work done on fleshed human cadavers (as is, for example, done by the San Luis Obispo County Fire Investigation Strike Team: SLOFIST, Inc.: https://www.slofist.org) is paramount in the advancement of the field. However, potential research does not end there. Dry bone research has a lot to offer also. As was explained earlier in this section, to comprehensively document the stages of alteration of bones and teeth, research must be in isolation from soft tissues.

A common criticism of experimental research involving the controlled burning of skeletal remains by using a furnace is that it fails to replicate "real cases." This is true for most cases, but the use of furnaces in forensic cases, some involving genocide, has also been reported in the literature (Kennedy, 1996; Mailänder, 2014; van Pelt, 2014), as was the case for the infamous Parkman-Webster case (Bemis, 1850; Snow, 1982). The concealment and destruction of bodies by using a furnace is certainly one of the most efficient ways of discarding a body and is often found to be the method of choice of murderers (Symes *et al.*, 2012). It is often reported by the media as the method of disposal used in crime cases, as a simple Google search will reveal. It is also recurrently used in popular TV shows such as "Ozark" and "Bones," thus showing that this kind of body disposal is present in people's imagination. However, case studies involving human remains processed at furnaces are rarely reported in scientific papers, which is surprising. Possibly, discarding bodies by using furnaces is so efficient that it hinders forensic investigations, making the success rate of identification of such cases so low. If that is indeed the case, it means that forensic anthropologists need to develop their skills to the next level to successfully address such cases.

No experimental set-up can replicate all "real cases," nor is it supposed to. To overcome the technical challenges posed by burnt human skeletal remains, a multi-stage and multi-approach effort must be undertaken. The experimentally burnt skeletons of the CEI/XXI Collection constitute one contribution, among others, to the advancement of the field and its amassing is carried out under the clear notion that no resource can respond to all scenarios and challenges posed by burnt human skeletal remains.

17.1.3 The 21st Century Identified Skeletal Collection

The CEI/XXI Collection is composed of 302 adult skeletons of both sexes, and is housed at the Laboratory of Forensic Anthropology, University of Coimbra (UC). Since its first presentation to the scientific community (Ferreira *et al.*, 2014), this collection has grown in the number of skeletons and new data is now available (Ferreira *et al.*, 2020). The skeletal remains are identified in terms of sex and age at death; all the individuals had Portuguese nationality. The CEI/XXI collection comprises skeletons donated to the UC by the municipality of Santarém (responsible for the public cemetery where they were inhumed) and their collection and curation are covered by the Portuguese legal framework. After a three-year burial, Portuguese law allows non-judicial exhumations (Decreto-Lei no. 411/98) so that the remains may be moved to a different location (e.g. another cemetery or a private family grave). This is often carried out in cemeteries with little space that frequently require the reutilization of graves. If, after exhumation, the corpse still displays soft tissues (which is the most common scenario in Portuguese cemeteries after only three years of burial), the grave is covered again and can be reopened only after two years. Non-judicial exhumations can only happen if the corpse is skeletonized (Ferreira and Cunha, 2013). Moreover, the constitution of this collection and the investigations carried out have received a positive legal decision from the Ethics Committee of the Faculty of Medicine of the University of Coimbra (reference number: CE_026.2016) (Ferreira *et al.*, 2020).

As mentioned in the previous paragraph, the collection consists only of adult individuals, mostly elderly, being representative of the adult Portuguese population mortality curve. The female individuals (n = 162; 53.64%) died at ages ranging from 28 to 101 years old (mean: 81.19; S.D.: 12.89), while males (n = 140; 46.36%) were aged between 25 and 96 years old at time of death (mean: 73.20; S.D.: 15.61). The CEI/XXI individuals died between 1982 and 2012 and were exhumed between 1999 and 2016 (Ferreira *et al.*, 2020). The bone representation in each skeleton is generally good, with only a few absent bones (usually corresponding to several hand bones), and the skeletal preservation is reasonable, with most of the skulls and long bones fully preserved (Ferreira *et al.*, 2020).

Like most identified collections, this one is also an excellent educational and scientific resource. Since the individuals died recently, this collection is an asset for the development of forensic anthropology in Portugal; its skeletons being more representative of the variability of the current cases that reach the forensic anthropologist at the autopsy table. Some of the skeletons are used in classes of the master's and doctoral courses, namely in subjects discussing forensic taphonomy, biological profile, trauma analysis, and the identification process in forensic anthropology. This enriches students' knowledge and helps them acquire a solid education. Moreover, several graduate and undergraduate students will have done internships at the Laboratory of Forensic Anthropology, working with this collection. Since the first studies back in 2009 (Curate, 2011; Ferreira, 2012), several investigations have been carried out on the collection, both within the scope of master's and doctoral theses (from students at the University of Coimbra, but also from other Portuguese and foreign institutions), as well as from other research projects such as the HOT project (Research Project of the CEI/XXI Burnt Skeletons), which has the objectives of improving our understanding of heat-induced changes to bone and teeth, and improving analytical methods that are specific to burnt skeletal remains. This umbrella project has so far been successful at attracting funding (e.g. SFRH/BPD/84268/2012; PTDC/IVC-ANT/1201/2014 & POCI-01-0145-FEDER-016766). This prolific scientific production can be consulted in Ferreira *et al.* (2020) and it is also important to highlight that some of these works have promoted the development of open-source web-based applications (accessed at http://www.osteomics.com). The compilation of the collection is the result of a collaborative task involving the Research Centre for Anthropology and Health, the Centre for Functional Ecology (which hosts the Laboratory of Forensic Anthropology), and the Directorate-General for Cultural Heritage. These and two other institutions (the Molecular Physical Chemistry R&D Unit and the ISIS Neutron and Muon Source) are the main research units involved in the investigation carried out on the collection.

17.1.4 Preparing the Skeletons

A preparation protocol of the experimentally burnt skeletons is systematically performed every time a new skeleton is added to the collection. This process is crucial to record comprehensive information before the skeleton is exposed to specific thermal conditions. It is summarized in Figure 17.3.

17.1.4.1 Skeleton Selection

Each skeleton of the CEI/XXI collection is placed inside individualized containers (Figure 17.4), but additional bones from other skeletons are sometimes present due to commingling during their inhumation period at the cemetery. Therefore, commingled skeletons do not undergo a burning process as this is one of the exclusion criteria. Besides that, other criteria are taken into consideration. The skeleton cannot present evidence of uncommon pathologies, trauma, medical procedures, and rare individualizing factors of some other nature. The skeletons selected for experimental burning have a high preservation index and are all above 60 years old; most are in fact more than 70 years old. As mentioned in Section 17.1.3, the collection is mainly composed of aged individuals, so younger ones are not eligible for burning as well.

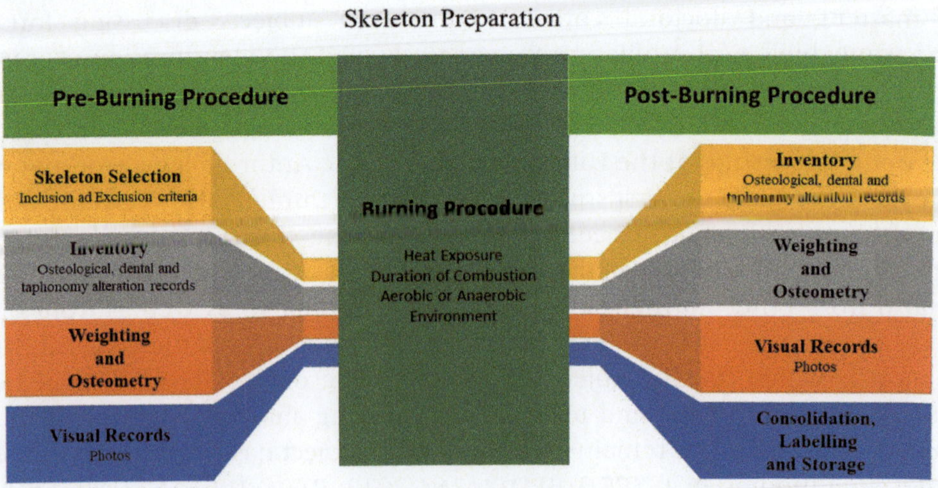

Figure 17.3 The diagram depicts a summary of the full process of skeleton preparation.

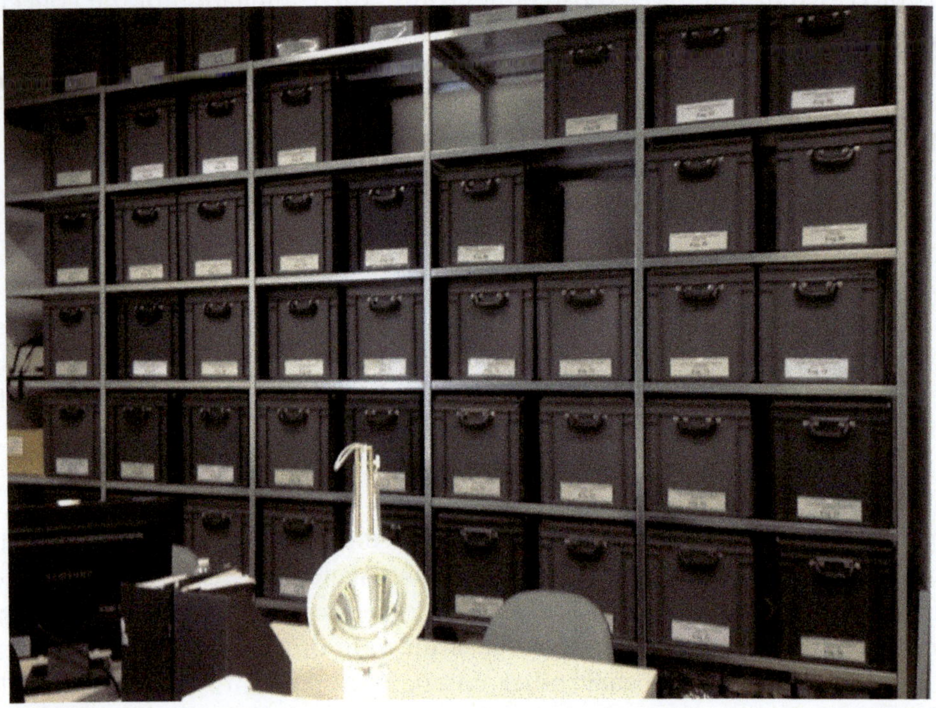

Figure 17.4 Containers of the CEI/XXI collection housed at the Laboratory of Forensic Anthropology.

17.1.4.2 Inventory and Record of Physical Properties

After being selected, an inventory of the skeleton is performed, recording all osteological and dental data (Smith, 1991; Buikstra and Ubelaker, 1994). The osteological data is recorded, based on the presence/absence and completion of each bone, and on its taphonomical alterations. Weights of all bones are recorded in a spreadsheet. Such data is relevant for the purpose of research about weight variation due to thermal alteration. The measurement of every bone is recorded according to Buikstra and Ubelaker (1994). Photos of the posterior and anterior anatomical views are taken for visual recording of the bones.

17.1.4.3 Burning Conditions

After the record of skeletal data, the next step is to experimentally burn the right bone antimeres. Only one of two antimeres is used so that an unburnt counterpart is available for future research. Until now, no complete skeleton has been exposed to thermal conditions. A small oven is used, which has a closed chamber that maintains equithermal exposure in the medium during the whole process. The oven is equipped with a type K probe (negative/nickel-aluminum, positive/nickel-chrome) following norm IEC 60584-2 which ensures quite precise temperature readings. The burning procedures adopted so far have varied greatly. Heat exposure ranged between 450°C and 1100°C. Its duration varied between 60 and 257 minutes. Both ventilated and non-ventilated conditions have been used. This wide variation provides better insight about the impact of heat-induced changes on bone.

After the burning process is completed and the antimeres under experiment are cooled down to room temperature, the inventory and the record of physical properties are again performed. The presence of any thermal alteration such as warping, fractures, color changes, and damage of the bone is recorded.

17.1.4.4 Post-burning Management

Due to their brittleness, bones are consolidated to allow their handling and ensure their preservation. The consolidation of each bone is done by using a 50% dilution of Primal SF-016 ER into ethanol. After the consolidation process is completed and bones dried, every bone, except for phalanges, is labeled with a pen marker in regions free of muscle attachments and joint surfaces. The experimentally burnt bones are stored in a container, placed onto polyurethane foam for protection against damage (Figure 17.5). This smaller container is then placed inside the larger container storing the remaining unburnt skeleton.

17.1.5 Composition of the Collection

The reference collection for the research of burnt human skeletal remains stemming from the CEI/XXI collection is composed of a total of 56 individuals (Table 17.1). The 32 female individuals (57.1%) present a mean age at death of 81.8 years (S.D.: 8.1), while the 24 males individuals (42.9%) had a mean age at death of 78.3 years (S.D.: 8.2). Therefore, although it is somewhat balanced in terms of sex distribution, this assemblage lacks young and middle-aged adults.

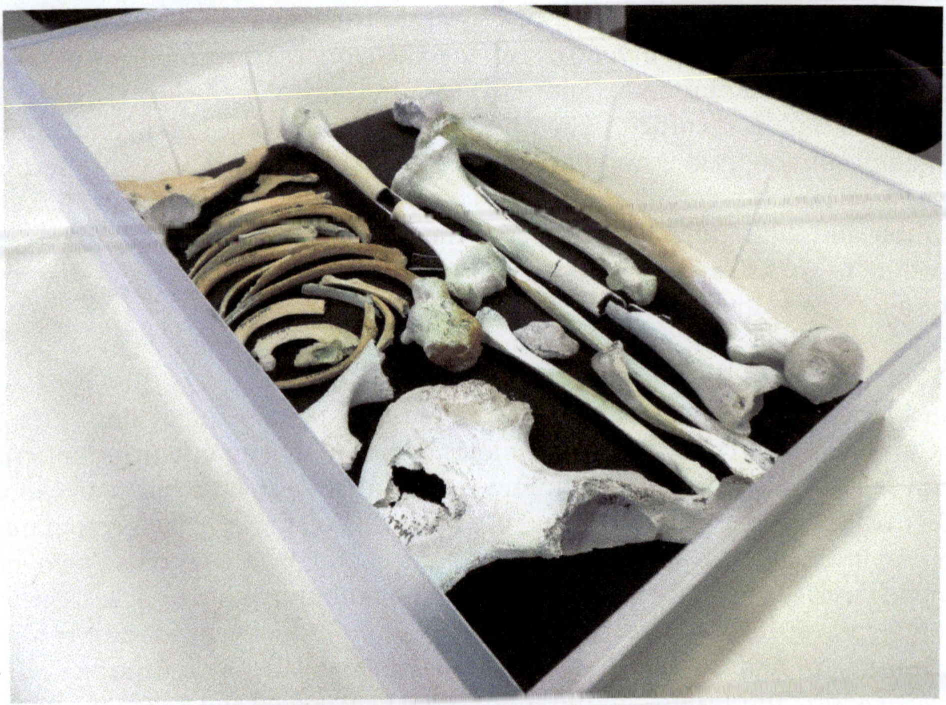

Figure 17.5 Burnt antimere of a skeleton stored in its container.

Table 17.1 Sex, age at death, and burn intensity of experimentally burnt skeletons of CEI/XXI (as of 27 January 2021).

Sex	n	Age at death	Maximum temperature (°C)	Duration (minutes)
Females	32	62–92	450–1100	90–257
Males	24	60–93	500–1050	60–257

The female skeletons were burnt at temperatures between 450°C and 1100°C, and the duration of the burning varied between 90 and 257 minutes. The male skeletons were burnt at temperatures between 500°C and 1050°C, and the duration of the burning varied between 60 and 257 minutes. The rate of heat increment ranged between 2.5°C and 9.2°C per minute for females from room temperature, while it varied between 2.5°C and 10.7°C in the male group.

17.2 Research Potential

The broad importance of this collection for the progress of research and the development of more consistent and reliable analytical methods for the anthropological examination of burnt human skeletal remains has been partially discussed in the introduction. However, it is also relevant to pinpoint some of the specific research topics that benefit directly from a collection such as this. The collection is still relatively small and the amount of experimentally burnt skeletons is far from what is commonly sought after for reference collections of known human individuals (Giraudi *et al.*, 1984; Hunt and Albanese, 2005; Cardoso, 2006; Cunha and Wasterlain, 2007; Dayal *et al.*, 2009). Predictably, the number of skeletons required to amass a collection that is representative of all possible burn configurations should be even higher than what is expected of a "normal" collection because the number of such possible configurations is limitless. Nonetheless, unprecedented research based on the collection is already underway.

One of the main focuses of research developed so far referred to the study of heat-induced microstructural changes in bone. This has been mainly composed of basic research to document how bone reacts to heat (Marques *et al.*, 2016; Piga *et al.*, 2016). Important information has been obtained from these kinds of studies, such as the confirmation of OH libration and OH stretching signals in bioapatite by inelastic neutron scattering (Marques *et al.*, 2016) and the description of hexagonal or polygonal large bone crystals of irregular edges by X-ray diffraction and transmission electron microscopy (Piga *et al.*, 2016). This, and other research about how heat exposure alters the microstructure and the composition of bones and teeth, increases knowledge regarding them.

Other research, more directed at practical applications, has also been carried out. Gonçalves *et al.* (2018a) tested the MassReg application to assess its accuracy in estimating the completeness of a human skeleton based on its mass. Pedrosa *et al.* (2020) explored the potential of vibrational spectroscopy, namely infrared analysis, for age-at-death estimation. Gonçalves *et al.* (2020) used the same technique to investigate the relationship between heat-induced microstructural changes and macroscopic metric changes to develop a method to estimate preburnt bone metric dimensions. Monteiro *et al.* (2020) have used dual-energy X-ray absorptiometry to document heat-induced changes in bone mineral density and assess how reliable osteodensitometric studies in burnt bones can be. Research using more traditional approaches has also been undertaken. Rodrigues *et al.* (2021) investigated how macroscopic heat-induced alterations – namely warping, metric changes, and fractures – affect the scoring of sexually dimorphic features used in the recommendations from Buikstra and Ubelaker (1994), Wasterlain (2000), Bruzek (2002), Gonçalves *et al.* (2013), and Curate *et al.* (2016).

There are many dilemmas for forensic anthropologists who are faced with burnt skeletal remains. The core of their duties, biological profiling, is especially impaired by heat-induced changes and research on this topic is, consequently, at the top of the list of priorities. It has been recurrently found that heat-induced changes affect the application of metric features but are somewhat innocuous to morphological diagnostic features (McKinley *et al.*, 2001; Fairgrieve, 2008; Gonçalves *et al.*, 2016; Thompson *et al.*, 2017). However, although the effect of heat exposure on metric features has indeed been often demonstrated (Dokladal, 1962; Gejvall, 1969;

Malinowski, 1969; Strzalko and Piontek, 1974; van Vark, 1974, 1975; Piontek, 1975, 1976; Herrmann, 1977; Rösing, 1977; Schutkowski, 1983; Schutkowski and Herrmann, 1983; Shipman *et al.*, 1984; Holck, 1986; Buikstra and Swegle, 1989; Wahl, 1996; van Vark *et al.*, 1996; Thompson, 2005; Gonçalves, 2011; Gonçalves *et al.*, 2013, 2015, 2020; Masotti *et al.*, 2013, 2019; Cavazzuti *et al.*, 2019), similar endeavors have rarely been undertaken in the case of morphological traits, the recent work of Veselka *et al.* (2021) being the only exception to our knowledge. Therefore, it appears that such long-held assumptions of the latter being rather immutable to heat-induced changes result merely from anthropologists' own perceptions of burnt skeletal remains. Prior to Veselka *et al.* (2021), to our knowledge, the only systematic study carried out was the recent work by Rodrigues *et al.* (2021). The results from this research indicate that the scenario is quite different from what has been assumed until now, since the scoring of sexually dimorphic morphological features before and after heat exposure presented considerable differences. This is not good news for anthropologists since it means that even the "safe haven" offered by morphological traits may be called into question; the paper by Veselka *et al.* (2021) suggests otherwise though, since the Falys-Prangle method provided promising results regarding age at death. These findings call for a more cautious approach to inferences made based on morphological features and reinforces the pressing need of a reference collection composed of experimentally burnt human skeletons.

More research, such as the one from Rodrigues *et al.* (2021), is needed so that a comprehensive portrait of the impact of heat exposure on skeletal remains can be obtained. The experimentally burnt skeletons from the CEI/XXI collection meet the conditions to investigate such matters since observations can be produced before and after the heat experiment. Since only one half of each skeleton is burnt, observations can also be carried out on the burnt antimere and compared with the unburnt antimere.

The study of large assemblages can help pinpoint usual trends such as the one observed for metric change, for which it has been clearly established that, at very high temperatures (usually higher than 600°C), bones tend to shrink (Shipman *et al.*, 1984; Buikstra and Swegle, 1989; Thompson, 2005; Gonçalves *et al.*, 2020). This is important information since it indicates that bones will become smaller and thus acquire more feminine metric dimensions. Inferences made about the sex of the individual must take this into account. It would be extremely useful to find specific trends for morphological features as well. For example, clear benefits would be obtained from knowing if the greater sciatic notch tends to become narrower, if the relief of the preauricular surface becomes smoother when exposed to heat, or if the porosity of the pubic symphysis increases. Documenting all these micro-phenomena may help predict them and this will be essential to develop analytical methods that are more adapted to burnt skeletal remains. Crossing that information with other variables such as age at death and sex is bound to bring additional advantages to such research in burnt skeletal remains.

This collection clearly benefits research on burnt human skeletal remains, but it is also relevant to discuss its limitations. As mentioned previously, skeletons are dry, so research focusing on topics for which soft tissues may be important cannot be undertaken. For example, investigation about the combustibility and burn patterns of the human body (Bohnert *et al.*, 1997; Symes *et al.*, 2008, 2014) cannot be replicated by using the experimentally burnt skeletons from the CEI/XXI Collection. The same can be said about the burn dynamics involved in our experimental conditions that do not reproduce those often seen in forensic settings. The latter frequently involve more on-and-off heat exposures (DeHaan, 2015) that are extremely difficult to investigate experimentally under strictly controlled conditions. Even the mere monitoring of such experiments in terms of bone heat exposure is quite challenging.

Another limitation of the collection is the fact that the skeletons have been subjected to an undeterminable amount of diagenetic change due to the inhumation period they have experienced, even though the latter had a short duration (6–7 years) for most skeletons. Although this has its own advantages, since it allows diagenetic studies to be carried out, it impedes investigations on unaltered bone. Of course, some problems may be counteracted, for example by removing exogenous carbonates with acetic acid (Snoeck *et al.*, 2014), but other issues are not as easily solved, as is the case of the potential increase of the crystallinity index (Stiner *et al.*, 2001). Therefore, research involving physical-chemical studies must take this limitation into account.

It can be argued that the above described situations are considered limitations only to a certain extent because no collection can reflect all possible variables. However, the current major drawback of the experimentally burnt skeletal assemblage is related to its very uneven age-at-death distribution. It closely reflects the skewed distribution of the CEI/XXI collection, which in turn reflects the mortality curves of the Portuguese population (Ferreira *et al.*, 2014, 2020). Only a very small portion of the population dies at younger ages. Therefore, this age-at-death distribution problem is difficult to overcome and, predictably, will not be easily solved in the coming years.

17.3 Final Comments

It is legitimate to ask how, realistically, will this collection change forensic anthropology's praxis regarding burnt skeletal remains. The authors feel confident that, although it is evident that not all problems will be solved by it, it is nevertheless a step in the right direction. For a long time, studies involving burnt human skeletal remains constituted only a small fraction of all bioanthropological work. During the twentieth century, few have demonstrated a systematic interest in these kinds of remains (e.g. Gejvall, 1969; Buikstra & Goldstein, 1973; Herrmann, 1976; Wahl, 1981; Schutkowski, 1983; McKinley, 1994b; van Vark *et al.*, 1996). Boosted by those resilient researchers, this field is currently experiencing a new wave of interest. This, added to the increasing investment on the application of more advanced techniques (e.g. vibrational spectroscopy and X-ray diffraction) and the eventual creation of reference collections of experimentally burnt skeletons, is a promising recipe to achieve new heights regarding the analysis of burnt skeletal remains.

Advanced techniques have been applied to burnt bones and teeth for a long time (e.g. Bonucci and Graziani, 1975; Harsanyi, 1975; Shipman *et al.*, 1984). However, this new wave has characteristics which set it apart from previous studies. The continuing progress of such techniques has improved their resolution, while requiring less amounts of sample. This means that there is less reluctance in providing samples for this kind of analysis. In addition, the critical mass simultaneously involved in the analysis of burnt skeletal remains appears to have increased dramatically. For example, the year 2020 has seen the publication of multiple papers covering analysis through Fourier-transform infrared spectroscopy (Gonçalves *et al.*, 2020; Iriarte *et al.*, 2020; Legan *et al.*, 2020; Leskovar *et al.*, 2020; Monteiro *et al.*, 2020; Pedrosa *et al.*, 2020). As a result, one may argue that only nowadays is the critical mass large enough to guarantee one requisite for scientific knowledge: experimental replication and subsequent validation. This condition is critical to ensure constructive findings and to gradually elevate our ability to analyze burnt human skeletal remains to a level that is closer to the one currently held by the analysis of their unburnt counterparts.

Acknowledgments

We would like to thank all who have been working on the preparation, analysis, and organization of the experimentally burnt skeletons of the 21st Century Identified Skeletal Collection, especially Ana Rita Vassalo, Catarina Rodrigues, Cristiana Monteiro, João d'Oliveira Coelho, Catarina Coelho, and David Navega. We are also grateful to the municipality of Santarém for their valuable aid on the constitution of this collection. Funding was given by the Fundação para a Ciência e Tecnologia (FCT) (SFRH/BPD/84268/2012; SFRH/BPD/110710/2015; PTDC/IVC-ANT/1201/2014) and COMPETE 2020 (POCI-01-0145-FEDER-016766). This work was carried out at the R&D Unit Center for Functional Ecology – Science for People and the Planet (CFE), with reference UIDB/04004/2020, financed by FCT/MCTES through national funds (PIDDAC). We are thankful to the reviewers for the comments and suggestions on the paper.

References

Bass, W.M. and Jantz, R.L. (2004) Cremation weights in East Tennessee. *Journal of Forensic Sciences*, **49**(5), 901–904.

Bemis, G. (1850) *Report of the Case of John W. Webster*. Charles C. Little and James Brown, Boston, MA.

Blumenbach, J.F. (1776) *De Generis Humani Varietate Nativa.* Vandenhoeck, Goettingae.

Bohnert, M., Rost, T., Faller-Marquardt, M., Ropohl, D., and Pollack, S. (1997) Fractures of the base of the skull in charred bodies, post-mortem heat injuries or signs of mechanical traumatisation? *Forensic Science International,* **87**, 55–62.

Bonucci, E. and Graziani, G. (1975) Comparative thermogravimetric, X-ray diffraction and electron microscope investigations of burnt bones from recent, ancient, and prehistoric age. *Atti Memorie Accademia Nazionale die Lincei Scienze, Fisiche, Matematiche Naturali, Series,* **8**(59), 517–534.

Bradtmiller, B. and Buikstra, J.E. (1984) Effects of burning on human bone microstructure, a preliminary study. *Journal of Forensic Sciences,* **29**(2), 535–540.

Bruzek, J. (2002) A method for visual determination of sex, using the human hip bone. *American Journal of Physical Anthropology,* **117**, 157–168.

Buikstra, J. and Goldstein, L. (1973) *The Perrins Ledge Crematory.* In: *Reports of Investigations.* Illinois State Museum, Springfield, IL.

Buikstra, J. and Swegle, M. (1989) Bone modification due to burning, experimental evidence. In: *Bone Modification* (eds. R. Bonnichsen and M.H. Sorg). Center for the Study of the First Americans, Orono, ME, pp. 247–258.

Buikstra, J. and Ubelaker, D. (1994) Standards for data collection from human skeletal remains, Proceedings of a Seminar at the Field Museum of Natural History. *Arkansas Archaeological Survey Report,* **44**.

Campbell, M.N. and Fairgrieve, S.I. (2011) Differentiation of traumatic and heat-induced dental tissue fractures via SEM analysis. *Journal of Forensic Sciences,* **56**(3), 715–719.

Cardoso, H.F.V. (2006) Brief communication: The collection of identified human skeletons housed at the Bocage Museum (National Museum of Natural History), Lisbon, Portugal. *American Journal of Physical Anthropology,* **129**, 173–176.

Cavazzuti, C., Bresadola, B., d'Innocenzo, C., Interlando, S., and Sperduti, A. (2019) Towards a new osteometric method for sexing ancient cremated human remains. Analysis of Late Bronze Age and Iron Age samples from Italy with gendered grave goods. *PLOS One,* **14**(1), e0209423.

Cunha, E. and Wasterlain, S. (2007) The Coimbra identified osteological collections. In: *Skeletal Series and Their Socio-economic Context* (eds. G. Grupe and J. Peters). Verlag Marie Leidorf, Rahden/Westf, pp. 23–33.

Curate, F. (2011) *O Perímetro do Declínio, osteoporose e fracturas de fragilidade em três amostras identificadas portuguesas – Séculos XIX e XX.* Departamento de Ciências da Vida. Unpublished doctoral dissertation, Universidade de Coimbra, Coimbra.

Curate, F., Cunha, E., Coelho, J.D.O., Gonçalves, D., Coelho, C., Ferreira, M.T., *et al.* (2016) A method for sex estimation using the proximal femur. *Forensic Science International,* **266**, 579–e1.

Dayal, M.R., Kegley, A.D.T., Štrkalj, G., Bidmos, M.A., and Kuykendall, K.L. (2009) The history and composition of the Raymond A. Dart collection of human skeletons at the University of the Witwatersrand, Johannesburg, South Africa. *American Journal of Physical Anthropology,* **140**, 324–335.

DeHaan, J.D. (2015) Fire and bodies. In: *The Analysis of Burned Human Remains* (eds. C. Schmidt and S. Symes). Academic Press, London, pp. 1–16.

Dokladal, M. (1962) Uber die Moglichkeiten der Identifikation von Knochen aus Leichenbranden. *Mitteilungen der Sektion Anthropoloqie,* **6**, 15.

Duday, H., Depierre, G., and Janin, T. (2000) Validation des paramètres de quantification, protocoles et stratégies dans l'étude anthropologique des sépultures secondaires à incinération. L'exemple des nécropoles protohistoriques du midi de la France. In: *Archéologie de La Mort, Archéologie de la Tombe au Premier Âge du -fer* (eds. B. Dedet, P. Gruat, G. Marchand, M. Py, and M. Schwaller). UMR, Lattes, France, pp. 7–29.

Ellingham, S. and Sandholzer, M.A. (2020) Determining volumetric shrinkage trends of burnt bone using micro-CT. *Journal of Forensic Sciences*, **65**(1), 196–199.

Ellingham, S.T.D., Thompson, T.J.U., Islam, M., and Taylor, G. (2015) Estimating temperature exposure of burnt bone, a methodological review. *Science and Justice*, **55**(3), 181–188.

Erickson, P.A. (1997) Morton, Samuel George (1799–1851). In: *History of Physical Anthropology, an Encyclopedia* (ed. F. Spencer). Garland, New York, pp. 689–690.

Etxeberria, F. (1994) Aspectos macroscópicos del hueso sometido al fuego, revisión de las cremaciones descritas en el País Vasco desde la arqueologia. *Munibe*, **46**, 111–116.

Fairgrieve, S. (2008) *Forensic Cremation, Recovery and Analysis*. CRC Press, Boca Raton, FL.

Ferreira, M.T. (2012) Para lá da morte, estudo tafonómico da decomposição cadavérica e da degradação óssea e implicações na estimativa do intervalo pós-morte. Departamento de Ciências da Vida. Unpublished doctoral dissertation, Universidade de Coimbra, Coimbra.

Ferreira, M.T. and Cunha, E. (2012) Será credível estimar o PMI em restos cadavéricos em avançado estado de decomposição? *Cadernos do GEEvH*, **1**(2), 7–20.

Ferreira, M.T. and Cunha, E. (2013) Can we infer post mortem interval on the basis of decomposition rate? A case from a Portuguese cemetery. *Forensic Science International*, **226**(1), 298.e291–298.e296.

Ferreira, M.T., Vicente, R., Navega, D., Gonçalves, D., Curate, F., and Cunha, E. (2014) A new forensic collection housed at the University of Coimbra, Portugal: The 21st century identified skeletal collection. *Forensic Science International*, **245**, 202.e201–202.e205.

Ferreira, M.T., Coelho, C., Makhoul, C., Navega, D., Gonçalves, D., Cunha, E., and Curate, F. (2020) New data about the 21st century identified skeletal collection (University of Coimbra, Portugal). *International Journal of Legal Medicine*. https://doi.org/10.1007/s00414-020-02399-6.

Gejvall, N.-G. (1969) Cremations. In: *Science in Archaeology* (eds. D. Brothwell, E. Higgs, and G. Clark). Thames and Hudson, London, pp. 468–479.

Giraudi, R., Fissore, F., and Giacobini, G. (1984) The collection of human skulls and post-cranial skeletons at the Department of Human Anatomy of the University of Torino (Italy). *American Journal of Physical Anthropology*, **65**, 105–107.

Godinho, R.M., Oliveira-Santos, I., Pereira, M.F.C., Maurício, A., Valera, A., and Gonçalves, D. (2019) Is enamel the only reliable hard tissue for sex metric estimation of burned skeletal remains in biological anthropology? *Journal of Archaeological Science, Reports*, **26**, 101876.

Gómez Bellard, F. (1996) El análisis antropológico de las cremaciones. *Complutum Extra*, **6**(2), 55–64.

Gonçalves, D. (2011) The reliability of osteometric techniques for the sex determination of burned human skeletal remains. *Homo – Journal of Comparative Human Biology*, **62**, 351–358.

Gonçalves, D. (2012) Cremains, the value of quantitative analysis for the bioanthropological research of burned human skeletal remains. Departamento de Ciências da Vida. Unpublished doctoral dissertation, Universidade de Coimbra, Coimbra.

Gonçalves, D. and Pires, A.E. (2017) Cremation under fire, a review of bioarchaeological approaches from 1995 to 2015. *Archaeological and Anthropological Sciences*, **9**, 1677–1688.

Gonçalves, D., Thompson, T.J.U., and Cunha, E. (2013) Osteometric sex determination of burned human skeletal remains. *Journal of Forensic and Legal Medicine*, **20**(7), 906–911.

Gonçalves, D., Thompson, T.J.U., and Cunha, E. (2015) Sexual dimorphism of the lateral angle of the internal auditory canal and its potential for sex estimation of burned human skeletal remains. *International Journal of Legal Medicine*, **129**(5), 1183–1185.

Gonçalves, D., d'Oliveira Coelho, J., Acosta, M.A., Coelho, C., Curate, F., Ferreira, M.T., *et al.* (2016) One for all and all for one: Linear regression from the mass of individual bones to assess human skeletal mass completeness. *American Journal of Physical Anthropology,* **160**(3), 427–432.

Gonçalves, D., Coelho, J.d.O., Amarante, A., Makhoul, C., Oliveira-Santos, I., Navega, D., *et al.* (2018a) Dead weight, validation of mass regression equations on experimentally burned skeletal remains to assess skeleton completeness. *Science and Justice,* **58**(1), 2–6.

Gonçalves, D., Vassalo, A.R., Mamede, A.P., Makhoul, C., Piga, G., Cunha, E., *et al.* (2018b) Crystal clear, vibrational spectroscopy reveals intrabone, intraskeleton, and interskeleton variation in human bones. *American Journal of Physical Anthropology,* **166**(2), 296–312.

Gonçalves, D., Vassalo, A.R., Makhoul, C., Piga, G., Mamede, A.P., Parker, S.F., *et al.* (2020) Chemosteometric regression models of heat exposed human bones to determine their pre-burnt metric dimensions. *American Journal of Physical Anthropology.* https://doi.org/10.1002/AJPA.24104.

Gouveia, M., Santos, I.O., Santos, A.L., and Gonçalves, D. (2017) Sample-specific odontometric sex estimation: A method with potential application to burned remains. *Science and Justice,* **57**(4), 262–269.

Harsanyi, L. (1975) Scanning electron microscopic investigation of thermal damage of the teeth. *Acta Morpholog Academ Sci Hungaricae,* **23**(4), 271–281.

Herrmann, B. (1976) Experimentelle und theoretische beiträge zur leichenbrand unterschung. *Homo,* **27**, 114–118.

Herrmann, B. (1977) On histological investigations of cremated human remains. *Journal of Human Evolution,* **6**, 101–102.

Herrmann, N.P. and Bennett, J.L. (1999) The differentiation of traumatic and heat-related fractures in burned bone. *Journal of Forensic Sciences,* **44**(3), 461–469.

Holck, P. (1986) Cremated bones, a medical-anthropological study of an archaeological material on cremation burials. In: *Antropologiske Skrifter* (ed. P. Holck). Anatomisk Institutt Universitetet, Oslo.

Holden, J.L., Phakey, P.P., and Clement, J.G. (1995) Scanning electron microscope observations of human femoral bone, a case study. *Forensic Science International,* **74**, 17–28.

Hunt, D.R. and Albanese, J. (2005) History and demographic composition of the Robert J. Terry anatomical collection. *American Journal of Physical Anthropology,* **127**(4), 406–417.

Huxley, A.K. and Kósa, F. (1999) Calculation of percent shrinkage in human fetal diaphyseal lengths from fresh bone to carbonized and calcined bone using Petersohn and Köhler's data. *Journal of Forensic Sciences,* **44**(3), 577–583.

Iriarte, E., García-Tojal, J., Santana, J., Jorge-Villard, S.E., Teira, L., Muñiz, J., *et al.* (2020) Geochemical and spectroscopic approach to the characterization of earliest cremated human bones from the Levant (PPNB of Kharaysin, Jordan). *Journal of Archaeological Science, Reports,* **30**, 102211.

Kennedy, K.A.R. (1996) The wrong urn: Commingling of cremains in mortuary practices. *Journal of Forensic Sciences,* **41**(4), 689–692.

Krap, T., Ruijter, J.M., Nota, K., Karel, J., Burgers, L., Aalders, M.C.G., *et al.* (2019) Colourimetric analysis of thermally altered human bone samples. *Scientific Reports,* **9**(8923), 1–10.

Lebon, M., Reiche, I., Bahain, J.-J., Chadefaux, C., Moigne, A.-M., Fröhlich, F., *et al.* (2010) New parameters for the characterization of diagenetic alterations and heat-induced changes of fossil bone mineral using Fourier transform infrared spectrometry. *Journal of Archaeological Science,* **37**, 2265–2276.

Legan, L., Leskovar, T., Črešnara, M., Cavalli, F., Innocenti, D., and Ropret, P. (2020) Non-invasive reflection FTIR characterization of archaeological burnt bones, Reference database and case studies. *Journal of Cultural Heritage,* **41**, 13–26.

Lepkowski, V. and Wachholtz, L. (1903) Über veränderung naturlicher und kunstlicher gebisse durch extreme temperatur und fäulnis. *Artzliche Sachverstandigenzeitugen*, **6**, 119–121.

Leskovar, T., Pajnič, I.Z., Geršak, Ž.M., Jermand, I., and Črešnare, M. (2020) ATR-FTIR spectroscopy combined with data manipulation as a pre-screening method to assess DNA preservation in skeletal remains. *Forensic Science International, Genetics*, **44**, 102196.

Mailänder, E. (2014) A specialist, the daily work of Erich Muhsfeldt, chief of the crematorium at Majdanek concentration and extermination camp, 1942–44. In: *Destruction and Human Remains, Disposal and Concealment in Genocide and Mass Violence* (eds. É. Anstett and J.-M. Dreyfus). Manchester University Press, Manchester, pp. 46–68.

Malinowski, A. (1969) Synthèse des recherches polonaises effectuèes jusqu'à présent sur les os des tombes à incinération. *Przegląd Antropologiczny*, **35**, 127–147.

Marques, M.P.M., Gonçalves, D., Amarante, A., Makhoul, C., Parker, S.F., and Carvalho, L.A.E.B.d. (2016) Osteometrics in burned human skeletal remains by neutron and optical vibrational spectroscopy. *RSC Advances*, **6**, 68638–66864.

Martiniaková, M., Grosskopf, B., Omelka, R., Vondráková, M., and Bauerová, a.M. (2006) Differences among species in compact bone tissue microstructure of mammalian skeleton, use of a discriminant function analysis for species identification. *Journal of Forensic Sciences*, **51**(6), 1235–1239.

Masotti, S., Pasini, A., and Gualdi-Russo, E. (2019) Sex determination in cremated human remains using the lateral angle of the pars petrosa ossis temporalis, is old age a limiting factor? *Forensic Science, Medicine and Pathology*, **15**(3), 392–398.

Masotti, S., Succi-Leonelli, E., and Gualdi-Russo, E. (2013) Cremated human remains, is measurement of the lateral angle of the meatus acusticus internus a reliable method of sex determination? *International Journal of Legal Medicine*, **127**(5), 1039–1044.

McKinley, J.I. (1994a) Bone fragment size in British cremation burials and its implications for pyre technology and ritual. *Journal of Archaeological Science*, **21**, 339–342.

McKinley, J.I. (1994b) The Anglo-Saxon Cemetery at Spong Hill, North Elmham. Part VIII, The Cremations. *East Anglian Archaeology*, **69**.

McKinley, J.I., Bond, J.M., Brothwell, D.R., and Pollard, A.M. (2001) Cremated bone. In: *Handbook of Archaeological Sciences* (eds. D.R. Brothwell and A.M. Pollard). Wiley, Hoboken, NJ, pp. 281–292.

McKinley, J.I. (2004) Compiling a skeletal inventory, cremated human bone. In: *Guidelines to the Standards for Recording Human Remains* (eds. M. Brickley and J.I. McKinley). British Association for Biological Anthropology and Osteoarchaeology/Institute of Field Archaeologists, Reading, UK, pp. 14–19.

Monteiro, C., Ferreira, M.T., Curate, F., and Gonçalves, D. (2020) Assessing the reliability of dual-energy X-ray absorptiometry analyses in burned bones. *Australian Journal of Forensic Sciences*. https://doi.org/10.1080/00450618.2020.1826579.

Mulhern, D.M. and Ubelaker, D.H. (2012) Differentiating human from nonhuman bone microstructure. In: *Bone Histology, an Anthropological Perspective* (eds. C. Crowder and S. Stout). CRC Press, Boca Raton, FL, pp. 109–134.

Munro, L.E., Longstaffe, F.J., and White, C.D. (2007) Burning and boiling of modern deer bone, effects on crystallinity and oxygen isotope composition of bioapatite phosphate. *Palaeogeography, Palaeoclimatology, Palaeoecology*, **249**(1–2), 90–102.

Oliveira-Santos, I., Gouveia, M., Cunha, E., and Gonçalves, D. (2017) The circles of life, age at death estimation in burnt teeth through tooth cementum annulations. *International Journal of Legal Medicine*, **131**(2), 527–536.

Pedrosa, M., Curate, F., Carvalho, L.A.E.B.d., Marques, M.P.M., and Ferreira, M.T. (2020) Beyond metrics and morphology, the potential of FTIR-ATR and chemometrics to estimate age-at-death in human bone. *International Journal of Legal Medicine*. https://doi.org/10.1007/s00414-020-02310-3.

Pfeiffer, S. and Pinto, D. (2012) Histological analyses of human bone from archaeological contexts. In: *Bone Histology, an Anthropological Perspective* (eds. C. Crowder and S. Stout). CRC Press, Boca Raton, FL, pp. 297–311.

Piga, G., Baró, M.D., Escobal, I.G., Gonçalves, D., Makhoul, C., Amarante, A., *et al.* (2016) A structural approach in the study of bones, fossil and burnt bones at nanosize scale. *Applied Physics A*, **122**, 1031.

Piga, G., Malgosa, A., Thompson, T.J.U., and Enzo, S. (2008) A new calibration of the XRD technique for the study of archaeological burned human remains. *Journal of Archaeological Science*, **35**, 2171–2178.

Piontek, J. (1975) Polish methods and results of investigations of cremated bones from prehistoric cemeteries. *Glasnik Antropološkog Društva Jugoslavije*, **12**, 23–34.

Piontek, J. (1976) Proces kremacji i jego wpływ na morfologię kości w świetle wyników badań eksperymentalnych. *Archeologia Polski*, **21**, 247–280.

Rodrigues, C.O., Ferreira, M.T., Matos, V., and Gonçalves, D. (2021) Sex change in skeletal remains: Assessing how heat-induced changes interferes with sex estimation. *Science & Justice*, **61**(1), 26–36.

Rösing, F.W. (1977) Methoden und Aussagemöglichkeiten der anthropologischen Leichenbrandbearbeitung. *Archäologie und Naturwissenschaft*, **1**, 53–80.

Schutkowski, H. (1983) Uber den diagnostischen Wert der Pars petrosa ossis temporalis fur die Geschlechtsbestimmung. *Zeitschrift für Morphologie und Anthropologie*, **74**, 129–144.

Schutkowski, H. and Herrmann, B. (1983) Zur Möglichkeit der metrischen geschlechtsdiagnose an der Pars petrosa ossis temporalis. *Zeitschrift für Rechtsmedizin*, **90**, 219–227.

Shipman, P., Foster, G., and Schoeninger, M. (1984) Burnt bones and teeth: An experimental study of colour, morphology, crystal structure and shrinkage. *Journal of Archaeological Science*, **11**(4), 307–325.

Smith, B.H. (1991) Standards of human tooth formation and dental age assessment. In: *Advances in Dental Anthropology* (eds. M.A. Kelly and C.S. Larsen). Wiley-Liss, New York, pp. 143–168.

Snoeck, C., Lee-Thorp, J.A., and Schulting, R.J. (2014) From bone to ash, compositional and structural changes in burned modern and archaeological bone. *Palaeogeography, Palaeoclimatology, Palaeoecology*, **416**, 55–68.

Snow, C.C. (1982) Forensic anthropology. *Annual Review of Anthropology*, **11**, 97–131.

Stiner, M.C., Kuhn, S.L., Surovell, T.A., Goldberg, P., Meignen, L., Weiner, S., *et al.* (2001) Bone preservation in Hayonim Cave (Israel): A macroscopic and mineralogical study. *Journal of Archaeological Science*, **28**, 643–659.

Strzalko, J. and Piontek, J. (1974) Wpływ spalania w warunkach zbliżonych do kremacji pradziejowych na morfologię kości. *Przegląd Antropologiczny*, **40**, 315–326.

Symes, S.A., Dirkmaat, D.C., Ousley, S., Chapman, E., and Cabo, L. (2012) *Recovery and Interpretation of Burned Human Remains*. U.S. Department of Justice, Rockville, MD.

Symes, S.A., L'Abbé, E.N., Pokines, J.T., Yuzwa, T., Messer, D., Stromquist, A., *et al.* (2014) Thermal alteration to bone. In: *Manual of Forensic Taphonomy* (eds. J.T. Pokines and S.A. Symes). CRC Press, Boca Raton, FL, pp. 367–402.

Symes, S.A., Rainwater, C., Chapman, E., Gipson, D.R., and Piper, A. (2008) Patterned thermal destruction of human remains in a forensic setting. In: *The Analysis of Burned Human Remains* (eds. C. Schmidt and S. Symes). Academic Press, London, pp. 15–54.

Thompson, T.J.U. (2004) Recent advances in the study of burned bone and their implications for forensic anthropology. *Forensic Science International*, **146S**, S203–S205.

Thompson, T.J.U. (2005) Heat-induced dimensional changes in bone and their consequences for forensic anthropology. *Journal of Forensic Sciences*, **50**(5), 185–193.

Thompson, T.J.U., Gauthier, M., and Islam, M. (2009) The application of a new method of Fourier Transform Infrared Spectroscopy to the analysis of burned bone. *Journal of Archaeological Science*, **36**, 910–914.

van Pelt, R.J. (2014) Sinnreich erdacht, machines of mass incineration in fact, fiction, and forensics. In: *Destruction and Human Remains, Disposal and Concealment in Genocide and Mass Violence* (eds. É. Anstett and J.-M. Dreyfus). Manchester University Press, Manchester, pp. 117–146.

van Vark, G.N. (1974) The investigation of human cremated skeletal material by multivariate statistical methods I. Methodology. *Ossa*, **1**, 63–95.

van Vark, G.N. (1975) The investigation of human cremated skeletal material by multivariate statistical methods II. Measures. *Ossa*, **2**, 47–68.

van Vark, G.N., Amesz-Voorhoeve, W., and Cuijpers, A. (1996) Sex-diagnosis of human cremated skeletal material by means of mathematical-statistical and data-analytical methods. *Homo*, **47**, 305–338.

Veselka, B., Hlad, M., Steadman, D.W., Annaert, H., Boudin, M., Capuzzo, G., *et al.* (2021) Estimating age-at-death in burnt adult human remains using the Falys–Prangle method. *American Journal of Physical Anthropology*, **175**(1), 128–136.

Wahl, J. (1981) Ein Beitrag zur metrischen Geschlechtsdiagnose verbrannter und unverbrannter menschlicher Knochenreste – ausgearbeitet an der pars petrosa ossis temporalis. *Zeitschrift für Rechtsmedizin*, **86**(2), 79–101.

Wahl, J. (2008) Investigations on pre-Roman and Roman cremation remains from southwestern Germany, results, potentialities and limits. In: *The Analysis of Burned Remains* (eds. C.W. Schmidt and S.A. Symes). Academic Press, London, pp. 145–161.

Wahl, J.K. (1996) Erfahrungen zur metrishen Geschlechtsdiagnose bei Leichenbränden. *Homo*, **47**(1–3), 339–359.

Walker, P.L., Miller, K.W.P., and Richman, R. (2008) Time, temperature and oxygen availability: An experimental study of the effects of environmental conditions on the color and organic content of cremated bone. In: *The Analysis of Burned Human Remains* (eds. C.W. Schmidt and S.A. Symes). Academic Press, London, pp. 129–137.

Warren, M.W. and Maples, W.R. (1997) The anthropometry of contemporary commercial cremation. *Journal of Forensic Sciences*, **42**(3), 417–423.

Wasterlain, S. (2000) Morphé. Análise das proporções entre os membros, dimorfismo sexual e estatura de uma amostra da colecção de esqueletos identificados do Museu antropológico da Universidade de Coimbra. Departamento de Antropologia. Unpublished doctoral dissertation, Universidade de Coimbra, Coimbra.

Welinder, S. (1908) *An Experiment with the Analysis of Sex and Gender of Cremated Bones*. Tor, Uppsala, Sweden.

White, T., Black, M.T., and Folkens, P.A. (2015) *Human Osteology*, 3rd edn. Academic Press, Amsterdam.

PART 4
Case Studies

CHAPTER 18

Analysis of Burnt Human Remains Statistical Perspectives from Casework in Forensic Anthropology

Douglas H. Ubelaker, PhD, D-ABFA; Cassandra M. DeGaglia, MA and Haley Khosrowshahi, MA

Department of Anthropology, National Museum of Natural History Smithsonian Institution, Washington, D.C.

Douglas H. Ubelaker, US Government employee, Curator, Department of Anthropology, National Museum of Natural History Smithsonian Institution, Washington, D.C.

18.1 Introduction

Analysis of burnt human remains represents a significant challenge in forensic anthropology. Thermal exposure leads to loss and alteration of soft tissue, followed by fragmentation and morphological distortion of bones and teeth. The forensic anthropologist analyzing such remains can find bone recognition difficult due to fragmentation, shrinkage, and other forms of morphological alteration. Current scientific methods greatly facilitate the extraction of useful information from burnt remains but even with recent advances, analysis remains challenging.

18.2 Materials and Methods

This chapter examines the experience of the first author in the analysis of burnt remains. Records of casework between 1975 and 2019 offer perspective on the impact of burnt remains in the long-term work of a forensic anthropologist. The cases examined from this 44-year period primarily originated from the Federal Bureau of Investigation (FBI) in the Washington D.C. area, although cases from other sources are also included. Following a long Smithsonian Institution/FBI tradition that began with the work of Smithsonian Curator Aleš Hrdlička (Ubelaker, 2000), the first author consulted and reported on cases submitted to the FBI that related to forensic anthropology. Non-FBI cases during this period originated from

Burnt Human Remains: Recovery, Analysis, and Interpretation, First Edition. Edited by Sarah Ellingham, Joe Adserias-Garriga, Sara C. Zapico and Douglas H. Ubelaker.

other law enforcement agencies, medicolegal units, and international organizations in need of anthropological opinion. Many of these cases involved some aspect of thermally altered remains. The first author assigned case numbers when they were received in his laboratory. The numbers relate to the individual submission and not necessarily to the number of individuals represented.

Between the years of 1975 and 2019, the first author was involved in 987 total forensic cases. This author maintains case files for 714 of these cases. The remaining 273 cases reflect work in which the first author participated but others were responsible for reports. Two notable examples relate to the first author's participation in the analysis of decedents resulting from the Gulf War in 1991 and the attack on the Pentagon in 2001. Although the first author contributed extensively to these efforts, reports were generated by others.

One hundred and sixteen (16%) of these 714 reports indicated thermal changes to the material submitted for analysis. This chapter uses these case files maintained by the first author to present temporal and geographic trends of cases, including burnt remains in comparison to broader trends of all cases reported on. Evidence submitted as cases was recovered from a variety of locations and displayed a range of thermal effects, including charring of soft tissue, charring of bone, and calcination of bone. The anatomical regions affected by thermal changes, as well as other taphonomic and traumatic factors affecting the remains, were also noted.

Five-year intervals were designated to assess the temporal trend of thermal affects in this sample. Most cases in this sample originated from the USA. Geographic regions from the US Census Bureau were used to classify these as originating from the West, Midwest, South, or Northeast. Cases relating to remains originating from outside the USA were categorized geographically as "other."

Evidence included in this sample was recovered from a wide range of environments. For this study, the designations "within," "outside," and "unknown" were used to classify recovery environments. Cases assigned the label "within" contained evidence found in an enclosed space. This classification included remains recovered from car crashes, airplane crashes, dumpsters, oil drums, cremated remains in containers, structural fires, and explosions inside structures. Cases assigned the label "outside" contained evidence found outside a structure or container. This classification included remains from surface sites, water, and burial recoveries, including archaeological sites.

Thermal alterations to hard and soft tissues, as well as effects on other organic and inorganic materials were noted.

The anatomical area, or areas, affected by thermal changes were also noted. The following body regions were designated: 1. Head (cranium and mandible); 2. Thorax (C-1 through T-12, hyoid, clavicles, scapulae, and ribs); 3. Upper extremities (humeri, ulnae, and radii); 4. Hands (carpals, metacarpals, and hand phalanges); 5. Abdomen/pelvis (L-1 through coccyx and os coxae); 6. Lower extremities (femora, patellae, tibiae, and fibulae); and 7. Feet (tarsals, metatarsals, and foot phalanges). Paired anatomical elements were further assigned their side. When remains of paired elements were too fragmentary to side, the category of "indeterminate" was assigned.

18.3 Results

Table 18.1 shows all cases in which the first author was involved according to five-year intervals. Table 18.2 shows the relationship of cases with evidence of thermal involvement in their reports to the sample of 714 cases with reports maintained by the first author. The first interval (1975–1979) contained only

Table 18.1 All cases by five-year interval.

	Number	% of 987 cases
1975–1979	62	6.28
1980–1984	100	10.13
1985–1989	110	11.14
1990–1994	277	28.06
1995–1999	118	11.96
2000–2004	88	8.92
2005–2009	101	10.23
2010–2014	90	9.12
2015–2019	41	4.15
Total	987	100.00

Table 18.2 Cases with reports by five-year interval.

	Number of cases	% of 714 cases	Number of burn cases	% burn cases of 714 cases
1975–1979	49	7	1	0.14
1980–1984	82	11	12	1.68
1985–1989	94	13	4	0.56
1990–1994	223	31	80	11.20
1995–1999	96	13	11	1.54
2000–2004	76	11	5	0.70
2005–2009	49	7	3	0.42
2010–2014	22	3	0	0.00
2015–2019	23	3	0	0.00
Total	714	100	116	16.25

one burn case, constituting less than 2% of the 714 cases with reports. The highest concentration of burn cases was in the 1990–1994 interval. Eighty (11% of the 714 cases with reports) were affected by heat. The high frequency of thermal effects in this interval reflects involvement of the Smithsonian and FBI in recovery efforts at the Branch Davidian complex in Waco, Texas (Ubelaker *et al.*, 1995). If the 57 cases from the Waco incident are omitted, the number of burn cases from the 1990–1994 interval is 23, which is still the highest frequency temporally, but by a less dramatic margin. The last two intervals included no burn cases, likely related to the FBI's 2009 shift to working with their own anthropologists.

Thermally affected cases originated from all geographic regions of the USA (Census Bureau) as well as from other countries. Of the cases in this sample, 77 (66% of the 116 burn cases) originated from the Southern USA, 13 (11% of the burn cases) originated from the Western USA, 9.5 (8% of the 116 burn cases) originated from the Midwestern USA, 9 (8% of the 116 burn cases) originated from the Northeastern USA, and 7.5 (6% of the 116 burn cases) originated from outside the USA (Other). Four of the cases with elements originating from outside the USA were recovered from the Middle East, two from Europe, one from Central America, and one from a Pacific island. Decimal values are listed for burn cases from the Midwest and Other because one case was split to reflect the fact that it contained elements recovered from both the Midwestern USA and outside the USA (Central America). The highest concentration of thermally affected cases was in the Southern USA (77 cases, 66% of the thermally affected sample). The geographic distribution is affected in a similar manner as the temporal distribution by the events in Waco. If the cases from Waco are omitted, the number of cases from the south is 20. While this is still higher than the number of cases from other geographic regions, the difference is less drastic. Table 18.3 shows the geographic distribution of the 987 total cases. Table 18.4 shows the geographic distribution of burn cases with reports in relation to the 714 total cases with reports and the 116 cases with noted thermal alterations.

Table 18.3 All cases by geographic region.

	Number	% of 987 cases
West USA	155	15.70
Midwest USA	73	7.40
South USA	377	38.20
Northeast USA	143	14.49
Other	220	22.29
Unknown	19	1.93
Total	987	100.00

Table 18.4 Cases displaying evidence of thermal changes with reports by geographic region.

	Number	% of 714 cases	% of 116 burn cases
West USA	13	1.82	11.2
Midwest USA	9.5	1.33	8.19
South USA	77	10.78	66.38
Northeast USA	9	1.26	7.76
Other	7.5	1.05	6.47
Unknown	0	0.00	0.00
Total	116	16.25	100.00

"Within" was the most common recovery designation, with 76 (66%) of the cases in this sample found within some sort of enclosed space or container. Twenty-six (22%) of the burn cases were found outside. Fourteen (12%) did not contain enough information in their reports to reliably assign to either "within" or "outside."

The area of the body most commonly affected by heat in this sample was the head (cranium and/or mandible), with 64 (16%) of burn cases involving the head. Following were the thorax with 59 cases (14%) and the pelvis with 54 cases (13%). The right leg (43 cases, 10%) was marginally more represented than the left leg (41 cases, 10%) and the right arm (30 cases, 7%) was slightly more common than the left arm (26 cases, 6%). Non-human elements were present in 18 (4%) of the burn cases, and included non-human animal remains as well as other organic and inorganic substances. Fourteen cases (3%) contained elements that were too burnt to be identified with certainty. Elements of hands and feet as well as arms and legs that were too compromised to be assigned to a side were present in the sample in low percentages. The total number of anatomical regions examined was 410, which is greater than the 116 cases that comprise the sample because many cases presented evidence of heat-related trauma on more than one area of the body. It should be noted that recovered evidence is often fragmentary and that material submitted to anthropologists is sometimes influenced by the nature of the request of the inquiring agency (e.g. a cranium and mandible being submitted for facial approximation without associated post-cranial elements). A complete summary of the frequency of anatomical elements affected by thermal changes is presented in Table 18.5.

Burn cases in this sample were frequently affected by a variety of other taphonomic and traumatic factors. Twelve cases (10%) displayed hallmarks of surface exposure, while four (3%) presented evidence of at least partial burial. Three cases (3%) contained sun-bleached elements and 2 (2%) presented indications of exposure to water.

Table 18.5 Anatomical regions with evidence of thermal alterations.

	Number	% of 410 body regions
Cranium/mandible	64	15.61
Thorax (incl. scapulae & hyoid)	59	14.39
Abdomen/pelvis (incl. sacrum & coccyx)	54	13.17
R. leg	43	10.49
L. leg	41	10.00
R. arm	30	7.32
L. arm	26	6.34
N-H	18	4.39
Unknown	14	3.41
L. foot	11	2.68
? leg	10	2.44
R. foot	9	2.20
? hand	8	1.95
R. hand	7	1.71
? arm	6	1.46
? foot	6	1.46
L. hand	4	0.98
Total	410	100.00

Despite the destructive effects, 29 (25%) of the 116 cases showed evidence of trauma. Fourteen burn cases displayed hallmarks of sharp force trauma (13%), ten (9%) showed evidence of projectile trauma, five (4%) contained evidence of blast related trauma, and none had indications of blunt force trauma.

18.4 Discussion

Overall, 116 (16%) of the 714 cases with reports presented evidence of burning. Generally, this indicates that evidence of burning is relatively common in forensic anthropology casework.

Temporal trends in cases involving burning largely reflect major events and investigative procedures. For example, the elevated number of burn cases in the 1990–1994 interval directly reflects first author involvement in the analysis of decedents related to events in Waco, Texas (Ubelaker *et al.*, 1995). The lack of burn cases since 2010 reflects a career shift by the first author to concentrate on radiocarbon interpretation and humanitarian and human rights issues.

The geographic regions from which the cases originated reflect similar factors. The elevated number from the south (38% of all cases and 66% of burn cases) relates to the Waco analysis. Numbers from all regions reflect administrative decisions relating to case acceptance and the availability of other forensic anthropologists. Frequencies of the burn cases in each time interval and geographic region reflect administrative policies, largely made by FBI officials, shaping the nature and distribution of cases submitted for analysis.

Most burn cases (66%) originated from within an enclosure. Most burn victims are recovered from the site where the burning event took place. Although the nature of these sites varies considerably (e.g. house structures, automobiles, etc.) the association indicates that it is less common for burnt victims to be transported to a different location.

In the analysis of the area of the body altered by burning, the head was commonly affected, followed by the thorax and pelvis. These data are not surprising since the head is usually completely exposed. The thorax and pelvis may be somewhat protected by clothing, but minimal soft tissue covering some parts of the skeleton in these areas produces vulnerability. Of course, position of the body, the nature of the fire, and other variables influence skeletal changes.

Skeletal analysis can reveal evidence of post-mortem alterations in addition to thermal effects. In the cases analyzed here, some presenting evidence of burning also displayed taphonomic indications of surface exposure, partial burial, sun bleaching, and water exposure.

Clearly, bone exposure to fire can produce dramatic morphological alterations and fragmentation. However, even in such cases, evidence of trauma can be preserved. Of the 116 burn cases examined, 25% retained evidence of trauma. These 29 cases included indicators of sharp force, projectile, and blast-related trauma. Of course, other evidence of trauma may not have been detected due to the thermal alterations.

Involvement at the Branch Davidian Complex:

The first author's involvement in recovery efforts of the 1993 events at the Branch Davidian complex in Waco, Texas, resulted in 65 case files. Fifty-seven of these contain indications of exposure to high temperatures, making up 71% of the burn cases in this temporal interval and 49% of the total number of burn cases. Case files from Waco noted evidence of thermal changes, ranging from charring of external soft tissue to calcination of bone. This subset of the sample heavily influenced the distribution of both the temporal and geographic analyses of this study. The average number of cases for a five-year interval in this sample was 109. The interval between 1990 and 1994, which includes the events at Waco, has the highest number of cases for any of the designated intervals, with 277.

Fifty-six of the individuals recovered from the complex were found inside a structure. The fifty-seventh did not have recovery information associated with the report and was assigned to the "unknown" category.

18.5 Conclusions

The analysis of burnt human remains represents a challenging but common component of forensic anthropology casework. Future anthropologists can expect burnt cases that originate from a variety of contexts to be presented for analysis. New methods facilitate such analysis allowing more information to be gleaned about the individuals represented.

Literature Cited

Ubelaker, D.H. (2000) A history of Smithsonian-FBI collaboration in forensic anthropology, especially in regard to facial imagery. *Forensic Science Communications*, **2**(4), *Gale Academic OneFile*, link.gale.com/apps/doc/A137921529/AONE?u=anon~54c1efa2&sid=googleScholar&xid=ed7e3e8b.

Ubelaker, D.H., Owsley, D.W., Houck, M.M., Craig, E., Grant, W., Woltanski, T., *et al.* (1995) The role of forensic anthropology in the recovery and analysis of Branch Davidian compound victims: Procedures and characteristics of the victims. *Journal of Forensic Sciences*, **40**(3), 335–340.

United States Census Bureau. (2021) https://www2.census.gov/geo/pdfs/maps-data/maps/reference/us_regdiv.pdf.

CHAPTER 19

The Challenge of Burnt Remains from the Brazilian "Microwave Oven"

Melina Calmon Silva[1], PhD; Eugénia Cunha[2], PhD, C-FASE, and Yara Vieira Lemos[3], MSc

[1] *Affiliated Researcher at the Doris Z. Stone Laboratory for Biological and Forensic Anthropology at Tulane University, New Orleans, LA; Executive Secretary of the Brazilian Association of Forensic Anthropology (ABRAF) 2020/2022*

[2] *Director of the National Institute of Legal Medicine and Forensic Sciences, Lisbon, Portugal; Full Professor at University of Coimbra, Centre for Functional Ecology, Department of Life Sciences, Laboratory of Forensic Anthropology, Coimbra, Portugal*

[3] *Medical Examiner of the Civil Police of Minas Gerais – Laboratory of Forensic Anthropology and Applied Thanatology, Brazil; Professor at the Medical Sciences College of Minas Gerais and the Criminology Institute, Brazil; President of the Brazilian Association of Forensic Anthropology (ABRAF) 2020/2022*

19.1 Introduction

The term commonly known in Brazil as the "microwave oven" death refers to the criminal act of execution, especially practiced amongst narcotraffickers, where an individual is placed inside a pile of tires before they are set on fire. The goal of this practice is to torture the victims and to hinder the ability of forensic practitioners to identify those individuals. This practice alludes to "necklacing," the burning of tires placed around a victim's neck, practiced in South Africa, among other countries, since the 1990s, against the supporters of the apartheid (Moosage, 2010).

The direct action of fire is the thermal agent most used to produce carbonization. Usually, a fuel agent is used, such as alcohol, diesel oil, kerosene, cooking gas, vehicular natural gas, or gasoline. The wick is what keeps the flame burning. The dressed human body works like a candle "inside out." Human fat (the fuel source) is on the inside, and the victim's clothing and rubber tire (the wick) is on the outside. As the human body is 60–65% water, the flame remains lit through tires, causing dehydration, dryness, and destroying the body in part or in whole. In addition, the burning of tires results in the melting of rubber and exposure of the steel frame originally inside the tire structure, and these materials can get entangled with the carbonized body, making it difficult to assess the individual

Burnt Human Remains: Recovery, Analysis, and Interpretation, First Edition. Edited by Sarah Ellingham, Joe Adserias-Garriga, Sara C. Zapico and Douglas H. Ubelaker.

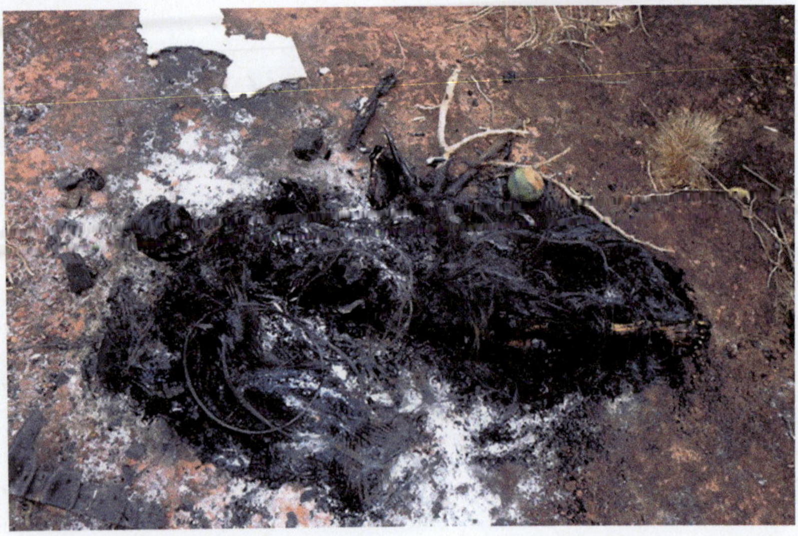

Figure 19.1 Crime scene comprised of an individual who was killed through a microwave oven death mechanism. Fotografia cedida pelo Instituto de Criminalística da Polícia Civil do Distrito Federal.

and identify and separate structures for medicolegal purposes and investigations (Figure 19.1).

The violence rates in Brazil are vastly reported in the news and scientific literature. The traumatic manner of death consolidates the increasing need for anthropological and odontological analysis of remains. "Microwave oven" death investigations are challenging in that, among other things, it becomes hard to distinguish between traumas caused by the direct action of fire and those traumatic injuries caused by other violent acts (Cunha, 2019). The interpretation of burnt bones is relatively common during the investigation of forensic cases, requiring the expertise of a forensic anthropologist. A forensic anthropological analysis on cases involving thermal alterations is needed to address a variety of issues that include, but are not limited to, recovery, reconstruction, trauma interpretation, bone recognition, taphonomic changes, and a successful DNA extraction.

Although such violent practice is not commonly seen across the world, Brazilian medicolegal institutions (MLIs) have become familiarized with "microwave oven" related deaths. This chapter strives to give an overview of the topic and provide real case studies from forensic investigations related to this particular manner of death.

19.2 Brazilian Homicide Rates

Homicide is the most serious outcome of interpersonal violence, with a total worldwide death toll of more than all wars combined since the year 2000. The global homicide rate is 6.7 per 100,000 inhabitants per year; however, in low-middle-income American countries it is 28.5 per 100,000 inhabitants per year, the highest rate worldwide (Mikton *et al.*, 2016).

In Brazil, the homicide rate is four times higher than the world average (26.2 per 100,000) (Murray *et al.*, 2013). Since 1980, the rate has been steadily increasing, but between 2004 to 2014 it has stagnated, with about 60,000 homicides per year (Waiselfisz, 2013; Mikton *et al.*, 2016). In 2019, there was a decrease in homicides, with a reported rate of 20.01 per 100,000, with a total of 41,726 homicides in that year alone (G1.globo.com/monitor-da-violencia).

Homicide rates in Brazil are higher in areas of greater income inequality (Gawryszewski and Costa, 2005; Araújo *et al.*, 2010; Murray *et al.*, 2013). Although the last decade has shown economical changes in Brazil, large regional and socio-economic inequalities remain. The best socio-economic indicators are seen in the south and south-east regions of the country, whereas the north and north-east regions show the worst indicators, while reporting the increasing homicide rates from 2004 to 2014 (Waiselfisz, 2016; World Bank, 2016). The hard-hit regions are also the ones comprising the most vulnerable populations. Around 10% of the Brazilian population lived below the poverty line (Campello and Neri, 2013) and 10% were illiterate in 2010 (Paim *et al.*, 2011).

Moreover, homicide rates in Brazil are 12 times higher in men; in particular, the group at highest risk of being victims of homicide are young black men with lower educational background (Araújo *et al.*, 2010; Murray *et al.*, 2013). According to Auger *et al.* (2016), the main causes for shorter life expectancy for Brazilian men are homicides and road traffic accidents. In 2017, a study showed that 59.1% of causes of death among Brazilian men aged 15–19 years old were designated as homicide (Cerqueira *et al.*, 2017). The primary means used to commit homicide in Brazil is by the use of firearms (Cerqueira *et al.*, 2017; Lemos *et al.*, 2019).

Although a multitude of variables must be considered when analyzing the data regarding homicides amongst Brazilians, for the purpose of the "microwave oven" death analysis, such practice is almost exclusively restricted to gangs and narcotraffickers, which are also more targeted towards young men. The correlation between violent deaths and illicit activities is well known and described in the 2017 study that shows a possible positive correlation between the increase of homicide rates in the north and north-east Brazilian regions with the narcotrafficker war between gangs in the same regions (Cerqueira *et al.*, 2017).

19.3 The Relationship between Homicide and Drugs

The association between violence and the consumption of psychoactive substances has been extensively studied worldwide (Briefing, 2006; Atkinson *et al.*, 2009). The World Health Organization defines violence as: "the intentional use of physical force or power, threatened or actual, against oneself, another person, or against a group or community, that either results in or has a high likelihood of resulting in injury, death, psychological harm, mal-development or deprivation" (Krug *et al.*, 2002). Degenhardt *et al.* (2013, 2014) suggested that the burden of disease attributable to illicit drug consumption should consider the consequences of violence associated with drug use.

Urban violence has grown into a major public concern in Brazil, but studies measuring its social and economic burden are scarce. Not surprisingly, a 2009 national survey estimated that 47.2% of Brazilians did not feel safe in the city where they lived (IBGE, 2010). The study by Abdalla *et al.* (2014) found that approximately 9.3% of the Brazilian population has been victim of at least one form of urban violence. This proportion increases to 19.7% among cocaine users and to 18.1% among individuals with alcohol use disorders (AUD). The results showed that nearly one in ten Brazilians reported having been a victim of at least one urban violence event, and more than one in twenty reported having been the perpetrator of at least one act of urban violence. The latest national report (Waiselfisz, 2014) placed Brazil as the seventh most violent country in the world. AUD were highly associated with being a victim and a perpetrator of urban violence, whilst binge drinking was associated with victimization. Cocaine use, on the other hand, was highly associated with perpetration.

Therefore, the identification of violence predictors and correlates are essential to elaborate preventive initiatives (Krug *et al.*, 2002). Combining the country's worrying rates of violence (Murray *et al.*, 2013), with the elevated alcohol and crack / cocaine use rates (Abdalla *et al.* 2014), it becomes essential to establish an understanding of the association between the use of these two drugs and urban violence in Brazil. Nevertheless, violence and drug correlations are particularly intense when related to the providers who fight for the control over drug distribution, and consumers who can be targeted if they owe money to drug dealers. The use of illicit drugs has a strong relationship with victimization by lethal violence and is frequently found in necropsies of homicide victims (Lemos *et al.*, 2019).

19.4 The "Microwave Oven" Modality of Death / Disposability of Human Remains

The "microwave oven" is a colloquial (slang) name given in Brazil to a criminal form of carbonization adopted mainly by drug dealers (Durão *et al.*, 2015). This illegal procedure is of extreme violence and includes torture and judgment of the enemy and condemnation to death in the "microwave" (Jaguaribe and Reis, 2009).

The microwave is an improvised crematorium, placed in an open space, usually on the top of the *favelas*. The place is made to incinerate people inside tires which are set on fire with any flammable substance, but more commonly gasoline (Figure 19.2). The process consists of two parts: the first is to insert the victim in a tire stack, followed by setting the structure on fire, aiming for the carbonization. It takes place in areas neglected by the state, dominated by the narcotraffickers, and it aims to destroy the forensic evidence, as it increases the challenge of identification and estimation of

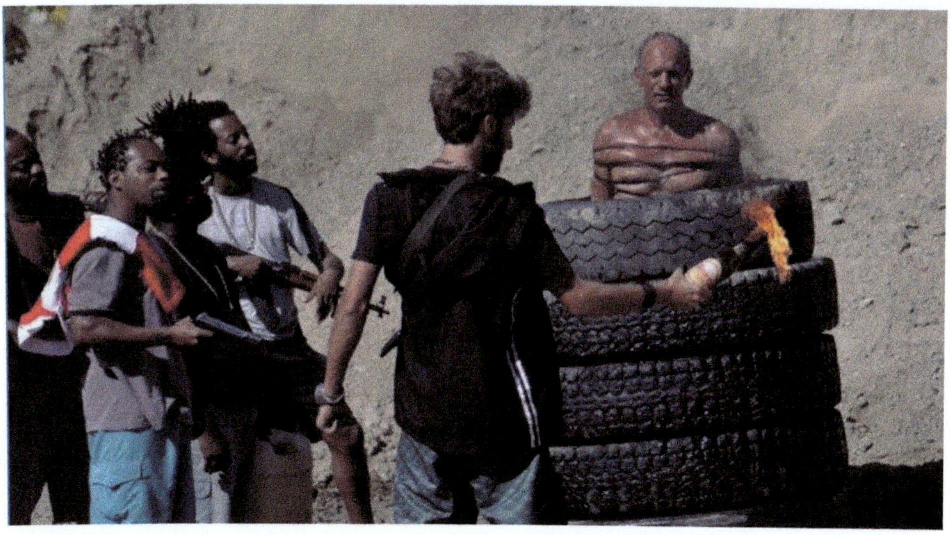

Figure 19.2 Soap opera "Vidas em Jogo" by Record, depicting the use of "microwave" execution. Photo made by Munir Chatack. Public domain.

cause of death, making it a much bigger task to address justice (Jaguaribe, 2009). The goal of this violent act is to intimidate rivals, to cause suffering and pain, and to hamper identification and cause of death.

The victim may be alive or already dead by several causes (gunshot wounds, stab wounds, etc.) when the process begins. Discovering if the victim was alive when exposed to fire is a major issue for the legal processes in Brazil, since it is considered a factor for penalty increase for the perpetrator (Brasil, 1940). Although tires don't catch fire spontaneously, they can quickly and easily become inflamed by a propellant, as they have combustible properties. Depending on the weather and surrounding conditions, the fire can become visibly intense (Coelho and Rezende, 2016).

Other countries, such as South Africa, Haiti, Sri Lanka, and Nigeria, have similar practices of lynching, called necklacing. In South Africa, necklacing came as a legacy from townships in the 1980s, as a form of punishment to those who were perceived as sell-outs to the white-minority rule, or sometimes to common criminals convicted by the "people's courts." In that practice, a single tire is put around the neck of the victim, sometimes the victim has their hands and feet tied, gasoline is poured over, and the victim is set on fire (Nomoyi and Schurink, 1998) (Figure 19.3).

A very emblematic Brazilian case of "microwave oven" death was that of the investigative journalist Tim Lopes, of Globo TV Channel. In June of 2002, he left the television company to visit one of the communities of the famous "Alemão Complex" *favela*, to proceed to record a piece at a "funk baile" – which is a party highly associated with increased drug use and the illegal presence of minors in the *favelas*. Tim Lopes was going to investigate and report underage sex and drug consumption during a party financed by drug dealers (Guedes, 2002). After being

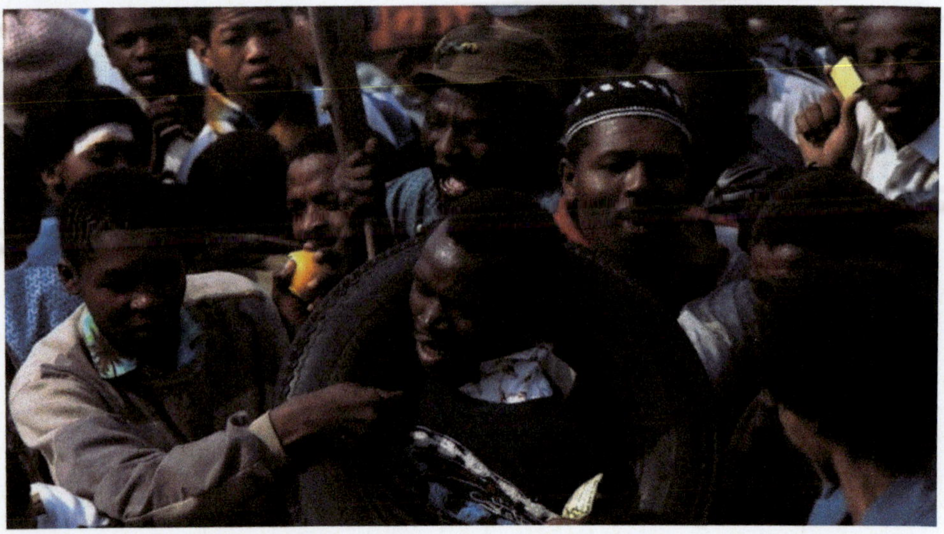

Figure 19.3 A man suspected of being a police informant is almost "necklaced" by an angry mob during a funeral in Duncan Village in South Africa. David Turnley/Corbis/VCG via Getty Images. Fair use.

discovered by the security of the narcotraffickers, they conducted a "people's court" to decide if they were going to kill him or spare his life. Unfortunately, the gang decided for the first. After being bulleted in the feet and tortured by a group of nine men, Tim Lopes was executed by a sword, dismembered, and burned inside tires (Jakobskind, 2003). Brazil is one of the 20 deadliest countries listed on the website of the Committee to Protect Journalists (Lauría, 2012).

Tim Lopes' death culminated in the discovery of clandestine graves in which murdered individuals were disposed of by the narcotraffickers. Many of the individuals found in those graves were people reported as missing persons. The graves contained many victims of the "microwave oven" death, and the reporting of those findings by the Brazilian media resulted in discussions regarding violation of human rights and the political inaction to tackle the issues of organized crime (Jakobskind, 2003).

19.4 Phases of Rubber Tire Combustion

Rubber tires are designed to absorb the heat created by the friction of road contact; therefore they do not ignite easily. However, rubber tires are composed of combustible compounds, such as oil, benzene, carbon, toluene, sulfur, and rubber (Noll *et al.*, 2014). The composition and heat absorption capacity of rubber tires make it difficult to extinguish fires once ignition takes place. The steel cords present in the tire structure, together with the carbon component, serve as a heat sink, storing the heat within the tire. Even if extinguishing the fire cools the tire from open flaming to a smoldering stage, the capacity of heat absorption can cause them to re-ignite.

Noll *et al.* (2014) describe stages of tire combustion, and by their observations we can separate four distinct phases, defined as:

Ignition and Propagation Phase: Production of flammable vapor at approximately 1000°F (538°C). A flame front that is hot and applied to a large area with constant heat flow can decompose the tires to temperatures as low as 410°F (210°C).

Compression Phase: Collapse of top layers of the tires with increase of smoke levels. High piles of tires will collapse within themselves within 30–60 minutes. The collapse of the pile creates a semi-solid mass of rubber, tire cords, and steel. The open flaming starts to slow down, and equilibrium starts to occur.

Equilibrium and Pyrolysis Phase: Equilibrium is reached when fuel conversion is equal to the amount of heat, fuel, and oxygen available. This phase shows a deep internal fire with temperatures reaching 2000°F (1100°C). Fuel is consumed slowly and completely.

Smoldering Phase: Production of a lot of smoke, resulted from combustion, and toxic chemicals. If tires are being free burned, the products of combustion are fewer and most of the toxic chemicals are consumed.

When tires are ignited in piles, the burning goes inwards into the middle of the pile. This is facilitated by the shape of the tire casings, which ensure a flow of air to provide oxygen from underneath as the heat and gases rise vertically. The steel cords present in the tire composition serve as a covering that breaks up water streams.

19.5 The Challenges of Investigating "Microwave Oven" Deaths

The determination of cause and manner of death of individual victims of thermal action is the first and foremost goal in forensic investigations. Many specific alterations are present when the human body is exposed to fire for a prolonged period of time. It is always challenging to determine the cause of death in a burnt body investigation; thus, it is crucial to analyze the remains beyond their burning injuries (Bohnert *et al.*, 1997, 1998). If bodies are relatively fresh, with no drastic injuries to internal organs, the presence of soot in the airways, esophagus, and stomach indicate that the victim was alive during the fire (Saukko and Knight, 2015). It might also be possible to detect carbon monoxide or cyanide levels in the body. These elements suggest that the death was caused by thermal action, which can sometimes result in the burning of the victims (Montenegro *et al.*, 2013). However, if the thermal action is extensive, damaging external soft tissue, muscles, internal structures, and bones, the investigation becomes more difficult and requires specialists to work in a holistic manner.

When a body becomes carbonized, there is a massive loss of soft and hard tissue, with changes in the structure and form of the body, resulting in partial or total charred remains. Based on Montenegro *et al.* (2013), the main alterations seen in carbonized remains are:

1. Loss of volume, weight, and stature.

2. Semi-flexion of the limbs (pugilistic position), due to the dehydration of the skin and contraction of flexor muscles, with fingers in claw position.
3. The body surface is blackened, the skin tense and retracted; it can present with straight continuity solutions, with regular, clean edges at the level of the joints, in the upper third of the arms and lower third of the thighs, without vital reaction. These skin continuity solutions can be misdiagnosed, like incised wounds. In areas protected by clothing, areas may remain intact.
4. There is amputation of the limbs, which in the upper limbs occurs at the level of the upper third of the humerus and in the lower limbs at the lower third of the femur.
5. The soft tissues are burned, lost, and present all degrees of burns.
6. The scalp in most cases is destroyed, leaving the calvaria exposed. The skull shows multiple fissures. Sometimes the skullcap ruptures, due to the pressure of the gases, externalizing the brain mass.
7. The brain tissue is cooked and exits through the destroyed cranial vault. There may be epidural hematoma after death, due to the rupture of the blood vessels of the diploe and venous sinuses.
8. The chest and abdomen can open, giving way to the heart and intestines, due to the great tension formed by gases and vapors. The heart, uterus, bladder, and prostate are very resistant to heat.
9. Particles of coal and soot in the respiratory tree are signs of burns ante-mortem.
10. The blood may have a chocolate color due to the formation of methemoglobin or a cherry-pink color due to the formation of carboxyhemoglobin, which are signs of burning in life.
11. The teeth are highly resistant to the action of fire, making it possible to recognize the enamel, dentin, and cement. The dental changes allow us to estimate the temperature of the fire.

Eckert *et al.* (1988) promoted a system for categorization of fire modification; their system delineates thermal alterations by amounts of surviving tissue. Therefore, the classification includes:

1. Charring – where the internal organs remain.
2. Partial cremation – where soft tissues remain.
3. Incomplete cremation – where bone fragments remain.
4. Complete cremation – where only ashes remain.

Conversely, the Glassman and Crow Scale (1996), defined thermal alterations in other categories:

1. Recognizable for identification – typical of smoke death, with possible epidermal blistering and singeing of the hair.
2. Possibly recognizable – with varying degrees of charring on elements such as the hands / feet, genitalia, and ears.

3. Non-recognizable – with major destruction / disarticulation of the head and extremities.
4. Extensive burn destruction – where the skull and extremities are severely fragmented or missing.
5. Cremation – where little or no tissue remains and osteological fragments are scattered and incomplete.

Classifications such as the ones presented above, describe the state of the soft and hard tissue after the effect of direct fire. One must acknowledge that it is possible that a body or a bone element presents multiple classifications concomitantly. Nevertheless, considering the already complex analysis of burnt or carbonized remains, the presence of rubber tires enveloping a body while burning only adds to creating an even more problematic environment that requires the careful work of highly skilled forensic experts.

19.6 The Role of Forensic Anthropology

Bone matrix contains water, blood vessels, fat, and other tissues. When bone is heated, its components are affected and respond in different manners, such as evaporating, charring, contracting, expanding, or burning. Bone itself dehydrates, shrinks, delaminates, calcinates, and fractures. The organic and inorganic matrices degrade and transform. Among many uncertainties regarding the exact process in which these transformations occur, researchers have been able to identify temperature ranges that can be associated with certain bone modifications (Holager, 1970; Civjan *et al.*, 1972; Bonucci and Graziani, 1975; Rootare and Craig, 1977; Shipman *et al.*, 1984; Thompson, 2004; Symes *et al.*, 2015; Marques *et al.*, 2018, 2021; Lemmers *et al.*, 2020).

Due to the modifications caused by fire and heat, anthropologists have become essential in the investigation of thermal alterations and physical evidence in human remains' cases, being responsible for analyses and interpretations of the bodies. The contextual reconstruction of an individual's death, and the subsequent positive identification of an individual, can be hindered by destructive thermal effects. Therefore, the involvement of a forensic anthropologist from crime scene investigation to recovery and laboratory analysis, is crucial to collect evidentiary data.

Taphonomical changes and post-mortem interpretations have gained space in the scope of forensic anthropologists working in forensic investigations. When dealing with "microwave oven" deaths, especially, perimortem trauma and postmortem taphonomic changes can become intertwined. The proper interpretation of the elements surrounding an individual's death have a vast impact on the criminal investigation of the case. Hence, a forensic anthropologist who is knowledgeable about taphonomic processes and perimortem bone trauma must be involved in such forensic cases to provide reliable information to assist in the cause and manner of death determination, as well as to assist in the positive identification of the deceased individual (Dirkmaat *et al.*, 2008; Symes *et al.*, 2014, 2015).

The following case studies shed light on the work of forensic anthropology in "microwave oven" death investigations in Brazil and were performed by the forensic anthropology laboratory of the Medico-Legal Institute André Roquette in Belo Horizonte, in the state of Minas Gerais.

19.6.1 Case Study 1

A forensic team was assigned to proceed with the examination of an unknown charred corpse, located in a small municipality (Figure 19.4). According to the police report, it was suspected that it was a certain individual who was allegedly executed due to drug debts to several drug dealers. Witnesses reported that he was tortured and intensely physically beaten, with a high-adhesion glue applied to his mouth. Then he would have been tied up, taken in the trunk of a vehicle to another place where he was beheaded by a machete, shot 4–5 times in the head and placed between tires, where the perpetrators of the crime added gasoline and set the tires on fire to hide the body.

Before proceeding with the examination of the remains, a radiological examination of all segments was carried out. It was possible to identify materials with high radiological density, such as ballistic elements, in the location close to the skull and the cervical region, in addition to the mentonian region. It was possible to observe materials with high radiological density in the location of a dental element, such as material commonly used in dental treatment. It was also possible to see multiple filaments of material of high radiological density surrounding the body, like the internal structure of tires (Figure 19.5).

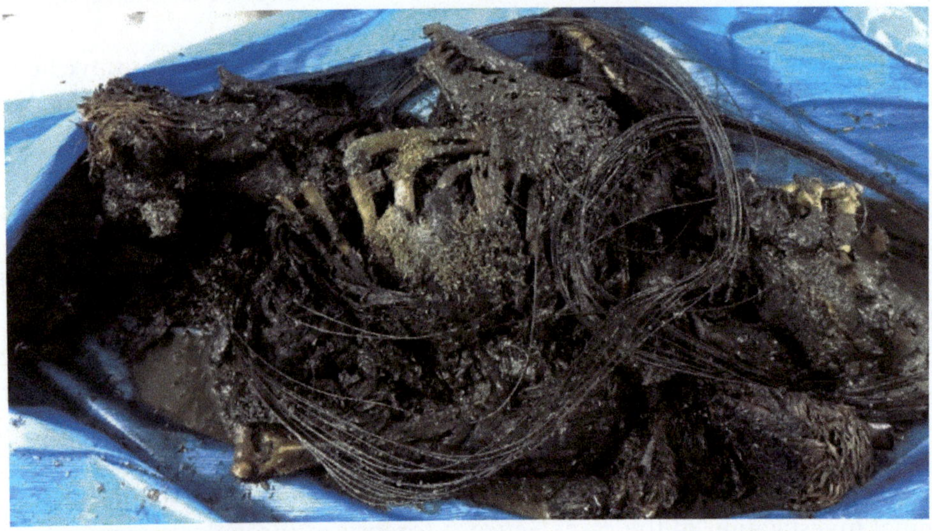

Figure 19.4 Human remains surrounded by multiple metallic filaments that involve the thoracoabdominal and cranial regions.

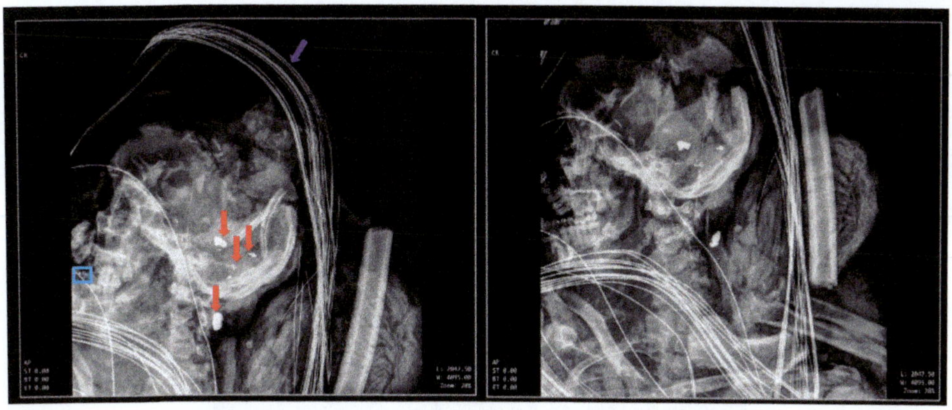

Figure 19.5 Radiological examination of the cadaver showing materials with high radiological density next to the remnants of the skull and cervical region (red arrows); material with high radiological density in a dental element (marked in blue); multiple filamentary materials around the skull and thorax of the corpse (purple arrow).

The anthropological report observed a carbonized human body showing destruction of the cutaneous and muscle-aponeurotic planes in a diffuse way. The body presented under the destructive transformative phenomenon of putrefaction, predominantly in the advanced decomposition phase, with focal areas of skeletonization, of interest, to the anterior segment of the left rib cage, the middle and distal third of the right humerus. Larvae were present next to the human remnants. There was carbonization of the face and head, with extensive areas of continuity solution in the viscerocranium and neurocranium, with exposure of cranial fossae and brain tissue, which was present in the collective stage of putrefaction. Male external genitalia were carbonized, which in cross section showed remnants of spongy bodies and urethra (Figure 19.6). Some skeletal elements were selected for preparation for the purpose of morphological study (Figures 19.7 and 19.8).

The reconstruction of the remains and the analysis of the complete bones available from the case, allowed the forensic team to recognize and address multiple traumas present in the skeleton (Figures 19.9, 19.10 and 19.11).

The biological profile of the case was performed, together with trauma and taphonomic analysis. Sex was estimated to be male, by the presence of male external genitalia. Ancestry estimation was hampered by the absence of bone elements essential for its determination. The stature was estimated through anthropometric indices as being around 164 cm, with a variation of + – 8.44 cm. The age was estimated to be 25–30.7 years, 95% confidence interval, range 19–53 years. The time of death was estimated to be greater than five days previously. However, chronothanatognosis (determination of the time of death) for cadavers that have not been buried and that have suffered the action of elements of destruction (fire) is hampered by the lack of precise elements for its calculation. The cause of death was addressed to be possibly due to head trauma by high-velocity impact (firearm

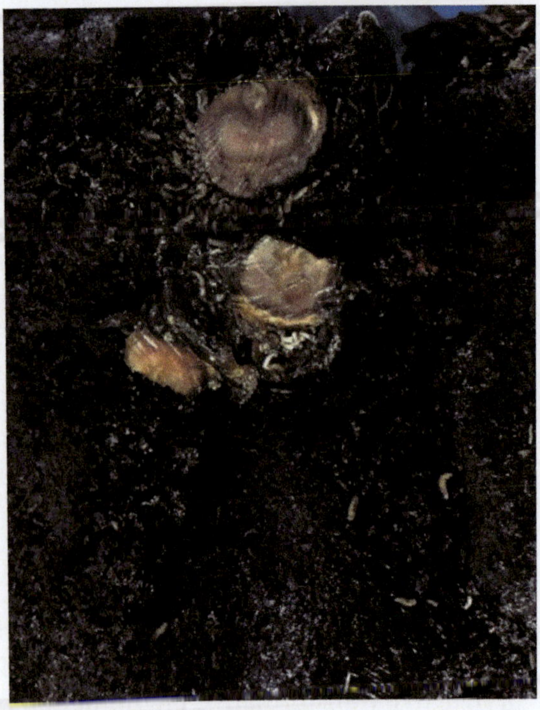

Figure 19.6 Cross section of the external genitalia, which showed remnants of spongy bodies and urethra.

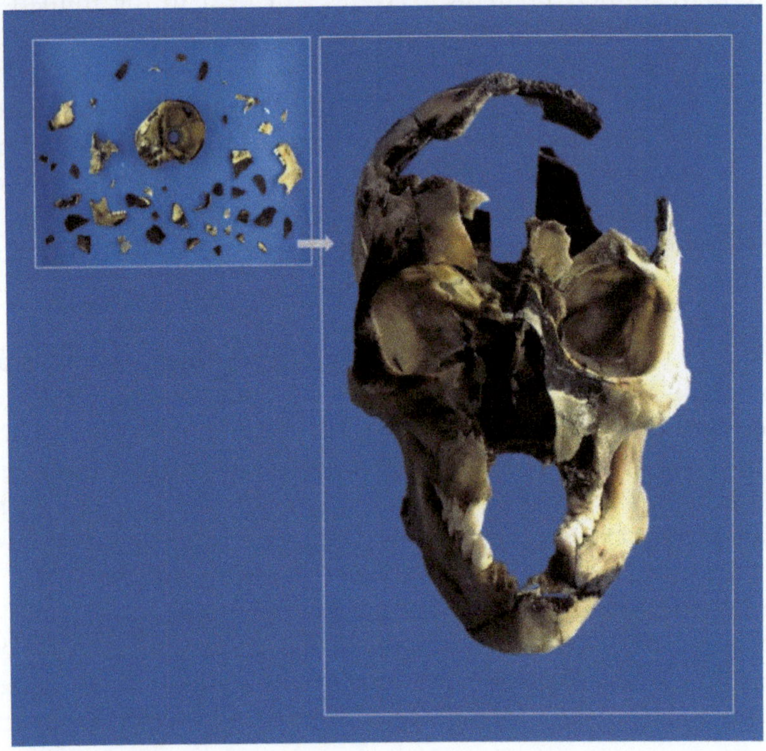

Figure 19.7 Cranial reconstruction (anterior view).

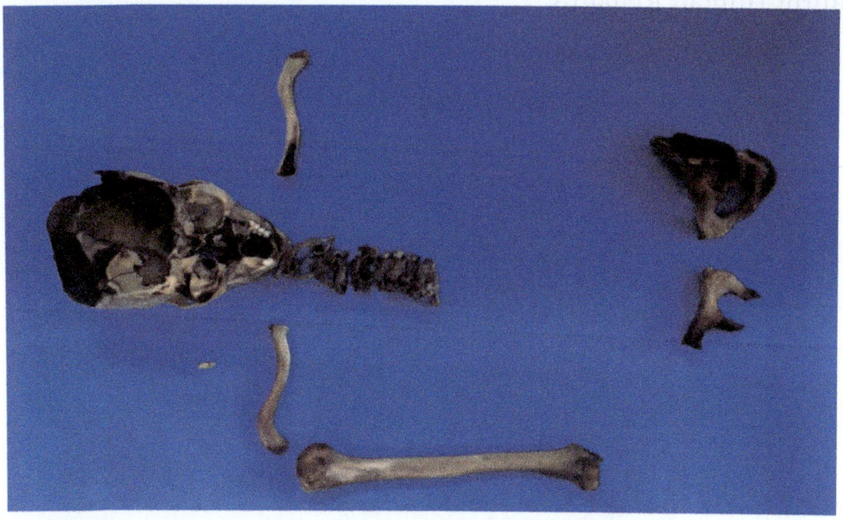

Figure 19.8 Skeletal elements cleaned to be used for analysis.

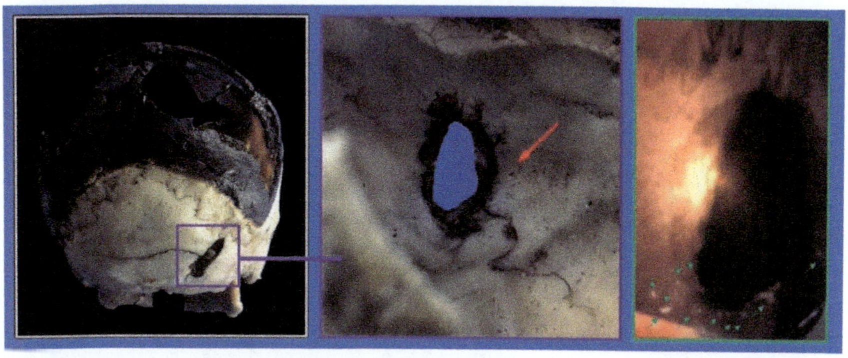

Figure 19.9 Posterior view of the skull after reconstitution (image on the right). Area of bone continuity solution in the occipital region in the form of a keyhole. Radiological image (periapical radiological film) showing fragments of high radiological density in the region adjacent to the predicted area of bone continuity solution (green arrows in the image on the right).

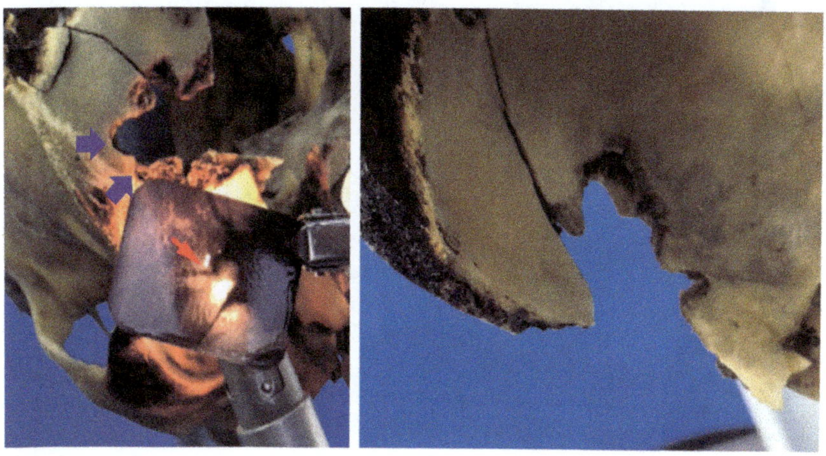

Figure 19.10 The adjacent areas (purple arrows) were of interest to the frontal bone. They had a conical section shape with their base showing irregular edges, with 28.85 mm in the largest diameter, facing the inside of the cranial cavity and the apex, with regular edges, with 25.49 mm in the largest diameter, facing the outside of the skull, Bonnet funnel sign. The radiological examination in periapical film showed images of high radiological density at its edges, reinforcing that it is an orifice related to the passage of a firearm projectile.

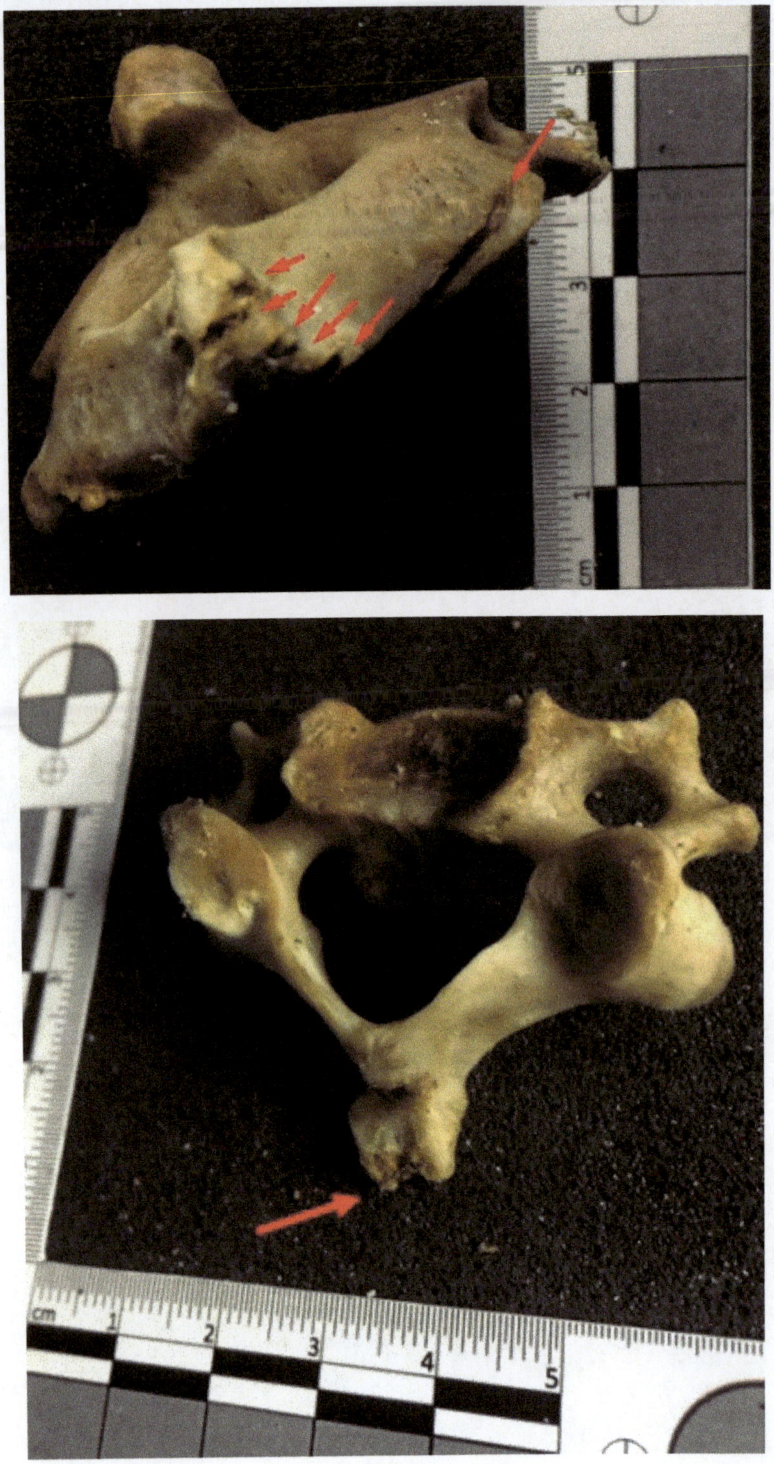

Figure 19.11 Detail of six areas of bone loss in C2 (left) with characteristics of having been produced by a sharp-blunt instrument. Detail of areas of bone loss in C4 (right) with characteristics of having been produced by a sharp-blunt instrument located in the spinous process.

projectiles) and cervical trauma by a sharp-blunt instrument. The individual was positively identified through DNA testing after a narrowing down of possible individuals by forensic anthropology and the witnesses accounts.

19.6.2 Case Study 2

The forensic anthropology team was assigned to a case referred by the Police Department of a small municipality. Police reports described the incident as a fire that started in a remote area of a farm. Witnesses said that they tried to extinguish the fire for more than a day, after the flames got out of control, resulting in damage on their property. While assessing the damages, the witnesses observed a partially carbonized body surrounded by the remains of rubber tires. The body was recovered and transferred to the laboratory for anthropological analysis.

The individual was partially carbonized and presented in a pugilistic position with protrusion of the tongue. A cross section of the external genitalia showed remnants of spongy bodies and urethra. Together with the human remains, metallic filaments were recovered, partially entangled around the thoracic region of the individual (Figure 19.12).

The search for signs that could help the identification of the body was carried out, with the careful removal of the upper layers of soot that were attached to the skin. Subsequently, the cutaneous segments that contained tattoos were prepared in the forensic anthropology laboratory, with hydration with glycerin and deionized water to provide a greater degree of detail. While analyzing the individual, areas of sharp-force traumas were observed on its back, three in the left scapular region, two in the left infra-scapular region, two in the para-vertebral region (one on the left and one on the right, one in the vertebral region) (Figure 19.13).

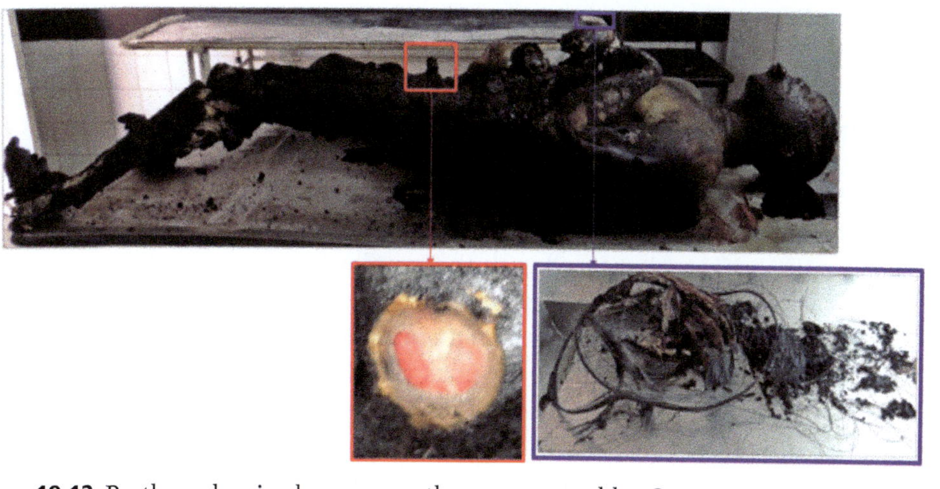

Figure 19.12 Partly carbonized corpse on the necropsy table. Cross section of the penis revealed spongy bodies and urethra (marked in red). Around the body there are multiple metallic ellipses, in the thoracic region, adhered to vestiges of vestments, which were removed for the beginning of the necroscopic examination (marked in purple).

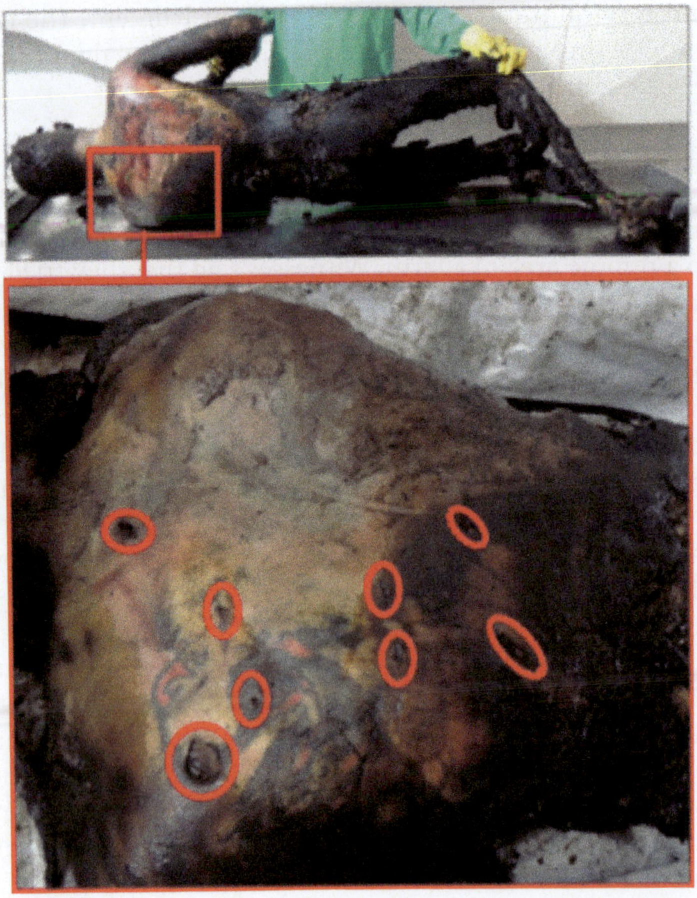

Figure 19.13 Sharp-force trauma wounds located in the dorsal region of the unknown individual (red circles).

The skull and mandible had multiple areas of bone loss, constituting 29 fragments. At the laboratory of forensic anthropology, anatomical reconstruction was carried out by juxtaposing the cranial and mandibular fragments with a multipurpose instant adhesive of medium viscosity, composed of ethyl cyanoacrylate. The frontal bone flap was reconstituted with thermoplastic glue. After drying and stabilizing the cranial and mandibular fragments, the skull and the respective mandible were anatomically positioned to perform an anthropological study (Figure 19.14).

The frontal bone showed various traumas and an area with quadrangular bone remodeling, with rounded edges and the presence of blue suture threads that tied the bone flap to the skull, passing through rounded holes in the skull (Figure 19.15).

The biological profile of the case was performed, together with trauma and taphonomic analysis. Sex was estimated to be male, by the presence of male external genitalia. The age at death was estimated to be compatible with a young adult individual aged 19–30 years, with an average of 24.5 years. The stature was

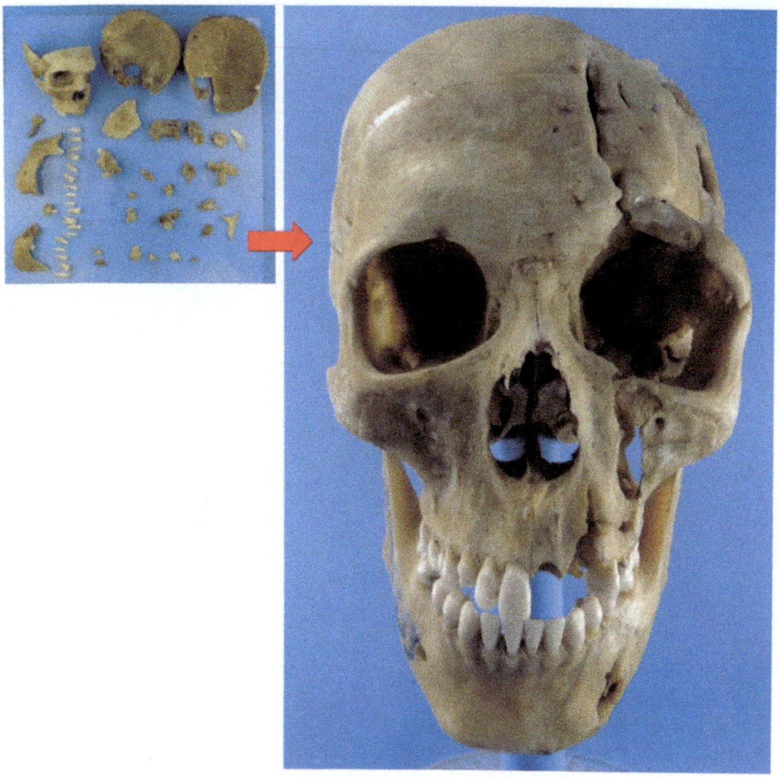

Figure 19.14 Skull and mandible in anterior view after reconstitution.

estimated through anthropometric indices as being 182.5–183.5 cm (+– 6.9 cm). The time of death was estimated to be of a minimum of seven days previously. The cause of death was assessed to be multiple sharp-force traumas.

During the forensic anthropological analysis, the positive identification of the individual was also pursued. A search on the missing persons' reports from the surrounding area was performed using the anthropological analysis as a narrowing down tool. During this step, a possible match was observed, and the family was contacted for an interview.

During the family interview conducted by the medical examiner responsible for the report, it was found that the missing person, aged 24, had last been seen about two weeks prior to the incident by his family members. The individual, a man of height around 180 cm, had several tattoos on different regions of the body and a medical history that included a motorcycle accident, that had happened five years previously. The motorcycle accident caused severe traumatic brain injury that required neurosurgical treatment and hospitalization. Due to this trauma, the individual had an extensive scar from the frontal to the parietal region. According to the family, his face was a little dented. He was admitted to a large hospital for about 15 days at the time of the accident and chose not to have other surgeries for aesthetic

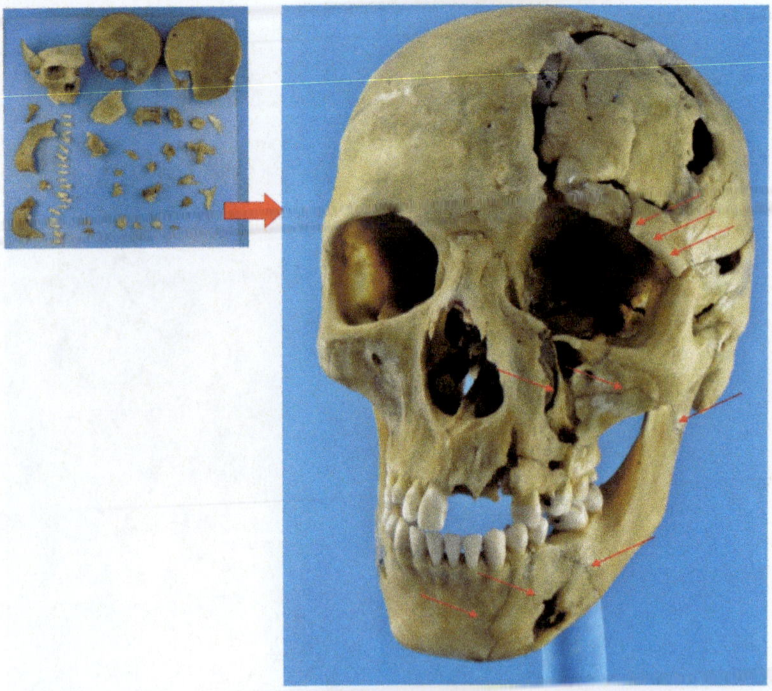

Figure 19.15 Skull and mandible in left antero-lateral view after reconstitution. The frontal bone showed an area with quadrangular bone remodeling, with rounded edges and the presence of blue colored threads that tied the bone flap to the skull. The presence of an area of continuity solution was observed, interested in the viscerocranium and the left mandible, with multiple fractures (red arrows).

correction. He had passed through the prison system, where he had one of his teeth extracted, but the family members did not know exactly which tooth it was.

The family members sent digital photographs of the missing young man and tomographic films dated from the time of the accident. In the images it was possible to observe a concave area in the frontal region on the left, parallel to the sagittal suture. The presence of a linear scar parallel to the coronoid suture was also noted (Figure 19.16).

The tomographic films sent by the family members (ante-mortem images) were analyzed and selected, considering those in which anatomical morphological characteristics of the skull were well evidenced for comparison with the tomographic images obtained from the skull of the unknown individual (post-mortem images). After proper preparation, tomographic examination, and photographic record of the deceased individual, the images referred to in this report as ante-mortem and those referred to as post-mortem were compared, looking for points of agreement and or disagreement between them. Multiple anatomical similarities were detected between post-mortem and ante-mortem images (Figures 19.17, 19.18, 19.19, 19.20). Additionally, there were multiple points of convergence between the outline of the tattoos shown on the unknown deceased individual and the images of the tattoos shown in the photographs of the missing person.

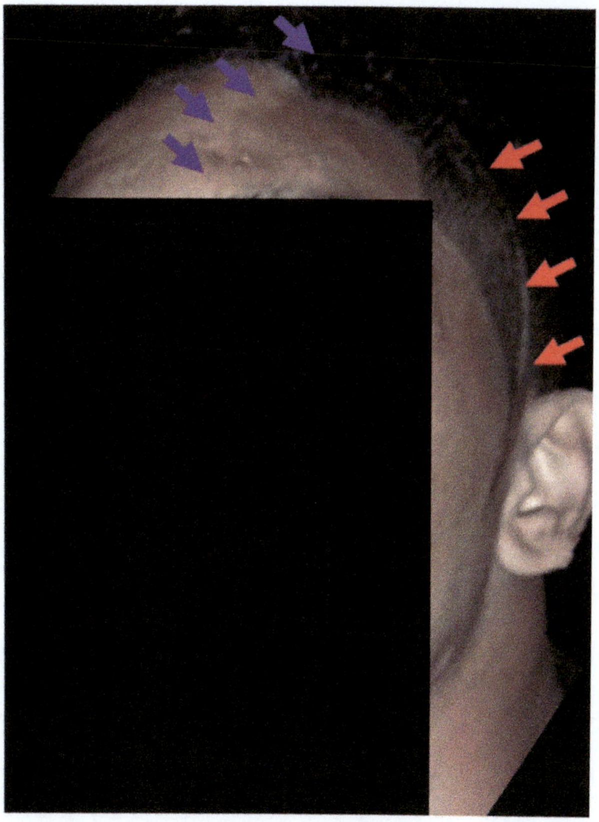

Figure 19.16 Adaptation of the photograph sent by the family members of the missing person showing, in the frontal region, an area with an indentation of the upper third of the left face (purple arrows) and the presence of a scar in the temporo-parietal region on the left.

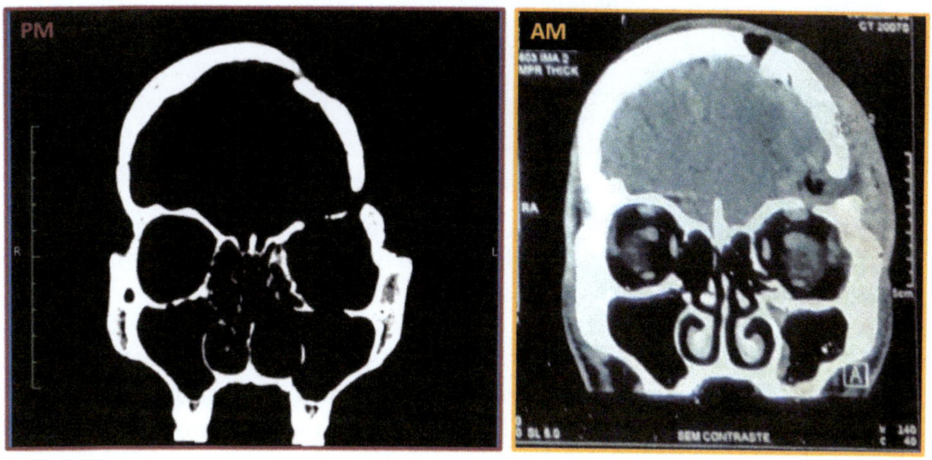

Figure 19.17 Sagittal section showing an area of remodeling corresponding to a similar neurosurgical procedure between the PM (post-mortem) and AM (ante-mortem) images in the left frontal bone.

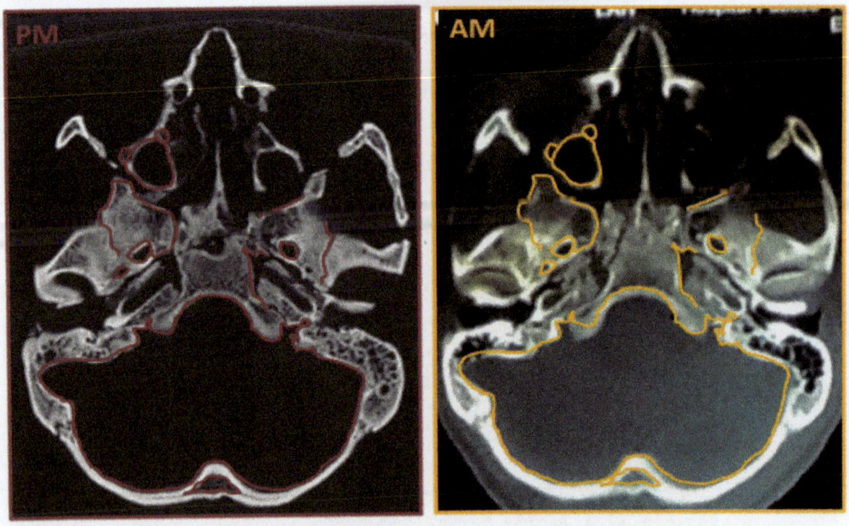

Figure 19.18 Points of similarity in right maxillary sinus; contour of the posterior fossa; contour of the sphenoids; and foramina.

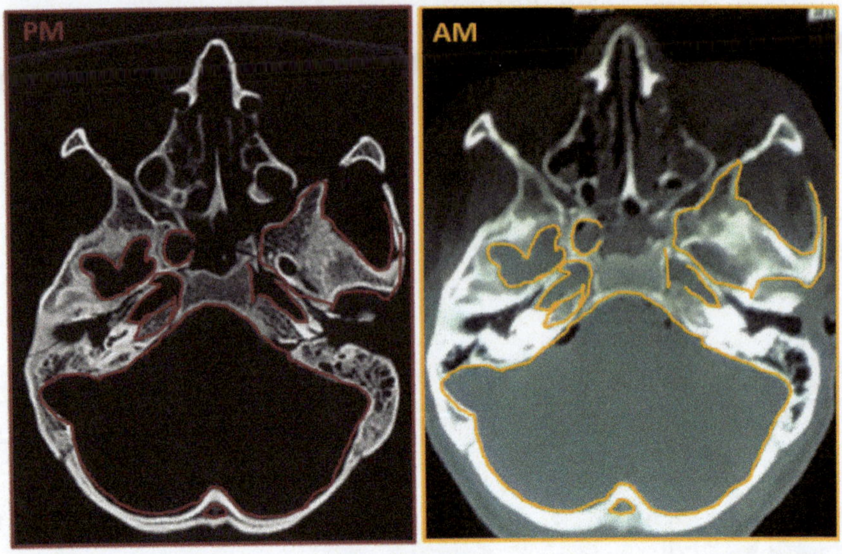

Figure 19.19 Coincident images in contour of the right temporal bone; segment of the right sphenoid sinus; morphology of the bony structure of the middle fossa; contour of the posterior fossa.

The evaluation of the biological profile represented by sex, stature, and age at death of the deceased individual fitted the profile of the missing person given by the family members, as well as the data submitted by ante-mortem documents. The ante-mortem photographs and tomographic images compared to the post-mortem images presented concordant and coincident points in addition to the absence of excluding points between the data observed. Therefore, the presence of matching individual anatomical elements, individualizing characteristics, and

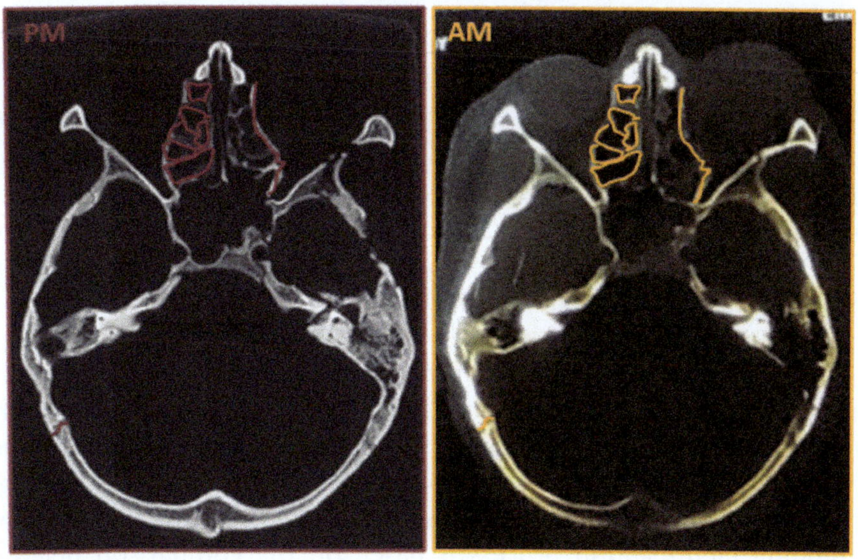

Figure 19.20 Coincident images in morphology of the ethmoidal cells on the right and their lateral wall on the left.

biological profile, resulted in the positive identification of the deceased individual as being the missing person reported by his family members.

19.7 Conclusion

Forensic anthropologists have become increasingly involved in situations in which fire has impacted human remains. Some of these damages are so significant that the heat and fire obstruct and hamper the analysis and interpretation of the physical evidence. Nevertheless, the analysis of the forensic scene also provides evidence to the understanding of the circumstances in which they occurred.

The "microwave oven" death is a type of criminal act of execution performed in Brazil, mostly by narcotraffickers, and distinct from other types of fire or heat means of death. The observation of the scene and human remains involved, provide enough evidence to identify its practice. Accurate interpretation and understanding of the scene and human remains are crucial for the criminal investigation and the positive identification of the deceased individual.

The "microwave oven" death results in a partial or complete carbonization of a human body, depending on the number of tires used and the time spent burning. The analysis of carbonized bodies of victims of this act is complex due to the damage caused by the fire and the melting of the rubber tires, causing human remains and iron and rubber to become intertwined. Additionally, the heat and fire damage can make it difficult to distinguish between types of traumas, manner of death, and to achieve the positive identification of the deceased individual, as this type of criminal act is generally used to hamper the identification.

Technological advances in the medical field have allowed for new methods to be implemented in forensic analysis. The critical observation, description, and comparison of features and structures have been used to aid in the positive identification of human remains extensively damaged from thermal destruction. The expertise of a knowledgeable forensic anthropologist is crucial to achieve reliable results in the analysis of victims of the "microwave oven" death.

The positive identification of individuals was demonstrated in this chapter by two case studies from the forensic anthropology laboratory at the Medico-Legal Institute André Roquette in Belo Horizonte, Minas Gerais, Brazil. The authors stress that the positive identification of individuals is a team effort, as demonstrated by the case studies. The analyses of a trained forensic anthropologist are imperative to compose the holistic process leading to a positive identification. The legally binding identification process is based on the comparison between the ante-mortem and post-mortem data, which involves the data from missing persons and unidentified remains, respectively, demonstrating enough valuable evidence that they relate to one single individual. Furthermore, although the "microwave oven" is used to impede identification and burden forensic analysis, the expertise of a forensic anthropologist will enhance the forensic team's capacity to provide accurate and reliable results for the criminal investigation.

Conflicts of Interest

The authors have no funding and conflicts of interest to disclose.

Ethical Approval

All procedures performed in this study involving human participants were conducted in accordance with the ethical standards of the institutional ethics committee (Approval No. 4.407.412) and the 1964 Declaration of Helsinki and its later amendments or comparable ethical standards.

Acknowledgments

The authors would like to thank the Superintendência de Polícia Civil de Minas Gerais and the radiologist, Adriana Zatti Lima, for performing tomographic images. No funds to disclose.

References

Abdalla, R.R., Madruga, C.S., Ribeiro, M., Pinsky, I., Caetano, R., and Laranjeira, R. (2014) Prevalence of cocaine use in Brazil: Data from the II Brazilian national alcohol and drugs survey (BNADS). *Addictive Behaviors*, **39**(1), 297–301.

Araújo, E.M.D., Costa, M.D.C.N., Oliveira, N.F.D., Santana, F.D.S., Barreto, M.L., Hogan, V., *et al.* (2010) Spatial distribution of mortality by homicide and social inequalities according to race/skin color in an intra-urban Brazilian space. *Revista Brasileira de Epidemiologia*, **13**(4), 549–560. pmid:21180845.

Atkinson, A., Anderson, Z., Hughes, K., Bellis, M.A., Sumnall, H., and Syed, Q. (2009) *Interpersonal violence and illicit drugs*. Center for Public Health, Liverpool John Moores University. (PDF) World Health Organization Centre for Violence Prevention, Liverpool, UK, 25 pages. https://www.who.int/publications/m/item/interpersonal-violence-and-illicit-drugs.

Auger, N., Le Serbon, E., Rasella, D., Aquino, R., and Barreto, M.L. (2016) Impact of homicide and traffic crashes on life expectancy in the largest Latin American country. *Journal of Public Health*, **38**(3), 467–473.

Bohnert, M., Rost, T., Faller-Marquardt, M., Ropohl, D., and Pollak, S. (1997) Fractures of the base of the skull in charred bodies – post-mortem heat injuries or signs of mechanical traumatisation? *Forensic Science International*, **87**(1), 55–62.

Bohnert, M., Rost, T., and Pollak, S. (1998) The degree of destruction of human bodies in relation to the duration of the fire. *Forensic Science International*, **95**(1), 11–21.

Bonucci, E. and Graziani, G. (1975) Comparative thermogravimetric, X-ray diffraction and electron microscope investigations of burnt bones from recent, ancient, and prehistoric age. Atti Memorie Accademia Nazionale die Lincei Scienze, Fisiche, *Matematiche Naturali Series*, **8**(59), 517–534.

Brasil. Criminal Code. (1940) *Article 121 Decree Law 2848/40*. https://www.jusbrasil.com.br/busca?q=Art.+121+do+Decreto+Lei+2848%2F40, accessed March 01, 2021.

Briefing, W.P. (2006) *Interpersonal violence and alcohol*. (((PDF) World Health Organization, Geneva. https://lx.iriss.org.uk/sites/default/files/resources/Interpersonal%20violence%20and%20alcohol.pdf.

Campello, T. and Neri, M.C. (2013) *Programa Bolsa Família: uma década de inclusão e cidadania*, 1st edn. (((9(PDF) Brasília. IPE, Nazareth, Brazil. http://repositorio.ipea.gov.br/bitstream/11058/2082/4/Livro-Programa_Bolsa_Familia-uma_década_de_inclusão_e_cidadania.pdf.

Cerqueira, D., Lima, R.S.D., Bueno, S., Valencia, L.I., Hanashiro, O., Machado, P.H.G., *et al.* (2017) *Atlas da Violência 2017-IPEA e FBSP*, pp. 69–69. https://www.ipea.gov.br/atlasviolencia/download/2/2017.

Civjan, S., Selting, W.J., De Simon, L.B., Battistone, G.C., and Grower, M.F. (1972) Characterization of osseous tissues by thermogravimetric and physical techniques. *Journal of Dental Research*, **51**(2), 539–542.

Coelho, H.A. and Rezende, E.N. (2016) A responsabilidade civil Ambiental na Inglaterra. *Revista do Direito*. Santa Cruz do Sul, **1**(48), 167–186.

Cunha, E. (2019) Devolvendo a identidade: A antropologia forense no Brasil. *Ciência e Cultura*, **71**(2), 30–34. https://dx.doi.org/10.21800/2317-66602019000200011.

Degenhardt, L., Whiteford, H., and Hall, W.D. (2014) The Global Burden of Disease projects: What have we learned about illicit drug use and dependence and their contribution to the global burden of disease? *Drug and Alcohol Review*, **33**(1), 4–12.

Degenhardt, L., Whiteford, H.A., Ferrari, A.J., Baxter, A.J., Charlson, F.J., Hall, W.D., *et al.* (2013) Global burden of disease attributable to illicit drug use and dependence: Findings from the Global Burden of Disease Study 2010. *The Lancet*, **382**(9904), 1564–1574.

Dirkmaat, D.C., Cabo, L.L., Ousley, S.D., and Symes, S.A. (2008) New perspectives in forensic anthropology. *American Journal of Physical Anthropology: The Official Publication of the American Association of Physical Anthropologists,* **137**(S47), 33–52.

Durão, C., Machado, M.P. and Júnior, E.D., 2015. Death in the "microwave oven": A form of execution by carbonization. *Forensic Science International,* **253**, e1–e3. https://doi.org/10.1016/j.forsciint.2015.05.012.

Eckert, W.G., James, S., and Katchis, S. (1988) Investigation of cremations and severely burned bodies. *The American Journal of Forensic Medicine and Pathology,* **9**(3), 188–200.

Gawryszewski, V.P. and Costa, L.S. (2005) Social inequality and homicide rates in Sao Paulo City, Brazil. *Revista de Saúde Pública,* **39**(2), 191–197.

Glassman, D.M. and Crow, R.M. (1996) Standardization model for describing the extent of burn injury to human remains. *Journal of Forensic Science,* **41**(1), 152–154.

Guedes, L.J. (2002) Corpo de Tim Lopes é identificado por exame de DNA, diz polícia. *Folha de São Paulo.* https://www1.folha.uol.com.br/folha/cotidiano/ult95u54153.shtml.

Holager, J. (1970) Thermogravimetric examination of enamel and dentin. *Journal of Dental Research,* **49**(3), 546–548.

IBGE – Instituto Brasileiro de Geografia e Estatística. (2010) *Características da vitimização e do acesso à justiça no Brasil 2009,* 1st edn. (PDF) PNAD, Rio de Janeiro, Brazil. https://biblioteca.ibge.gov.br/visualizacao/livros/liv47311.pdf.

Jaguaribe, B. and Reis, R. (2009) The violence of the real: A conversation with Rogério Reis. *Public Culture,* **21**(2), 229–233.

Jakobskind, M.A. (2003) *Dossiê Tim Lopes*. Europa, Rio de Janeiro, Brazil.

Krug, E.G., Mercy, J.A., Dahlberg, L.L., and Zwi, A.B. (2002) The world report on violence and health. World Health Organization, Geneva. *The Lancet,* **360**(9339), 1083–1088.

Lauría, C. (2012) Colombia, Mexico, and Brazil: The deadliest countries in the hemisphere for journalists. *NACLA Report on the Americas,* **45**(3), 35.

Lemmers, S.A., Gonçalves, D., Cunha, E., Vassalo, A.R., and Appleby, J. (2020) Burned fleshed or dry? The potential of bioerosion to determine the pre-burning condition of human remains. *Journal of Archaeological Method and Theory,* **27**(4), 972–991.

Lemos, Y.V., Wainstein, A.J.A., Savoi, L.M., and Drummond-Lage, A.P. (2019) Epidemiological and toxicological profile of homicide victims in a legal medicine unit in Brazil. *Journal of Forensic and Legal Medicine,* **65**, 55–60, ISSN 1752-928X, https://doi.org/10.1016/j.jflm.2019.05.008.

Marques, M.P.M., Gonçalves, D., Mamede, A.P., Coutinho, T., Cunha, E., Kockelmann, W., *et al.* (2021) Profiling of human burned bones: Oxidising versus reducing conditions. *Scientific Reports,* **11**(1), 1–13.

Marques, M.P.M., Mamede, A.P., Vassalo, A.R., Makhoul, C., Cunha, E., Gonçalves, D., *et al.* (2018) Heat-induced bone diagenesis probed by vibrational spectroscopy. *Scientific Reports,* **8**(1), 1–13.

Mikton, C.R., Butchart, A., Dahlberg, L.L., and Krug, E.G. (2016) Global status report on violence prevention 2014. *American Journal of Preventive Medicine,* **50**(5), 652–659. https://doi.org/10.1016/j.amepre.2015.10.007.

Montenegro, J.B., Leal, J.L.F., Cruz, D.B., de Carvalho, M.V.D., de Souza, E.H.A., and do Egito Vasconcelos, B.C. (2013) Perícia nas vítimas de carbonização. *Derecho y Cambio Social,* **10**(32), 29.

Moosage, R. (2010) A prose of ambivalence: Liberation struggle discourse on necklacing. *Kronos,* **36**(1), 136–157.

Murray, J., de Castro Cerqueira, D.R., and Kahn, T. (2013) Crime and violence in Brazil: Systematic review of time trends, prevalence rates and risk factors. *Aggression and Violent Behavior,* **18**(5), 471–483. https://doi.org/10.1016/j.avb.2013.07.003.

Noll, G.G., Hildebrand, M.S., Schnepp, R., and Rudner, G.D. (2014) *Hazardous Materials: Managing the Incident*. Jones & Bartlett Publishers, Burlington, MA.

Nomoyi, N. and Schurink, W. (1998) An exploratory study of insider accounts of necklacing in three Port Elizabeth townships. *Violence in South Africa*, 147–174.

Paim, J., Travassos, C., Almeida, C., Bahia, L., and Macinko, J. (2011) The Brazilian health system: History, advances, and challenges. *The Lancet*, **377**(9779), 1778–1797.

Rootare, H.M. and Craig, R.G. (1977) Vapor phase adsorption of water on hydroxyapatite. *Journal of Dental Research*, **56**(12), 1437–1448.

Saukko, P. and Knight, B. (2015) *Knight's Forensic Pathology*, 4th edn. CRC Press, London.

Shipman, P., Foster, G., and Schoeninger, M. (1984) Burnt bones and teeth: An experimental study of color, morphology, crystal structure and shrinkage. *Journal of Archaeological Science*, **11**(4), 307–325.

Symes, S.A., L'abbé, E.N., Pokines, J.T., Yuzwa, T., Messer, D., Stromquist, A., *et al.* (2014) Thermal alteration to bone. In: *Manual of Forensic Taphonomy* (eds. J.T. Pokiness and S.A. Symes). CRC Press, Baton Rouge, LA, pp. 367–402.

Symes, S.A., Rainwater, C.W., Chapman, E.N., Gipson, D.R., and Piper, A.L. (2015) Patterned thermal destruction in a forensic setting. In: *The Analysis of Burned Human Remains* (eds. C.W. Schmidt and S.A. Symes). Academic Press, Cambridge, MA, pp. 17–59.

Thompson, T. (2004) Recent advances in the study of burned bone and their implications for forensic anthropology. *Forensic Science International*, **146**, S203–S205.

Waiselfisz, J.J. (2013). *Mapa da Violencia 2013: Homicidios e Juventude no Brasil*, 1st edn. (PDF) Secretaria-Geral da Presidência da República, Brasília. http://flacso.org.br/files/2020/03/mapa2013_homicidios_juventude.pdf.

Waiselfisz, J.J. (2014). *Mapa da Violência 2014: os jovens do Brasil.* ((PDF) *Secretaria- Geral da Presidência da República, Secretaria Nacional de Juventude, Secretaria de Políticas de Promoção da Igualdade Racial, Brasília.* http://www.vias-seguras.com/os_acidentes/estatisticas/estatisticas_nacionais/estatisticas_do_ministerio_da_saude/mapa_da_violencia_2014_os_jovens_do_brasil.

Waiselfisz, J.J. (2016). *Mapa da Violencia 2016. Homicidios por arma de fogo no Brasil*, 1st edn. (PDF) Rio de Janeiro: FLACSO/CEBELA, Brazil. http://flacso.org.br/files/2016/08/Mapa2016_armas_web-1.pdf.

World Bank. (2016) Official Website. http://www.worldbank.org/en/country/brazil/overview#1.

CHAPTER 20

Recovery and Identification of Fatal Fire Victims from the 2018 Northern California Camp Fire Disaster

Colleen Milligan[1], PhD, D-ABFA; Alison Galloway[2], PhD, D-ABFA; Ashley Kendell[3], PhD; Lauren Zephro[4], PhD; P. Willey[5], PhD, D-ABFA and Eric Bartelink[6], PhD, D-ABFA

[1] *Chair and Anthropology Advisor, Anthropology Department, California State University, Chico, California*

[2] *Professor emerita, University of California, Santa Cruz, California*

[3] *Assistant Professor of Anthropology, California State University, Chico, California*

[4] *Forensic Services Director, Santa Cruz County Sherriff's Office, Santa Cruz, California*

[5] *Professor emeritus at California State University, Chico, California*

[6] *Professor of Anthropology, California State University, Chico, California*

20.1 Overview of the Camp Fire

Wildfires are uncontrolled and unplanned conflagrations that occur in rural areas and most often spread in the presence of dry fuel sources, high winds, lack of precipitation, and higher temperatures (Westerling *et al.*, 2003). Sources of ignition for wildfires span from both natural and man-made, including natural lightning strikes, sparks from cars and trailers, and failures of equipment and infrastructure, such as power lines. This means that multiple different avenues may be involved in determining what becomes a major wildfire incident. One avenue is the conditions that create fuel sources for wildfires. Prolonged periods of drought and increases in average temperature contribute to an abundance of dry vegetation, the main fuel source for wildfires (Westerling *et al.*, 2003; Marlon *et al.*, 2012; McEvoy *et al.*, 2019). Another avenue is the opportunities for fires to start. With increasing development in fire-prone areas, especially rural or remote locations, the number of opportunities that could cause ignition of a fire multiplies. In addition, an aging infrastructure has the potential to fail under stress, further increasing the opportunities for ignition (Mitchell, 2013).

In 2018, California was emerging from a major drought period encompassing severe and exceptional drought conditions over the previous six years (National Drought Mitigation Centre). California's natural weather cycle includes cool and

Burnt Human Remains: Recovery, Analysis, and Interpretation, First Edition. Edited by Sarah Ellingham, Joe Adserias-Garriga, Sara C. Zapico and Douglas H. Ubelaker.

wet winters and hot and dry summers, reflecting the state's Mediterranean climate. Typically, seasonal rains start in the late fall for most of California and end during the late spring / early summer (Schoenherr, 2017). Drought conditions are highly dependent on the amount of precipitation that comes with these seasonal rains. Too little rainfall or snow accumulation means less water held in natural and man-made reservoirs, resulting in dryer vegetation (Schoenherr, 2017).

In addition, both Northern California and Southern California see seasonal wind patterns that develop from high pressure ridges to low pressure troughs across the mountain ranges. In the south, these winds are called the Santa Ana winds (Fovell and Cao, 2017). In the north, they are commonly called the Diablo or Diablo-like winds (Liu *et al.*, 2020). The winds occurring with these seasonal patterns involve speeds that exceed typical wind conditions (Brewer and Clements, 2020). They also carry increasingly dry air as the wind accelerates downslope from higher pressure ridges, which means the air has less humidity (The Camp Fire Public Report, 2020). From 2017 to 2019, dangerous seasonal wind conditions occurred before the seasonal rains began in late fall in California (Brown *et al.*, 2020). As a result, the potential for extreme fire behavior increased from late summer to late fall when the time since the last rain was longest.

The area around the point of ignition of the Camp Fire shows seasonal fall Diablo-like winds that flow through the Feather River Canyon. As illustrated in the previous paragraph, the winds move from a high-pressure ridge to lower pressure with accelerating speed due to a gap wind effect as the air moves down the canyon on the western face of the Sierra Nevada Mountains (Gaberšek and Durran, 2006; Keeley and Syphard, 2019). The 2018 Camp Fire started in Pulga, California, near the Poe Dam in the Jarbo Gap Canyon. The three Butte County communities affected by the Camp Fire: Concow, Paradise, and Magalia, are all affected by these seasonal "Jarbo Gap" winds.

The fire that started on November 8, 2018, near Camp Creek Road, and was subsequently called the Camp Fire, combined a prolonged dry period with a high wind event in the Jarbo Gap and an infrastructure failure of Pacific Gas & Electric (PG&E) high voltage line equipment. It followed what was already the most destructive fire season on record for the State of California. Wildfires in 2018 were declared a National Disaster on August 4, after 33 larger fires had ignited since the previous February, many of which were associated with the Carr Fire in July of 2018 (Lareau *et al.*, 2018). After that declaration, the active fire season continued with ten fires in the remainder of August, six fires in September, five fires in October, and four fires that started during wind effects on November 8 in both Northern and Southern California (Cal Fire). The November 8 event was preceded by a Red Flag Warning issued by the National Oceanic and Atmospheric Administration (NOAA) on November 7. Red Flag Warnings are issued when the weather conditions exist for potential wildfires that could spread rapidly by high winds and low humidity. The Red Flag Warning issued for the Butte County area on November 7 predicted 20–30 mph winds with gusts up to 30–55 mph, and daytime humidity at 5–15% (NOAA).

The Camp Fire started from a failure of an iron hook holding a high voltage line on a PG&E transmission tower sometime between 6:15 am and 6:20 am (The Camp Fire Public Report, 2020). The failure caused the line to arc against the steel tower sending sparks and molten metal into the brush below and igniting the fire. Jarbo Gap Remote Automated Weather Station recorded sustained winds exceeding 20 mph with gusts between 41 to 52 mph the night before and morning when the fire began (Brewer and Clements, 2020; The Camp Fire Public Report, 2020). These winds quickly spread the fire beyond the capacity of local resources to contain it. By 6:40 am, the Cal Fire units, responding quickly, switched priorities from combating the fire to evacuation of residents in the Pulga and Concow areas. Within the next hour, the fire spread more than seven miles, jumping across the Feather River Canyon, to the town of Paradise (The Camp Fire Public Report, 2020).

From the beginning, the fire grew rapidly, with winds sending softball-sized embers well in advance of the fire front. By 10:45 am, infrared images showed that the southern portion of the town of Magalia had fire activity as well as the northern and eastern portions of the town of Paradise (The Camp Fire Public Report, 2020). The fire progressed down the Paradise ridge to the eastern border of the city of Chico that evening before forward progression was stopped. Full containment occurred ten days later (Cal Fire). In total, 153,336 acres burned in the Camp Fire, an area equivalent to the combined area of the cities of San Francisco and Oakland (Figure 20.1). Within the three primary communities affected, Concow, Paradise, and Magalia, 18,804 structures were destroyed,

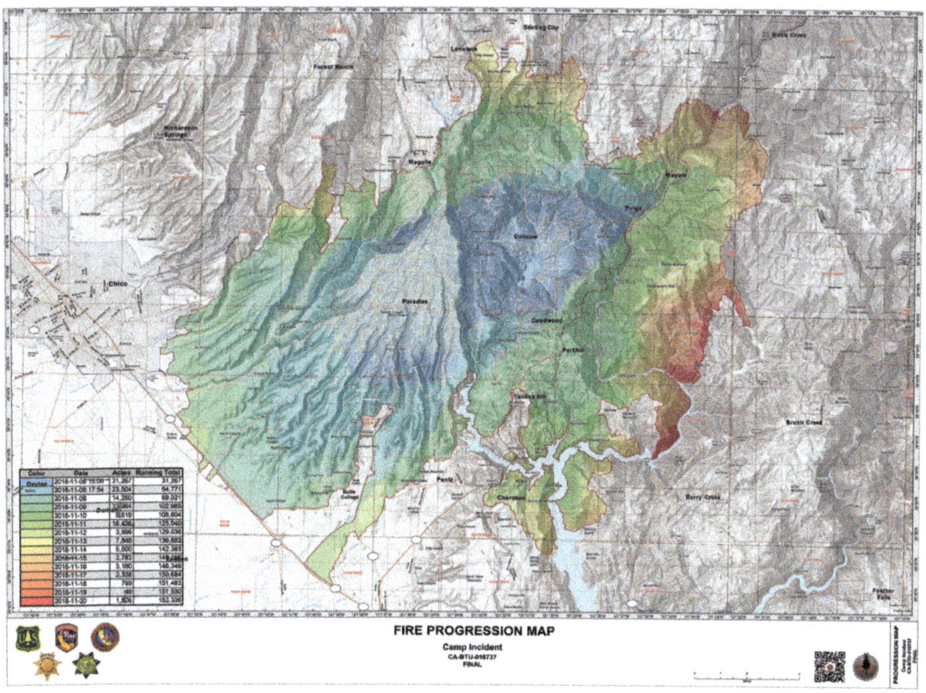

Figure 20.1 Cal Fire map of final progression of 2018 Camp Fire.

with 13,696 of those being residences (The Camp Fire Public Report, 2020). Sadly, there were also 85 victims of the fire. The Camp Fire is both the most destructive and the deadliest fire on record in the State of California. The subsequent sections will focus specifically on the victim recovery and identification.

20.2 Wildfire Burn Environments and Condition of Remains

Wildfire temperatures can greatly exceed that recorded for structure and vehicle fires and are comparable to cremation retort temperatures. For example, wildfires frequently exceed 800°C, even reaching temperatures as hot as 1200°C for large-scale fire events (Gabbert, 2011). Similarly, average cremation temperatures typically range from 871 to 927°C, but may reach as high as 1150°C (Schultz *et al.*, 2008; Van Deest *et al.*, 2011). In contrast, structure fires typically reach temperatures around 800–900°C (DeHaan, 2008), but generally do not sustain temperatures found in commercial cremations or wildfire events for any period of time. Skeletal elements exposed to fire begin initial carbonization and loss of unbound water at temperatures ranging from 20 to 350°C, and complete combustion of the organic portion can occur at temperatures that exceed 350°C (Schurr *et al.*, 2008). Warping and shrinkage of skeletal remains happens at 700–800°C from pyrolization of the organic content in skeletal remains (Ubelaker, 2009). Given the lack of fire suppression during the initial hours of the Camp Fire, trees, structures, and automobiles were left to completely burn, resulting in much more thermal destruction of human remains compared to most structure fires, where fire suppression efforts often occur soon after the fire is reported to authorities.

Human remains recovered from wildfire contexts often show a range of thermal patterns (even within the same individual), due to both intrinsic and extrinsic factors. Intrinsic factors include the sex, age, and body size of the victim, as well as their body location within the structure or vehicle. For example, a 150 lb elderly female found alongside a 250 lb young male would show more complete thermal destruction due to less soft tissue protection and less bone mass. Extrinsic factors include the size, temperature, and duration of the wildfire; the location of the residence or vehicle within the path of the fire; presence and type of combustible materials in proximity to the body; the wind direction and speed; and the location where the fire victim died (e.g. bathroom, bedroom, front seat of automobile, etc.). As an example, fire victims found in bathtubs may show protection of some parts of the body from complete thermal destruction. Typical fatal wildfires find fire victims recovered in various states of thermal destruction. For the Camp Fire, most victims were either completely calcined (similar to a commercial cremation prior to pulverization) or were predominately calcined, with some charred bone and / or soft tissue found in the more protected areas of the body such as the thorax, pelvic region, and thigh. In a few cases, bodies were recovered partially intact, with a charred torso and charred to calcined appendicular elements. Due to the extent of thermal destruction, extra care was required for recovering as much of the human remains as possible from each fire scene. Charred remains were more likely to yield DNA than calcined bone and showed a higher-than-expected success rate (Gin *et al.*, 2020).

20.3 Field to Morgue: What's Important for Identification Efforts?

Anthropologists played two principal roles in the Camp Fire: searches and field recoveries, and identification of victims as part of morgue operations. The anthropologists' roles in search and recovery evolved as the 2018 incident progressed, becoming more efficient during the 21-day period of intense recovery operations. The most effective approach occurred when an anthropologist was embedded in the Incidence Command (IC) and non-anthropologists conducted most of the structure searches.

After searching locations where missing persons were believed to be, search and rescue teams, Cal Fire units, and the National Guard went structure to structure, removing overburden debris and searching properties for remains (Figures 20.2–20.3). Most non-anthropologist searchers had little or no training in identifying burnt remains, requiring a system of daily briefings to prepare search teams for the day ahead. Anthropologists were on call to deploy to locations when searchers identified possible remains. Their discovery was reported to the IC, and the IC deployed an anthropologist and / or a team consisting of both anthropologists and coroners to the scene to determine the significance of possible remains. Coroners controlled recovery of relatively intact bodies, maintained paperwork, photography, and other documentation, and established transfer of custody.

The anthropologist's role at the scene consisted of locating, identifying, and recovering burnt remains. Identification involved a series of steps. First, the discovered material was assessed for whether it was bone or not bone. Many non-bone materials appeared similar to bone in color and shape. As examples, burnt drywall and bed mattresses looked similar to fragmented human cranial bones, and burnt insulation appeared similar to trabecular bone. If suspected material was bone, then it was identified as human or nonhuman. Examples of nonhuman bone included deer mounts (e.g. cranial and antler remains), most often found along walls and in front of fireplaces, dozens of pets (mostly dogs and cats), wildlife (e.g. deer, squirrels), beef and pig bones for dogs, and meat cuts located near refrigerators and stoves. If the bones were identified as human, they were assessed for medicolegal significance, suggesting they had resulted from the fire. Examples of non-fire-related human remains included an archaeological Native American

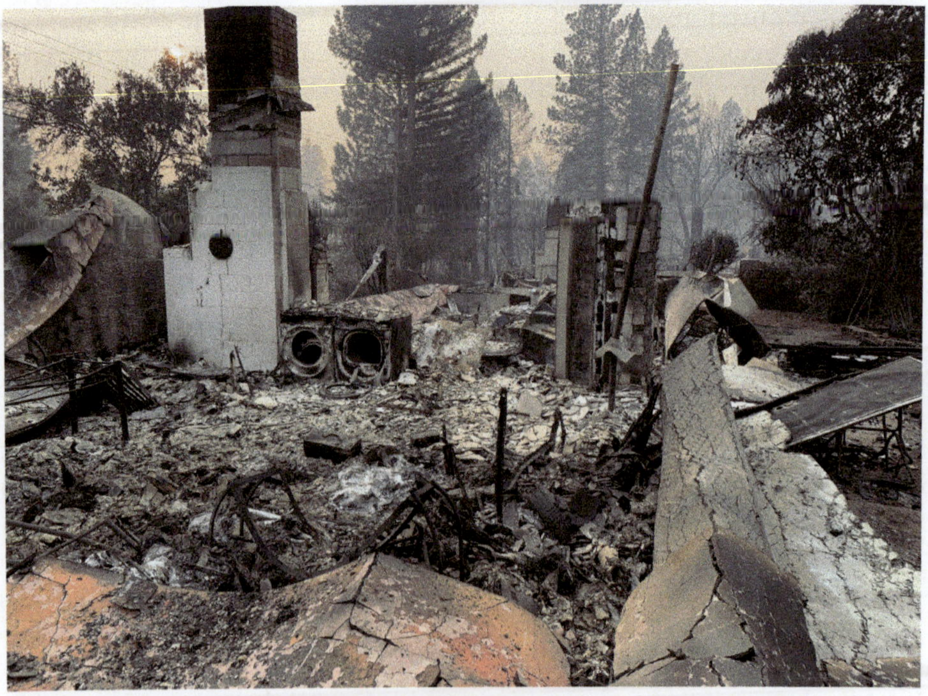

Figure 20.2 Burnt residential structure from the 2018 Camp Fire.

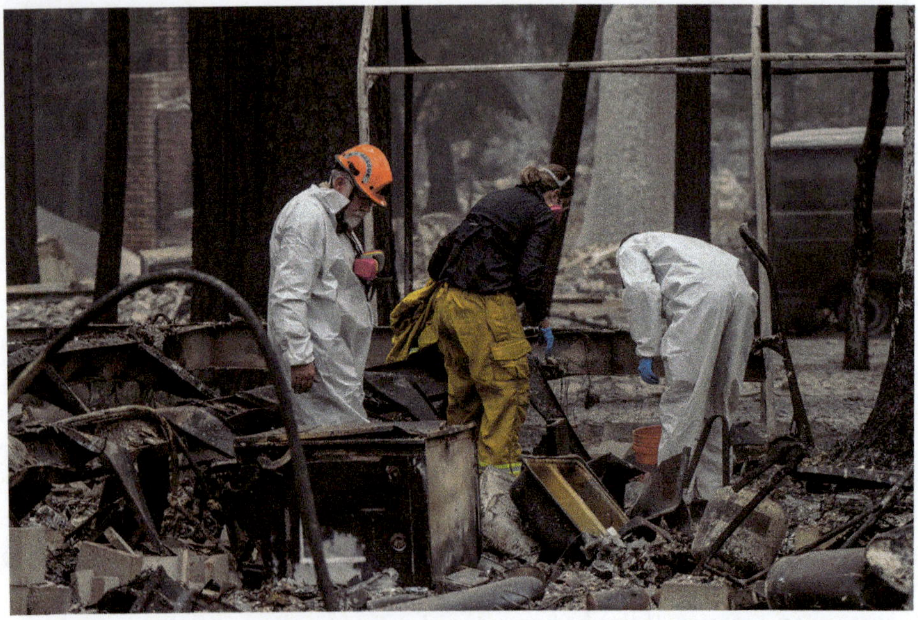

Figure 20.3 Debris removal from a fire scene context from the 2018 Camp Fire.

skull found in a residence and an anatomical cranium found in the residence of a dentist.

When Camp Fire-related human remains were located, modified archaeological procedures were used to expose and recover victims (Figure 20.4). An individual's remains tended to be concentrated in one spot, allowing for a systematic recovery process. Excavation started with exposed, identifiable elements, working outward from the core area to ensure the recovery of as much skeletal material as possible. Simple tools, including trowels, dustpans, large screens, small hand sieves, and occasionally shovels, were employed in the recovery efforts. Following the first substantial rain, debris clumped together, making dry screening difficult if not impossible. At that point in the recovery process, fire engines and their crews provided low velocity streams of water for wet screening (Figure 20.5).

In addition to human remains, fieldwork also emphasized recovery of associated personal effects and medical devices in the hope that they would aid in personal identification. Just as individuals' remains tended to be concentrated, so, too, did associated personal effects and medical devices. Examples of potentially identifiable artifacts included surgical implants, dental implants and devices, and jewelry.

Several challenges hindered the search and recovery effort. As previously mentioned, the first challenge involved sorting burnt structural material, nonhuman bones, and human remains not related to Camp Fire losses from the victims' remains. Additional challenges arose from the overall context of the structures that victims were found in and around. Multi-level structures proved difficult in

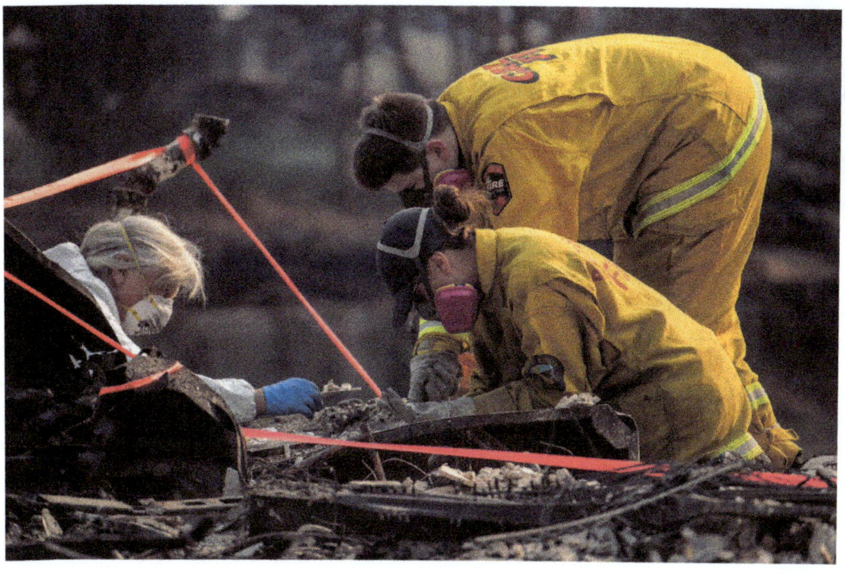

Figure 20.4 Excavation in progress from the 2018 Camp Fire.

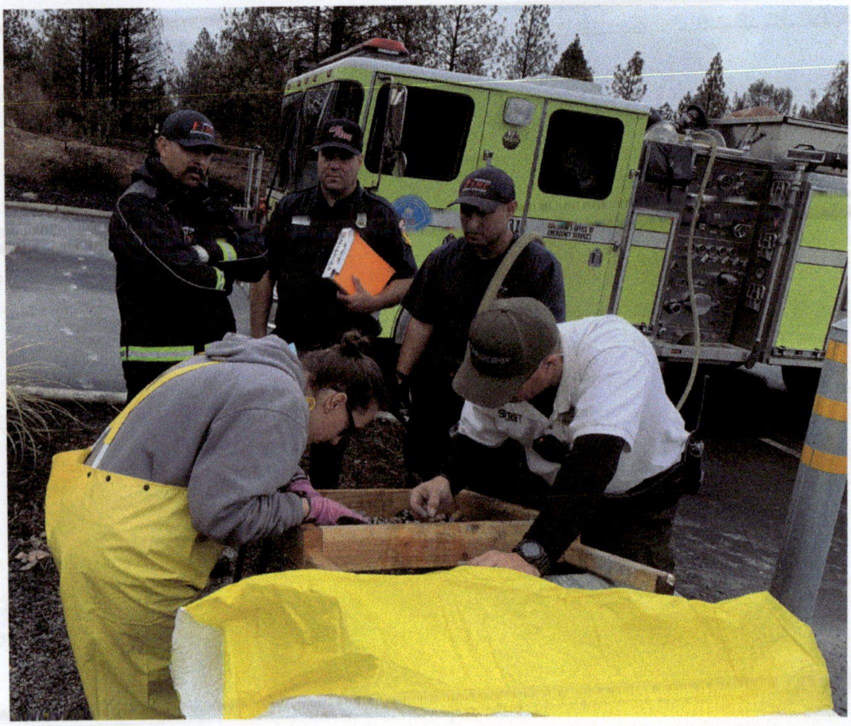

Figure 20.5 Use of wet screening to separate burnt remains from debris from the 2018 Camp Fire.

large part because of the depth of burnt debris covering the remains. One two-story home was searched three times because the human remains were so fragmentary that anthropologists could not locate any duplicated elements. Commingling in situations such as that posed immense challenges both in the field and in the morgue. When a case was commingled, anthropologists in the field attempted to identify portions of individuals in situ with the hope of recovering individuals separately. When separation of individuals proved impossible in the field, note was made of commingling and anthropologists at the morgue were tasked with separation.

In addition to search and recovery challenges during the Camp Fire, difficulties occurred with transport of remains. Butte County lacked a dedicated morgue. As a result, Sacramento County Morgue offered their facility for the duration of the incident. Once remains were excavated and placed in a body bag, they were transferred to mortuary services for transport to Sacramento County Morgue. Although the distance and two-hour drive from Butte County to Sacramento County constituted hurdles, working relations between the field and morgue were generally good. The next section will focus on the mortuary operations.

20.4 Morgue Identification

While anthropology teams were needed for the morgue operations as soon as victim recoveries began, the immediate needs for field recovery delayed the implementation of this phase. A team was dispatched to the Sacramento morgue approximately ten days after the onset of the fire and consisted of one anthropologist who had been diverted from the field and one recruited from a law enforcement agency. By this time, pathologists had already begun to work on the remains and the stations for processing were established.

Upon arrival, the anthropologists finalized the Anthropology Reporting Form to be included in the overall review package. The process for documentation was also reviewed so that the anthropologists knew where they fitted within the processing format. Cameras were provided by the coroner's unit and all photographs compiled on the facility computers.

Remains were brought out to a two-station section of the morgue set aside for the anthropologists. Typically, two case numbers were brought out together, one for each anthropologist. These were processed separately and then the anthropologists switched tables to cross-check each other's work. When there was agreement on the findings, the body could be returned to the coolers.

Bodies arrived in a range of conditions and in a variety of containers. Some bodies were only lightly charred and needed only minimal anthropological analysis. However, many were severely burned and highly fragmented. Containers included body bags, wrapped sheets, cardboard boxes, plastic buckets, and paper bags. In some cases, non-human bones were found with the human remains, usually remnants of the pets commingled with their human owners. In many cases, non-osseous material was also present. This included drywall, insulation, and wiring along with molten glass and aluminum, the latter of which often melted and solidified around bone fragments.

One immediate observation was that the normal approach to dealing with forensic cases was not appropriate for this work. A normal forensic approach would be to lay out bone fragments by element and side. However, the few elements that could be identified, often could not be reliably sided and the resulting allocation of bones was so small that it was unproductive. Instead, large panels of paper were spread on the gurney and divided into categories of head, teeth, pectoral girdle, upper limb, hand, ribs, vertebrae, pelvic girdle, lower limb, and foot.

Normal findings of the biological profile (sex, age, ancestry, stature, identifying features) were often unobtainable due to the fragmentary nature of the remains and the shrinkage of bone caused by the fire, rendering most measurement-based techniques unproductive. Occasionally small segments of the pubic bones or sciatic notch area could be found, but frequently the assessment of sex was based on gracility or robusticity of the bones. Age was also hampered by loss of most joints used in estimation. Again, occasionally bones with ample features were found, but these were rare. Instead, most individuals were aged based on the presence or absence of age-related pathologies, particularly osteoarthritis, osteophytosis, and vertebral collapse due to osteoporosis. Ancestry assessment was virtually impossible on the severely burnt remains and was only conducted in one instance. Stature was also not attempted because most bodies were received with calcined long bones where shrinkage prevented use of bone lengths to estimate living stature.

Additional issues that arose in the mortuary analysis were due to incomplete recovery of remains, split recovery, and commingled remains. Incomplete recovery was more common in the first days of recovery when torsos were collected by non-anthropologist personnel, but small bones were often overlooked, often hands and feet. Split recoveries and commingled recoveries required additional information to identify, specifically the location of where the remains were recovered. When two bags from one address were noted, they were analyzed together, and the findings compared. Split recoveries were found when body segments from one bag did not duplicate those from the other and there was consistency in size and biological profile. This often happened when there was a multistory building, and the remains were dispersed over a wider area when the structure collapsed.

The most difficult situation was the commingling of remains. Because several victims huddled together during the fire, the remains were found together with debris from the collapsed structure. Separation in the field was impossible and bodies were placed as best as possible into the appropriate body bags. However, at the morgue it became apparent that, while skulls may have been divided correctly, the remainder of the bodies were often fully mixed in each bag from the location. Even determining the number of remains required hours of work.

The final observation from the morgue is the pace of analysis. The purpose of this work was to identify the dead, but many times it was not possible to obtain any information on biological profile. Therefore, devoting hours to simply sorting bones into the appropriate categories did nothing to advance the identification. The balance between the desire to maximize identification of the bones in the remains and maximizing the number of cases that could be examined was one that was hard to accommodate. In the end, bodies were sorted for elements that could provide information on biological profile and answered the question as to whether there was incomplete, split, or commingled recovery. The result was that each anthropologist was usually able to work 5–8 case numbers in an eight-hour shift.

The collective efforts of the identification teams resulted in the identification of 85 individuals who died from the Camp Fire. Rapid DNA was used in the identification of 58 fire victims, followed by 15 by dental records, five by fingerprints, two by orthopedic devices, two by visual identification, and two by personal effects and circumstantial evidence (Gin *et al.*, 2020). Despite the tremendous success of this identification effort, there remains one outstanding identification. Identification of this recovered individual is further complicated given that there are no remaining missing persons. There are ongoing efforts to extract DNA from these remains to resolve this final case.

20.5 Conclusions

Wildfires provide a unique professional context for forensic anthropologists both in the field and the morgue. One of the strongest lessons learned from the 2018 Camp Fire was the value of embedding anthropologists within both contexts. A good working relationship between the Butte County Sheriff's Office and the Chico State Human Identification Laboratory was at the core of successfully bringing nearly 70 anthropologists to aid in the recovery and identification of victims. However, no professionals working mass disasters work in isolation. The recovery was completed, with all victims accounted for, three weeks after the start of the fire. This was a colossal feat given that the search area covered 153,336 acres and included 18,804 structures. The search for victims required hundreds of personnel from sheriff-coroner offices, Search and Rescue teams, the National Guard, Cal Fire, and anthropologists from California and Nevada. The mortuary operations likewise required teams of pathologists, anthropologists, dentists, and medicolegal investigators.

All the personnel involved had a role to play in the operations. During the apex of the recovery operations, a day in the field started early, with briefings for all search personnel groups. Coroner groups and anthropologists were paired into teams to begin working through priority addresses, while other teams of anthropologists were staged on standby for calls from the Search and Rescue and Cal Fire teams. One anthropologist was in the Incident Command Trailer daily to coordinate all the teams in the field. The standby anthropology groups deployed across the burnt area during the day to determine if marked materials were human remains, nonhuman remains, burnt debris, or non-forensically significant human material. When human remains were found, the coroner / anthropology teams recovered the remains and worked to resolve commingling issues in the field. Regardless, the remains were packaged and sent to the mortuary at the end of each day with location information and notes on the minimum number of individuals represented in the remains. Simultaneously, the teams at the mortuary began the identification process for the previous day's victims. Gin *et al.* (2020) provide a good overview of the multidisciplinary nature of identifications. Communication between the field and the mortuary was essential to the operations. Anthropologists responding to wildfires have a complex and multifaceted role. Recognizing, recovering, and identifying burnt human remains is an essential skill for anthropologists responding to fatal wildfires. So, too, is the ability to work alongside all disaster response workers.

References

Brewer, M.J. and Clements, C.B. (2020) The 2018 Camp Fire: Meteorological analysis using in situ observations and numerical simulations. *Atmosphere*, **11**(1), 47.

Brown, T., Leach, S., Wachter, B., and Gardunio, B. (2020) The Extreme 2018 Northern California Fire Season. *Bulletin of the American Meteorological Society*, **101**(1), S1–S4.

The Camp Fire Public Report: A summary of the Camp Fire Investigation. Butte County District Attorney's Office. Released June 16, 2020.

DeHaan, J.D. (2008) Fire and bodies. In: *The Analysis of Burned Human Remains* (eds. W. Schmidt and S.A. Symes). Academic Press, Burlington, MA, pp. 1–13.

Fovell, R.G. and Cao, Y. (2017) The Santa Ana winds of Southern California: Winds, gusts, and the 2007 Witch fire. *Wind and Structures*, **24**, 529–564.

Gabbert, B. (July, 2011) At what temperature does a forest fire burn? Wildfire Today. https://wildfiretoday.com/2011/02/26/at-what-temperature-does-a-forest-fire-burn.

Gaberšek, S. and Durran, D.R. (2006) Gap flows through idealized topography. Part II: Effects of rotation and surface friction. *Journal of the Atmospheric Sciences*, **63**, 2720–2739.

Gin, K., Tovar, J., Bartelink, E.J., Kendell, A., Milligan, C., Willey, P., *et al.* (2020) The 2018 California wildfires: Integration of rapid DNA to dramatically accelerate victim identification. *Journal of Forensic Sciences*, **65**(3), 791–799.

Keeley, J.E. and Syphard, A.D. (2019) Twenty-first century California, USA, wildfires: Fuel-dominated vs. wind-dominated fires. *Fire Ecology*, **15**, 24. https://doi.org/10.1186/s42408-019-0041-0.

Lareau, N.P., Nauslar, N.J., and Abatzoglou, J.T. (2018) The Carr Fire vortex: A case of pyrotornadogenesis? *Geophysical Research Letters*, **45**(23), 13–107.

Liu, Y.-C., Di, P., Chen, S.-H., Chen, X., Fan, J., DaMassa, J., *et al.* (2020) Climatology of diablo winds in Northern California and their relationships with large-scale climate variabilities. *Climate Dynamics*, **56**(3), 1335–1356.

Marlon, J.R., Bartlein, P.J., Gavin, D.G., Long, C.J., Scott Anderson, R., Briles, C.E., *et al.* (2012) Long-term perspective on wildfires in the western USA. *Proceedings of the National Academy of Sciences*, **109**(9), E535–E543.

McEvoy, D.J., Hobbins, M., Brown, T.J., VanderMolen, K., Wall, T., Huntington, J.L., *et al.* (2019) Establishing relationships between drought indices and wildfire danger outputs: A test case for the California-Nevada drought early warning system. *Climate*, **7**(4), 52.

Mitchell, J.W. (2013) Power line failures and catastrophic wildfires under extreme weather conditions. *Engineering Failure Analysis*, **35**, 726–735.

National Drought Mitigation Center, University of Nebraska-Lincoln. https://droughtmonitor.unl.edu/Data/Timeseries.aspx, accessed September 7, 2020.

Schoenherr, A.A. (2017) *A Natural History of California*. University of California Press, Oakland, CA.

Schultz, J.J., Warren, M.W., and Krigbaum, J.S. (2008) Analysis of human cremains: Gross and chemical methods. In: *The Analysis of Burned Human Remains* (eds. W. Schmidt and S.A. Symes). Academic Press, Burlington, MA, pp. 75–94.

Schurr, M.R., Hayes, R.G., and Cook, D.C. (2008) Thermally induced changes in the stable carbon and nitrogen isotope ratios of charred bones. In: *The Analysis of Burned Human Remains* (eds. W. Schmidt and S.A. Symes). Academic Press, Burlington, MA, pp. 95–108.

Ubelaker, D.H. (2009) The forensic evaluation of burned skeletal remains: A synthesis. *Forensic Science International*, **183**(1–3), 1–5.

Van Deest, T.L., Murad, T.A., and Bartelink, E.J. (2011) A re-examination of cremains weight: Sex and age variation in a Northern California sample. *Journal of Forensic Sciences*, **56**(2), 344–349.

Westerling, A.L., Gershunov, A., Brown, T.J., Cayan, D.R., and Dettinger, M.D. (2003) Climate and wildfire in the Western United States. *Bulletin of the American Meteorological Society*, **84**(5), 595–604.

CHAPTER 21

Recovery and Identification of Burnt Remains in a Military Theatre of Operations The Warrior Six

Julie Roberts, PhD, ChFA
Scientific Advisor, Alecto Forensic Services, United Kingdom
Visiting Research Fellow, John Moores University, Liverpool, United Kingdom

21.1 Introduction

This chapter presents a case study involving the deaths of six British soldiers during Operation Herrick, the British military operation in Afghanistan which took place between 2002 and 2014. A total number of 441 British soldiers were killed during the Operation, with the majority of deaths being caused by improvised explosive devices (IED) (Evans, 2013; Russell *et al.*, 2016). Operation Herrick was divided into 19 deployments and the incident which resulted in the deaths of the soldiers, who subsequently became known as "the Warrior Six," occurred in 2012 during Herrick 15.

The focus of this case study is on the methods used to recover the burnt and commingled remains of the soldiers from the Warrior armoured vehicle and preliminary examinations of them in the temporary mortuary at Camp Bastion, Afghanistan. It demonstrates how the skills of the forensic anthropologist / archaeologist can be utilized when remains are extensively fragmented and burnt, and it emphasizes the importance of utilizing expert advice within the scene. The study also illustrates how the expert can be successfully integrated within a team of investigators to produce the best possible outcome in terms of recovery and repatriation of the deceased.

In consultation with the Royal Military Police (RMP), a decision was made to retain the anonymity of the casualties in this case study. Their names can be found in the public domain, but details of the levels of disruption and damage to the bodies of each soldier have not been published. As such, they will be referred to throughout as Soldiers A, B, C, D, E, and F. Similarly, the chapter will not contain any pictures of the large body parts, although fragments of burnt bone are shown. These have

Burnt Human Remains: Recovery, Analysis, and Interpretation, First Edition. Edited by Sarah Ellingham, Joe Adserias-Garriga, Sara C. Zapico and Douglas H. Ubelaker.

been included to illustrate the effects of burning (particularly calcination), the high levels of fragmentation, and the methodological challenges which the working environment and the condition of the remains posed. All figures and images, with the exception of Figure 21.3 were taken or provided by the RMP. Figure 21.3 was produced by the author in the field, using a template provided by the RMP.

21.1.1 Improvised Explosive Devices and Blast Injuries

An IED may be defined as "any device that uses modified conventional, or unconventional munitions to exert their effect" (Edwards and Clasper, 2016:98). IEDs can take multiple forms and they are designed to cause maximum devastation (*ibid*). During an explosion, damage to the human body may occur as a result of either blast or fragmentation mechanisms and in the clinical literature injuries are divided into four categories: primary, secondary, tertiary, and quaternary blast injuries (Dussault *et al.*, 2014; Delannoy *et al.*, 2019). Physical manifestations range from blast lung, bowel, and tympanic membrane (primary injuries only), through to complete disruption of the body, amputations, penetration, and crush injuries (Eskridge *et al.*, 2012). The traumatic injuries caused by blast are complex and multifactorial. In addition to the size and nature of the device itself, injuries are greatly influenced by the external environment, for example the proximity of the victim to the device, whether the blast occurred in an enclosed or outdoor space, and presence of any intervening barriers (Edwards and Clasper, 2016). Research in Israel during the 1990s demonstrated that explosions in confined spaces were associated with both a higher incidence of primary blast injuries and a higher mortality rate than those which took place in the open air (Leibovici *et al.*, 1996). Certain parts of the body are more susceptible to injury than others and, in a military context, body armour plays a crucial role in mitigating severity of injuries, often determining whether or not a casualty will survive (Eskridge *et al.*, 2012; Breeze *et al.*, 2016; McGuire *et al.*, 2019).

During operations in Afghanistan and Iraq, anti-vehicular (AV) mines and IEDs became the most common cause of death amongst coalition troops and local security forces (Ramasamy *et al.*, 2009).

21.1.2 The Effects of Heat on Bone

The effects of heat on bone are well documented. They occur as a result of dehydration and oxidation of the organic component of the bone, and eventual recrystallization of the mineral component at very high or sustained temperatures (Holden *et al.*, 1995; DeHaan and Nurbakhsh, 2001; DeHaan, 2015; Thompson, 2015; Ellingham *et al.*, 2018). Predictable color changes ranging from orange-brown through to black, light gray, and white, reflect the amount of organic material left in the bone (Shipman *et al.*, 1984; Devlin and Herrmann, 2008; Symes *et al.*, 2015; Krap *et al.*, 2019). Burning will also cause delamination and patination (flaking and "checking"), curved cracking, thumbnail fractures, and step fractures, in bones which still contain some collagen (Gonçalves *et al.*, 2014;

Symes *et al.*, 2015). As the elasticity of bone is lost due to the combustion process it becomes much more fragile and susceptible to mechanical damage from a range of factors such as collapse of building structures, unfavourable weather conditions, and even just movement of the body itself (Mayne Correia, 1997; Waterhouse, 2013). This can result in high levels of fragmentation which affect both the recovery and the identification of burnt remains.

In terms of the impact on forensic casework and human identification, the most significant effects of burning are degradation and destruction of DNA, which occurs during carbonization and calcination, the point at which the bone turns from black to gray (Imaizumi *et al.*, 2014). Similar results have been found in teeth and it has been demonstrated that burnt samples which were brown, black, or gray in color provided low or undetectable DNA quantification results (Federchook *et al.*, 2019). This means that standard primary methods of identification can often not be applied to extensively burnt remains (Mamede *et al.*, 2018).

21.2 Background to the Case

At approximately 18.30 hours (local time) on March 7, 2012, a Warrior armoured vehicle carrying six British soldiers was hit by an IED whilst on patrol in Helmand Province, Afghanistan (see Figure 21.1).

The turret was blasted off in the explosion and the vehicle was thrown onto its side (see Figure 21.2). It set on fire and all six soldiers onboard were killed. The soldiers inside had been carrying a large amount of ammunition; therefore the fire inside the vehicle was instant and intense. The bodies of Soldiers A, B, and C, were ejected from the main part of the vehicle at the time of the incident and those of Soldiers D, E, and F remained within the vehicle.

RMP Special Investigation Branch (SIB) officers attended the scene and found Soldier A partially buried beneath the turret, Soldier B still inside the inverted turret, and Soldier C lying adjacent to the vehicle with the appearance of having fallen out of the aperture left by the turret. They made a rapid recovery of those bodies and body parts into body bags, and then loaded the vehicle and turret with the remains still inside onto a recovery truck for transportation back to Camp Bastion. The bodies of Soldiers A, B, and C, which were the least disrupted, were transferred to the mortuary at the Role 3 Camp Bastion Hospital. The Warrior vehicle and the turret were secured in an area known as "K Compound" and the insides of both were preserved untouched pending advice from the SIB forensic team in the UK.

On the same evening that the incident took place the RMP contacted Cellmark Forensic Services (CFS), to request assistance with the identification of the deceased. Subsequent strategy meetings were held between senior officers, the UK RMP forensic team, the forensic anthropologist and DNA scientists employed

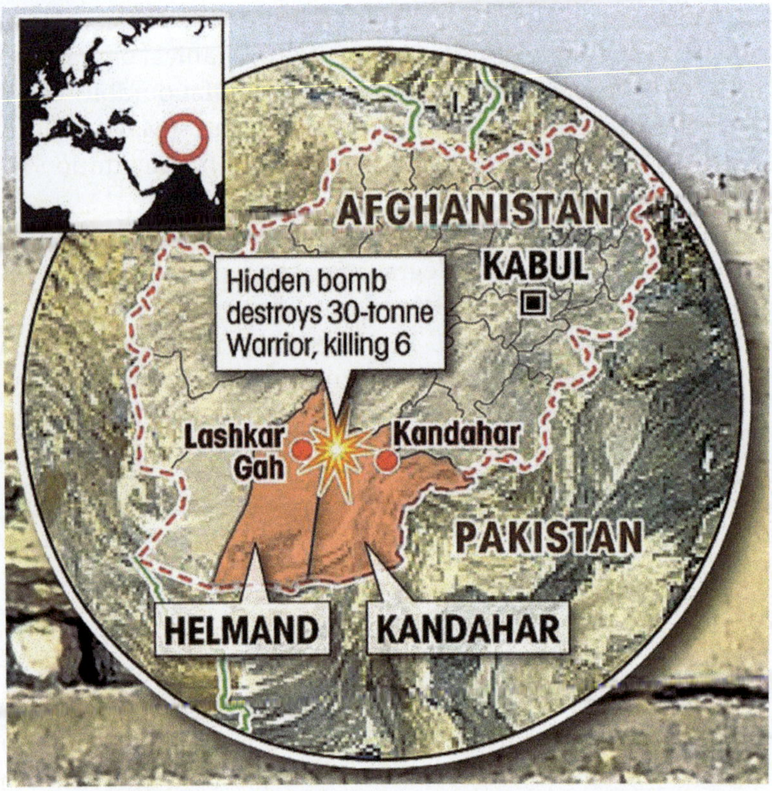

Figure 21.1 Location of incident within Helmand Province.

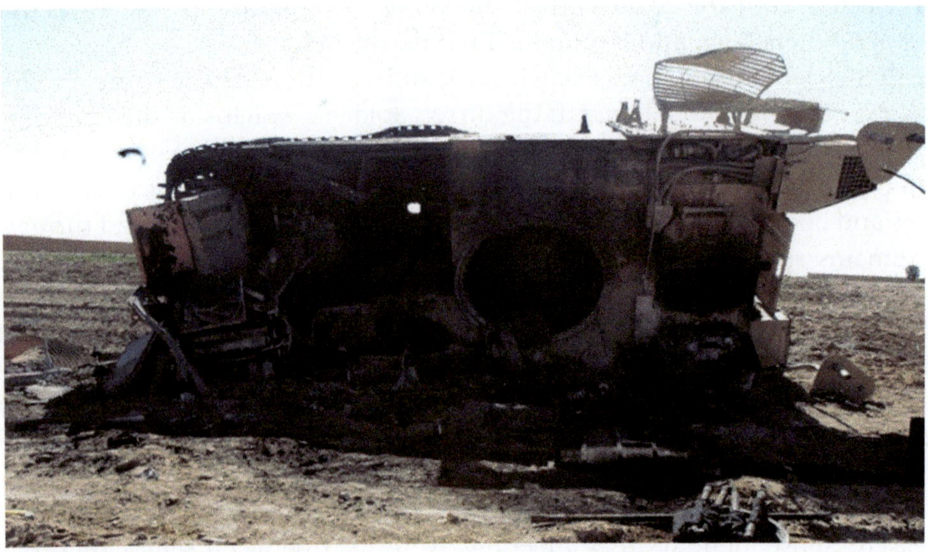

Figure 21.2 The Warrior vehicle blasted onto its side at the site of the explosion.

by CFS, and the Home Office Forensic Pathologist, regarding the best way to proceed. Having also reviewed some images from the scene, it was agreed that as the bodies of three of the soldiers and the commingled fragments of potentially all six soldiers were still inside the warrior vehicle and the turret, it would be advantageous for a forensic anthropologist to deploy to Afghanistan. The rationale for this was that an anthropologist could:

- Assist with formulating a recovery strategy for the remains that would maximize the chances of identification of all six soldiers.
- Excavate the vehicle and the turret using archaeological techniques in accordance with the strategy devised.
- Undertake preliminary re-assignation of burnt fragments to larger body parts, where it could be seen that this would not be possible by DNA analysis in the UK.
- Make a preliminary record of any individuating features or closely associated personal effects that might assist in the identification of the deceased.
- Package the burnt fragile fragments of bone in a way that would minimize the possibility of damage during transit.

As part of planning and preparation for deployment there was close liaison with the Service Police team in Afghanistan who were leading the investigation. Members of the team had recently completed a training course delivered by the deploying forensic anthropologist, which had provided them with instruction on the recovery and identification of fragmented and commingled human remains. As such, they were able to provide expert assistance and support throughout the excavation of the vehicle and examination of the remains. The forensic anthropologist deployed to Afghanistan (the author) is also a forensic archaeologist with extensive experience of excavating and identifying burnt, commingled remains and working in hostile environments.

21.3 Assessment of the Vehicle and Recovered Remains

On arrival at Camp Bastion the forensic anthropologist was provided with a comprehensive briefing by the RMP Senior Investigating Officer (SIO) and Deputy SIO (DSIO). This included information on the circumstances of the attack, the condition of the vehicle and the casualties, and details of the recovery of the vehicle and the human remains from the scene. Immediately following the briefing, a preliminary inspection of the exterior of the vehicle was made. Figure 21.3 is a picture of an undamaged Warrior vehicle showing where troops would normally be located. In this instance, Soldiers A and B had been sitting in the Gunner's and Commander's elevated seats, Soldier D had been sitting in the driver's compartment, and Soldiers C, E, and F had been sitting in the area labeled "Troop Seating." Figure 21.4 shows the exterior of the Warrior vehicle struck by the IED.

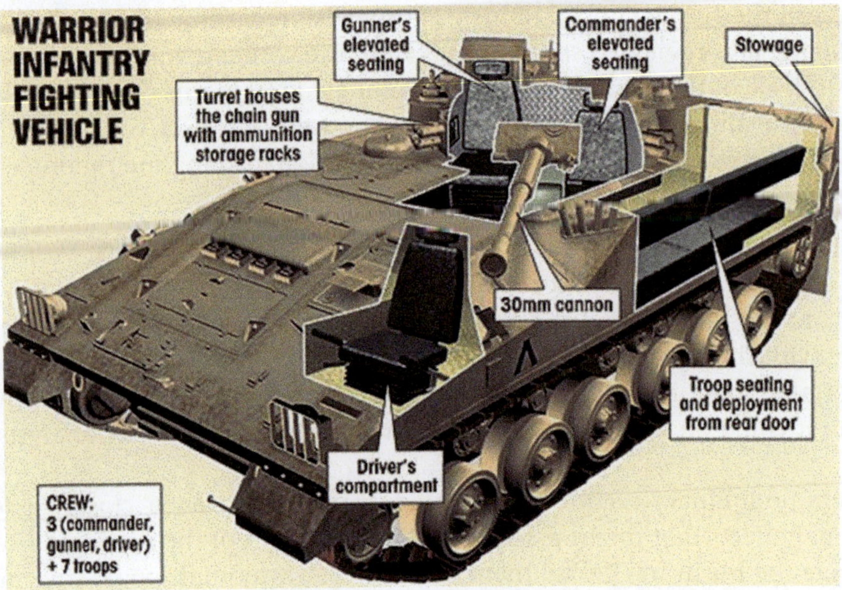

Figure 21.3 Design of a Warrior fighting vehicle showing position of troops.

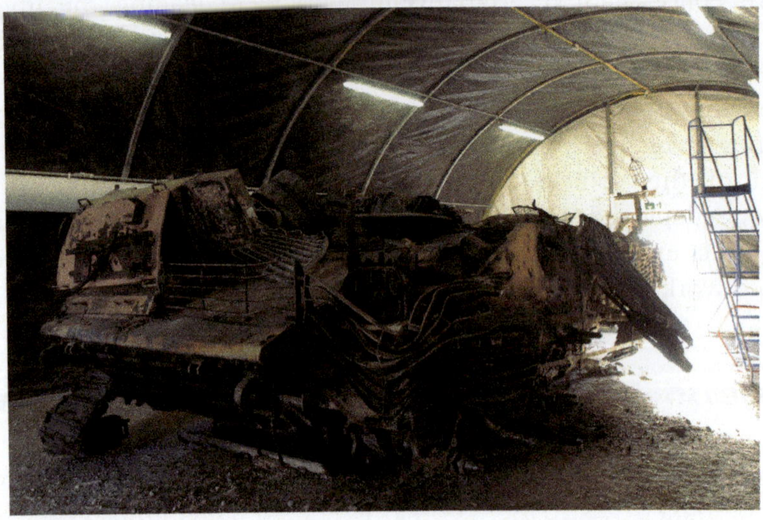

Figure 21.4 Exterior of Warrior vehicle struck by IED.

The interior of the Warrior vehicle could be viewed by standing on its roof and looking through the aperture left by the ejection of the turret in the blast (see Figure 21.5). From this position it was possible to see that the interior of the vehicle was completely burnt out, filled with debris and burnt human remains. The majority of the disassociated bone fragments appeared to be completely calcined. As such, it was immediately apparent that it would not be possible to identify and re-associate these fragments with the main body parts of the soldiers by DNA analysis, and that other methods would have to be employed.

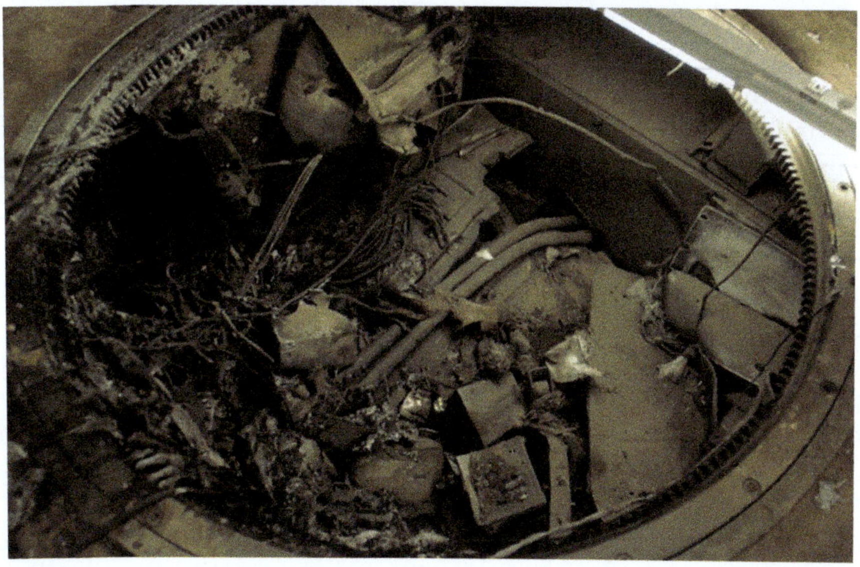

Figure 21.5 Inside the vehicle, viewed through aperture left by ejection of the turret.

During the preliminary assessment it was possible to see only two large body parts clearly. One (Soldier D) was in the driver's compartment and the other (Soldier E) was lying in the central region of the back of the vehicle. A possible third soldier (Soldier F) was partially visible, covered in rubble and lodged underneath one of the rear seats. An inspection of the inside of the detached turret revealed that there were multiple fragments of burnt bone inside it which would also require excavation.

In addition to the fragments and body parts inside the Warrior vehicle there were three body bags which contained burnt bone, soft tissue, and earth recovered from the scene. The contents of Bag Z had been collected from directly underneath the turret and beneath the bodies of Soldiers A and B, so a preliminary assumption was made that the fragments within it belonged to them. Also recovered from the same location was a collection of 18 bones which had been exhibited separately. As these had fallen out of the turret when it was lifted, they were subsequently re-bagged as one collection, labeled Z2, and noted as also probably belonging to soldiers A and B. The other two body bags had not been assigned a letter, so they were labeled Bags X and Y by the anthropologist. These bags contained bone fragments that had spilled out of the vehicle through the aperture left by the turret. They had been closely associated with Soldier C but could also have originated from the commingled remains of Soldiers E and F in Zones 4, 5, and 6 (see Figure 21.6).

Prior to finalizing the excavation strategy, the three incomplete bodies of Soldiers A, B, and C were examined in the Role 3 Hospital, so that a record of all missing body parts could be made. This information was also used to assist with the calculation of duplicated skeletal elements and re-assignment of fragments at the end of the excavations and examinations in Camp Bastion.

21.4 Excavation Strategy and Methodology

The excavation strategy was formulated with the aim of reconciling as many of the burnt fragments as possible, to specific named individuals. Four criteria were used to provisionally reassign the fragments to the six main body parts of varying sizes, labeled Soldier A, B, C, D, E, or F:

1. The occurrence of a "mechanical fit," whereby the two broken ends of a bone could be fitted together, and a fragment could be physically re-joined to a main body part.
2. The identification of isolated bones or parts of bones, which were already present in the articulated remains of five out of the six soldiers. For example, if Soldiers A, B, C, D, and E were in possession of all their thoracic vertebrae, any additional disarticulated thoracic vertebrae must belong to Soldier F, whether they were in direct association with him or not.
3. The occurrence of fragments in areas of the vehicle where it was believed commingling could not have taken place.
4. The position of the fragments and any direct association with a main body-part, for example fragments of cranium that could be co-joined, located at the top of the neck of a body.

The first three criteria were taken as conclusive evidence that a fragment belonged to a main body part. The fourth provided strong support but could only be confirmed by DNA analysis where this was possible. All preliminary assignments of fragments to bodies in Afghanistan, was subject to approval by the coroner following the post-mortem examinations in the UK.

As part of the excavation strategy a considerable number of potential hazards and risks, including large pieces of jagged metal, substances that might cause irritation to the skin and eyes, and the presence of unexploded ammunition within the vehicle, had to be considered. This was done in close consultation with senior members of the military police team and ammunition technology officers (ATO).

A systematic approach for the excavations was of paramount importance in order to maximize recovery of the remains and ensure that the location of the fragments could be recorded accurately. To facilitate this the vehicle was divided into eight zones which corresponded to existing divisions such as partitions, shelving, and seating. The placing of the zones also took into account the damage caused by the blast and the location of the main body parts. Figure 21.6 is a drawing which illustrates the zones and the incomplete bodies / body parts within the vehicle, produced prior to excavations commencing. The descriptions below the figure provide further detail of the zones.

Zone 1: The driver's cabin which formed a separate unit at the front of the Warrior vehicle. There was a small tunnel behind the driver's seat which would normally allow access from the driver's cabin to the rear of the vehicle.

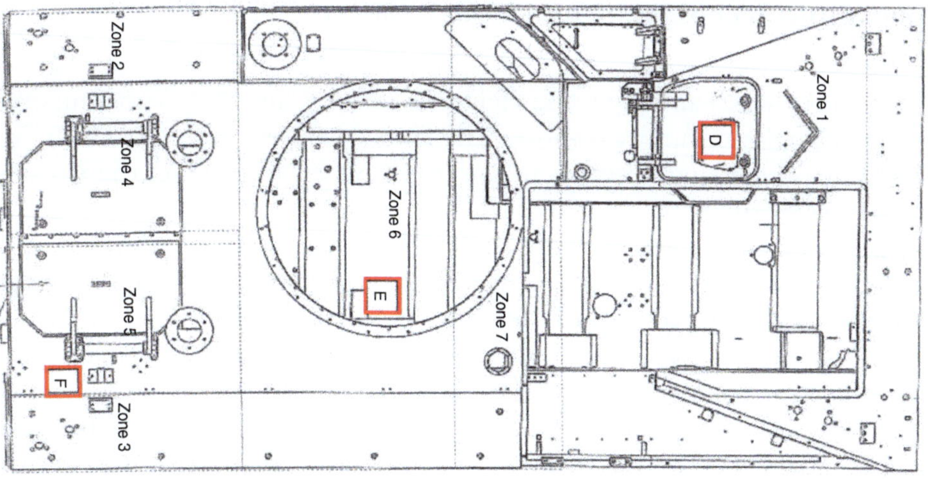

Figure 21.6 Plan drawing of the Warrior vehicle showing zones and location of main body parts for Soldiers D, E, and F.

This was largely blocked by the driver's seat and usual access into the cabin would be through a door in the roof above the seat. The effects of the blast had caused the entrance of the tunnel to become blocked, which meant that the cabin was effectively a sealed unit through which no fragments could pass in or out.

Zone 2: The area which extended along the top of the rear seats on the left-hand (driver) side of the vehicle. It included the side of the vehicle up to the level of the roof. The interior had been burnt away to expose recesses which formed metal shelves in the side of the vehicle.

Zone 3: The area above the rear seats on the right side of the vehicle, which extended up to the roof. It corresponded to Zone 2 on the opposite side, and it, too, was burned out, exposing metal shelves.

Zone 4: The floor at the rear of vehicle on the left side, beneath the seats and Zone 2. It extended as far as the end of the seats and inwards towards the middle of the vehicle where it met with Zone 5.

Zone 5: The floor at the rear of the vehicle underneath the seats on the right and Zone 3. It extended as far as the end of the seats and inwards towards the middle of the vehicle where it met with Zone 4.

Zone 6: The floor area in the centre of the vehicle beneath where the turret had been. It started at the ends of the seats on both sides where Zones 4 and 5 finished, and extended forwards for the full width of the vehicle as far as the edge of the breach in the floor caused by the explosion.

Zone 7: The interface between Zone 6 and Zone 1, this was a somewhat arbitrary area extending from the other side of the breached metal floor, across the full width of the vehicle, to the rear wall of the driver's cabin and Zone 1.

Zone 8: The interior of the turret which had been blasted off the roof of the Warrior vehicle.

The vehicle was examined and declared safe by an ATO who remained on standby throughout the excavations. The zones were excavated from the rear of the vehicle, progressing forwards to the front. Access to conduct the excavations was via the aperture in the roof, as it was not possible to open the rear doors because of damage caused to them by the blast and the large amounts of debris and seating which were blocking them. The sheer volume of small fragments of burnt bone, and the constraints of time and space, meant that utilization of Interpol DVI documentation was not practical in this situation. Instead, the same rigorous and systematic process described below was applied in each Zone.

The large pieces of debris were removed from the top layer of rubble and preserved in a designated area within "K Compound." Following pre-excavation photography of the zone, the larger fragments of bone were recovered individually by hand and transferred to the temporary mortuary. The smaller fragments of bone which could not be separated from the dust and debris were removed by trowel and put into trays which were labeled according to zone. This material was then sieved by RMP and RAF police officers who had undertaken training in the recovery and identification of fragmented remains (a sieving station had been set up adjacent to the vehicle). It was agreed that a 4-mm mesh would achieve optimum recovery of identifiable fragments, whilst still allowing the pace of the excavations to be maintained. All bone fragments recovered from the sieving were taken to the temporary mortuary for examination by the forensic anthropologist and the sieved material was retained. Figure 21.7 shows the excavation in progress.

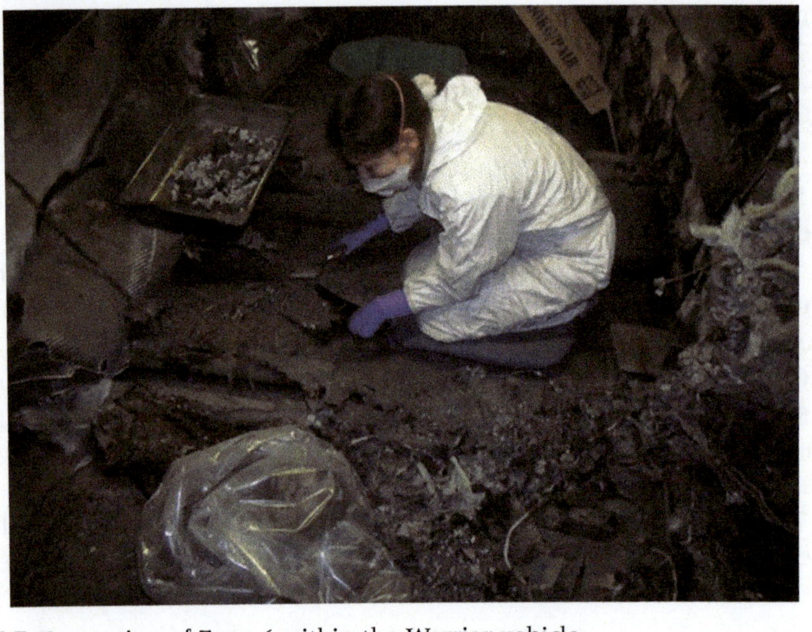

Figure 21.7 Excavation of Zone 6 within the Warrior vehicle.

The body armour from each zone was collected, produced as a separate exhibit, and labeled according to zone to increase the chances of it being reconciled with the correct wearer. As previously discussed, studying the damage caused to body armour in conjunction with the remains of the deceased has been of vital importance in improving the chances of subsequent casualties surviving blast incidents. This has been particularly true of the research conducted on body armour from military operations in Iraq and Afghanistan (Breeze *et al.*, 2016). Personal effects such as ID tags and pocketknives were collected and exhibited separately if they were not being worn or carried by the deceased, and no personal effects were removed from any of the bodies in Afghanistan.

The large body parts of Soldiers D, E, and F were recovered from the vehicle as soon as this could be achieved without causing damage to the remains. Whilst the excavation was in progress nylon bags were placed over their neck and head regions to minimize damage to any dentition which could potentially be used to assist with their identification. It was a relatively straightforward procedure to carefully lift the main body parts of Soldiers E and F once the surrounding debris had been removed and the areas around them had been processed. The recovery of Soldier D, however, was far more challenging. The body was more complete and access into and out of the driver's cabin was problematic. Prior to commencing excavation of Zone 1, a number of options were considered regarding how best to lift the body, which was lying prone along the seat facing backwards, out. Removing the body through the trap door in the roof was discounted as it was felt that this would cause too much disruption to the fragile remains, particularly the cranium, which had sustained perimortem fractures. Ultimately, the forensic anthropologist and DSIO were able to carefully lift Soldier D from the seat without causing any damage and he was passed through the tunnel to the rear of the chair, which had been cleared and lined with bubble wrap to protect the remains. The body was then placed on a stretcher in the rear of the vehicle, lifted out through the aperture left by the loss of the turret, and transferred to the temporary mortuary.

It took approximately four days to complete the excavations in the main vehicle and then work in the turret (Zone 8) commenced. The space within the inverted turret was extremely limited and visibility was poor. The seating was removed to create a larger working area, but only one person at a time could gain partial access. As in the main part of the vehicle, the larger fragments of bone were removed individually by hand and the debris containing smaller fragments was recovered by trowel and placed in trays for sieving. Much of the work had to be carried out in an inverted position and use of a head torch improved visibility. The turret was found to contain multiple commingled calcined foot bones and fragments of lower limb, some of which were quite large. The remains of a right foot were identified, partially fused to the metal floor of the turret on the left side where the right foot of the gunner would have been placed. To the immediate right of this foot was a burnt left foot, also partially fused to the floor, in the location where the commander of the vehicle would have been sitting. The right foot was provisionally assigned to Soldier B and the left foot was assigned to Soldier A. It was thought that the commingled fragments within Zone 8 were most likely attributable to Soldiers A and B, but the possibility that some fragments might also belong to Soldier C could not be excluded entirely.

21.5 Examination of the Remains in the Temporary Mortuary

A temporary mortuary was constructed by RMP officers within "K Compound" immediately following the incident and prior to the arrival of the forensic anthropologist in Afghanistan (Figure 21.8). Mortuary facilities were available at the Role 3 Hospital but that was located a considerable distance away (Camp Bastion being 35 square kilometres in size) and, as an operational field hospital, it focused on treating large numbers of live casualties. The temporary mortuary was situated adjacent and to the rear of the tent which housed the Warrior vehicle and the sieving stations. Logistically this meant that it was easy for the forensic anthropologist and Service Police team to work between the two locations, and the distance for transferring the remains was minimal.

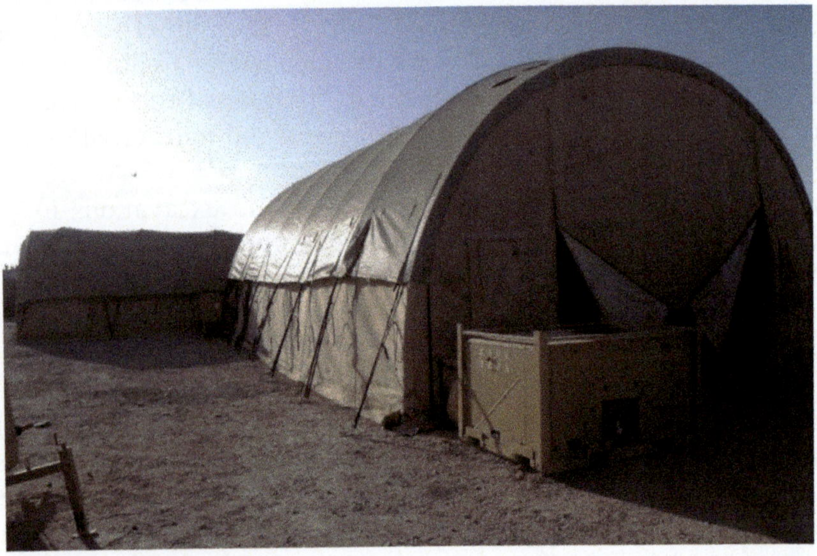

Figure 21.8 Tent housing the Warrior vehicle with temporary mortuary to the rear, "K Compound," Camp Bastion.

Six examination tables had been set up and only minor changes were made by the forensic anthropologist to the organization of the mortuary following the initial assessment of the vehicle and remains within it. These changes consisted of relabeling the examination tables according to zone rather than body number, on the basis that no assumptions could be made about the identity of the soldiers until all the examinations had been completed.

Full anthropological examination of the remains was difficult due to their burnt and fragmented condition and as the remains were so fragile, handling of all the body parts was kept to a minimum to prevent further damage prior to full post-mortem examination in the UK. All the fragments and associated items were photographed on arrival in the temporary mortuary by the designated RMP photographer who also acted as exhibits officer (see Figure 21.9).

Excavations in the Warrior vehicle had to continue in conjunction with the fragments being received and examined in the mortuary, as there was considerable pressure to repatriate the remains as quickly as possible. To address this and enable progress to continue in both areas, a member of the Service Police team who had completed the specialist training in human remains was appointed as triage officer in the temporary mortuary. The triage officer was responsible for transferring the fragments from the photography station to the correct examination table and dividing them into skeletal elements. The forensic anthropologist periodically reviewed these preliminary identifications in advance of conducting the full examinations. Figure 21.10 shows some of the smaller fragments being laid out on the examination tables, together with body armour and other associated personal effects.

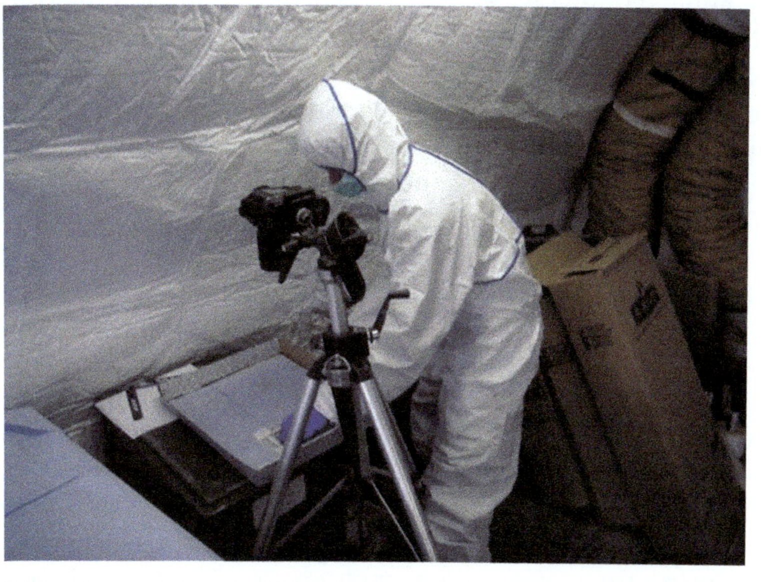

Figure 21.9 RMP photographer / exhibits officer within temporary mortuary.

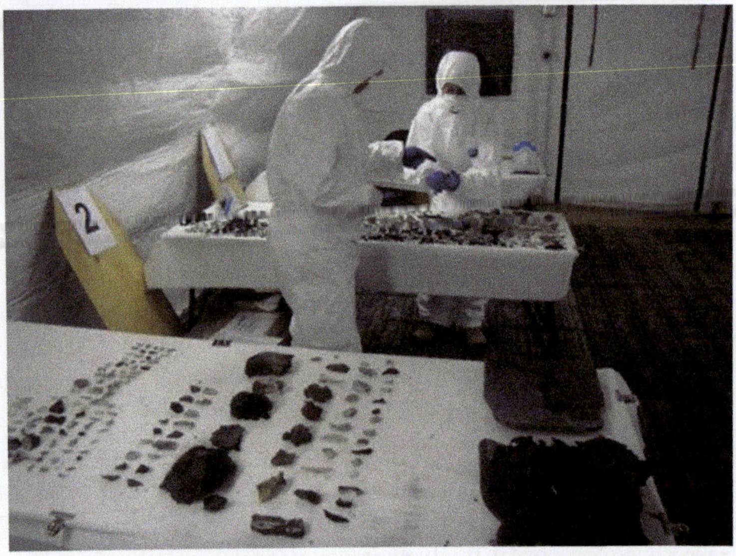

Figure 21.10 Examination of smaller fragments and personal effects in the temporary mortuary.

Each fragment of bone greater than 4 mm in size was examined individually and, where possible, identified according to skeletal element or tooth. Fragment identification was aided by reference to White and Folkens (2005) and dental casts (ESP Adult Teeth Model Set). Observations relating to fragment size, color, and extent of burning were also recorded. The biological sex and ancestry of all six soldiers was already known. Age estimation was based on Scheuer and Black (2000) and Buikstra and Ubelaker (1994). Where available, the appearance of the pubic symphyses (Brooks and Suchey 1990) and the sternal ends of the ribs (İşcan *et al.*, 1985) were also assessed. Information relating to age at death was in fact of limited use, as all the soldiers except for one had been within the same age range of 19–21 years. It was not possible to estimate the statures of any of the deceased due to fragmentation and distortion of the long bones caused by the fire. Where there was good preservation of soft muscle tissue on the larger body parts, an assessment could be made of body build. Any dentition was preserved for the specialist attention of a forensic odontologist rather than cleaned and examined. Figures 21.11 and 21.12 show a typical example of a larger fragment of bone and a tooth root (respectively) which were recovered individually.

All body parts and fragments were reviewed for the presence of individuating features. Ante-mortem data, including information from medical notes, had been recorded prior to leaving the UK. These showed that five of the deceased had indicators such as scars, tattoos, and minor healed fractures, which might have assisted in their identification. Unfortunately, due to the severity of the burns and disruption to the remains these were no longer observable. The medical notes proved to be useful in the case of only one soldier who had suffered from a heart defect that had been surgically repaired during childhood. Evidence of this was seen on the CT scans performed on the incomplete bodies of Soldiers A, B, and C, at the Role 3 Bastion hospital mortuary immediately following their recovery. It was possible

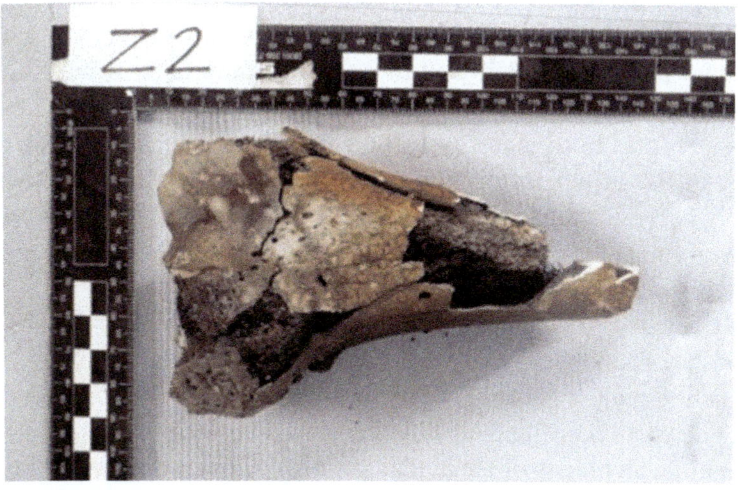

Figure 21.11 Calcined distal end of femur.

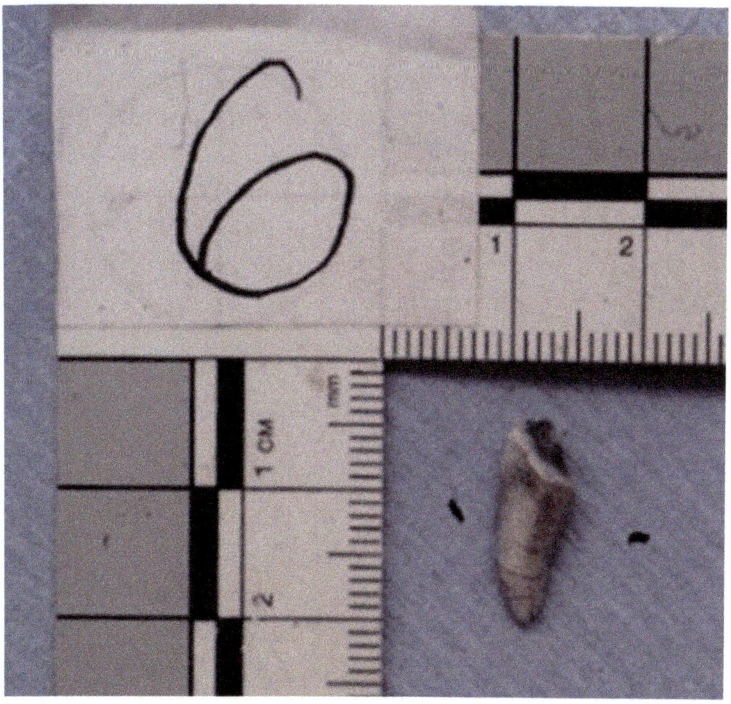

Figure 21.12 Calcined tooth root.

for the forensic pathologist in the UK to view these images remotely and for a positive identification to be made on that basis.

21.6 Examinations in the Role 3 Hospital

Once all the body parts and fragments had been recovered from the vehicle and the turret, they were transferred from the temporary mortuary in "K Compound" to the mortuary at the Role 3 hospital. As with Soldiers A, B, and C, the incomplete bodies of Soldiers D, E, and F were CT scanned on arrival. A full review of all the fragments and body parts was then made. This included an assessment of whether any of the larger fragments could be physically fitted to the main body parts, and any corresponding joint surfaces could be articulated. The next sections give a short summary of the remains of each soldier following this process.

21.6.1 Soldier A

The lower limbs of Soldier A were missing from mid-thigh level downwards, but the rest of the body was complete. Some body parts were extensively charred, and sections of bone were missing from the left elbow and the front of the ribs. Muscle tissue containing fragments of tibial plateau and shaft of tibia and fibula had been placed within the same body bag as Soldier A at the scene. From the excavations in the turret, the incomplete left foot which had been fused to the metal floor was attributed to Soldier A. Also returned to him from the turret were fragments of the right and left distal tibia (including a large piece of the proximal joint surface), the right and left patella, and the distal ends of the right and left femur. These assignations were based on similarities in size and morphology, articulations, positions within the turret, and observations from photographs taken at the scene. Fragments of distal shafts and ends of the right and left fibula were thought also to belong to Soldier A, but Soldier B could not be completely excluded, so those identifications were tentative.

21.6.2 Soldier B

The lower limbs of Soldier B were partially missing from just above the level of the knees. The right and left femur were articulated at the hips and covered by soft tissue, but both were fractured across the lower ends of the shafts just above the knees. It was not possible to see the upper parts of the knee joints, but the lower parts (the intact proximal ends of the tibia and fibula) were present on both sides, held in place by soft tissue. The right and left tibia were broken off at the upper third of the shaft and the middle and distal sections and feet were missing. The rest of the body was largely intact, but it was extensively burnt and there were some areas of damage to the skeleton. There was disruption to the left elbow, some of the bones from the right hand were missing and there was damage to the ribs on the right side. The incomplete right foot which had been fused to the metal floor in the turret was returned to Soldier B. It was also possible to achieve mechanical fits of the following fragments to the body: the proximal end of the right radius, three fragments of shaft of right femur, a piece of the outer table of the cranial vault. Articulations could be made between the partial right foot, a right talus, and the distal end of the right tibia, which had all been recovered from the turret.

21.6.3 Soldier C

The body of soldier C comprised the base of the cranium, the neck, torso, incomplete arms, and thighs, which were all joined and covered by soft tissue. The cranial base included the mastoid processes and petrous temporal bones, but the mandible and dentition were not visible. Only the proximal part of the upper arm was present on the right side, but more of the left arm appeared to have survived. It was not possible to record the latter accurately due to the position of the body and the requirement to minimize movement of the remains in their fragile state. The thighs were intact to the level of the lower shafts of the femora. An additional piece of burnt tissue and two calcined fragments of shaft of tibia, recovered from the scene, had been included within the body bag of Soldier C.

The location of Soldier C, both before and after death, meant that there was a high probability any disassociated remains from him were extensively commingled with those from Soldier E and, to a lesser extent, Soldier F. It was felt that the majority of the fragments belonging to Soldier C would be in Zones 6 and Bags X and Y, but the possibility of them being more widely dispersed could not be excluded due to the disturbance of the vehicle. A collection of disassociated cranial fragments were tentatively assigned to Soldier C, based on the fact that other, repeated, pieces of crania found in the rear of the vehicle were in close association with Soldiers E and F.

21.6.4 Soldier D

The articulated head, neck, torso, upper arms, and upper thighs of Soldier D had survived. The body was extensively burnt, there was no soft tissue surviving on the cranium, and the mandible was partially disarticulated. The left side of the face was badly fragmented and there was also a large defect in the cranial vault. There was some damage to the torso in the mid-thoracic region on the left side and there was slight damage to the sacrum. The distal half of the right and left humerus, and the entire right and left forearms and hands were missing. The right and left lower limbs were missing from the mid-shaft of the femur downwards.

At the time of recovery, the body had been in a prone position in the driver's chair, with the tops of the upper arms pointing downwards either side of it. Fragments of right distal humerus, radius, ulna, metacarpals, and phalanges had collected in the gap between the outer wall of the vehicle and the left side of the chair. Similarly, on the other side of the chair, fragments of left distal humerus, radius, ulna, metacarpals, and phalanges, had collected in the gap between the right side of the seat and the wall partitioning the cabin from the engine. This strongly suggested that the forearms and hands had become disassociated from the rest of the body whilst it was lying in the same prone position in the chair, and that the body (and the fragments) had not moved when the vehicle had been turned onto its side. In addition to the upper limb bone, fragments of right and left femur, tibia, fibula, the patellae, numerous tarsals and metatarsals (some of which were intact), and phalanges, were found in front of the driver's seat in the footwell area.

As there was no evidence of commingling of body parts from different individuals in Zone 1 and the fragments recovered corresponded to the missing body parts from Soldier D, both in terms of skeletal element and position within the cabin, they were assigned to him with a high level of confidence. Multiple loose teeth recovered from Zone 1 were also attributed to Soldier D.

21.6.5 Soldier E

The body of Soldier E comprised an articulated incomplete skull, neck, torso, the proximal halves of the upper arms, and the upper part of the right thigh. The body was severely burnt with deeply charred muscle tissue and the spine and neck were hyperextended. Parts of the mandible and maxilla, including dentition, had survived. There was some damage to the right and left shoulder girdle and to the ribs, the right side of the pelvis appeared to be intact, but the left os coxae was entirely missing. The arms had broken off in the region of the upper third of the humerus on both sides.

The location of Soldier E meant that there was a high probability any disassociated remains from him were extensively commingled with those from either Soldier F or Soldier C. It was felt that many of the fragments in Zone 6 (the central part of the rear of the vehicle) could have originated from Soldier E, but there was also a chance that they could have been in Zones 4, 5, 7, or Bags X and Y. It was possible to physically fit a small number of the recovered fragments from those zones to the body of Soldier E. These included most of the left clavicle and three fragments of the left humeral shaft. A number of cranial fragments, which were closely associated with the top of his neck and basi-cranium, could also be re-joined with each other.

21.6.6 Soldier F

Soldier F was the most severely burnt and disrupted of the six soldiers. His main body part consisted of only an incomplete head, neck, shoulders, and top of the thoracic spine (T1). The base of the cranium was largely intact and some of the facial bones including the right and left zygoma, the maxilla, and the posterior part of the mandible were present. It was also possible to see some dentition in situ.

The location of Soldier F meant that there was a high probability that any disassociated remains from him were extensively commingled with those from Soldier E and possibly Soldier C. However, the sheer level of disruption he had sustained meant that there were many bones no longer present in his body which were present in the other five soldiers. This meant that disarticulated duplicated fragments could be assigned to him with confidence. Duplicated elements which could only have belonged to him included eight thoracic vertebrae, five lumbar vertebrae, and some fragments from the left and right os coxae. Multiple fragments of ribs, limbs, and hand and foot bones, also found in Zones 2, 4 and 5, could not be assigned to Soldier F with any degree of confidence because other soldiers were also missing these body parts.

It was possible to physically fit some fragments recovered from the rear of the vehicle to Soldier F. These included part of the left scapula and shaft of the left humerus, and the left and right clavicles. It was also possible to make some tentative reassignments based on observations of the remains in situ during the excavations. The removal of the seat at the rear of the vehicle on the right-hand side had revealed the remains of Soldier F lying on top of the debris; immediately around the cranium and the neck had been a collection of cranial fragments arranged in the correct anatomical positions together with some some loose dentition. These fragments were lifted individually but labeled as probably belonging to Soldier F.

Following completion of a written and photographic summary, the burnt fragments were packaged in bubble wrap either individually or in groups depending on their size and condition. They were then placed in plastic bags which were labeled according to skeletal element and zone. The bags were put into boxes which were also labeled by zone, and each box was produced as an exhibit. This methodology was adopted to minimize damage during transit, to maintain continuity, and to facilitate re-association of the fragments in the UK. The body bags and boxes of associated fragments were then placed in coffins and an attempt was made to organize them so that there was one soldier per coffin. The large number of fragments which could not be attributed to an individual soldier had to be accommodated, however, so those boxes were placed in coffins with smaller body parts where there was space available. The repatriation service at Camp Bastion began at approximately 03.30 hours on 20 March 2012 and the flight transporting the remains left for the UK at 05.30 hours. The remains of the soldiers were escorted by RMP officers, funeral directors from Albin International Repatriation, and the forensic anthropologist.

21.7 Post-mortem Examinations and Positive Identification in the UK

All fallen British service personnel from operational environments are repatriated to the UK for coroners' inquests. They are flown into RAF Brize Norton in Oxfordshire; therefore they are subject to the jurisdiction of the Oxfordshire coroner.

The "Warrior Six" arrived back in the UK on March 20, 2012 and their post-mortem examinations commenced that same evening at the John Radcliffe

Infirmary in Oxford. They were managed by the RMP forensic team and led by two Home Office forensic pathologists highly experienced in the examination of casualties from Iraq and Afghanistan. Also present were the RAF dental team who were trained in forensic odontology and experienced in the examination of burnt and disrupted remains.

The deploying forensic anthropologist attended the examinations in the UK and provided the other experts with contextual information relating to the excavation, location, and condition of the remains, plus details of the packaging and labeling of body parts and fragments in Afghanistan. Additional anthropological assistance included further identification of the fragments of burnt bone and physical reconstruction of some of the body parts, together with a second anthropologist who joined the team. The second forensic anthropologist also peer reviewed the decisions made in Afghanistan.

As part of the wider peer review process, the deploying forensic anthropologist explained the rationale for the presumptive assignations to the forensic pathologists and the coroner with the following outcomes:

1. Decisions made in relation to Soldiers A, B, and D were accepted. Attempts were made to confirm the identity of some of the reassigned fragments by DNA analysis but these failed due to the calcined state of the remains. A written justification for the reassignments was produced by the forensic anthropologist and this was approved by the coroner.
2. The decisions relating to the re-assignation of fragments to Soldier F (based on mechanical fits and duplicated skeletal elements) were accepted by the forensic pathologists and coroner. The cranial fragments associated with Soldier F were successfully reconstructed and, as it was possible to obtain a full DNA profile from one of the fragments, the entire cranium could then be repatriated to Soldier F.
3. Closer examination of Soldier E and his CT imagery gave a precise indication of which parts of the pelvic girdle were missing. This enabled decisions to be made regarding some of the pelvic fragments which could have belonged to either Soldier E or Soldier F. These decisions were accepted by the forensic pathologists, but later rejected by the coroner.
4. Some of the more tentative assignations made in Afghanistan, particularly in relation to Zone 6, were not accepted by the forensic pathologists. It was therefore agreed that some of the commingled fragments which had been assigned to Soldiers C, D, and E on a preliminary basis, should remain as commingled "common tissue." This was because it was felt there was simply not enough evidence to state conclusively that the fragments could only have come from one of the three individuals.

Full DNA profiles which matched those of the six soldiers were obtained from each of the incomplete bodies and large body parts.

21.8 Conclusions

The strategy adopted for the excavation of the remains from the Warrior vehicle in Afghanistan maximized the chances of full recovery of all the body parts belonging to the six soldiers. It also facilitated the repatriation of a significant number of calcined fragments to the main body parts, which would not have been possible by DNA analysis. This reduced the overall number of fragments that had to be labeled "common tissue" and it also meant that as much of each body as possible could be returned to the families of the deceased.

The temporary mortuary facility in Camp Bastion and the specialist knowledge of the Service Police team enabled the fragments and body parts to be processed and examined in a controlled manner. This meant that the chances of further damage to the fragile remains and the opportunity for errors surrounding photographs and exhibits was greatly reduced.

The recovery, examination, and identification of commingled burnt fragments can be extremely complex and challenging even in normal circumstances. When undertaken in a military theatre of operation under severe time constraints, the magnitude of these challenges is amplified. This case study illustrates that even in a hostile environment, best practice can still be employed providing the correct expertise is utilized at the scene and in the mortuary. It also demonstrates how scientists and police teams can successfully work together to achieve optimum results.

Acknowledgments

I would like to thank the Officer Commanding, Captain Hugh Parsons, and his team of 62 Section SIB RMP for all their expert support and assistance in Afghanistan.

I would also like to thank Provost Marshal (Army) for granting me permission to write this chapter for publication, with particular thanks to Major Bob Grant for his assistance in facilitating the review.

References

Breeze, J., Lewis, E.A., Fryer, R., Hepper, A.E., Mahoney, P.F., and Clasper, J.C. (2016) Defining the essential anatomical coverage provided by military body armour against high energy projectiles. *BMJ Military Health*, **162**(4), 284–290.

Brooks, S. and Suchey, J.M. (1990) Skeletal age determination based on the os pubis: A comparison of the Acsádi-Nemeskéri and Suchey-Brooks methods. *Human Evolution*, **5**(3), 227–238.

Buikstra, J.E. and Ubelaker, D.H. (1994) Standards for data collection from human skeletal remains. *Arkansas Archaeological Survey Research Series*, **44**.

DeHaan, J.D. (2015) Fire and bodies. In: *The Analysis of Burnt Human Remains*, 2nd edn. (eds. C.W. Schmidt and S.A. Symes). Elsevier, Ltd, Academic Press, San Diego, CA, pp. 1–15.

DeHaan, J.D. and Nurbakhsh, S. (2001) Sustained combustion of an animal carcass and its implications for the consumption of human bodies in fires. *Journal of Forensic Sciences*, **46**(5), 1076–1081.

Delannoy, Y., Delabarde, T., Plu, I., Legrand, I., Taccoen, M., Tracqui, A., *et al.* (2019) Terrorist explosive belt attacks: Specific patterns of bone traumas. *International Journal of Legal Medicine*, **133**, 565–569.

Devlin, J.B. and Herrmann, N.P. (2008) 6 – Bone color as an interpretive tool of the depositional history of archaeological cremains. In: *The Analysis of Burned Human Remains* (eds. C.W. Schmidt and S.A. Symes). Academic Press, San Diego, CA, pp. 109–x.

Dussault, M.C., Smith, M., and Osselton, D. (2014) Blast injury and the human skeleton: An important emerging aspect of conflict related trauma. *Journal of Forensic Sciences*, **59**(3), 606–612.

Edwards, D.S. and Clasper, J. (2016) Blast injury mechanism. In: *Blast Injury Science and Engineering: A Guide for Clinicians and Researchers* (eds. A.M.J. Bull, J. Clasper, and P.F. Mahoney). Springer, New York, pp. 135–143.

Ellingham, S.T.D., Thompson, T.J.U., and Islam, M. (2018) Scanning Electron Microscopy–Energy Dispersive X-Ray (SEM/EDX): A rapid diagnostic tool to aid the identification of burnt bone and contested cremains. *Journal of Forensic Sciences*, **63**(2), 504–510.

Eskridge, S., Macerab, C.A., Galarneaua, M.R., Holbrook, T.L., Woodruff, S.I., MacGregor, A.J., *et al.* (2012) Injuries from combat explosions in Iraq: Injury type, location, and severity. *Injury. International Journal of the Care of the Injured*, **43**, 1678–1682.

Evans, B. (2013) Six soldiers who died when roadside bomb exploded under their Warrior vehicle 'could not have been saved', says army officer. *Daily Mail*. https://www.dailymail.co.uk/news/article-2465366/Six-soldiers-died-bomb-exploded-unlawfully-killed.html.

Federchook, T.J., Pokines, J.T., Crowley, K., and Grgicak, C.M. (2019) Recovery of DNA from teeth exposed to variable temperatures. *Forensic Anthropology Journal*, **2**(3), 143–151.

Gonçalves, D., Cunha, E., and Thompsom, T.J.U. (2014) Estimation of the pre-burning condition of human remains in forensic contexts. *International Journal of Legal Medicine*, **29**, 1137–1143.

Holden, J.L., Phakey, P.P., and Clement, J.G. (1995) Scanning electron microscope observations of heat-treated human bone. *Forensic Science International*, **74**, 29–45.

Imaizumi, K., Taniguchi, K., and Ogawa, Y. (2014) DNA survival and physical and histological properties of heat-induced alterations in burnt bones. *International Journal of Legal Medicine*, **128**, 439–446.

İşcan, M.Y., Loth, S.R., and Wright, R.K. (1985) Age estimation from the rib by phase analysis: White females. *Journal of Forensic Science*, **30**(3), 853–863.

Krap, T., Ruijter, J.M., Nota, K., Karel, J., Leike Burgers, A., Aalders, M.C.G., *et al.* (2019) Colourimetric analysis of thermally altered human bone samples. *Nature: Scientific Reports*, (9), 8923. https://doi.org/10.1038/s41598-019-45420-8.

Leibovici, D., Gofrit, O.N., Stein, M., Shapira, S.C., Noga, Y., Heruti, R.J., *et al.* (1996) Blast injuries: Bus versus open-air bombings – A comparative study of injuries in survivors of open-air versus confined-space explosions. *Journal of Trauma-Injury Infection & Critical Care*, **41**(6), 1030–1035.

Mamede, A.P., Gonçalves, D., Marques, M.P.M., and Batista de Carvalho, L.A.E. (2018) Burned bones tell their own stories: A review of methodological approaches to assess heat-induced diagenesis. *Applied Spectroscopy Reviews*, **5**(8), 603–635.

Mayne Correia, P. (1997) Fire modification of bone: A review of the literature. In: *Forensic Taphonomy: The Postmortem Fate of Human Remains* (eds. W.D. Haglund and M.H. Sorg). CRC Press, Boca Raton, FL, pp. 275–294.

McGuire, R., Hepper, A., and Harrison, K. (2019) From Northern Ireland to Afghanistan: Half a century of blast injuries. *J R Medical Corps*, **165**, 27–32.

Ramasamy, A., Hill, A.M., Hepper, A.E., Bull, A.M.J., and Clasper, J.C. (2009) Blast mines: Physics, injury mechanisms and vehicle protection. *BMJ Military Health*, **155**(4), 258–254.

Russell, R.J., Hunt, N.C.A., and Delaney, R. (2016) The mortality review panel: A report on the deaths on operations of UK service personnel 2002–2013. In: *Blast Injury Science and Engineering: A Guide for Clinicians and Researchers* (eds. A.M.J. Bull, J. Clasper, and P.F. Mahoney). Springer, New York, pp. 135–143.

Scheuer, L. and Black, S. (2000) *Developmental Juvenile Osteology*. Elsevier Academic Press, San Diego, CA.

Shipman, P., Foster, G., and Scheoninger, M. (1984) Burnt bones and teeth: An experimental study of color, morphology, crystal structure and shrinkage. *Journal of Archaeological Sciences*, **11**, 307–325.

Symes, S.A., Rainwater, C.W., Chapman, E.N., Gipson, D.R., and Piper, A.L. (2015) Patterned thermal destruction of human remains in a forensic setting. In: *The Analysis of Burnt Human Remains*, 2nd edn. (eds. C.W. Schmidt and S.A. Symes). Elsevier, Ltd, Academic Press, San Diego, CA, pp. 17–59.

Thompson, T.J.U. (2015) The analysis of heat-induced crystallinity change in bone. In: *The Analysis of Burnt Human Remains*, 2nd edn. (eds. C.W. Schmidt and S.A. Symes). Elsevier, Ltd, Academic Press, San Diego, CA, pp. 323–339.

Waterhouse, K. (2013) The effect of victim age on burnt bone fragmentation: Implications for remains recovery. *Forensic Science International*, **231**, 409e1–409e7.

White, T.D. and Folkens, P.A. (2005) *The Human Bone Manual*. Elsevier Academic Press, San Diego, CA, pp. 359–400.

CHAPTER 22

Volcanoes, Bones, and Heat

The Case of the AD 79 Victims of Vesuvius

Pier paolo Petrone, MSc

Head of Laboratory of Human Osteobiology and Forensic Anthropology, Departmental Section of Legal Medicine, Department of Advanced Biomedical Sciences, University of Naples Federico II, Naples, Italy

22.1 Introduction

The study of the victims of past natural disasters is able to influence the perspectives of anthropological studies and analysis (Petrone, 2012, 2019b). The human remains found in the Roman towns buried in AD 79 by the Plinian eruption of Vesuvius are clear evidence of this. For some years, field investigations and studies in situ and in the laboratory of what are called "living fossils" have allowed scholars to acquire information of absolute novelty and value both from a historical and scientific standpoint, depending on the type of approach and method of study adopted. This "field laboratory" has developed into a paleo-forensic and bioarchaeological investigation of a mass volcanic catastrophe (Petrone and Fedele, 2002; Petrone *et al.*, 2014). Field and laboratory research carried out initially on the victims of Herculaneum (Mastrolorenzo *et al.*, 2001b) was later extended to the victims found in the surge deposits in Pompeii (plaster casts), and those discovered in the Villa B of Oplontis (Mastrolorenzo *et al.*, 2010). More recent research finally revealed in detail the heat effects suffered by the victims and the cause of death in Herculaneum (Petrone *et al.*, 2018).

The multidisciplinary analysis based on the taphonomic and bio-anthropological study of skeletal remains in their original context, alongside the geo-archaeological and anthropological investigations concerning the relationships between human remains and volcanic ash deposits, proved to be fundamental for an interpretation of events that occurred in each eruptive phase at gradually increasing distances from the volcano. This approach provided alternative new hypotheses on the effects of the eruption on people and structures, and, ultimately, the causes of death of the resident population in the towns of Herculaneum and Pompeii, as

Burnt Human Remains: Recovery, Analysis, and Interpretation, First Edition. Edited by Sarah Ellingham, Joe Adserias-Garriga, Sara C. Zapico and Douglas H. Ubelaker.

well as in several villas and suburban settlements up to a distance of 20 kilometers away from the volcano (Mastrolorenzo *et al.*, 2001a, 2000b, 2004; De Natale *et al.*, 2004; Petrone, 2019b).

22.2 The AD 79 Eruption of Vesuvius

The Somma-Vesuvius volcanic complex is an active volcano, one of the most dangerous on Earth. Almost three million people live nearby in metropolitan Naples and surroundings, in the area immediately threatened by possible future eruptions (Mastrolorenzo *et al.*, 2006; Linde *et al.*, 2017). The eruptive history of Vesuvius, based on stratigraphic evidence, shows that the volcano tends to have on average a major (Plinian) eruption approximately every 2000 years (Sheridan *et al.*, 1981; NASA Earth Observatory, 2006; Lockwood and Hazlett, 2010). Plinian eruptions are highly destructive volcanic events that produce severe and long-lasting damage over thousands of squared kilometers of the territory surrounding volcanoes (Blong, 1984; McCormick *et al.*, 1995). These kinds of events are particularly lethal, since they generate catastrophic pyroclastic density currents (PDCs), rapid gravity-driven currents of volcanic ash, and hot gases produced by the collapse of the eruptive column, known as pyroclastic surges and flows (Sigurdsson *et al.*, 1985).

In AD 79 a sudden Plinian event with volcanic pumice fallout and subsequent ash avalanches affected an extensive area, causing total devastation and thousands of victims (Sigurdsson *et al.*, 1985; Petrone, 2019b). The initial phase of pumice fallout, driven by the dominant southerly and south-easterly winds (Sigurdsson *et al.*, 1985), was dispersed up to a distance of tens of kilometers (Sigurdsson *et al.*, 1985; Barberi *et al.*, 1990). The later pyroclastic surges and flows reached up to 30 kilometers west, south-west, and south of Vesuvius (Sigurdsson *et al.*, 1982, 1985; Mastrolorenzo *et al.*, 2004).

In the early phase of the eruption the first fatalities occurred in Pompeii because of roofs and floors collapsing due to pumice accumulation (Giacomelli *et al.*, 2003). In the next hours, the remaining inhabitants of Herculaneum (ca. 4000–5000) (Maiuri, 1977), Pompeii (ca. 20,000) (Maiuri, 1958), and those from nearby settlements (e.g. Villa B at Oplontis) (Nunziante *et al.*, 2003; Thomas, 2015), who did not escape in time, were overwhelmed by a series of hot surge clouds (Dobran *et al.*, 1994).

At Herculaneum (Figure 22.1), about 350 people who had taken refuge in 12 waterfront chambers were suddenly engulfed by the abrupt collapse of the rapidly advancing first pyroclastic ash surge (Figure 22.2) (Mastrolorenzo *et al.*, 2001b; Petrone, 2019b). In a few hours the towns of Herculaneum, Pompeii, and Stabiae, situated respectively about 7, 10, and 16 kilometers from the vent, were permanently buried by subsequent pyroclastic currents (Sigurdsson *et al.*, 1985), whose eruptive deposits reached a maximum thickness of about 20 meters, as on the ancient seashore at Herculaneum where most of the victims were discovered

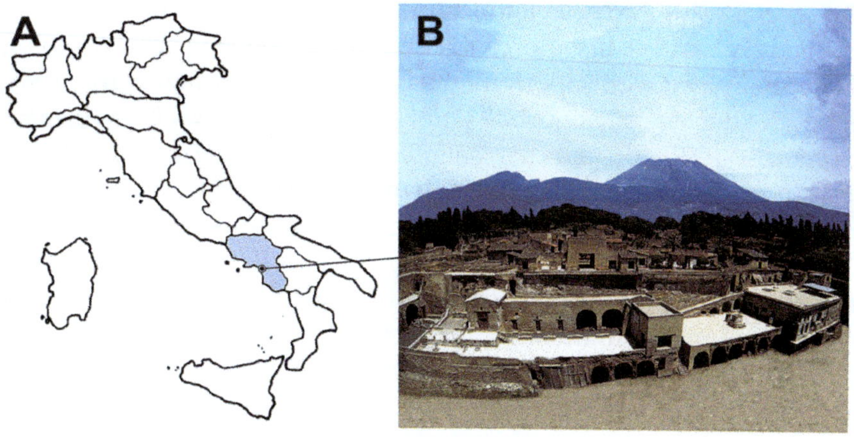

Figure 22.1 The archaeological site of Herculaneum. A. Location of the site in Campania, Italy. B. Image of the Herculaneum excavations.

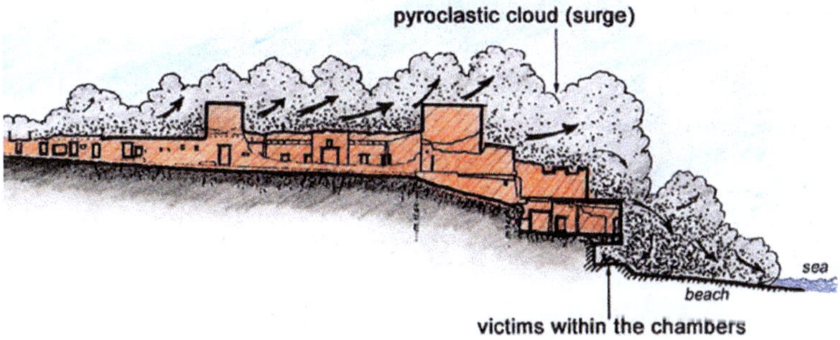

Figure 22.2 Sectional view of the town. Representation of the passage of pyroclastic flows.

(Sigurdsson *et al.*, 1982; Mastrolorenzo *et al.*, 2001b; Petrone, 2019b). In the Vesuvius area, the archaeological investigations of the last three centuries has brought to light several Roman settlements and hundreds of human victims, with devastating effects even at a distance of 20 kilometers as far as Stabiae and suburban villas in Gragnano, nearby (Ruggiero, 1881; De Carolis *et al.*, 1998).

Recent global eruptions show that pyroclastic density currents are the dominant hazard in densely populated areas (Baxter, 1990; Druitt, 1998). Dilute PDCs or surges are typically intensely hot (200–500°C), fast-moving clouds (100–300 km/hr) of fine ash, in an environment low in free oxygen content and rich in superheated steam and other volcanic gases (Sigurdsson *et al.*, 1985; Baxter, 1990). In such condition survival is likely to be impossible, particularly in areas closer to the vent (Baxter *et al.*, 2017). In PDCs, thermal injury may be at least as important as asphyxia in causing immediate death (Baxter, 1990).

In the main proximal body of a surge the temperature may be as high as 400–500°C, but with temperatures of 200–300°C being more common in distal regions (Baxter,

1990; Baxter *et al.*, 2017). These temperatures are analogous to those of the AD 79 pyroclastic surges that hit first Herculaneum, at the foot of the volcano, and later Pompeii, as determined with various methods, including thermoremanent magnetization (TRM) on lithic clasts (Kent *et al.*, 1981), bone analysis vs. heating experiments (Mastrolorenzo *et al.*, 2010), and charcoal reflectance (Caricchi *et al.*, 2014).

Pyroclastic surges are responsible for emplacement of the largest widespread ash deposit in the suburban area of Herculaneum (Sigurdsson *et al.*, 1982, 1985). Rapid deposition of extremely fine-grained ash into thermally stratified volcanic deposit (Sparks, 1976) on the beach and within the waterfront chambers, and abrupt entrapment and burial of the victims' corpses by the hot ash surge (Sigurdsson *et al.*, 1985; Mastrolorenzo *et al.*, 2001b) could have protected them from being altered by diagenetic processes (Allison and Briggs, 1991). The final result was the exceptional preservation of fully articulated skeletons (Figure 22.3) (Baxter, 1990; Petrone *et al.*, 2018; Petrone, 2019b).

22.3 The Date of the Eruption

The date of the Plinian event of AD 79 has long been debated. The controversy was recently reawakened following the discovery of a charcoal writing on the wall of a room of the "House with Garden" in Pompeii, which refers to the date of

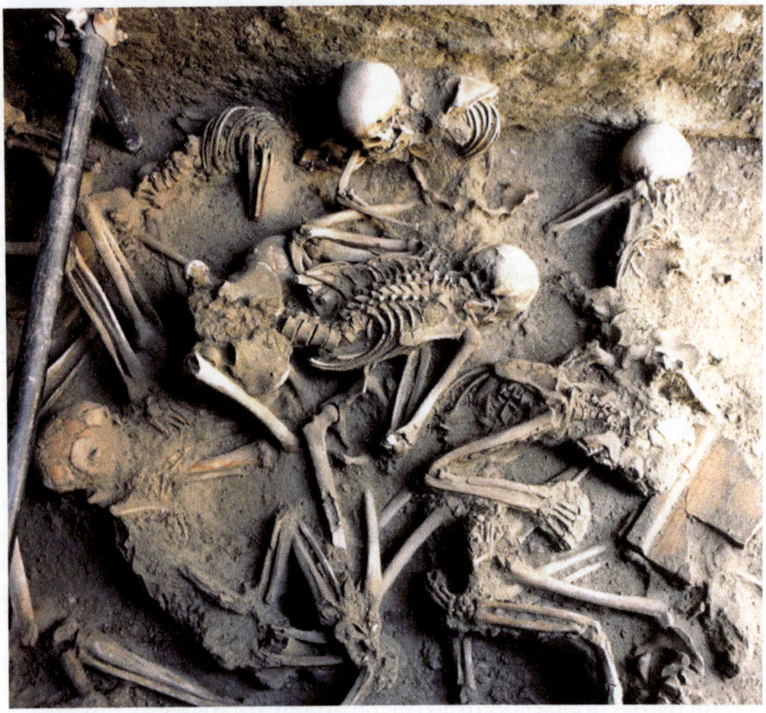

Figure 22.3 Human victims crowding one of the waterfront chambers (chamber 12).

October 17 (sixteen days before the Calends of November), but without any specific indication of the year (ANSA.it NEWS, 2018).

There are several interpretations of literary sources. The date of August 24, which has always been the most accredited, refers to that indicated in the letter of Pliny the Younger (nephew of Pliny the Elder, admiral of the Roman fleet based in Misenum) to Tacitus (Sigurdsson *et al.*, 1982; Gilman, 2007). However, medieval transcripts of Pliny's letter report several different dates, such as 1 and 23 November, and also 24 and 30 October (Pappalardo, 2019). The latter came back particularly in vogue after the recent discovery of the wall inscription mentioned previously. The date of October 24 would seem plausible, also considering the interpretation of a coin found in the "House of the Golden Bracelet," and two epigraphic testimonies (Stefani, 2006; Rolandi *et al.*, 2007). A date later in the autumn would also be confirmed by other archaeological finds, such as the discovery of wine amphorae, presumably used for fermentation, and fall-ripening fruits such as figs, pomegranates, dates, plums, chestnuts, and grapes (Pappalardo, 1990; Borgongino and Stefani, 2002; McCoy, 2014).

Interestingly, during a recent survey of the victims' skeletal remains from Herculaneum made by the author, a fair number of charred remains of grape seeds and chewed grape berries were found (Figure 22.4). The presence of both grape seeds and berries may well be considered as the remains of a fleeting meal, even if in the absence of more detailed analyses it is not possible to exclude they were raisins.

22.4 Historical and Archaeological Context of the Discovery

The Roman towns buried by the AD 79 eruption represent a unique historical and an archaeo-anthropological heritage. The first ever discovery of the buried city of

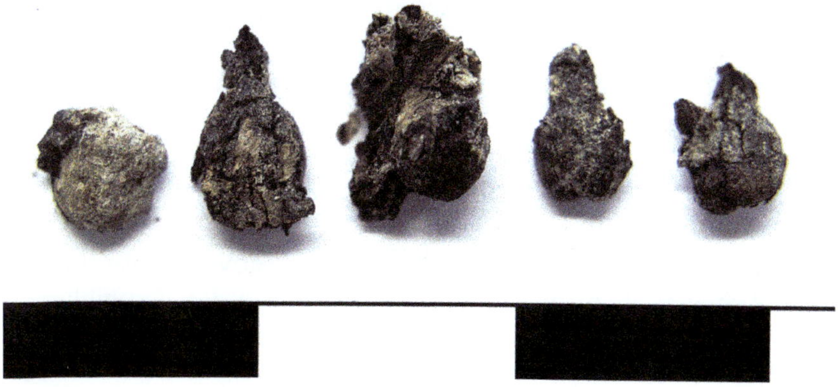

Figure 22.4 Remains of the last meal? Charred grapes and grape pips found close to one of the victims.

Herculaneum was the theatre, during the excavation of a well in 1710 (Ruggiero, 1885). The first discovery of human victims of the eruption dates to the early Bourbon exploration of the town by tunnels and is dated November 18, 1739 (Ruggiero, 1885). In 1831, during open-air excavations, a single victim was discovered inside the "House of the Skeleton," followed in 1932 by six victims found in the *apodyterium* of the men' sector of the Central Baths (Pagano, 2003). In all, the eighteenth-century excavations of the tunnels uncovered 12 victims, followed by seven other corpses in the open pit investigations during the following century, and 19 around the middle of the twentieth century (De Carolis and Patricelli, 2013).

In the first half of the twentieth century, a large part of the town of Herculaneum was unearthed thanks to open-air excavations led by Amedeo Maiuri, erstwhile director of the archaeological site (Camardo and Notomista, 2017). The details were revealed of how a whole urban settlement, including its remaining doomed inhabitants, was buried, at the time of the catastrophe and then preserved for almost two millennia (Pagano, 2000). The remarkable state of preservation was achieved through rapid burial by volcanic deposits tens of meters thick. Buildings are often preserved up to the second floor, as well as wooden furniture, frescoes, mosaics, statues, pitchers, or even organic matter. But, above all, the most exceptional discovery of the last decades of the past century has been the victims' bodies, found in great number in the suburban area.

The discovery of well-preserved archaeological structures of the Roman age has never been a novelty in Italy, but the integral preservation of an entire town, including aspects of daily life, private houses, and public buildings, and even the finding of victims' bodies is an absolute *unicum*. The discovery in the 1980s and, later, in the 1990s of hundreds of victims inside 12 chambers on what used to be the ancient seafront of Herculaneum (Pagano, 2000) proved to be of extraordinary value for historical and archaeological reconstructions. This finding has proven particularly important for scientific studies that have arisen about the devastating effects on a population struck by a sudden natural catastrophe (Sigurdsson *et al.*, 1982, 1985; Bisel, 1987; Budetta, 1993; Mastrolorenzo *et al.*, 2001b, 2010; Giacomelli *et al.*, 2003; Guidobaldi, 2007; Baxter *et al.*, 2017; Petrone *et al.*, 2018; Petrone, 2019b).

In Herculaneum, a new campaign of excavations started in the early 1980s (Guidobaldi, 2007). After removing huge amounts of tuff deposits, the seafront area of the town was reached, leading to the exceptional discovery of a huge number of human skeletons. On the beach and in six of the twelve waterfront chambers some 150 victims of the eruption were uncovered, buried by volcanic debris (Sigurdsson *et al.*, 1985; Bisel, 1987). Once removed, these skeletons were the subject of several bioanthropological studies (for a detailed bibliography see Petrone, 2019b). Further archaeological investigations conducted by the Superintendent of Pompeii in the early 1990s in the other chambers brought to light an additional large group of human victims, left untouched within the volcanic ash surge deposit for some years (Budetta, 1993). These human remains were then the subject of a new archaeological investigation, carried out by the author from 1997 to 1999, by means of an improvement project based on a new approach (Petrone, 2012, 2019a), aimed at enhancing this exceptional archaeological and anthropological context through the making of casts from glass fiber (Petrone and Fedele, 2002). After documentation, excavation, and recovery of a hundred skeletons (Petrone and Fedele, 2002; Petrone, 2012, 2019b), the casts of the victims were finally placed in the original context of discovery as they appear on the site today (Figure 22.5).

The archaeological investigations all together brought to light some 350 victims who had taken refuge in the waterfront chambers and on the beach (Figure 22.6). The few victims found in the town and the temporary shelter of people in the seafront area suggests that most residents had managed to escape in time in the Naples direction, north-west, due the south-east direction of the initial pumice fallout caused by the prevailing winds. This is testified by literary, archaeological, and epigraphic evidence of recovery in Neapolis and nearby towns of many who escaped the eruption (Taylor, 2015).

22.5 Bioarchaeological and Taphonomic Study

The human remains from Herculaneum, exceptionally preserved over time, can be considered "time capsules," capable of revealing the details of an unexpected and sudden catastrophe (Petrone and Fedele, 2002; Petrone, 2012, 2019b). During the campaign of excavation which started in June 1997, two years of site investigation identified key information on the direct and indirect effects caused by the surge on people, and the way they died. Particular attention was given to the relationship between archaeological stratigraphy, human remains, and volcanic

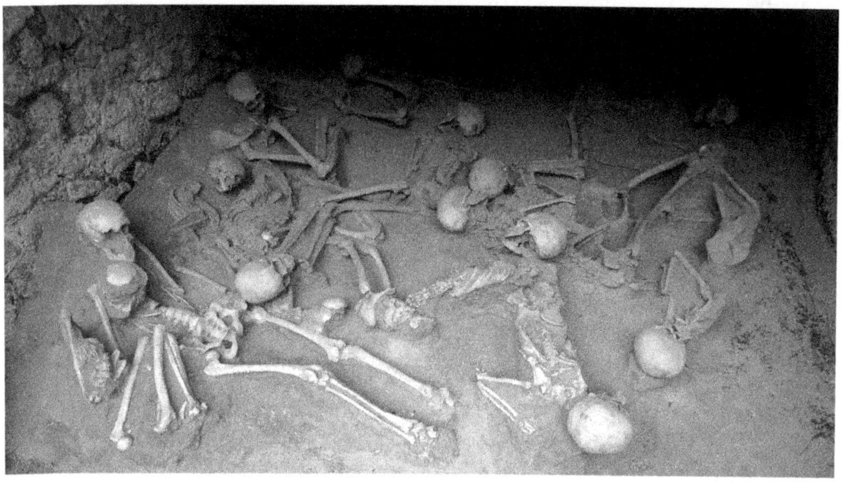

Figure 22.5 Fiberglass cast of the skeletons of victims found in the 1990s (chamber 11).

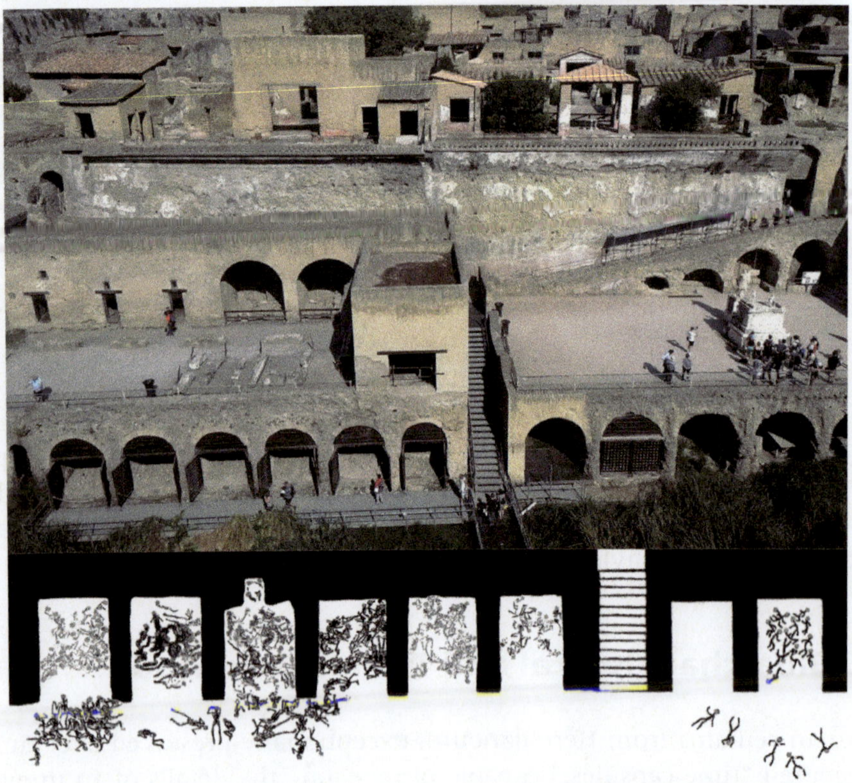

Figure 22.6 The waterfront chambers on the sea-shore area. Representation of the human victims discovered on the beach and inside the chambers.

deposit, by means of a multidisciplinary survey (Mastrolorenzo *et al.*, 2001b, 2010; Petrone and Fedele, 2002; Petrone, 2012, 2019b; Petrone *et al.*, 2014, 2018).

Unlike previous investigators, the idea was to answer questions, such as: what made the integral preservation of victims' postures and skeletal joints possible? What mechanism could explain the floating of bodies within the ash bed deposit? Or why did so many skeletons show cracking of skulls and long bones, or contracted hands and feet? What were those reddish residues found on the bones and in the ash filling the skulls, or impregnating the ash deposit in which the bodies were buried? And finally, how could the vital attitude of the victims be explained? All these questions were answered by site and laboratory investigation, as summarized below.

The posture of the victims, of particular importance for a reconstruction of the taphonomic processes related to the rapid deposition of the volcanic products, proved to be essential to assess the causes of death of people at Herculaneum by engulfment from hot pyroclastic flows. The overall evidence showed for the first surge a temperature of about 500°C, a particularly high temperature for a pyroclastic current (Sigurdsson *et al.*, 1985; Baxter, 1990), hot enough to cause instant death of the inhabitants (Mastrolorenzo *et al.*, 2001b; Petrone, 2019b). The exudation of boiling blood from the sagittal venous sinus, testified in some victims' skulls by evidence of heat hematoma (Figure 22.7), and the increase in pressure resulting from bleeding in the brain, caused instantaneous death. Hands, feet, and the whole body underwent an instantaneous thermal-induced muscular contraction, and the positions of their bodies were fixed by the sudden deflation of the ash bed occurring soon after its emplacement. Their skulls shattered, their bones and teeth broke, and the soft tissues vanished, causing body tissues to be rapidly replaced by the ash. The temperature decrease caused the ash bed to cool and harden, thus preserving the skeletons in the postures in which they died (Mastrolorenzo *et al.*, 2001b, 2010; Petrone *et al.*, 2018; Petrone, 2019b). The cooling of the ash deposit at Herculaneum does not appear to have lasted long (Giordano *et al.*, 2018), as has also been recently noted through reflectance of charcoal, which showed a maximum temperature of 520°C (Petrone *et al.*, 2020a).

With regard to the passage and emplacement of pyroclastic flows, no appreciable evidence of substantial mechanical effects on the victims was detectable in Herculaneum, both in the city and in the suburban area. Instead, the general evidence shows that once the town was hit by the first scorching ash cloud of the deadly wave, people would have died within a fraction of a second, as testified by

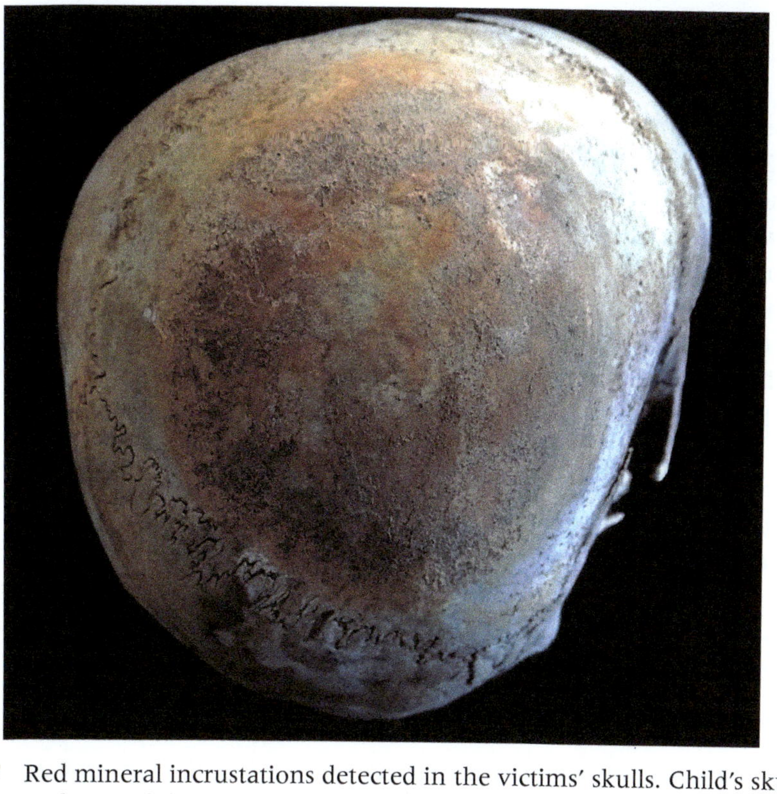

Figure 22.7 Red mineral incrustations detected in the victims' skulls. Child's skull showing a round area of thick red mineral residues encrusting the right parietal bone.

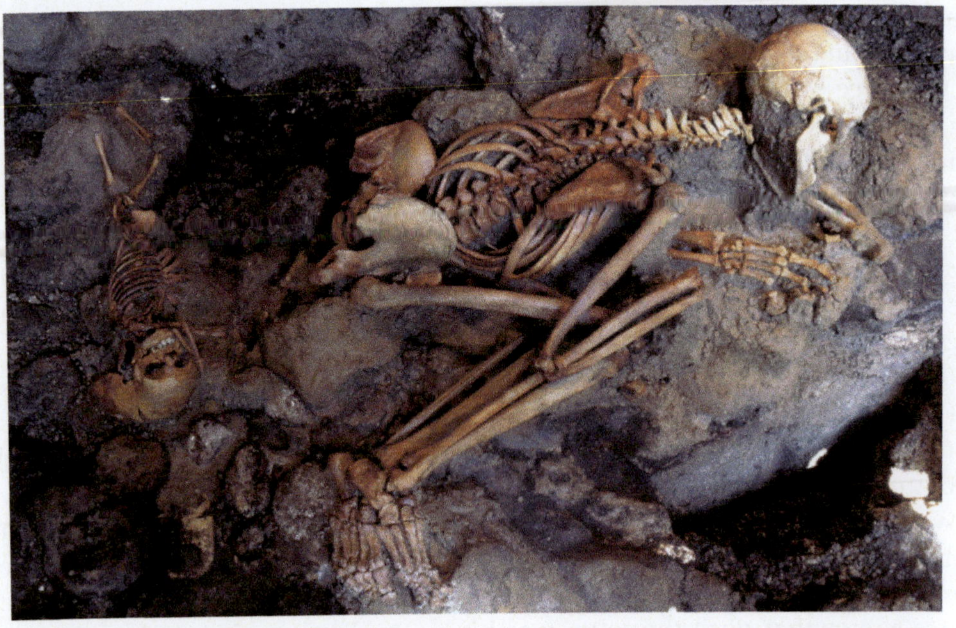

Figure 22.8 Skeletons showing "life-like" stance: a child (left) and young adult male (right) unearthed from the ash surge deposit (chamber 10). The child's corpse displays flexure only of the upper limbs, indicative of an incipient "pugilistic attitude." Full exhibit of this heat-induced stance is never found in the Herculaneum victims.

the vital attitude of the victims' corpses as if suspended in the last instant of life (Figure 22.8) (Mastrolorenzo *et al.*, 2001b; Petrone *et al.*, 2018; Petrone, 2019b).

Our study of the heat effects on corpses was later extended to the victims found in the surge deposits in Pompeii and Oplontis. As in Herculaneum, most of the victims showed postures preserved in "suspended" actions, most likely indicative of sudden death (Baxter, 1990; Mastrolorenzo *et al.*, 2010; Petrone, 2019b). The apparent defensive position seen in the Pompeii victims, repeatedly cited by various scholars in support of a slow death and terrible suffering, was actually due to the fixed flexion of extremities and limbs induced by heat due to protein coagulation and shortening of the muscles around the time of death, a posture known as "pugilistic attitude" (Baxter, 1990) (Figure 22.9).

In order to estimate the temperature reached by the lethal pyroclastic surge, macroscopic analyses, optical microscopy, histochemistry, and scanning electron microscopy (SEM) of bone samples from the Vesuvian sites were performed (Mastrolorenzo *et al.*, 2010). The results were then compared with those from several modern bone samples (human hand phalanx) heated to temperatures from 100°C to 800°C. The comparison between structural changes detected in the victims' bone and recent bones treated in the laboratory suggested that people were exposed to temperatures of about 500°C in Herculaneum, around 600°C in Oplontis and 250–300°C in Pompeii, at about 6, 7, and 10 kilometers from the volcano, respectively.

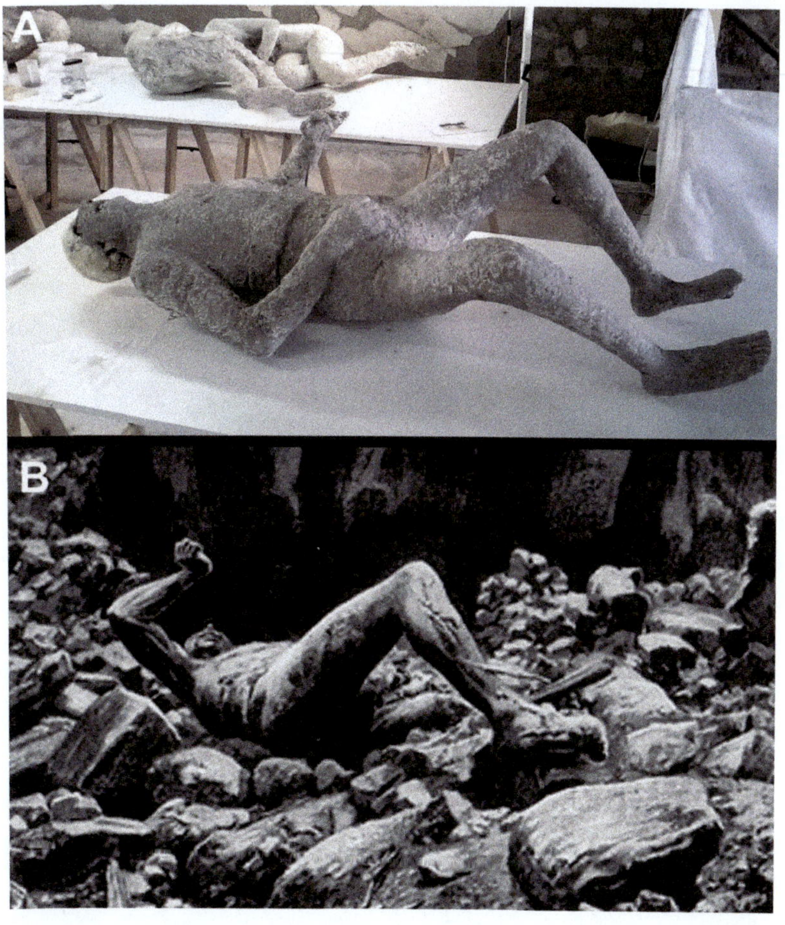

Figure 22.9 Pugilistic attitude of victims from historical eruptions. A. Pompeii, AD 79. B. Mont Pelée, 1902.

The appearance of vital postures in most of the AD 79 victims suggests that all residents within 10–20 kilometers from the volcano were killed instantly by the pyroclastic currents, including those who had survived the initial fallout phase of the eruption while sheltering inside buildings, both in Herculaneum and in Pompeii. These results are comparable with the study of a previous Plinian eruption of Vesuvius that overwhelmed the Campanian plain in the Early Bronze Age (3945 ± 10 cal BP, San Paolo Belsito, Naples, South Italy) (Mastrolorenzo *et al.*, 2006; Sevink *et al.*, 2011). The Avellino Pumice event is manifested by exceptional discoveries, such as fully preserved villages, with abandoned huts, objects, animals, and, above all, human casualties. In this case, evidence of survival at about 15 kilometers from the volcano is documented by the footprints of thousands of people fleeing in a northwesterly direction during the eruption (Figure 22.10) (Mastrolorenzo *et al.*, 2006). The most recent field and laboratory research conducted on the sites buried by the Avellino and Pompeii Plinian eruptions shows the hazard facing the three million

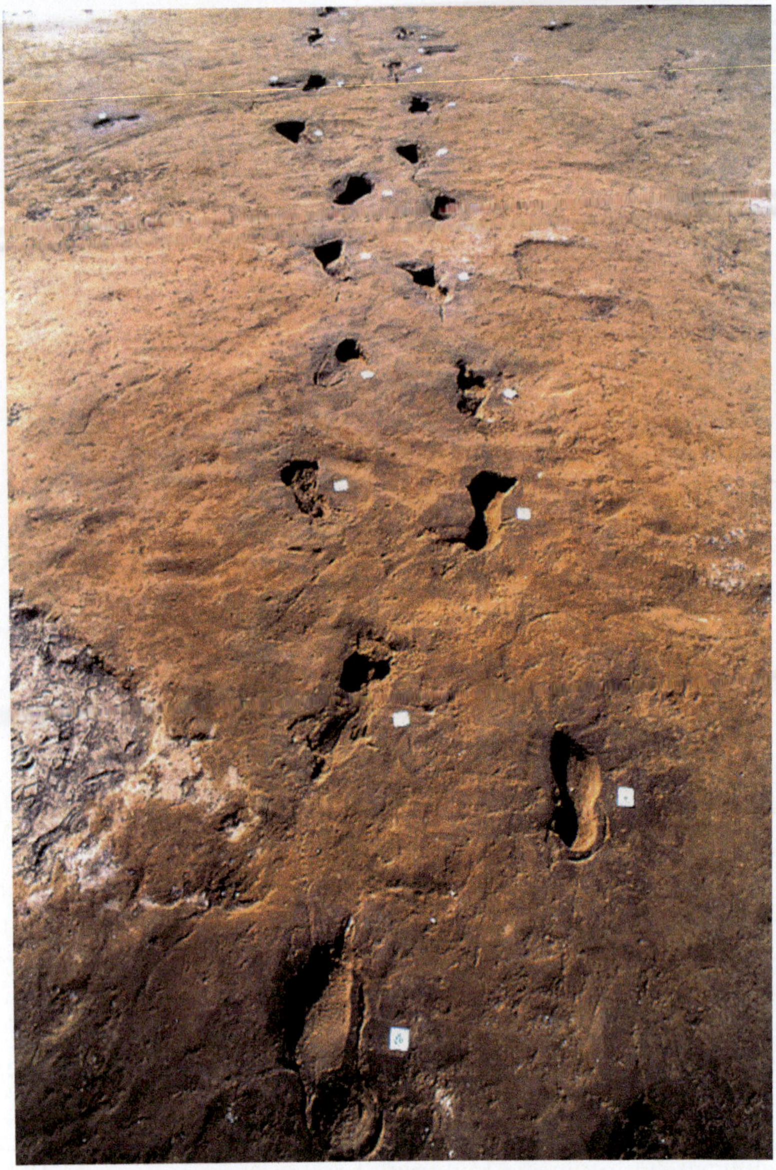

Figure 22.10 Footprints in volcanic ash of fugitives during the Bronze Age Avellino eruption of Vesuvius (ca. 4000 BP).

residents in metropolitan Naples and surroundings in the event of a future Vesuvius eruption (Mastrolorenzo *et al.*, 2006; NASA Earth Observatory, 2006; Hall, 2007).

22.6 The Causes of Death

The effects of the eruption on the inhabitants of Herculaneum and the other urban settlements close to the volcano have been the subject of several studies

(Baxter, 1990; Capasso, 2000, 2001; Mastrolorenzo *et al.*, 2001a, 2001b, 2004, 2010; De Carolis and Patricelli, 2003, 2013; Giacomelli *et al.*, 2003; Luongo *et al.*, 2003b; Petrone, 2012, 2019b; Petrone *et al.*, 2018, 2020a, 2020b). Apart from the casualties of the initial pumice fallout phase by building collapse in Pompeii (De Carolis and Patricelli, 2003, 2013; Luongo *et al.*, 2003a, 2003b), studies on the causes of death mostly refer to the effects of heat associated with the emplacement of pyroclastic surge clouds in both Herculaneum (Capasso, 2000; Mastrolorenzo *et al.*, 2001b, 2010; Hansell *et al.*, 2006; Petrone *et al.*, 2014, 2018; Schmidt *et al.*, 2015; Petrone, 2019b; Martyn *et al.*, 2020) and Pompeii (Baxter, 1990; Luongo *et al.*, 2003a).

Although hot surges have been mostly accepted as a major cause of mortality in the AD 79 eruption, there are some differences in interpretation depending on the distance from the volcano and, within the same site, on the place where victims were found. As regards Herculaneum, more recent studies agree on the instant death of people discovered in the seashore area (Schmidt *et al.*, 2015; Petrone *et al.*, 2018; Petrone, 2019b), although some authors hypothesized a gradient of heat-induced effects (Martyn *et al.*, 2020). Thus, even if nearly every skeleton had some evidence of bone thermal exposure (changes in color, charring, fracturing) (Capasso, 2000; Mastrolorenzo *et al.*, 2001b; Schmidt *et al.*, 2015; Petrone *et al.*, 2018; Petrone *et al.*, 2020a), the few victims found on the beach were assumed to show greater thermal effects compared to those sheltering inside the chambers (Capasso, 2001; Schmidt *et al.*, 2015; Martyn *et al.*, 2020). Based on the previous assumption, it was also hypothesized that death was instantaneous only for people found on the beach, while those taking refuge in the chambers would have died of asphyxiation (Capasso, 2000, 2001; Martyn *et al.*, 2020). However, a comparative analysis of the full skeletal sample has not yet been performed since the victims, coming from different excavation surveys (Maiuri, 1961; Bisel, 1987; Petrone and Fedele, 2002; Petrone, 2019b), were studied and stored separately. With regard to previous interpretations on the causes of death, particularly at a greater distance than in Pompeii, death by asphyxiation in both pumice fallout and pyroclastic surge phases has long remained the most accredited hypothesis (De Carolis and Patricelli, 2003; Giacomelli *et al.*, 2003; Luongo *et al.*, 2003a; Maiuri, 1961).

The latter accounts are at variance with the search for volcanological evidence of PDCs (Sigurdsson *et al.*, 1982, 1985) and a first forensic interpretation concerning the victims found in the surge deposit (Baxter, 1990), as well as with more recent multidisciplinary studies. Taphonomic, bio-anthropological and volcanological site investigations, and laboratory evidence (Mastrolorenzo *et al.*, 2001b; Petrone *et al.*, 2018, 2020a; Petrone, 2019b), coupled with results from heating experiments on recent human bone samples (Mastrolorenzo *et al.*, 2010), have shown that Herculaneum's residents were instantly killed by the extremely high temperature of the emplacing first pyroclastic surge, although it had been previously believed that death had occurred by slow suffocation from ash inhalation. Skull and bone charring and cracking, as well as instant hand and foot contraction (flexor reflex by the nociceptive C fibers) (LaMotte and Campbell, 1978) and spine hyperextension, have been described as thermally induced major effects on the victims' skeletons unearthed from both the beach and the sea-front chambers (Capasso, 2000, 2001; Mastrolorenzo *et al.*, 2001b; Schmidt *et al.*, 2015; Petrone *et al.*, 2018; Petrone, 2019b). Histological and ultra-structural investigation has revealed linear and polygonal cracking of the intra- and inter-osteonic structure associated with incipient recrystallization (Mastrolorenzo *et al.*, 2010; Petrone, 2019b), bone changes typically induced by intense heat (Shipman *et al.*, 1984; Fernández Castillo *et al.*, 2013).

Evidence of sudden death, as a consequence of increase of the intracranial pressure (testified by skull cracking) resulting from thermally-induced brain bleeding and boiling (testified by bone staining and charring), is also provided by the victims' corpses appearing to be suspended in their last vital action, a posture known as "lifelike stance." The lack of a voluntary self-protective reaction or agony indicates that any vital activity had to stop within a time shorter than the conscious reaction time, a state known as fulminant shock (Brinkmann *et al.*, 1979). The vital aspect shown by the victims in Herculaneum, Pompeii, and the other Vesuvian sites shows that people were alive at the time of the postural stiffening, and its widespread presence indicates that the entire resident population was exposed to the same lethal conditions. As also observed in the other sites buried by the AD 79 eruption, the overall evidence suggests the occurrence of thermally-induced instant death of the inhabitants in the Vesuvius area up to at least 20 kilometers from the vent (Baxter, 1990; Mastrolorenzo *et al.*, 2001b, 2010; Petrone *et al.*, 2018).

22.7 The Most Recent Studies

Recent multidisciplinary research on the lethal effects of the pyroclastic ash surge induced by the AD 79 eruption in the Vesuvius area showed that in the vicinity of Pompeii heat was the main cause of death of those who had previously been thought to have died of ash suffocation (Mastrolorenzo *et al.*, 2010). This was also posited for the victims of Herculaneum, specifically for those who had taken refuge in waterfront chambers along the beach and were then sheltered from direct mechanical impact, but not from heat of the emplacing first ash surge (Mastrolorenzo *et al.*, 2001b, 2010; Schmidt *et al.*, 2015; Petrone *et al.*, 2018).

Key features of body exposure to intense heat are provided by recurrent skull cracking, as detected by recurrent clear-cut fractures, with sharp margins like those seen in cremated bones (Figure 22.11). In several cases, fracture lines radiate from a common center, thus showing a "stellate" appearance. A single skull may also be affected by multiple fracture centers. Dark staining is typically associated with these cracked areas, whose exposed surface is charred as well. Interestingly, fractures are always limited to the charred bone areas. A recurrent feature is the dark staining of the inner table beside a zone of unchanged color, with a distinct blackened/non-blackened pattern, often associated with a typical effect of dark

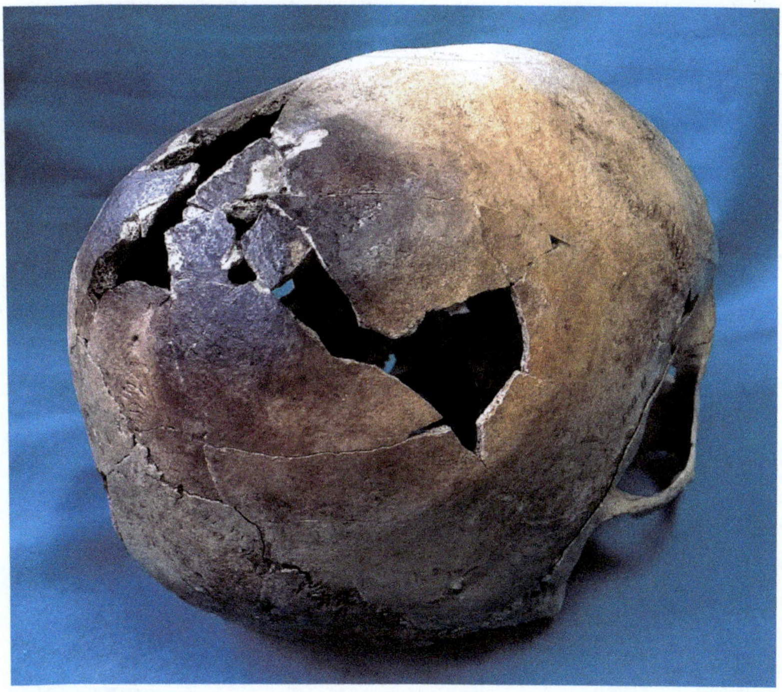

Figure 22.11 Thermal effects in victim's skeleton. Skull of an old-aged adult male showing a dark stained and cracked parietal bone.

staining "exuding" from open sutures. This evidence is concomitant with the pattern of bone cracking, since dark stained areas often exhibit fissure fractures, or may even be shattered, while those of unchanged color are never affected by such major heat effects. Bone that is black in color represents carbonized skeletal material in direct contact with heat or flames (Hermann, 1970; Symes *et al.*, 2015). Dark colors, particularly black, are related to the carbonization of collagen (Shipman *et al.*, 1984; Symes *et al.*, 2014). Heating can be related to combustion (with oxygen) or charring (without oxygen), both of which require the formation of char (Braadbaart *et al.*, 2007). The heating process also depends on temperature, heating rate (°C/min), and exposure time (Jiang *et al.*, 2014).

A significant feature associated with the charring of the inner cranial table is the brown coloration of the vascular grooves (*sulci arteriosi* and *sulci venarum*) (Figure 22.12). As in other cases, dark staining of the intracranial cavity appears to be gradual, the bone progressively appearing natural/pale yellow (α), bright brown (β), dark brown and black (γ) (Munsell Soil Colour Charts, 1954). Pale yellow is indicative of minor thermal exposure (≤ 200°C), whereas darker bone coloration matches with higher temperatures (300 to 400–500°C) (Shipman *et al.*, 1984; Braadbaart *et al.*, 2007; Mastrolorenzo *et al.*, 2010; Symes *et al.*, 2014, 2015).

At Herculaneum, the direct contact of the soft tissues with the pyroclastic surge indicates that the charring was caused by hot-emplaced volcanic ash (Jiang *et al.*,

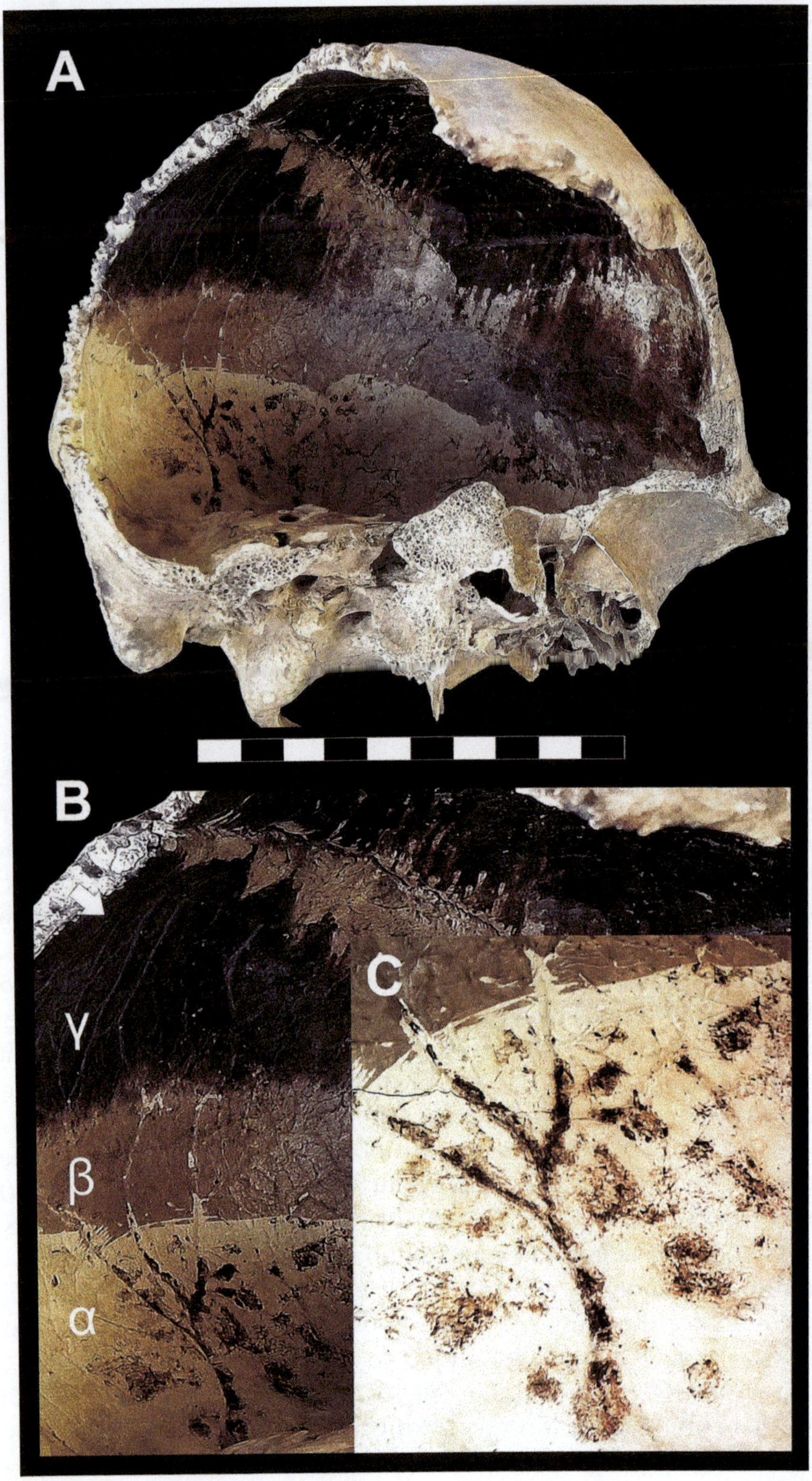

Figure 22.12 Thermal effects on the cranial cavity. A. Skull showing dark staining of the intracranial bone table. B. The inner bone surface progressively changes from pale yellow to black (α–γ). C. Brown residues encrusting the vascular grooves (scale bar in cm).

2014), a characteristic uncommon for victims of pyroclastic density currents, whose bodies are mostly preserved (Baxter, 1990). In the AD 79 eruption, assuming environmental reducing conditions (lack or low content of oxygen) at the surge emplacement (Sigurdsson *et al.*, 1985; Baxter, 1990), the dark staining of bones is likely to be due to a charring process affecting the victims engulfed within the hot ash cloud (Sharma *et al.*, 2015; Reidsma *et al.*, 2016). This particular condition seems to be confirmed by the results of experimentally heated bone vs. victims' bones from the AD 79 volcanic context (Mastrolorenzo *et al.*, 2010), as well as by other heating experiments in reducing (i.e. charring) (Reidsma *et al.*, 2016) and aerobic (i.e. combustion) conditions (Krap *et al.*, 2019; van Hoesel *et al.*, 2019). The soft tissues of a corpse act as a physical barrier against the heat and keep bones in anaerobic conditions (Imaizumi, 2015). The latter process and the unevenness of soft tissue thickness in the body and an unequal distribution of heat during exposure itself, possibly due to the different distribution of corpses in the chambers (Figure 22.6), may explain the difference in color alterations and the varying degrees of charred bones in the same individual or even on a single bone (Dehaan, 2008).

As regards the thermal origin of cracking detected on the skull of the AD 79 eruption victims, heat-induced fractures are always limited to the charred areas, since developing heat fractures do not have the energy to radiate out of charred areas into the uncharred bone (Symes *et al.*, 2015). This evidence is particularly significant since it demonstrates the perimortem origin of the skull fractures induced by the hot ash surge, excluding post-mortem causes like the weight of the ash deposit or the direct impact of the surge itself, as previously hypothesized (Capasso, 2001; Schmidt *et al.*, 2015; Martyn *et al.*, 2020). In such cases, the skeletons would have been at least partly dismembered or crushed, which they were not, as demonstrated by complete preservation of the victims' skeletons and their anatomical joints (Figure 22.8).

An extraordinary find concerns skulls filled with ash, which indicates that after vanishing, the brain was replaced by ash (Figure 22.13). The presence of such an ash cast in all victims, even those showing minor heat effects, provides evidence that the pyroclastic surge was sufficiently hot and fluid to penetrate the intracranial cavity soon after soft tissues and organic fluids vanished, as supported by the intracranial micro stratigraphy showing lamination by successive apposition of thin ash layers.

A recent re-examination of the Herculaneum victims' skeletons and their ash burial context has revealed the preservation of atypical red mineral residues encrusting the bones, which also impregnate the volcanic ash filling the skulls and the ash-bed deposit (Figure 22.14). Analysis by inductively coupled plasma mass spectrometry (ICP-MS) revealed an extremely high amount of iron in the class of red incrustations detected from the cranial and postcranial bones, the ash filling the intracranial cavity, and the ash bed. In contrast, samples of ash (surge deposit) and sand (chamber bottom) not impregnated by red residues showed a negligible amount of iron (Petrone *et al.*, 2018). These findings indicate that the extremely high content of iron could not be ascribed to volcanic ash or other volcanic products, suggesting that it might have originated from the victims' body fluids.

This question was further investigated by searching for the possible presence of heme-containing protein residues by means of protein approaches. The red incrustation areas from several iron-containing samples were submitted to trypsin

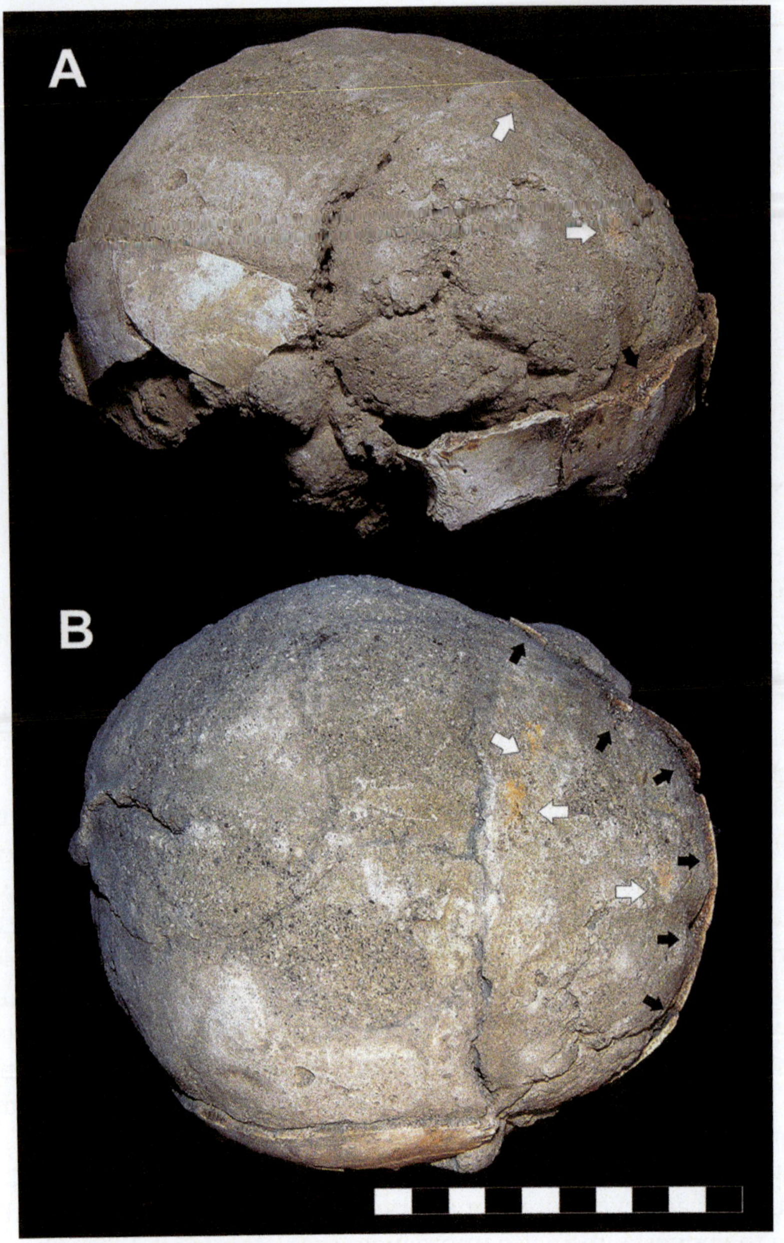

Figure 22.13 Brain ash casts from the victims' skulls. A. Shattered skull of a child filled by ash, from one of the rare skeletons preserved from the early 1900s' excavations of the town (Weaver's house). B. Perfect replica of the brain shape is apparent from the imprint of the coronal and sagittal open sutures (B). The ash is impregnated by red mineral residues (B, C, white arrows), which also encrust the exposed bone margins (A, B, black arrows) and the outer bone surface (A, right supraorbital region) (scale bar in cm).

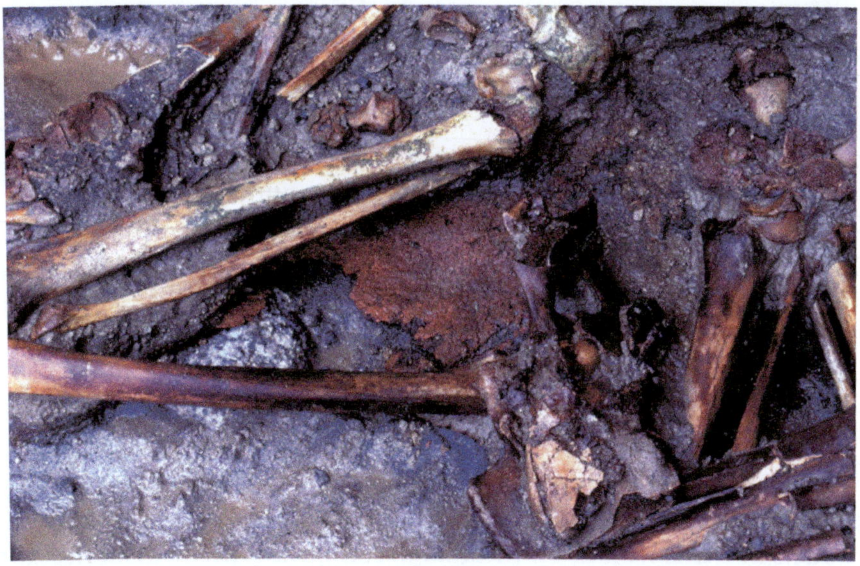

Figure 22.14 Thick layer of red mineral residues at the contact surface of the skeleton with the volcanic ash deposit in which the victims were embedded.

digestion after different extraction procedures, and the putative protein digests were analyzed by liquid chromatography-tandem mass spectrometry (LC-MS/MS) (Vinciguerra *et al.*, 2016). No peptides originating from tissue proteins could be detected in the samples. However, although sampling did not notch into the bone, but only the incrustation was taken, in several cases it was possible to detect a few reliable peptides from human collagen proteins alpha-1(I) and alpha-2(I) (Petrone *et al.*, 2018). These results suggest that only proteins protected by the inorganic scaffold of the bones survived the unbearable temperature experienced, while proteins less protected by the thin hard tissue were mostly degraded. This latter evidence suggests that the persistence of collagen in some victims' bones reported by some authors (Martyn *et al.*, 2020) is not sufficient to support the hypothesis that the temperature inside the waterfront chambers must have been substantially lower than previously established through analysis of victims' bones and heating experiments on recent bones (Mastrolorenzo *et al.*, 2010; Petrone *et al.*, 2018).

Of particular note in this regard is a recent extensive proteomic investigation which shows that heat intensity is a negligible factor in preserving organic matter in the 79 AD victims (Ntasi *et al.*, 2022). Research results reveals that the bone proteomes from Pompeii are more degraded than in Herculaneum, despite here corpses were exposed to much higher temperatures than those experienced at Pompeii. The specimens from Pompeii shows lower content of non-collagenous proteins, higher deamidation level and higher extent of collagen modification. In Pompeii, the slow decomposition of corpses' soft tissues in the natural dry-wet hydrogeological soil cycles damaged their bone proteome more than what was experienced at Herculaneum. Here, the rapid vanishing of body tissues due to the intense heat and the resulting bones buried in an environment permanently waterlogged with groundwater inhibited the destructive action of microbes.

This matter was further addressed by Raman microspectroscopic investigation on representative samples to identify or exclude various iron-containing compounds (Petrone *et al.*, 2018). Special attention was paid to detect and discriminate the possible preservation heme or heme-degradation products within the red mineral residues (Neugebauer *et al.*, 2012). For this purpose, a number of samples were selected based on iron content data provided by ICP-MS and analyzed using a Raman microspectroscopy with 514 and 647 nm excitation. Microscopically heterogeneous residues showing spots of different colors were sampled several times in different areas. Twelve samples did not provide any Raman band, while eleven samples showed Raman features. Among the latter, some of them taken from red encrusted material showed iron-related bands, consistent with ICP-MS analysis. The large amounts of iron and iron oxides detected by inductively coupled plasma mass spectrometry and Raman microspectroscopy showed such residues to be the final products of heme iron upon thermal decomposition. The evidence of preservation of significant putative evidence of hemoprotein thermal degradation from the eruption victims suggested the rapid vanishing of body fluids and soft tissues of victims at death, resulting from exposure to the hot ash avalanches.

Evidence of a heat-induced process of rapid body flesh disappearing is given by the incipient "pugilistic attitude" testified by rare flexure of the upper limbs, but not yet evident in the lower limbs (Figure 22.8). This heat-induced posture results from denaturation of proteins and muscle fiber dehydration which cause rapid muscle contraction, with consequent abduction of the limbs to the body (Saukko and Knight, 2004). Since a body shows a pugilistic attitude soon after exposure to pyroclastic surge temperatures of around 200–250°C (Baxter, 1990) or burning for about ten minutes in a crematorium at temperatures between 670°C and 810°C (Redsicker and O' Connor, 1997), the lack of a complete pugilistic pose in the victims' corpses at Herculaneum may indicate that the muscles disappeared more quickly than they contracted. This also seems attested by the "lifelike" stance observed in the victims' corpses resulting from the extraordinarily well-preserved skeletal joints fixing the body shape in three-dimensional space (Figure 22.8) that could only be explained by very rapid replacement of flesh by volcanic ash. In contrast, the widespread occurrence of pugilistic attitude in the Pompeii victims is attributable to the long-lasting persistence of body flesh, apparent from the shape of the plaster casts, as a consequence of exposure to a lower temperature estimated to be around 250–300°C (Petrone *et al.*, 2018), enough to cause muscle contraction, but insufficient for soft tissues to vanish rapidly.

As to the mechanism of death at Herculaneum, evidence such as the red residues rich in iron oxides detected from the ash filling the intracranial cavity and encrusting the inner and the outer table, as well as the brown coloration of the venous sinuses, strongly suggests massive heat-induced hemorrhage (Black and Graham, 2002) and a rise in intracranial pressure, as appears clearly from recurrent skull explosive fracture (Saukko and Knight, 2004). In forensic cases of skull bursting, particularly in children, the expelled brain matter may form a circular pattern around the head (Knight, 1991), a feature also occurring in a few Herculaneum skulls (Figure 22.7). Examination of fire victims has also shown the presence of heat hematoma (Kawasumi *et al.*, 2013), with brown bone color being associated with hemoglobin (Saukko and Knight, 2004). This is a heat-induced coagulation lying between the bone and the dura, caused by exudation from the venous sinuses of boiling blood, which becomes spongy and brown. The bone table overlying the hematoma is usually charred (Goyal *et al.*, 2010), as repeatedly seen in the victims' skulls at Herculaneum. An increase in pressure caused by bleeding in the various compartments of the brain is considered the most common mechanism of sudden death (Bohnert *et al.*, 1998). The detection of iron-containing compounds from the ash filling the endocranial cavity, coupled with brown coloration of venous sinuses, bone blackening and cracking, strongly suggests a widespread pattern of heat-induced hemorrhage, intracranial pressure increase, and bursting, all concurrent factors in causing the instantaneous death of the inhabitants in Herculaneum.

A summary of the last minutes of people's life in Herculaneum may be as follows. The bleeding and boiling of the brain caused instantaneous death (Petrone, 2012; Petrone *et al.*, 2018) and the cease of any vital activity before the victims had time to display a defensive reaction. Hands, feet, and the whole body underwent an instantaneous thermal-induced contraction. The increase in intracranial pressure caused skulls to shatter, bones, and teeth to break, and soft tissues to disappear rapidly and be replaced by volcanic ash. The temperature then reduced, causing the volcanic ash deposit to cool and harden in a time of the order of some tens of minutes (Mastrolorenzo *et al.*, 2001b). Thus the bodies were fixed in the postures in which they died (Mastrolorenzo *et al.*, 2010; Petrone *et al.*, 2018). Evidence shows that, once the town was hit by the first scorching ash cloud, all the people would have died in a fraction of a second, as testified by the stance of the corpses as if "frozen" in the last instant of life.

22.8 An Exceptional Discovery

In the 1960s, in the Collegium Augustalium at Herculaneum, a human victim was found lying on a wooden bed, buried by volcanic ash (Figure 22.15). During a recent paleoforensic survey, a unique discovery was made. In this victim's skull, remains that were vitrified instead of saponified were discovered, apparently derived from his brain (Figure 22.16). This vitrified material also encrusted the surface of the skull bone. This glassy material was undetectable elsewhere in the skeleton or in the adjacent volcanic ash, nor was it found in other locations at the archaeological site (Petrone *et al.*, 2020b). Vitrification is a natural process that occurs when a liquid drops below its glass transition temperature turning into glass or a glaze, which depends largely on the cooling rate and the viscosity of the liquid (Schmelzer and Tropin, 2018). The preservation of this vitrified material implies that the brain was not destroyed during exposure to the hot pyroclastic flows and that time was allowed for its rapid cooling and transformation into glass before the final burial beneath further meters of hot pyroclastic debris. This

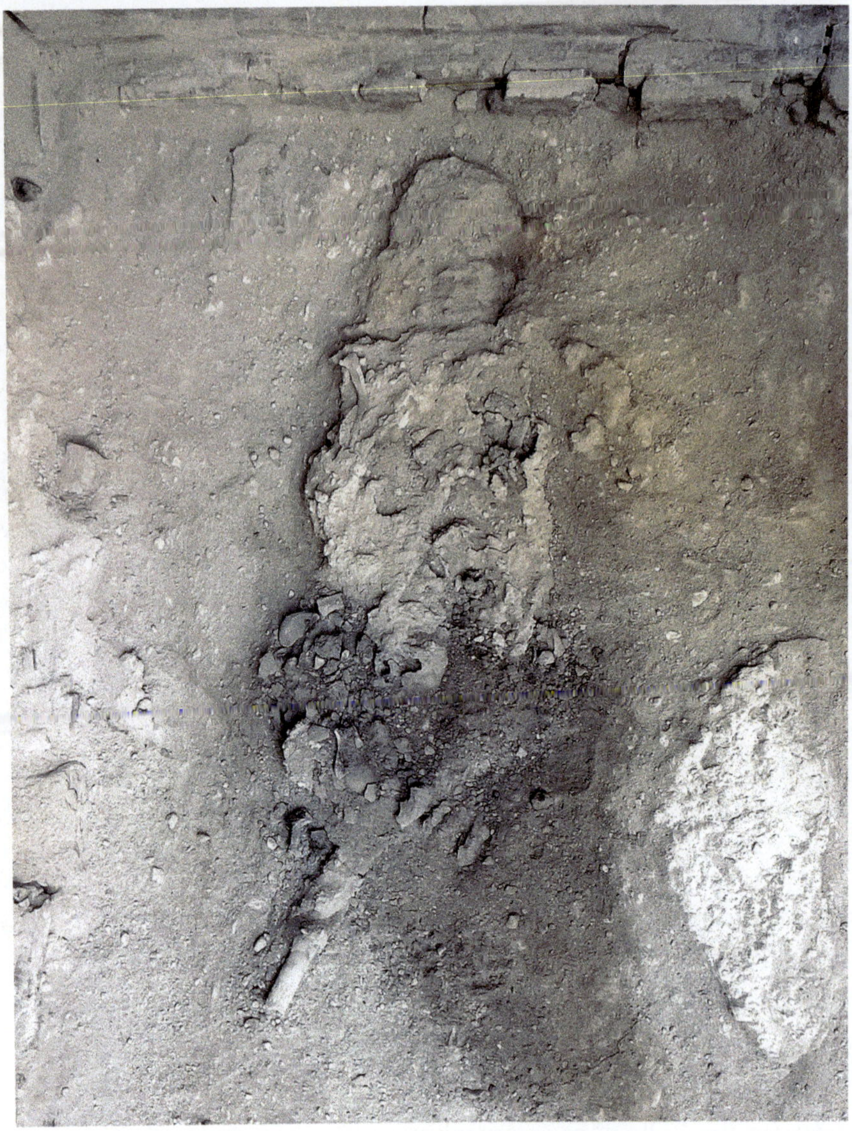

Figure 22.15 The AD 79 human victim found in the Collegium Augustalium (Herculaneum).

indicates that some time gaps must have occurred during the sequence of pyroclastic flow events that progressively hit and buried the town, as also recently suggested at Pompeii (Scarpati *et al.*, 2020).

Cerebral tissue from archaeological human remains are uncommon finds (Papageorgopoulou *et al.*, 2010). Under certain taphonomic conditions that prevent soft tissue decomposition, brain remains are typically mummified or mostly saponified, meaning that their triglycerides have been converted to glycerol and fatty acid salts, or soap (Ubelaker and Zarenko, 2011). However, ancient brains reported in the literature show only poor preservation of neuronal structures (Doran *et al.*, 1986; O'Connor *et al.*, 2011). Proteomics and mass spectrometry

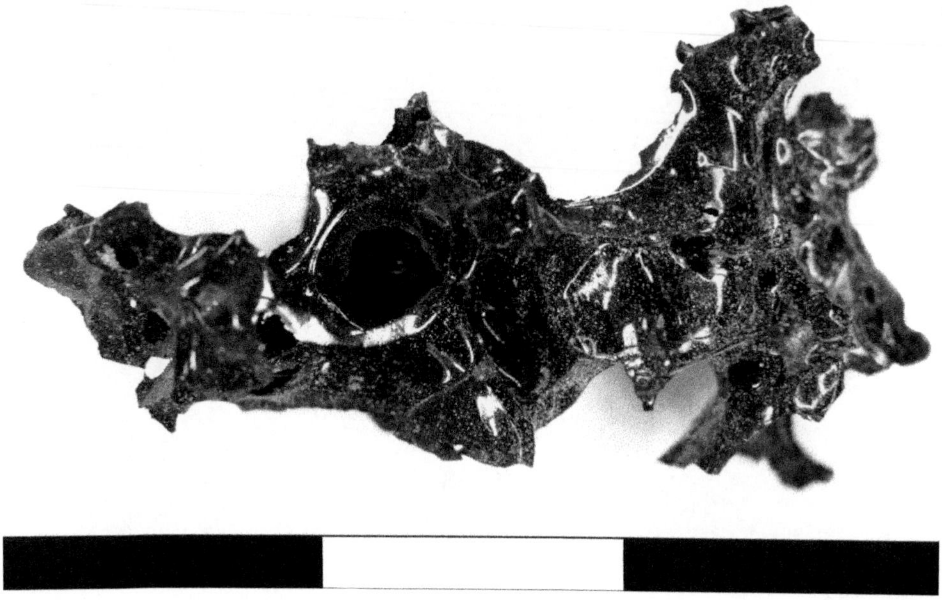

Figure 22.16 Vitrified fragment of human brain from an AD 79 eruption victim (scale bar 3 cm).

investigation of the glassy material inside the skull identified several proteins highly expressed in human brain tissues and adipic and margaric fatty acids, components of human hair fat (Weitkamp *et al.*, 1947; Delplancke *et al.*, 2018), thus indicating preservation of vitrified human brain tissue. A maximum temperature of 520°C was detected on charred wood from the Collegium, as also detected for the victims discovered in a series of waterfront chambers (Mastrolorenzo *et al.*, 2010; Petrone *et al.*, 2020b). This suggests that extreme radiant heat was able to ignite body fat and vaporize soft tissues (Petrone *et al.*, 2018), which was followed by a rapid drop in temperature as testified by the vitrification process that affected the victim's brain and some charcoal as well (Petrone *et al.*, 2020a). The detection of the glassy material from the victim's head, of proteins expressed in human brain, and of fatty acids of human hair origin indicates that the tissue was thermally-induced preservation of vitrified human brain.

Using SEM and a specific image-processing tool based on a neural network, several typical central nervous system (CNS) ultrastructures from the victim's vitrified brain (Figure 22.17) and spinal cord tissue were discovered (Petrone *et al.*, 2020b). These remains are unique for the excellent quality of tissue preservation, giving an opportunity to examine in detail the ultrastructure of a 2000-year-old human brain. Due to a natural process of vitrification, at Herculaneum the CNS was "frozen" in its native condition, preserving intact remnant cell structures in the neuronal tissue. The conversion of human tissue to glass (vitrification) occurred as a result of the rapid cooling of the volcanic ash deposit after exposure to the hot ash cloud at a temperature of about 500°C (Caricchi *et al.*, 2014; Giordano *et al.*, 2018; Pensa *et al.*, 2019). Previous heating bone experiments showed analogous

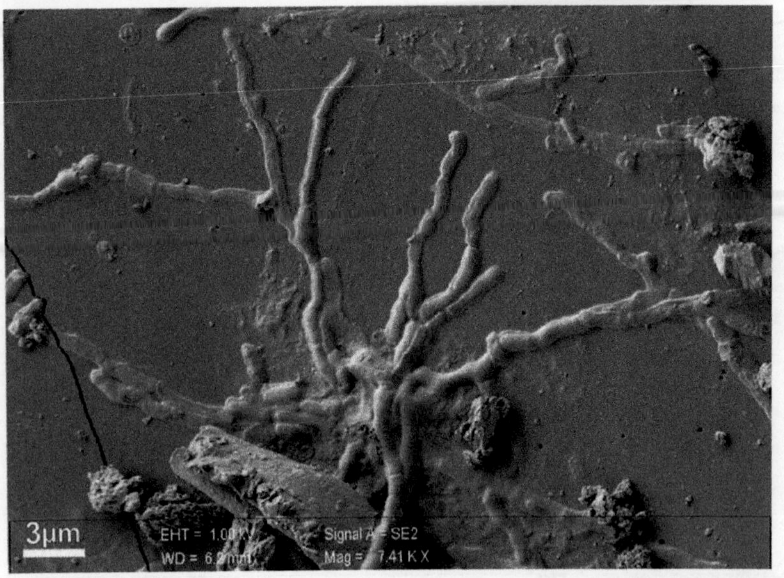

Figure 22.17 SEM image of brain axons from the vitrified cerebral tissue of an AD 79 human victim.

temperatures (Mastrolorenzo *et al.*, 2010) that were also confirmed by recent reflectance analysis on carbonized wood from Herculaneum (Petrone *et al.*, 2020a).

22.9 Conclusions

The multidisciplinary site investigations and the lines of research carried out on the victims of the AD 79 eruption proved to be of fundamental significance for the biological, archaeological, and historical reconstruction of the population living at the foothills of Mt. Vesuvius. Scientific studies continue unabatedly, and new ongoing research promises to reveal key information of absolute novelty regarding the biological kinship and the social mobility of Herculaneum's inhabitants, within the economic and social relationships of this rich Roman town with other countries in the Mediterranean basin. As an integral part of the most recent major archaeological discoveries, the AD 79 victims can be considered as "time capsules," being an entire cross section of a living Roman society, suspended in time and place because of a huge, unexpected natural catastrophe, which incredibly preserved intact entire urban settlements, including aspects of daily life. The skeletal population of Herculaneum and its archaeological context represent a unique testimony among the known archaeological sites for its exceptional finds so far and those awaiting discovery in the near future. These findings have important implications in the field of bioanthropological and volcanological research, which may open a new line of biogeoarchaeological investigations on previously undetected evidence. This is particularly true for the sites buried by the Vesuvius eruptions, given the high-risk scenario for three million people living close to the volcano today.

References

Allison, P.A. and Briggs, D.E.G. (eds.). (1991) *Taphonomy: Releasing the Data Locked in the Fossil Record*. Plenum Press, New York.

Barberi, F., Macedonio, G., Pareschi, M.T., and Santacroce, R. (1990) Mapping the tephra fallout risk: An example from Vesuvius, Italy. *Nature*, **344**, 142–144.

Baxter, P.J. (1990) Medical effects of volcanic eruptions, I. Main causes of death and injury. *Bulletin of Volcanology*, **52**, 532–544.

Baxter, P.J., Jenkins, S., Seswandhana, R., Komorowski, J.C., Dunn, K., Purser, D., *et al.* (2017) Human survival in volcanic eruptions: Thermal injuries in pyroclastic surges, their causes, prognosis and emergency management. *Burns*, **43**, 1051–1069.

Bisel, S.C. (1987) Human bones at Herculaneum. *Rivista di Studi Pompeiani*, **I**, 123–131.

Black, M. and Graham, D.I. (2002) Sudden unexplained death in adults caused by intracranial pathology. *Journal of Clinical Pathology*, **55**, 44–50.

Blong, R.J. (1984) *Volcanic Hazards. A Sourcebook on the Effects of Eruptions*. Academic Press, Sydney.

Bohnert, M., Rost, T., and Pollak, S. (1998) The degree of destruction of human bodies in relation to the duration of the fire. *Forensic Science International*, **95**, 11–21.

Borgongino, M. and Stefani, G. (2002) Intorno alla data dell'eruzione del 79 d.C. *Rivista di Studi Pompeiani*, **12–33**, 177–215 (in Italian).

Braadbaart, F., Wright, P.J., van der Horst, J., and Boon, J.J. (2007) A laboratory simulation of the carbonization of sunflower achenes and seeds. *Journal of Analytical and Applied Pyrolysis*, **78**, 316–327.

Brinkmann, B., Kleiber, M., Koops, E., and Püschel, K. (1979) Vitale reaktionen bei akutem verbrühungstod. *Zeitschrift fur Rechtsmedizin*, **83**, 1–16.

Budetta, T. (1993) I nuovi scavi nell'area suburbana di Ercolano. In: *Ercolano 1738–1988. 250 anni di ricerca archeologica* (ed. L. Franchi Dall'Orto). L'Erma di Bretschneider, Roma, pp. 677–690 (in Italian).

Camardo, D. and Notomista, M. (2017) *Ercolano: 1927–1961*. L'impresa archeologica di Amedeo Maiuri e l'esperimento della città museo. Studi e Ricerche del Parco Archeologico di Pompei, **34**. L'ERMA di Bretschneider, Roma (in Italian).

Capasso, L. (2000) Herculaneum victims of the volcanic eruptions of Vesuvius in 79 AD. *The Lancet*, **356**, 1344–1346.

Capasso, L. (2001) *I fuggiaschi di Ercolano. Paleobiologia delle vittime dell'eruzione vesuviana del 79 d.C.* L'Erma di Bretschneider, Roma, (in Italian).

Caricchi, C., Vona, A., Corrado, S., Giordano, G., and Romano, C. (2014) AD 79 Vesuvius PDC deposits' temperatures inferred from optical analysis on woods charred in-situ in the Villa dei Papiri at Herculaneum (Italy). *Journal of Volcanology and Geothermal Research*, **289**, 14–25.

De Carolis, E. and Patricelli, G. (2003) Le vittime dell'eruzione. In: *Storie da un'eruzione* (eds. A. d'Ambrosio, P.G. Guzzo, and M. Mastroroberto). Pompei Ercolano Oplontis, Milano, pp. 56–72.

De Carolis, E. and Patricelli, G. (2013) Rinvenimenti di corpi umani nel suburbio pompeiano e nei siti di Ercolano e Stabia. *Rivista di Studi Pompeiani*, **24**, 11–32 (in Italian).

De Carolis, E., Patricelli, G., and Ciarallo, A. (1998) Rinvenimenti di corpi umani nell'area urbana di Pompei. *Rivista di Studi Pompeiani*, **9**, 75–123.

Dehaan, J.D. (2008) Fire and bodies. In: *The Analysis of Burned Human Remains* (eds. C.W. Schmidt and S.A. Symes). Academic Press, London, pp. 1–13.

Delplancke, T.D.J., de Seymour, J.V., Tong, C., Sulek, K., Xia, Y., Zhang, H., *et al.* (2018) Analysis of sequential hair segments reflects changes in the metabolome across the trimesters of pregnancy. *Scientific Reports*, **8**, 36.

De Natale, G., Pappalardo, L., Petrone, P., Ricciardi, I., Rossano, S., and Troise, C. (2004) *Ricerca Scientifica e Mitigazione del Rischio Vulcanico – Vesuvio dentro il vulcano, parte 1*, Vol. **1**. Osservatorio Vesuviano – INGV, Napoli, pp. 1–29 (in Italian).
Dobran, F., Neri, A., and Todesco, M. (1994) Assessing the pyroclastic flow hazard at Vesuvius. *Nature*, **367**, 551–554.
Doran, G.H., Dickel, D.N., Ballinger, W.E., Jr., Agee, O.F., Laipis, P.J., and Hauswirth, W.W. (1986) Anatomical, cellular and molecular analysis of 8,000-yr-old human brain tissue from the Windover archaeological site. *Nature*, **323**, 803–806.
Druitt, T.H. (1998) Pyroclastic density currents. In: *The Physics of Explosive Volcanic Eruptions*, Vol. **145**, (eds. G.S. Gilbert and R.S.J. Sparks). Geological Society London Special Publication, London, pp. 145–182.
Fernández Castillo, R., Ubelaker, D.H., Acosta, J.A., de La Rosa, R.J., and Garcia, I.G. (2013) Effect of temperature on bone tissue: Histological changes. *Forensic Science International*, **226**, 33–37.
Giacomelli, L., Perrotta, A., Scandone, R., and Scarpati, C. (2003) The eruption of Vesuvius of 79 AD and its impact on human environment in Pompeii. *Episodes*, **26**, 234–237.
Gilman, B. (2007) *Ashen Sky: The Letters of Pliny the Younger on the Eruption of Vesuvius*. Getty Publications, Los Angeles, CA.
Giordano, G., Zanella, E., Trolese, M., Baffioni, C., Vona, A., Caricchi, C., *et al.* (2018) Thermal interactions of the AD 79 Vesuvius pyroclastic density currents and their deposits at Villa dei Papiri (Herculaneum archaeological site, Italy). *Earth and Planetary Science Letters*, **490**, 180–192.
Goyal, M.K., Kochar, S.R., and Asawa, S.S. (2010) Heat induced morphological changes in the brain. *Journal of Indian Academy of Forensic Medicine*, **32**, 75–77.
Guidobaldi, M.P. (2007) *Ercolano. Guida agli scavi*. Electa, Napoli (in Italian).
Hall, S. (September 2007) Vesuvius. Asleep for Now. National Geographic, **20**, 114–133. http://www.nationalgeographic.com/magazine/2007/09/vesuvius-volcano-dormant-eruption-pompeii.
Hansell, A.L., Horwell, C.J., and Oppenheimer, C. (2006) The health hazards of volcanoes and geothermal areas. *Occupational and Environmental Medicine*, **63**, 149–156.
Hermann, B. (1970) Anthropologische bearbeitung der leichenbranden von Berlin-Rudow. *Ausgrabungen in Berlin*, **1**, 61–71.
Imaizumi, K. (2015) Forensic investigation of burnt human remains. *Research and Reports in Forensic Medical Science*, **5**, 67–74.
Jiang, B., Harlow, G.E., Wohletz, K., Zhou, Z., and Meng, J. (2014) New evidence suggests pyroclastic flows are responsible for the remarkable preservation of the Jehol biota. *Nature Communications*, **5**, 3151.
Kawasumi, Y., Usui, A., Hosokai, Y., Sato, M., and Funayama, M. (2013) Heat haematoma: Post-mortem computed tomography. *Clinical Radiology*, **68**, e95–e97.
Kent, D.V., Dragoslav, N., Pescatore, T., and Sparks, S.R.J. (1981) Paleomagnetic determination of emplacement temperature of Vesuvius A.D. 79 pyroclastic deposits. *Nature*, **290**, 393–396.
Knight, B. (1991) *Forensic Pathology*. Edward Arnold, London.
Krap, T., Ruijter, J.M., Nota, K., Karel, J., Burgers, A.L., Aalders, M.C.G. *et al.* (2019) Colourimetric analysis of thermally altered human bone samples. *Scientific Reports*, **9**, 8923.
LaMotte, R.H. and Campbell, J.N. (1978) Comparison of responses of warm and nociceptive C-fiber afferents in monkey with human judgments of thermal pain. *Journal of Neurophysiology*, **41**, 509–528.
Linde, N., Ricci, T., Baron, L., Shakas, A., and Berrino, G. (2017) The 3-D structure of the Somma-Vesuvius volcanic complex (Italy) inferred from new and historic gravimetric data. *Scientific Reports*, **7**, 8434.

Lockwood, J.P. and Hazlett, R.W. (2010) *Volcanoes: Global Perspectives*. Wiley-Blackwell, Oxford.

Luongo, G., Perrotta, A., and Scarpati, C. (2003a) Impact of the AD 79 explosive eruption on Pompeii, I. Relations amongst the depositional mechanisms of the pyroclastic products, the framework of the buildings and the associated destructive events. *Journal of Volcanology and Geothermal Research*, **126**, 201–223.

Luongo, G., Perrotta, A., Scarpati, C., De Carolis, E., Patricelli, G., and Ciarallo, A. (2003b) Impact of the AD 79 explosive eruption on Pompeii, II. Causes of death of the inhabitants inferred by stratigraphical and areal distribution of the human corpses. *Journal of Volcanology and Geothermal Research*, **126**, 169–200.

Maiuri, A. (1958) Pompeii. *Scientific American*, **198**, 70.

Maiuri, A. (1961) Last moments of the Pompeians. *National Geographic*, **120**, 651–669.

Maiuri, A. (1977) Herculaneum. Rome… *Episodes-Newsmagazine of the International Union of Geological Sciences*, **26**(3), 235–238.

Martyn, R., Craig, O.E., Ellingham, S.T.D., Islam, M., Fattore, L., Sperduti, A., *et al.* (2020) A re-evaluation of manner of death at Roman Herculaneum following the AD 79 eruption of Vesuvius. *Antiquity*, **94**, 76–91.

Mastrolorenzo, G., Pappalardo, L., Ricciardi, I., and Petrone, P.P. (2004) Active volcanism and related events in Campania: Primary and secondary effects of explosive volcanic eruptions on the environment and people. 32nd International Geological Congress, Florence, Italy, Post-Congress P67, 6, P55–PW06.

Mastrolorenzo, G., Petrone, P., Pagano, M., Incoronato, A., Baxter, P.J., Canzanella, A., *et al.* (2001a) The 79 AD Vesuvius Plinian eruption at Herculaneum and its impact on the people. In: *Tephras, Chronology, Archaeology* (eds. E. Juvigné and J.P. Raynal). CDERAD, Laussonne, France, pp. 183–189.

Mastrolorenzo, G., Petrone, P.P., Pagano, M., Incoronato, A., Baxter, P.J., Canzanella, A., *et al.* (2001b) The Herculaneum victims of Vesuvius in A.D. 79. *Nature*, **410**, 769–770.

Mastrolorenzo, G., Petrone, P.P., Pappalardo, L., and Guarino, F.M. (2010) Lethal thermal impact at the periphery of pyroclastic surges: Evidences at Pompeii. *PloS ONE*, **5**(6), e11127/1–12. https://doi.org/10.1371/journal.pone.0011127.

Mastrolorenzo, G., Petrone, P., Pappalardo, L., and Sheridan, M.F. (2006) The Avellino 3780 yr B.P. catastrophe as a worst-case scenario for a future eruption at Vesuvius. *Proceedings of the National Academy of Sciences of the United States of America*, **103**, 4366–4370.

McCormick, M.P., Thomason, L.W., and Trepte, C.R. (1995) Atmospheric effects of the Mt Pinatubo eruption. *Nature*, **373**, 399–404.

McCoy, M.T. (2014) The responses of the Roman Imperial Government to natural disasters 29 BCE–180 CE. Theses and Dissertations. https://scholarworks.uark.edu/etd/2148.

Munsell Soil Colour Charts. (1954). Munsell Color Company Inc, Baltimore, MD.

NASA Earth Observatory. (2006) Mount Vesuvius, Naples, Italy: Image of the Day. https://earthobservatory.nasa.gov/IOTD/view.php?id=6403.

Neugebauer, U., März, A., Henkel, T., Schmitt, M., and Popp, J. (2012) Spectroscopic detection and quantification of heme and heme degradation products. *Analytical and Bioanalytical Chemistry*, **404**, 2819–2829.

Ntasi, G., Rodriguez Palomo, I., Marino, G., Dal Piaz, F., Sirano, F., Cappellini, E. *et al.* (2022) Written in bone proteins: molecular signatures in the 79 AD victims' skeletal remains from Herculaneum and Pompeii. Scientific Reports, doi.org/10.1038/s41598-022-12042-6 (in press).

Nunziante, L., Fraldi, M., Lirer, R., Petrosino, P., Scotellaro, S., and Cicirelli, C. (2003) Risk assessment of the impact of pyroclastic currents on the towns located around Vesuvio: A non-linear structural inverse analysis. *Bulletin of Volcanology*, **65**, 547–561.

O'Connor, S., Ali, E., Al-Sabah, S., Anwar, D., Bergström, E., Brown, K.A., *et al.* (2011) Exceptional preservation of a prehistoric human brain from Heslington, Yorkshire, UK. *Journal of Archaeological Science*, **38**, 1641–1654.

Pagano, M. (ed.). (2000) *Gli antichi ercolanesi. Antropologia, società, economia. Guida alla mostra*. Electa, Milano (in Italian).

Pagano, M. (2003) L'apodyterium delle Terme del Foro, settore maschile. In: *Storie da un'eruzione. Pompei, Ercolano, Oplontis* (eds. A. d'Ambrosio, P.G. Guzzo, and M. Mastroroberto (a cura di)). Mondadori Electa, Milano, pp. 120–121 (in Italian).

Papageorgopoulou, C., Rentsch, K., Raghavan, M., Hofmann, M.I., Colacicco, G., Gallien, V., *et al.* (2010) Preservation of cell structures in a medieval infant brain: A paleohistological, paleogenetic, radiological and physico-chemical study. *Neuroimage*, **50**, 893–901.

Pappalardo, U. (1990) L'eruzione pliniana del Vesuvio nel 79 d.C.: Ercolano. In: *Volcanology and Archaeology*, Vol. **25** (eds. C. Albore Livadie and F. Widemann). PACT, Strasbourg, France, pp. 197–215 (in Italian).

Pappalardo, U. (2019) Eruzione del 79 d.C. Riordinando le date. *Archeologia Viva*, **193**, 8–9 (in Italian).

Pensa, A., Capra, L., and Giordano, G. (2019) Ash clouds temperature estimation. Implication on dilute and concentrated PDCs coupling and topography confinement. *Scientific Reports*, **9**, 5657.

Petrone, P. (2012) Human corpses as time capsules: New perspectives in the study of past mass disasters. *Journal of Anthropological Sciences*, **89**, 3–6.

Petrone, P. (2019a) Ercolano 79 A.D.: Corpi umani come capsule del tempo. *Cronache Ercolanesi*, **49**, 283–296 (in Italian).

Petrone, P. (2019b) The Herculaneum victims of the 79 AD Vesuvius eruption: A review. *Journal of Anthropological Sciences*, **97**, 1–22.

Petrone, P. and Fedele, F. (eds.). (2002) *Vesuvio 79 A.D. Vita e morte ad Ercolano*. Fridericiana Editrice Universitaria, Napoli.

Petrone, P., Pucci, P., Niola, M., Baxter, P.J., Fontanarosa, C., Giordano, G., *et al.* (2020a) Heat-induced brain vitrification from the 79 AD Vesuvius eruption. *The New England Journal of Medicine*, **382**, 383–384.

Petrone, P., Giordano, G., Vezzoli, E., Pensa, A., Castaldo, G., Graziano, V., *et al.* (2020b) Preservation of neurons in an AD 79 vitrified human brain. *PLoS ONE*, **15**(10), e0240017.

Petrone, P., Niola, M., Di Lorenzo, P., Graziano, V., Paternoster, M., and Buccelli, C. (2014) A new forensic approach to past mass disasters: The human victims of Vesuvius. *Austin Journal of Forensic Science and Criminology*, **1**, 1–2.

Petrone, P., Pucci, P., Niola, M., Baxter, P.J., Fontanarosa, C., Giordano, G., *et al.* (2020b) Heat-induced brain vitrification from the 79 AD Vesuvius eruption. *The New England Journal of Medicine*, **382**, 383–384.

Petrone, P., Pucci, P., Vergara, A., Amoresano, A., Birolo, L., Pane, F., *et al.* (2018) A hypothesis of sudden body fluid vaporization in the 79 AD victims of Vesuvius. *PloS ONE*, **13**(9), e0203210.

Pompei, un'iscrizione sposta la data dell'eruzione da agosto ad ottobre. ANSA.it NEWS, Cultura, Arte, 16 ottobre 2018 (in Italian). http://www.ansa.it/sito/notizie/cultura/arte/2018/10/16/pompei-iscrizione-eruzione-a-ottobre_078f0fa1-b347-4017-9284-d76475f16eb9.html.

Redsicker, D.R. and O' Connor, J.J. (1997) *Practical Fire and Arson Investigations*. Elsevier, New York.

Reidsma, F.H., van Hoesel, A., van Os, B.J.H., Megens, L., and Braadbaart, F. (2016) Charred bone: Physical and chemical changes during laboratory simulated heating under reducing conditions and its relevance for the study of fire use in archaeology. *Journal of Archaeological Science*, **10**, 282–292.

Rolandi, G., Paone, A., Di Lascio, M., and Stefani, G. (2007) The 79 AD eruption of Somma: The relationship between the date of the eruption and the southeast tephra dispersion. *Journal of Volcanology and Geothermal Research*, **169**, 87–98.

Ruggiero, M. (1881) *Degli scavi di Stabia dal MDCCXLIX al MDCCLXXXII*. Tipografia dell'Academia reale delle scienze, Napoli, Italy (in Italian).

Ruggiero, M. (1885) *Storia degli scavi di Ercolano ricomposta su' documenti superstiti*. Tipografia dell'Accademia reale delle scienze, Napoli, Italy (in Italian).

Saukko, P. and Knight, B. (2004) *Knight's Forensic Pathology*. Edward Arnold Ltd, London.

Scarpati, C., Perrotta, A., Martellone, A., and Osanna, M. (2020) Pompeian hiatuses: New stratigraphic data highlight pauses in the course of the AD 79 eruption at Pompeii. *Geological Magazine*, **157**, 695–700.

Schmelzer, J.W.P. and Tropin, T.V. (2018) Glass transition, crystallization of glass-forming melts, and entropy. *Entropy*, **20**, 103.

Schmidt, C.W., Oakley, E., D'Anastasio, R., Brower, R., Remy, A., and Viciano, J. (2015) Herculaneum. In: *The Analysis of Burned Human Remains* (eds. C.W. Schmidt and S.A. Symes). Academic Press, Cambridge, MA, pp. 149–161.

Sevink, Y., Van Bergen, M.J., Van Der Plicht, J., Feiken, H., Anastasia, C., and Huizinga, A. (2011) Robust date for the Bronze Age Avellino eruption (Somma-Vesuvius): 3945±10 calBP (1995±10 calBC). *Quaternary Science Reviews*, **30**, 1035–1046.

Sharma, A., Pareek, V., and Zhang, D. (2015) Biomass pyrolysis – A review of modelling, process parameters and catalytic studies. *Renewable & Sustainable Energy Reviews*, **50**, 1081–1096.

Sheridan, M.F., Barberi, F., Rosi, M., and Santacroce, R. (1981) A model for plinian eruption of Vesuvio. *Nature*, **289**, 282–285.

Shipman, P., Foster, G., and Schoeninger, M. (1984) Burnt bones and teeth: An experimental study of color, morphology, crystal structure and shrinkage. *Journal of Archaeological Science*, **11**, 307–325.

Sigurdsson, H., Carey, S., Cornell, W., and Pescatore, T. (1985) The eruption of Vesuvius in A.D. 79. *National Geographic Research*, **1**, 332–387.

Sigurdsson, H., Cashdollar, S., and Sparks, R.S.J. (1982) The eruption of Vesuvius in A.D. 79: Reconstruction from historical and volcanological evidence. *American Journal of Archaeology*, **86**, 39–51.

Sparks, R.S.J. (1976) Grain size variation in ignimbrites and implications for the transport of pyroclastic flows. *Sedimentology*, **23**, 147–188.

Stefani, G. (2006) La vera data dell'eruzione. *Archeo*, **10**, 10–13 (in Italian).

Symes, S.A., L'Abbé, E.N., Stull, K.E., LaCroix, M., and Pokines, J.T. (2014) Taphonomy and the timing of bone fractures in trauma analysis. In: *Manual of Forensic Taphonomy* (eds. J.T. Pokines and S.A. Symes). CRC Press, Boca Raton, FL, pp. 341–366.

Symes, S.A., Rainwater, C.W., Chapman, E.N., Gipson, D.R., and Piper, A.L. (2015) Patterned thermal destruction of human remains in a forensic setting. In: *The Analysis of Burned Human Remains* (eds. C.W. Schmidt and S.A. Symes). Academic Press, Cambridge, MA, pp. 149–161.

Taylor, R. (2015) Roman Neapolis and the landscape disaster. *Journal of Ancient History*, **3**, 282–326.

Thomas, M.L. (2015) Oplontis B: A center for the distribution and export of Vesuvian wine. *Journal of Roman Archaeology*, **28**, 403–411.

Ubelaker, D.H. and Zarenko, K.M. (2011) Adipocere: What is known after over two centuries of research. *Forensic Science International*, **208**, 167–172.

van Hoesel, A., Reidsma, F.H., van Os, B.J.H., Megens, L., Braadbaart, F. (2019) Combusted bone: Physical and chemical changes of bone during laboratory simulated heating under oxidising conditions and their relevance for the study of ancient fire use. *Journal of Archaeological Science: Reports*, **28**, 102033.

Vinciguerra, R., De Chiaro, A., Pucci, P., Marino, G., and Birolo, L. (2016) Proteomic strategies for cultural heritage: Form bones to paintings. *Microchemical Journal*, **126**, 341–348.

Weitkamp, A.W., Smiljanic, A.M., and Rothman, S. (1947) The free fatty acids of human hair fat. *Journal of the American Chemical Society*, **69**, 1936–1939.

Index

Note: **Bold** page numbers refer to tables and *italic* page numbers refer to figures.

Burnt Human Remains: Recovery, Analysis, and Interpretation, First Edition. Edited by Sarah Ellingham, Joe Adserias-Garriga, Sara C. Zapico and Douglas H. Ubelaker.